Clinical Applications of Cardiac CT
Second Edition

Filippo Cademartiri • Giancarlo Casolo •
Massimo Midiri
Editors

Clinical Applications of Cardiac CT

Second Edition

In collaboration with:
Erica Maffei
Sara Seitun
Chiara Martini
Giuseppe Tarantini
Francesco Prati

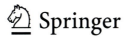

Editors:
Filippo Cademartiri
Cardiovascular Imaging Unit,
"Giovanni XXIII" Hospital,
Monastier di Treviso (TV), Italy

Giancarlo Casolo
Cardiology Unit,
Versilia Hospital,
Lido di Camaiore (LU), Italy

Massimo Midiri
DIBIMEF, Department of Radiology,
"P. Giaccone" University Hospital,
Palermo, Italy

In collaboration with:
Erica Maffei
Sara Seitun
Chiara Martini
Giuseppe Tarantini
Francesco Prati

ISBN 978-88-470-2521-9   e-ISBN 978-88-470-2522-6

DOI 10.1007/978-88-470-2522-6

Springer Milan Dordrecht Heidelberg London New York

Library of Congress Control Number: 2011942914

© Springer-Verlag Italia 2012

This work is subject to copyright. All rights are reserved, whether the whole or part of the material is concerned, specifically the rights of translation, reprinting, reuse of illustrations, recitation, broadcasting, reproduction on microfilm or in any other way, and storage in data banks. Duplication of this publication or parts thereof is permitted only under the provisions of the Italian Copyright Law in its current version, and permission for use must always be obtained from Springer. Violations are liable to prosecution under the Italian Copyright Law.

The use of general descriptive names, registered names, trademarks, etc. in this publication does not imply, even in the absence of a specific statement, that such names are exempt from the relevant protective laws and regulations and therefore free for general use.

Product liability: The publishers cannot guarantee the accuracy of any information about dosage and application contained in this book. In every individual case the user must check such information by consulting the relevant literature.

9 8 7 6 5 4 3 2 1   2012 2013 2014

Cover design: Ikona S.r.l., Milan, Italy
Typesetting: Graphostudio, Milan, Italy
Printing and binding: Arti Grafiche Nidasio, Assago (MI), Italy

Printed in Italy

Springer-Verlag Italia S.r.l. – Via Decembrio 28 – I-20137 Milan
Springer is a part of Springer Science+Business Media (www.springer.com)

Preface to the Second Edition

The second edition of Clinical Applications of Cardiac CT is the result of 2 years of hard work. The first edition was released in 2008 and there are several reasons for having a second edition planned and published after 3 years. Without doubt the main reason is related to the rapid development of the technology comprising the subject matter of this book. Since we finalized the first edition several things in the field of CCT (Cardiac Computed Tomography) have changed.

The technology has developed allowing for more robust and reliable scanning with significant radiation dose reduction; newer applications have been introduced such as myocardial perfusion; consistent data on the prognostic value of CCT have been published. Large trials have been undertaken with the aim of better defining the clinical role of CCT in different contexts. We have better insight into clinical applications, we know CCT is useful in many more fields than in the past, and we also expect CCT to grow in functional imaging and begin to replace other imaging modalities.

For all these reasons CCT is no longer the same, nor is the way we teach CCT. We therefore decided to update the first edition on the basis of all these considerations and also in an attempt to improve the structure and layout of the educational content. In doing so we have tried to better focus the first section of the book on the clinical aspects related to CCT applications.

The next three sections, targets of coronary and non coronary imaging, CT semeiology and technique respectively, have been revised and enriched with up-to-date information, while the last two sections have been revised to take into account the changing clinical scenario for CCT.

We contacted several new authors from the Italian and international arena to further enrich the contents of the book. We are happy and proud of the result and we think that, in addition to updating the book, there has been an improvement in the overall content and layout.

November 2011

Filippo Cademartiri
Giancarlo Casolo
Massimo Midiri

Acknowledgements

General Acknowledgements

A book, whether it is new or the second edition of an earlier one, is always a journey, sometimes the journey is long and sometimes it is also arduous. But wherever it takes you it always allows you to learn a lot about the topic you are dealing with. A good book is also the result of the cooperation between individuals and the expression of a certain network of knowledge.

As with the first edition, this volume is the result of a great deal of hard work by all of the authors and many others. Over the past two years many people have been involved who contributed in numerous ways to its completion.

In particular we would like to thank Springer-Verlag Italia in the persons of Antonella Cerri, Donatella Nebulone and Elisa Geranio for having supported us with the utmost professionalism in this project.

Many others provided ideas, energy and assistance and to them we would like to express our most sincere gratitude.

Filippo Cademartiri
Giancarlo Casolo
Massimo Midiri

Personal Acknowledgements

As usual for me, I would like to thank Prof. Gabriel P. Krestin, who has been the architect of my abilities in the subject matter of this volume. Without the fortunate meeting which allowed me to work alongside him I would never have achieved the desired results. My personal thanks are also due to the Erasmus Medical Center in Rotterdam, in the persons of Maja Thijse-Stemerdink, Nico Mollet, Pim de Feyter, Koen Nieman, Annick Weustink and many others who contributed to the training of many of the authors who participated in this volume.

I would then like to thank my co-editors (Massimo Midiri and Giancarlo Casolo) who are exceptional individuals and professionals who share my same vision of the subject matter.

Thanks from the bottom of my heart to all of the "fellows" who had the patience to bear with me in Rotterdam, in Parma, and in Monastier and then to participate in this undertaking.

Thanks to cardiologists, cardiac surgeons and all the clinicians for their collaboration and critical appraisal which always serves for improvement. Thanks also to the open minded professionals who started appreciating the role and importance of CCT.

Thanks to my closest collaborators Erica Maffei and Chiara Martini, because they are still following me and helping me with several projects.

Filippo Cademartiri

Foreword to the First Edition

For a very long time, radiologists have considered examination of the moving heart as the "holy grail" of noninvasive imaging. Echocardiography – with its high spatial and temporal resolution – has opened an entire avenue of possibilities for evaluating myocardial contractility or heart valve function. However, echocardiography does not allow alterations of the coronary arteries to be visualized. Similarly, magnetic resonance imaging and myocardial scintigraphy have proven to be valuable techniques in assessing myocardial perfusion and function, even in complex diseases. Despite these advances, invasive catheter angiography has remained the gold standard for visualization of the coronary artery lumen. Introduction of multislice CT was a real breakthrough, approaching the capabilities of catheter angiography with its unprecedented technological development from simultaneous data acquisition of 4 slices, through 16, 64, to over 300 slices in a single gantry rotation. With temporal resolutions under 100 milliseconds currently feasible, multislice CT comes close to catheter angiography for coronary lumen visualization.

That this technology could be implemented and optimized, that its value as well as its role in the clinical workup of patients with suspected coronary artery disease could be assessed in less than one decade, has only been possible due to the enthusiasm and hard work of many radiologists, cardiologists, and image processors in close collaboration with industrial engineers and developers. Many of the pioneers of this technology have been members of multidisciplinary teams. Their natural curiosity, spirit of innovation, mutual understanding in a supportive environment, and – last but not least – strong desire to benefit patients by improving healthcare have been the key to their success.

In many institutions, the introduction of multislice coronary CT-angiography for research and clinical purposes was overshadowed by turf battles between different specialties. At Erasmus MC, the "Rotterdam Model" was developed and proved to be a fruitful ground for the advancement of this technology. Under the leadership of Professor Pim de Feijter, a well-recognized cardiologist and expert in cardiac imaging, the Departments of Radiology and Cardiology built a communal, multidisciplinary group of medical specialists, research fellows, trainees and radiographers. Over the years this group has hosted more than 50 radiologists and cardiologists from all over the world and in all different stages of training.

The year 2000 witnessed the start of a very prized and meaningful collaboration with the imaging community in Italy when Filippo Cademartiri, one of the editors of this book, arrived at Erasmus MC. Since then, an entire generation of Italian residents and fellows have spent a year in Rotterdam learning about and doing research on coronary CT angiography. These scientists from Palermo, Rome, Parma, Trieste, Verona, Ferrara and Genoa have contributed with enthusiasm and hard work to the output of this very successful enterprise. Eight of these residents, as well as some of their Dutch colleagues, have co-authored chapters in this book. The exchange of scientific personnel over the years has led to strong ties and collaborations with many of their mentors and colleagues, some of whom have also contributed to this book. On behalf of the entire Erasmus MC as well as on a personal level, I am very proud and pleased to have established these ties, many of which have become long lasting friendships.

I would like to congratulate all the editors and authors of Clinical Applications of Cardiac CT for having produced a comprehensive overview of the technique and clinical application of this new diagnostic tool. It is a multifaceted, highquality work that will provide both present and future generations with an insight into this exciting and still developing area of medical imaging.

Rotterdam, July 2008

Prof. Gabriel P. Krestin
Chairman, Department of Radiology
Erasmus MC
University Medical Center Rotterdam
The Netherlands

Contents

Section I - Epidemiology and Clinical Assessment

1 Epidemiology of Coronary Artery Disease 3
Tessa S.S. Genders and M.G. Myriam Hunink

2 Physiology and Pathophysiology of Coronary Circulation 7
Andrea I. Guaricci, Luigi Di Biase, and Giancarlo Casolo

3 Subclinical Atherosclerosis and Primary Prevention 15
Giuseppe Tarantini, Paolo Buja, and Michela Facchin

4 Chronic (Stable) Coronary Artery Disease 29
Giancarlo Casolo

5 Acute Coronary Syndrome: Clinical Assessment 35
Paolo Buja and Giuseppe Tarantini

Section II - Targets of Coronary and non Coronary Imaging

6 Coronary Plaques 47
Antonio L'Abbate, Massimo Lombardi, and Gualtiero Pelosi

7 Myocardial Ischemia & Viability 59
Paolo G. Camici and Ornella Rimoldi

8 Left and Right Ventricular Function, Contractility, Geometry, and Mass 69
Andrea I. Guaricci, Natale Daniele Brunetti, Roberta Romito, Giancarlo Casolo,
and Matteo Di Biase

9 Pulmonary Veins and Cardiac Veins 79
Maurizio Del Greco, Flavia Ravelli, and Massimiliano Marini

Section III - CT Semeiology

10 Heart Anatomy 93
Ludovico La Grutta, Giovanni Gentile, Giuseppe Runza, Massimo Galia,
Filippo Cademartiri, and Massimo Midiri

11 Calcium Score and Coronary Plaque 115
Sara Seitun, Erica Maffei, Chiara Martini, Margherita Castiglione Morelli,
Anselmo A. Palumbo, and Filippo Cademartiri

12 Coronary Artery Stenosis on Cardiac CT 139
Sara Seitun, Erica Maffei, Chiara Martini, Margherita Castiglione Morelli,
and Filippo Cademartiri

13 Coronary Artery Stents 147
Francesca Pugliese, Katarzyna Gruszczynska, Ian Baron, Ceri L. Davies,
and Steffen E. Petersen

14 Evaluation of Bypass Grafts 153
Riccardo Marano, Giancarlo Savino, Carlo Liguori, and Lorenzo Bonomo

15 Myocardial Viability and Stress Perfusion 165
Tust Techasith, Brian Ghoshhajra, and Udo Hoffmann

16 Evaluation of Cardiac Volumetric and Functional Parameters 175
Giancarlo Messalli, Giuseppe Runza, Ludovico La Grutta, Erica Maffei, Chiara Martini,
Massimo Midiri, Jan Bogaert, and Filippo Cademartiri

17 Cardiac Veins and Pulmonary Veins 185
Maurizio Centonze, Giulia Casagranda, Maurizio Del Greco, Andrea Laudon,
Alessandro Cristoforetti, and Giandomenico Nollo

18 Collateral Findings on Cardiac CT 201
Roberto Malagò, Camilla Barbiani, Andrea Pezzato, Ugolino Alfonsi, Erica Maffei,
Roberto Pozzi Mucelli, and Filippo Cademartiri

19 Reporting in Cardiac CT 207
Erica Maffei, Chiara Martini, Udo Hoffmann, and Filippo Cademartiri

20 Training and Implementation in Cardiac CT 213
Erica Maffei, Chiara Martini, and Filippo Cademartiri

Section IV - Technique

21 CT and CT Angiography - Basics 219
Erica Maffei, Chiara Martini, and Filippo Cademartiri

22 CT of the Heart: Scan Technique 227
Erica Maffei, Chiara Martini, and Filippo Cademartiri

23 Patient Preparation for Cardiac CT 235
Erica Maffei, Chiara Martini, and Filippo Cademartiri

24 Contrast Material Administration in Cardiac CT 241
Erica Maffei, Chiara Martini, and Filippo Cademartiri

25 Principles of Cardiac CT Scan Protocol Optimization 247
Erica Maffei, Chiara Martini, and Filippo Cademartiri

26 Management of Radiation Dose in Cardiac CT 251
Erica Maffei, Chiara Martini, and Filippo Cademartiri

27 Artifacts in Cardiac CT 259
Roberto Malagò, Andrea Pezzato, Camilla Barbiani, Ugolino Alfonsi, Erica Maffei,
Filippo Cademartiri, and Roberto Pozzi Mucelli

Contents xiii

Section V - Clinical Applications

28 Diagnostic and Prognostic Value 281
Joanne D. Schuijf, Jacob M. van Werkhoven, Jeroen J. Bax, and Ernst E. van der Wall

29 Screening and High CV Risk Patients 289
Giancarlo Casolo

30 Thoracic Aortic Diseases 293
Vincenzo Russo, Francesco Buia, Giovanni Rinaldi, Giangaspare Mineo,
and Rossella Fattori

31 Clinical Indications of Cardiac CT 301
Erica Maffei, Chiara Martini, Sara Seitun, and Filippo Cademartiri

Section VI - Other Diagnostic Modalities

32 Stress ECG 313
Pompilio Faggiano, Giacomo Faden, and Livio Dei Cas

33 Rest and Stress Echocardiography 325
Fausto Rigo, Lauro Cortigiani, Elisabetta Grolla, and Eugenio Picano

34 Nuclear Medicine – SPECT/PET 349
Alberto Cuocolo

35 Cardiac Magnetic Resonance 357
Erica Maffei, Chiara Martini, Carlo Tedeschi, Andrea I. Guaricci, Giuseppe Tarantini,
Giancarlo Casolo, and Filippo Cademartiri

36 Invasive Imaging of Coronary Atherosclerotic Plaques 363
Francesco Prati, Michele Occhipinti, and Luca Di Vito

37 Future Developments in Cardiac CT 371
Filippo Cademartiri, Erica Maffei, Chiara Martini, Sara Seitun, and Giuseppe Tarantini

Index 375

Contributors

Ugolino Alfonsi Department of Radiology, "G.B. Rossi" University Hospital, Verona, Italy

Camilla Barbiani Department of Radiology, "G.B. Rossi" University Hospital, Verona, Italy

Ian Baron Department of Radiology and Nuclear Medicine, Medical University of Silesia, Katowice, Poland

Jeroen J. Bax Department of Cardiology, Leiden University Medical Center, Leiden, The Netherlands and The Interuniversity Cardiology Institute of The Netherlands, Utrecht, The Netherlands

Jan Bogaert Department of Radiology, Gasthuisberg University Hospital, Catholic University of Leuven, Leuven, Belgium

Lorenzo Bonomo Department of Bioimaging and Radiological Sciences, Institute of Radiology, "A. Gemelli" Hospital, Catholic University, Rome, Italy

Natale Daniele Brunetti Department of Cardiology, University of Foggia, Foggia, Italy

Francesco Buia Cardio-Thoraco-Vascular Department, Cardiovascular Radiology Unit, "Sant'Orsola" University Hospital, Bologna, Italy

Paolo Buja Interventional Cardiology Division, Department of Cardiac, Thoracic and Vascular Sciences, University of Padua, Padua, Italy

Filippo Cademartiri Cardiovascular Imaging Unit, "Giovanni XXIII" Hospital, Monastier di Treviso (TV), Italy

Paolo G. Camici Department of Cardiac, Thoracic and Vascular Sciences, "San Raffaele" University Hospital, Milano, Italy

Giulia Casagranda Radiology Unit, "Santa Chiara" Hospital, Trento, Italy

Giancarlo Casolo Cardiology Unit, Versilia Hospital, Lido di Camaiore (LU), Italy

Margherita Castiglione Morelli Department of Diagnostic and Interventional Radiology, "San Martino" University Hospital – IST – IRCCS, Genova, Italy

Maurizio Centonze Radiology Unit, "San Lorenzo" Hospital, APSS Trento, Trento, Italy

Lauro Cortigiani "Campo di Marte" Hospital, Lucca, Italy

Alessandro Cristoforetti Department of Physics, University of Trento, Trento, Italy

Alberto Cuocolo Departments of Biomorphological and Functional Sciences, University of Naples "Federico II", Naples, Italy

Ceri L. Davies Centre for Advanced Cardiovascular Imaging, Barts & The London NIHR Biomedical Research Unit/Department of Cardiology, Queen Mary University of London, London, UK

Livio Dei Cas Department of Cardiology, Spedali Civili University Hospital, Brescia, Italy

Maurizio Del Greco Cardiology Unit, "Santa Chiara" Hospital, Trento, Italy

Luigi Di Biase Department of Cardiology, University of Foggia, Foggia, Italy and Texas Cardiac Arrhythmia Institute – St. David's Medical Center, Austin, Texas, USA

Matteo Di Biase Department of Cardiology, University of Foggia, Foggia, Italy

Luca Di Vito Department of Cardiology, "A. Gemelli" Hospital, Catholic University, Rome, Italy

Michela Facchin Interventional Cardiology Division, Department of Cardiac, Thoracic and Vascular Sciences, University of Padua, Padua, Italy

Giacomo Faden Department of Cardiology, Spedali Civili University Hospital, Brescia, Italy

Pompilio Faggiano Department of Cardiology, Spedali Civili University Hospital, Brescia, Italy

Rossella Fattori Cardio-Thoraco-Vascular Department, Cardiovascular Radiology Unit, "Sant'Orsola" University Hospital, Bologna, Italy

Massimo Galia DIBIMEF, Department of Radiology, "P. Giaccone" University Hospital, Palermo, Italy

Tessa S.S. Genders Departments of Epidemiology and Radiology, Erasmus University Medical Center, Rotterdam, The Netherlands

Giovanni Gentile DIBIMEF, Department of Radiology, "P. Giaccone" University Hospital, Palermo, Italy

Brian Ghoshhajra Cardiac MR/PET/CT Program, Massachussetts General Hospital, Boston, CA, USA

Elisabetta Grolla "Campo di Marte" Hospital, Lucca, Italy

Katarina Gruszczynska Department of Radiology and Nuclear Medicine, Medical University of Silesia, Katowice, Poland

Andrea I. Guaricci Department of Cardiology, University of Foggia, Foggia, Italy

Udo Hoffmann Cardiac MR/PET/CT Program, Massachusetts General Hospital and Harvard Medical School, Boston, MA, USA

M.G. Myriam Hunink Departments of Epidemiology and Radiology, Erasmus University Medical Center, Rotterdam, The Netherlands and Department of Health Policy and Management, Harvard School of Public Health, Harvard University, Boston, MA, USA

Antonio L'Abbate "Sant'Anna" School of Advanced Studies, Pisa, Italy

Ludovico La Grutta DIBIMEF, Department of Radiology, "P. Giaccone" University Hospital, Palermo, Italy

Andrea Laudon Radiology Unit, "San Lorenzo" Hospital, APPS Trento, Trento, Italy

Carlo Liguori Department of Bioimaging and Radiological Sciences, Institute of Radiology, "A. Gemelli" Hospital, Catholic University, Rome, Italy

Massimo Lombardi Cardiovascular MR Unit, Fondazione CNR/Regione Toscana "G. Monasterio", Pisa, Italy

Erica Maffei Cardiovascular Imaging Unit, "Giovanni XXIII" Hospital, Monastier di Treviso (TV), Italy

Roberto Malagò Department of Radiology, "G.B. Rossi" University Hospital, Verona, Italy

Riccardo Marano Department of Bioimaging and Radiological Sciences, Institute of Radiology, "A. Gemelli" Hospital, Catholic University, Rome, Italy

Massimiliano Marini Cardiology Unit, "Santa Chiara" Hospital, Trento, Italy

Chiara Martini Cardiovascular Imaging Unit, "Giovanni XXIII" Hospital, Monastier di Treviso (TV), Italy

Giancarlo Messalli Department of Radiology, SDN-IRCCS, Naples, Italy

Massimo Midiri DIBIMEF, Department of Radiology, "P. Giaccone" University Hospital, Palermo, Italy

Giangaspare Mineo Cardio-Thoraco-Vascular Department, Cardiovascular Radiology Unit, "Sant'Orsola" University Hospital, Bologna, Italy

Giandomenico Nollo Department of Physics, BIOtech Research Centre, University of Trento, Trento, Italy

Michele Occhipinti CLI Foundation, Rome, Italy

Anselmo A. Palumbo Department of Radiology, University Hospital, Parma, Italy

Gualtiero Pelosi CNR, Institute of Clinical Physiology, Pisa, Italy

Steffen E. Petersen Centre for Advanced Cardiovascular Imaging, Barts & The London NIHR Biomedical Research Unit, The William Harvey Research Institute, Queen Mary University of London, London, UK

Andrea Pezzato Department of Radiology, "G.B. Rossi" University Hospital, Verona, Italy

Eugenio Picano CNR, Institute of Clinical Physiology, Pisa, Italy

Roberto Pozzi Mucelli Department of Radiology, "G.B. Rossi" University Hospital, Verona, Italy

Francesco Prati Interventional Cardiology Unit, "San Giovanni" Hospital, Rome, Italy

Francesca Pugliese Centre for Advanced Cardiovascular Imaging, Barts & The London NIHR Biomedical Research Unit, The William Harvey Research Institute, Queen Mary University of London, London, UK

Flavia Ravelli Department of Physics, University of Trento, Trento, Italy

Fausto Rigo Cardiology Division, "dell'Angelo" Hospital, Mestre-Venice, Italy

Ornella Rimoldi CNR, IBMF, Milano, Italy

Giovanni Rinaldi Cardio-Thoraco-Vascular Department, Cardiovascular Radiology Unit, "Sant'Orsola" University Hospital, Bologna, Italy

Roberta Romito Department of Emergency Cardiology, "Giovanni XXIII" University Hospital, Bari, Italy

Giuseppe Runza DIBIMEF, Department of Radiology, "P. Giaccone" University Hospital, Palermo, Italy

Vincenzo Russo Cardio-Thoraco-Vascular Department, Cardiovascular Radiology Unit, "Sant'Orsola" University Hospital, Bologna, Italy

Giancarlo Savino Department of Bioimaging and Radiological Sciences, Institute of Radiology, "A. Gemelli" Hospital, Catholic University, Rome, Italy

Joanne D. Schuijf Department of Cardiology, Leiden University Medical Center, Leiden, The Netherlands and The Interuniversity Cardiology Institute of The Netherlands, Utrecht, The Netherlands

Sara Seitun Department of Diagnostic and Interventional Radiology, "San Martino" University Hospital – IST – IRCCS, Genova, Italy

Giuseppe Tarantini Interventional Cardiology Division, Department of Cardiac, Thoracic and Vascular Sciences, University of Padua, Padua, Italy

Tust Techasith Cardiac MR/PET/CT Program, Massachussetts General Hospital, Menlo Park, CA, USA

Carlo Tedeschi Cardiology Division, "San Gennaro" Hospital, Naples, Italy

Ernst E. van der Wall Department of Cardiology, Leiden University Medical Center, Leiden, The Netherlands and The Interuniversity Cardiology Institute of The Netherlands, Utrecht, The Netherlands

Jacob M. van Werkhoven Department of Cardiology, Leiden University Medical Center, Leiden, The Netherlands and The Interuniversity Cardiology Institute of The Netherlands, Utrecht, The Netherlands

Section I

Epidemiology and Clinical Assessment

Epidemiology of Coronary Artery Disease

1

Tessa S.S. Genders and M.G. Myriam Hunink

1.1 Introduction

Coronary artery disease is defined as a pathologic process affecting the coronary arteries, although it is most often used to indicate atherosclerotic changes in the coronary arteries. This is also referred to as coronary heart disease (CHD). According to the American Heart Association [1], coronary heart disease includes the diagnoses of acute myocardial infarction, angina pectoris and all other forms of acute and chronic ischemic heart disease (ICD/10 I20-I25).

This chapter will discuss the epidemiology of CHD, including estimates on incidence, prevalence, mortality, and risk factors. Patients who suffer from CHD often present with either angina pectoris or an acute myocardial infarction (MI). Since cardiac computed tomography can play an important role in evaluating such patients, we will discuss the epidemiology of angina pectoris and acute MI separately as well.

1.2 Coronary Heart Disease

1.2.1 Incidence

Based on observations in the Framingham Heart Study, the lifetime risk at age 40 of developing CHD is estimated to be 49% in men, and 32% in women [2]. For both men and women, the risk of CHD increases with age [3] (Table 1.1)

The incidence in men is substantially higher compared to premenopausal women. However, the morbidity incidence in women increases dramatically beyond menopause [4], thereby reducing the differences

Table 1.1 Incidence (cases/1000 person years) of coronary heart disease* by age and sex based on the Framingham Heart Study, 1980-2003 [4]

Age	Men	Women
45-54	8.0	1.8
55-64	16.4	6.4
65-74	21.8	11.0
75-84	32.8	17.1
85-94	38.0	22.8

* Myocardial infarction, angina pectoris, coronary insufficiency, or fatal coronary heart disease.

between men and women. In support of this, a large Finnish cohort study of over 14 000 individuals found that the CHD incidence was 3 times higher in men compared to women. It was demonstrated that risk factor levels were more favorable in women, although the differences in the risk factors between men and women decreased with advancing age [6].

The National Health and Nutrition Examination Survey (NHANES) Epidemiologic Follow-up study in the United States (US) compared the CHD incidence in two historical cohorts. They found that the age-standardized incidence of CHD decreased from 133.3 per 10 000 person years for the 1971-1982 cohort to 113.5 per 10 000 person years for the 1982-1992 cohort [7].

1.2.2 Prevalence

According to the NHANES 2003-2006, the prevalence of CHD is 7.9% in US adults aged 20 and older. For men and women separately, the prevalence is 9.1% and 7.0% [1].

1.2.3 Mortality

Although total mortality from cardiovascular diseases (which includes stroke) has declined over the past years, it remains the most common cause of death both in Europe [8] and the US [1]. CHD accounts for approxi-

M.G.M. Hunink (✉)
Departments of Epidemiology and Radiology,
Erasmus University Medical Center, Rotterdam, The Netherlands
and Department of Health Policy and Management,
Harvard School of Public Health,
Harvard University, Boston, MA, USA

F. Cademartiri, G. Casolo, M. Midiri (eds.), *Clinical Applications of Cardiac CT,*
© Springer-Verlag Italia 2012

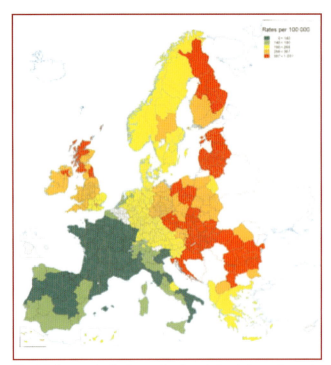

Fig. 1.1 Age-standardized mortality from ischemic heart disease in European regions (men; age group 45–74 years; year 2000). (Reproduced from [9], with permission)

mately 50% of all deaths due to cardiovascular diseases [1, 8]. In Europe, 1.92 million CHD related deaths occur every year. The age-standardized mortality rate for men varies considerably across Europe [9] (Fig. 1.1), with lower mortality rates in Central, Southern, and Western Europe. The highest mortality rates are observed in Eastern Europe. A similar pattern was observed for women. On average, it is estimated that over one in six women and over one in five men will die from CHD [8].

In the US from 1980 through 2000, the age-adjusted death rate for CHD decreased from 543 to 267 deaths per 100 000 population among men. Among women, the rate decreased from 263 to 134 deaths per 100 000. It is estimated that approximately half of the decrease is attributable to improvements in diagnosis and treatment and the other half to changes in risk factors [10, 11].

1.2.4 Risk Factors

The Framingham Heart Study [12] has provided valuable insight into the epidemiology and risk factors of cardiovascular diseases. The most important modifiable risk factors associated with an increased cardiovascular disease risk include: smoking, dyslipidaemia, high blood pressure, diabetes, and obesity [13]. Other factors proven to increase the risk of cardiovascular disease include: psychosocial factors [14], a low physical activity [15], a lack of daily consumption of fruit and vegetables [16] and a lack of regular alcohol intake [17].

A recent case-control study across 52 countries demonstrated that over 90% of all acute MIs as initial coronary event can be attributed to currently established risk factors [17].

1.3 Angina Pectoris

1.3.1 Incidence

Based on data from the NHLBI ARIC (National Heart, Lung, and Blood Institute - Atherosclerosis Risk in Communities) cohort (1987-2001), the age-adjusted incidence of angina pectoris as determined by the Rose Questionnaire was 10.8 cases per 1000 person years in men, and 13.4 in women. The highest incidence (17.9 per 1000 person years) was observed in black women.

A large Finnish prospective cohort study focused on the incidence of angina defined as a nitrate prescription or angina with positive diagnostic findings. The age-standardized annual incidence was 2.03 per 100 in men and 1.89 per 100 in women. In this study, no sex difference in prognosis (i.e. absolute coronary event rate at 4 years) was observed. The Euro Heart Survey studied over 3000 patients with a new clinical diagnosis by a cardiologist of stable angina and found that the rate of death and non-fatal MI at 1 year was 2.3 per 100 patient years [18]. They also demonstrated that of those patients with a new clinical diagnosis of stable angina, women with confirmed coronary artery disease have a 2-fold increased rate of death and nonfatal MI within the first year as compared to men [19].

1.3.2 Prevalence

According to a systematic review of existing healthy population based studies, the prevalence of angina as assessed by the Rose Angina Questionnaire, is estimated to be 5.7% in men and 6.7% in women, which varied widely (0.7-15%) across countries [20].

1.4 Acute Myocardial Infarction

More than 50% of all acute coronary events occur in patients without any history of CHD [21] and only 18% is preceded by longstanding angina symptoms [1].

1.4.1 Incidence

An analysis of US patients hospitalized between 1999 and 2008 revealed an age- and sex-adjusted incidence rate of acute MI of 208 cases per 100 000 person years [22]. Reports indicate that the incidence rate of ST elevation MI declined over the past decades [22, 23]. However, results also suggest that the true (larger) decline in incidence rate may be masked by an increased detection by using increasingly sensitive biomarkers in the diagnosis of acute MI [23].

Few data are available on CHD incidence rates for the European region [8]. Results from the WHO MONICA (World Health Organization - monitoring trends and determinants in cardiovascular disease) Project studied the trends over 10 years in CHD across 21 European countries, starting in the early 1980s. A coronary event included non-fatal events satisfying the criteria for definite MI, and fatal events classified as definite, possible, and unclassifiable coronary deaths. Observed annual event rates were 434 per 100 000 in men, and 103 per 100 000 in women. In this study, an annual decline in coronary events of approximately 2.1% for men and 1.4% for women was observed [24].

The Rotterdam study, a population-based cohort of 5148 men and women aged 55 and older in the Netherlands, revealed a documented MI incidence rate of 8.4 and 3.1 per 1000 person years for men and women, respectively. Furthermore, the rate of additional unrecognized infarctions was estimated to be 4.2 for men and 3.6 per 1000 person years for women, which implies that a substantial proportion (approximately 50%) of myocardial infarctions remain clinically unrecognized [25].

1.4.2 Prevalence

According to NHANES data, the prevalence of MI between 1988 and 1994 among US adults aged 35-54 was 2.5% for men and 0.7% for women [26]. The prevalence among men decreased over time (2.5% to 2.1%) but the prevalence among women increased (0.7% to 1.0%), as observed in the period between 1999 and 2004.

1.4.3 Prognosis

It is well recognized that patients who experienced a coronary event are at increased risk for future cardiovascular events. The absolute risk however, depends largely on the clinical presentation and the presence of other car-

diovascular risk factors.

In 2002, the Euro Heart Survey of acute coronary syndromes found a 30-day mortality rate of 8.4%, 3.5% and 13.3% for patients with ST elevation MI (STEMI), non ST elevation MI (NSTEMI) and undetermined electrocardiogram acute coronary syndrome, respectively [27]. The OPERA-registry demonstrated a similar 30-day mortality rate for STEMI and NSTEMI, but an increased 1-year mortality rate for NSTEMI as compared to STEMI (11.6% vs. 9.0%) [28]. The GUSTO-IIB trial investigated the prognosis of over 12 000 patients after an acute coronary syndrome. Results indicated that the 30-day mortality was higher for STEMI compared to NSTEMI patients (6.1% vs. 3.8%), whereas the cumulative mortality rate after one year was not significantly different (9.6% vs. 8.8%) [29]. Furthermore, a US population-based study of nearly 3000 acute MI patients found that the rate of sudden cardiac death after MI was constant at 1.2% per year, and that the 5-year cumulative incidence was 6.9% [30].

The National Registry of Myocardial Infarction in the US evaluated nearly 2 million patients that were hospitalized for acute MI from 1994 to 2006 and showed that the overall in-hospital mortality decreased from 10.4% in 1994 to 6.3% in 2006 [31].

Since a large part of the myocardial infarctions remain clinically unrecognized, it is important to investigate the clinical significance of such an event. A US based Cardiovascular Health Study database of patients 65 years and older allowed for the comparison of the prognosis between patients with unrecognized and recognized MIs. It was revealed that the six-year mortality rate was not significantly different between the two groups [32].

1.5 Conclusions

The CHD incidence and mortality decreased over the past decades due to improved medical treatments and changes in risk factors. CHD accounts for approximately 50% of all deaths due to cardiovascular diseases. In spite of the declining incidence and mortality, CHD manifestations such as angina pectoris and acute myocardial infarction are common. A substantial proportion of acute myocardial infarctions remain clinically unrecognized, but carry a similar prognosis as compared to recognized acute myocardial infarctions. More than 50% of all acute myocardial infarctions occur in patients without any history of coronary heart disease.

References

1. American Heart Association (2010) Heart Disease and Stroke Statistics – 2010 Update. Dallas, Texas: American Heart Association
2. Lloyd-Jones DM, Larson MG, Beiser A, Levy D (1999) Lifetime risk of developing coronary heart disease. Lancet 353:89-92
3. Wilson PW, D'Agostino RB, Levy D et al (1998) Prediction of coronary heart disease using risk factor categories. Circulation 97:1837-1847
4. National Heart, Lung, and Blood Institute (2006) Incidence and Prevalence: 2006 Chart Book on Cardiovascular and Lung Diseases. Bethesda, MD: National Heart, Lung, and Blood Institute
5. Gordon T, Kannel WB, Hjortland MC, McNamara PM (1978) Menopause and coronary heart disease. The Framingham Study. Ann Intern Med 89:157-161
6. Jousilahti P, Vartiainen E, Tuomilehto J, Puska P (1999) Sex, age, cardiovascular risk factors, and coronary heart disease: a prospective follow-up study of 14 786 middle-aged men and women in Finland. Circulation 99:1165-1172
7. Ergin A, Muntner P, Sherwin R, He J (2004) Secular trends in cardiovascular disease mortality, incidence, and case fatality rates in adults in the United States. Am J Med 117:219-227
8. European Heart Network (2011) European cardiovascular disease statistics: University of Oxford. http://www.ehnheart.org/cvd-statistics.html. Accessed 12 October 2010
9. Muller-Nordhorn J, Binting S, Roll S, Willich SN (2008) An update on regional variation in cardiovascular mortality within Europe. Eur Heart J 29:1316-1326
10. Ford ES, Ajani UA, Croft JB et al (2007) Explaining the decrease in U.S. deaths from coronary disease, 1980-2000. N Engl J Med 356:2388-2398
11. Wijeysundera HC, Machado M, Farahati F et al (2010) Association of temporal trends in risk factors and treatment uptake with coronary heart disease mortality, 1994-2005. JAMA 303:1841-1847
12. National Heart Lung and Blood Institute (2010) Framingham Heart Study. National Heart Lung and Blood Institute. http://www.framinghamheartstudy.org/. Accessed 13 October 2010
13. D'Agostino RB Sr, Vasan RS, Pencina MJ et al (2008) General cardiovascular risk profile for use in primary care: the Framingham Heart Study. Circulation 117:743-753
14. Haynes SG, Feinleib M, Levine S et al (1978) The relationship of psychosocial factors to coronary heart disease in the Framingham study. II. Prevalence of coronary heart disease. Am J Epidemiol 107:384-402
15. Kannel WB (1967) Habitual level of physical activity and risk of coronary heart disease: the Framingham study. Can Med Assoc J 96:811-812
16. Bazzano LA, He J, Ogden LG et al (2002) Fruit and vegetable intake and risk of cardiovascular disease in US adults: the first National Health and Nutrition Examination Survey Epidemiologic Follow-up Study. Am J Clin Nutr 76:93-99
17. Yusuf S, Hawken S, Ounpuu S et al (2004) Effect of potentially modifiable risk factors associated with myocardial infarction in 52 countries (the INTERHEART study): case-control study. Lancet 364:937-952
18. Daly CA, De Stavola B, Sendon JL et al (2006) Predicting prognosis in stable angina—results from the Euro heart survey of stable angina: prospective observational study. BMJ 332:262-267
19. Daly C, Clemens F, Lopez Sendon JL et al (2006) Gender differences in the management and clinical outcome of stable angina. Circulation 113:490-498
20. Hemingway H, Langenberg C, Damant J et al (2008) Prevalence of angina in women versus men: a sysematic review and meta-analysis of international variations across 31 countries. Circulation 117:1526-1536
21. Tunstall-Pedoe H, Morrison C, Woodward M et al (1996) Sex differences in myocardial infarction and coronary deaths in the Scottish MONICA population of Glasgow 1985 to 1991. Presentation, diagnosis, treatment, and 28-day case fatality of 3991 events in men and 1551 events in women. Circulation 93:1981-1992
22. Yeh RW, Sidney S, Chandra M et al (2010) Population trends in the incidence and outcomes of acute myocardial infarction. N Engl J Med 362:2155-2165
23. Parikh NI, Gona P, Larson MG et al (2009) Long-term trends in myocardial infarction incidence and case fatality in the National Heart, Lung, and Blood Institute's Framingham Heart study. Circulation 119:1203-1210
24. Tunstall-Pedoe H, Kuulasmaa K, Mahonen M et al (1999) Contribution of trends in survival and coronary-event rates to changes in coronary heart disease mortality: 10-year results from 37 WHO MONICA project populations. Monitoring trends and determinants in cardiovascular disease. Lancet 353:1547-1557
25. de Torbal A, Boersma E, Kors JA et al (2006) Incidence of recognized and unrecognized myocardial infarction in men and women aged 55 and older: the Rotterdam Study. Eur Heart J 27:729-736
26. Towfighi A, Zheng L, Ovbiagele B (2009) Sex-specific trends in midlife coronary heart disease risk and prevalence. Arch Intern Med 169:1762-1766
27. Hasdai D, Behar S, Wallentin L et al (2002) A prospective survey of the characteristics, treatments and outcomes of patients with acute coronary syndromes in Europe and the Mediterranean basin; the Euro Heart Survey of Acute Coronary Syndromes (Euro Heart Survey ACS). Eur Heart J 23:1190-1201
28. Montalescot G, Dallongeville J, Van Belle E et al (2007) STEMI and NSTEMI: are they so different? 1 year outcomes in acute myocardial infarction as defined by the ESC/ACC definition (the OPERA registry). Eur Heart J 28:1409-1417
29. Armstrong PW, Fu Y, Chang WC et al (1998) Acute coronary syndromes in the GUSTO-IIb trial: prognostic insights and impact of recurrent ischemia. The GUSTO-IIb Investigators. Circulation 98:1860-1868
30. Adabag AS, Therneau TM, Gersh BJ et al (2008) Sudden death after myocardial infarction. JAMA 300:2022-2029
31. Rogers WJ, Frederick PD, Stoehr E et al (2008) Trends in presenting characteristics and hospital mortality among patients with ST elevation and non-ST elevation myocardial infarction in the National Registry of Myocardial Infarction from 1990 to 2006. Am Heart J 156:1026-1034
32. Sheifer SE, Gersh BJ, Yanez ND 3rd et al (2000) Prevalence, predisposing factors, and prognosis of clinically unrecognized myocardial infarction in the elderly. J Am Coll Cardiol 35:119-126

Physiology and Pathophysiology of Coronary Circulation

2

Andrea I. Guaricci, Luigi Di Biase, and Giancarlo Casolo

2.1 Introduction

The heart supplies blood to itself through two coronary arteries that support the coronary circulation. Both arteries lie outside of the heart muscle running along the atrioventricular groove and branch off into a system of smaller vessels that supply the muscle cells. Because of the high oxygen requirements of the myocardium, capillary density is very high, (accounting for ~15 percent of the total cardiac mass). After giving off its oxygen and nutrients in the capillaries, the venous blood flows through coronary veins draining directly into the right atrium. Other drainage is by means of thebesian veins, which drain directly into the right heart, and anterior cardiac veins that empty into the right atrium. Small intramural collateral vessels represent functionally important elements that connect the coronaries and can enlarge after coronary obstruction, providing near-normal flow at rest to the distal segment of the diseased artery. When the heart needs to work harder than during basal conditions, the coronary arteries dilate, thus varying the resistance to the blood flow and increasing the oxygen supply to the heart. The blood flow may increase by five to six times in order to satisfy the oxygen needs of the hyperfunctioning heart muscle. Hence, myocardial contraction is closely connected to coronary flow and oxygen delivery. When oxygen demand and supply are altered by diseases affecting the coronary arteries and the circulation, the effect is the development of *ischemia*. The coronary circulation is able to partially compensate an imbalanced state owing to a pathologic condition. Thus, knowledge of the regulation of coronary blood flow in physiologic and pathophysiologic conditions, other than the relationship between ischemia and contraction, is essential for understanding and managing many cardiovascular disorders.

2.2 Myocardial Oxygen Consumption

The principal function of the coronary arteries is to provide oxygen and nutrients to the myocardium. The primary determinant of coronary blood flow is myocardial oxygen consumption (MVO2) which is calculated as the product of coronary blood flow and the arteriovenous (A-V) O2 difference which represents the arterial oxygen content minus the coronary sinus oxygen content. The coronary oxygen extraction is almost maximal at rest and the coronary sinus oxygen saturations are typically 30% or less (or PO2<20 mmHg). Since myocardial oxygen extraction is at rest already near maximum (75-80% up to a maximum of 90%), MVO2 can increase only by varying the coronary blood flow. In addition to coronary flow, oxygen delivery is directly determined by arterial oxygen content (PaO2) and consequently anemia results in proportional reductions in oxygen delivery. The main determinants of MVO2 are heart rate, inotropic state (contractility), and intramyocardial wall stress. MVO2 can be approximated clinically by the product of systolic blood pressure and heart rate (called the *rate-pressure product*).

2.2.1 Heart Rate

Heart rate is probably the factor that mostly affects MVO2. Heart rate increases by about threefold during intense exercise because of an adrenergic stimulation from both neural and circulating catecholamines [1]. During intense exercise, heart rate accounts for approximately 30% of the increase in coronary flow. During tachycardia, due to a higher rate or to the decreased diastolic time of coronary perfusion, there is increased oxygen consumption.

A.I. Guaricci (✉)
Department of Cardiology,
University of Foggia,
Foggia, Italy

F. Cademartiri, G. Casolo, M. Midiri (eds.), *Clinical Applications of Cardiac CT*,
© Springer-Verlag Italia 2012

2.2.2 Myocardial Contractility

The increase in the contractile state of the myocardium is critical for adjustments to intense exercise. In that state, the rate of change of left ventricular (LV) systolic pressure on time, an index of contractility, can also increase four- to fivefold. The significant increase in systolic pressure enables stroke volume to increase despite increases in heart rate. The corresponding increment of MVO2 requires an appropriate increase in coronary blood flow.

2.2.3 LV Wall Stress

LV systolic wall stress correlates directly with MVO2 since any increase in the workload of the heart increases MVO2. Accordingly to mathematical formula, LV wall stress is directly proportional to the LV pressure and to the LV diameter or volume, and it is inversely proportional to the LV wall thickness. Therefore, during chronic pressure overload, when LV concentric hypertrophy occurs, the wall stress is normalized by increased wall thickness. For that reason, baseline myocardial blood flow per gram of tissue remains essentially at normal levels, 1.0 mL/min/g, in LV hypertrophic conditions. When wall thickness is reduced by LV dilation, considering LV hypertrophy at constant value, thus, chronic volume overload causes eccentric hypertrophy, MVO2 will increase much more than in a condition of normalized wall stress. As a consequence, the increased oxygen requirement implies a recruitment of the coronary flow reserve already at rest.

2.3 Autoregulation of Coronary Blood Flow

During rest, normal coronary blood flow is approximately 60 to 100 mL/min per 100 g of myocardium and can increase by up to fivefold between the basal state and the maximal perfusion in order to match the metabolic demand regardless of the perfusion pressure [2]. Regional coronary blood flow remains constant as coronary artery pressure is reduced below aortic pressure over a wide range when the determinants of myocardial oxygen consumption are kept constant [3]. This process is called autoregulation and it is a mechanism intrinsic to myogenic tone. Coronary blood flow is closely correlated with the diastolic pressure-time index, which is the product of the average difference between aortic and left ventricular cavity pressure and the duration of diastole (i.e. it is the area between diastolic aortic pressure and left ventricular pressure). Coronary blood flow is decreased by systemic hypotension (by decreasing aortic diastolic pressure), increased LV end-diastolic pressure, and tachycardia (by shortening diastole). Hence, coronary blood flow can be augmented by increased systemic pressure, decreased left ventricular end-diastolic pressure, and slowing of the heart rate. At rest, therefore, coronary blood flow is maintained at a fairly constant level over a range of aortic pressures. The vascular smooth muscle cells are rich in stretch-operated ion channels activated by shear stress that stimulate cell contraction. The contractile activity of the smooth muscle cells causes a high myogenic tone which translates into a high resistance to flow [4]. As aortic pressure decreases, coronary blood flow is maintained by the dilation of the arterioles. With the increase in aortic pressure the same result is gained by the constriction of the arterioles. Therefore, during normal resting conditions, the coronary blood flow is pressure-independent. At low perfusion pressures, 40 mmHg, the resistance vessels are dilated maximally and any additional decrease in blood pressure results in a linear decrease in the blood flow leading to the onset of subendocardial ischemia. Hence, the coronary blood flow becomes pressure-dependent. Subepicardial flow occurs throughout the cardiac cycle and is maintained until very low perfusion pressure is reached. At approximately 20 mmHg, blood flow ceases owing to the compressive effects of extravascular intramyocardial pressure The difference existing between the myocardial layers is caused by increased oxygen consumption in the subendocardium, requiring a higher resting flow level, as well as the more pronounced effects of systolic contraction on subendocardial vasodilator reserve. Therefore, the susceptibility of the subendocardium to ischemia in the presence of a coronary stenosis is partially explained. At very high perfusion pressures, more than 140 mmHg, vasoconstriction is maximal and an additional increase in pressure results in a linear increase in blood flow.

2.4 Coronary Blood Flow Control

Resistance to coronary blood flow can be divided into three major components: (1) epicardial arteries, (2) arterioles and microcirculatory resistance arteries and (3) extravascular resistance [2]. There is no measurable pressure drop in the epicardial arteries although in the presence of hemodynamically significant epicardial artery narrowing (more than 50% diameter reduction), the resistance at this level contributes as an important component to the total coronary resistance. The diameter of epicardial arteries (>400 ηm) is mainly regulated by shear stress, and it contributes little pressure drop (<5%) over a wide range of coronary flow. The second component of coronary resistance is present at the level of resistance arteries (100 to 400 ηm) and arterioles (>100 ηm), which are able to regulate their tone, the former in response to local shear stress and luminal pressure changes (myogenic response) and the latter in response to changes in local tissue metabolism and directly control perfusion of the low-resistance coronary capillary bed. The capillary density of the myocardium averages $3500/mm^2$ and is greater in the subendocardium than the subepicardium. Cardiac contraction provides the third component of coronary resistance. Mechanical factors have an important effect on coronary blood flow. During myocardial contraction, intramyocardial pressure increases and the squeezing forces cause compression of small vessels and the reduction of coronary blood flow. At that time, the intraventricular pressure that opposes coronary flow is roughly equal to the aortic perfusion pressure. Hence, the myocardium is perfused mainly during the diastolic phase. During early diastole, a drop in intraventricular pressure occurs simultaneously to the decrease of aortic pressure; the former is bigger than the latter, allowing optimal coronary perfusion. Approximately 80% of coronary blood flow occurs during diastole in the left coronary artery. The situation is different in the proximal right coronary artery. The right ventricle wall is just a few millimeters thick and, during its performance, the compression on the vascular network is low owing to the low pressure values. Blood flow in the proximal right coronary artery during systole is approximately equal to that during diastole. In the distal right coronary artery diastolic flow is again more effective than systolic flow since it supplies the inferior wall of the LV.

The myocardial compressive effects are greater in the subendocardial layer than in the subepicardial layer. In a normal heart, the blood flow to the subendocardium is approximately 125 percent of that in the epicardium [5]. Nevertheless, this ratio drops in conditions of reduced perfusion pressure and particularly during coronary artery constriction or occlusion and in the presence of well-developed coronary collaterals. Hence, when coronary blood flow is reduced, as from an epicardial coronary artery stenosis, the subendocardial layer is the first region of the myocardium to suffer from oxygen depletion. A reversed subendocardial-to-subepicardial flow ratio is the hallmark of myocardial ischemia. Another condition in which the subendocardial coronary flow will decrease, but not to the same extent as in ischemia, is in hypertrophied left ventricle where the normal coronary arteries use their mechanism of autoregulation because of the higher energy demand, the larger compressive forces especially in the subendocardium. Although flow may be adequate at rest, subendocardial ischemia may occur with exercise or stress.

2.5 Coronary Tone and Resistances

2.5.1 Role of the Endothelium

The endothelium is formed by a single layer of cells on the vascular surface and is the largest organ in the body. Although the endothelium functions as a semipermeable membrane, it plays a pivotal role in coronary artery physiology and physiopathology. The integrity of endothelium is essential for guaranteeing normal function since it has the role of maintaining normal coronary blood flow.

The endothelium continuously produces substances to modulate vascular tone, including nitric oxide, prostacyclin, and endothelial-derived contracting factors such as endothelin. Several factors, including acetylcholine, histamine, bradykinin, substance P, and other platelet-derived substances stimulate endothelial cells to produce nitric oxide. Shear stress in a vessel's lumen also stimulates the release of nitric oxide and contributes to flow-mediated dilation that occurs with changes in coronary blood flow states. The strongest vasoactive constrictor peptide that directly stimulates receptors on smooth muscle cells, the endothelin, is produced by endothelium cells. Some factors such as thrombin, transforming growth factor-β, interleukin-1, epinephrine, antidiuretic hormone, and angiotensin II stimulate the release of endothelin. Moreover, the endothelium converts angiotensin to angiotensin II through tissue-bound angiotensin-converting enzyme (ACE), which also causes vasoconstriction (Table 2.1).

In normal conditions, epicardial arteries do not contribute significantly to coronary vascular resistance, even though their diameter is influenced by most of the above-mentioned factors, including platelet derived factors, circulating neurohormonal agonists, neural tone and local vascular shear stress. Some studies demonstrated that coronary resistance arteries also get endothelial modulation of diameter and that their size influences the response to physical forces such as shear stress, as well as paracrine mediators [6].

2.5.2 Vascular Control Mechanism

Metabolic mediators of coronary resistance control and local vascular control mechanisms are physiologically balanced to adjust regional tissue perfusion to the distal microcirculation. There is a differential expression of mechanisms among different sizes and classes of coro-

Table 2.1 Endothelium-dependent and effects of neural stimulation and autacoids on coronary tone in coronary resistance arteries

Substance	Endothelium-dependent	Normal response	Pathologic conditions (atherosclerosis)
Acetylcholine resistance	Nitric oxide, EDHF	Dilation	Attenuated dilation
Norepinephrine			
Alpha1		Constriction	Constriction
Beta2	Nitric oxide	Dilation	Attenuated dilation
Platelets			
Thrombin	Nitric oxide	Dilation	Constriction
Serotonin resistance	Nitric oxide	Dilation	Constriction
ADP	Nitric oxide	Dilation	Attenuated dilation
Thromboxane	Endothelin	Constriction	Constriction
Paracrine Agonists			
Bradykinin	Nitric oxide, EDHF	Dilation	Attenuated dilation
Histamine	Nitric oxide	Dilation	Attenuated dilation
Substance P	Nitric oxide	Dilation	Attenuated dilation
Endothelin (ET)			
ET-1	Nitric oxide	Net Constriction	Increased Constriction

nary resistance vessels, which coincides with their function.

2.5.3 Myogenic Regulation

The myogenic response consists in the capability of vascular smooth muscle to oppose changes in coronary arteriolar diameter. As a result of distending pressure decrease the vessels relax whereas they constrict when distending pressure is elevated. Myogenic tone is a property of vascular smooth muscle and occurs across a large size range of coronary resistance arteries. This kind of mechanism occurs primarily in arterioles smaller than 100 ηm and it seems to be an essential tool of coronary autoregulation [7].

2.5.4 Flow-Dependent Dilation

Coronary arteries regulate their diameter in response to changes in local shear stress. Some studies demonstrating that flow-induced dilation in isolated coronary arterioles has an endothelium-dependent mechanism mediated by NO while, in isolated atrial vessels this mechanism is mediated by endothelium-dependent hyperpolarizing factor (EDHF) [8-10]. The mechanisms appear to vary as a function of age, species and vessel size. Other studies demonstrating that hyperpolarization acts on the epicardial conduit arteries and NO predominates in the resistance vasculature [11]. Therefore, NO production is also increased by shear stress and is an excellent mediator of autoregulation in conditions of increased cardiac output, such as during exercise. This mechanism is the molecu-

lar basis of flow-dependent coronary vasodilation. The increased shear stress in consequence of the increased flow represents a stimulus for NO production that is followed by coronary dilation and subsequent lowering of shear stress. Studies showed that following a temporary coronary artery occlusion during the reactive hyperemia phase, the large coronary arteries dilated (termed *reactive dilation*) being entirely dependent on the increase in coronary blood flow [12].

2.5.5 Metabolic Factors

The most important metabolic factors include adenosine, acidosis and hypoxia. Of the agents released from myocardial cells, adenosine is probably the most important. Adenosine is produced from the breakdown of high-energy phosphates (adenosine triphosphate [ATP]). The breakdown product, adenosine monophosphate (AMP) accumulates and is converted to adenosine. Adenosine primarily dilates vessels smaller than 100 ηm and, from a functional point of view, experimental data demonstrate that it is not required for adjusting coronary flow to increases in metabolism or autoregulation [13]. Nevertheless, adenosine participates in vasodilation during hypoxia and during acute exercise-induced myocardial ischemia distal to a stenosis [14]. Substantially unresolved is the role of local hypoxia in the regulation of arteriolar tone, although it has strong properties as a potent coronary vasodilator. It is known that coronary flow increases proportionally to reduced PO2 or anemia and there is a two-fold increase in perfused capillary density in response to hypoxia, but this could simply reflect the close coupling between myocardial metabolism and flow. As regarding acidosis, it has been demonstrated to produce coronary vasodilation independent of hypoxia particularly in the setting of acute ischemia [5].

2.5.6 Autonomic Factors

The contribution of the autonomic nervous system to the control of blood flow may not be as relevant as the mechanical and metabolic effect. Changes in coronary blood flow with either sympathetic or parasympathetic stimulation are due predominantly to the accompanying changes in loading conditions and contractility even though a direct effect is present.

2.5.6.1 Parasympathetic Receptor Control
Vagal stimulation has a vasodilatory effect in the normal coronaries, inducing NO release by acetylcholine stimulation, thus increasing coronary blood flow. This happens both in resistance and conduit arteries. In conduit arteries the net vasodilation results from a direct muscarinic constriction of vascular smooth muscle and by an endothelium-dependent vasodilation owing to the direct stimulation of NO synthase. The increased flow-mediated dilation from concomitant resistance vessel vasodilation adds its effect to the abovementioned mechanisms. When coronary artery disease occurs, above all with the production of significant stenosis, the acetylcholine-mediated dilation upon resistance vessels is decreased. The effect on the epicardial conduit artery can be vasoconstriction considering the reduction in flow-mediated NO production. In addition to a direct effect on the coronary bed, the parasympathetic tone reduces heart rate, arterial pressure and inotropy, which together reduce the oxygen demand of the myocardium [15].

2.5.6.2 α-Adrenergic Receptor Control
The effect of sympathetic stimulation is to modulate the coronary tone by norepinephrine released from myocardial sympathetic nerves, as well as by circulating norepinephrine and epinephrine [16]. Stimulation of the a-receptors induces a vasoconstrictive response in conduit arteries. An important consequence of the a-adrenergic mediated vasoconstriction in a context of increased workload and particularly during exercise is an increase in oxygen extraction [17]. The vasoconstriction resulting from α-adrenergic receptor stimulation is increased in patients with coronary artery disease, probably reflecting the partial use of the coronary flow reserve in that situation [18]. The α-adrenergic tone of the coronary arteries can be activated by stimulation of reflex pathways, such as carotid baroreceptors upon carotid sinus hypotension, as well as by direct sympathomimetic stimulation.

2.5.6.3 β-Adrenergic Receptor Control
Coronary vasodilation is achieved by stimulation of the b-adrenergic receptors. Binding of the receptors in the coronary vessel itself will stimulate a Gs protein-mediated relaxation of the vascular smooth muscle cells [19]. In addition, binding of the receptors on the cardiac cells will stimulate a Gs protein-mediated increase in contractility, which, together with the increase in heart rate, will increase the metabolic demand and activate the recruitment of the coronary flow reserve through adenosine release. Whereas the $\beta2$ receptors are mainly responsible for the direct vasodilatory mechanism, the contribution of the $\beta1$ receptor predominates for the metabolic effect resulting from increased workload [20]. Therefore, in conduit arteries, sympathetic stimulation leads to $\beta2$-mediated vasodilation and the concomitant flow-mediated vasodilation from metabolic vasodilation of coronary resistance vessels enhances the dilation. Relatively to the coronary resistance vessel tone, the sum effect of $\beta1$-mediated increment in myocardial oxygen consumption of direct $\beta2$-mediated coronary vasodilation and of $\alpha1$-mediated coronary constriction is responsible for constriction or dilation predominance. Under normal conditions, exercise-induced $\beta2$-adrenergic dilation predominates with the effect of increment of blood flow proportionally to MVO2.

2.6 Coronary Flow Reserve

The ability to increase flow above resting values in response to pharmacologic vasodilation is termed coronary reserve. The coronary flow reserve (CFR) is the difference between coronary flow at rest and coronary flow during maximal perfusion. During exercise, the metabolic demands of the myocardium increase and the way to satisfy the MVO2 is to adequately increase coronary blood flow. Hence, the coronary flow reserve represents how much the system is able to augment blood flow with stress. It can be measured by employing both invasive tools and noninvasive techniques such as intracoronary Doppler during pharmacologic stress (e.g. adenosine test).

The physiologic condition which recruits the coronary flow reserve is exercise, while it can be already recruited at rest under different condition including the ischemic heart disease. During exercise, flow-mediated dilation and NO release, metabolic dilation by adenosine, and β-adrenergic vasodilation decrease coronary resistance. During tachycardia CFR is reduced by 10 percent for every 15 heartbeats owing to increased basal flow. It has been demonstrated experimentally that exercise is also accompanied by a vasoconstrictive a-adrenergic stimulation in order to balance an excessive decrease in coronary resistance, gaining a better myocardial oxygen extraction too [21]. In addition, the aortic perfusion pressure also increases, thereby improving the flow through large coronary arteries. CFR may be reduced in patients with essential hypertension and normal coronary arteries and in patients with aortic stenosis and normal coronary arteries [22-24]. Aging may induce a variability of CVR in unobstructed arteries [25]. The correction formula for age has shown that only patients with diabetes have a significant decrease of the traditional CVR and corrected CVR, whereas hypertension and current smoking have no influence on corrected CVR [26]. Other conditions determining impaired microcirculation are vasculitis syndromes, recurrent ischemia, abnormal myocardial metabolism and, of course, myocardial infarction [27].

2.7 Altered Coronary Physiology

2.7.1 Obstructive Coronary Disease

Atherosclerosis is the main cause of coronary stenosis and the coronary circulation has to overcome the fall of pressure across the obstruction in order to guarantee the normal perfusion to the myocardium. According to the laws of hydrodynamics, the drop in perfusion pressure across the stenosis is inversely proportional to the fourth power of the minimal luminal diameter. In other words, even a slight decrease in diameter will result in a major loss of pressure. Moreover, the length of the stenosis has its influence above all when it is a well represented parameter of the stenosis. Hence, the effects of coronary obstruction on blood flow depends mainly on the extent of the stenosis. Therefore, although minor luminal irregularities have little effect on the hemodynamics of the blood flow, a coronary stenosis obstructing at least 40 percent of the vessel diameter causes a drop in perfusion pressure, which requires a matching decrease of coronary resistance to maintain the normal flow at rest [28]. In parallel with resistance to flow, viscous friction, flow separation forces, and flow turbulence at the site of the stenosis produce energy loss at the stenosis. The energy loss has the effect of reducing pressure distal to the stenosis, producing significant trans-stenotic pressure gradients. The decreased resistance is mediated by adenosine release by recruiting the *coronary blood flow reserve* already at rest. The physiologic consequence of this phenomenon is reduced exercise capacity. If the degree of the obstruction progresses, the coronary blood flow reserve will progressively decrease and when it occludes at least 80% of the vessel diameter, the coronary reserve will be totally recruited at rest.

Chronic obstructive coronary disease produces a broadening of collateral circulation. Collateral vessels provide communication between the major coronary arteries and their branches. If stenosis of an epicardial coronary artery produces a pressure gradient across such a vessel, the collateral channel can dilate with time and provide an alternative avenue for blood flow [29]. Such functional collaterals can develop between the terminal extensions of two coronary arteries, between the side branches of two arteries, between branches of the same artery, or within the same branch (via *vasa vasorum*) Notably, the patients with well-developed collateral vessels have a low risk of developing acute myocardial infarction upon abrupt closure of the culprit coronary artery [30].

2.7.2 Paracrine Mediators in Coronary Artery Disease

With atherosclerotic plaque rupture and development of thrombus in epicardial arteries, some paracrine mediators are released. These factors modify epicardial tone in vascular regions close to eccentric ulcerated plaques. Moreover, by stimulating the release of NO and EDHF, paracrine mediators can have different effects on downstream vessel vasomotion which are dependent on vessel size as well as on the presence of a functionally normal endothelium. Some of most important paracrine substances are serotonin, thrombin, thromboxane A2 and ADP. Under normal conditions, serotonin dilates coronary resistance vessels (<100 ηm) and increases blood flow by stimulating the endothelium-dependent release of NO. When NO production is impaired as in atherosclerosis, the final effect is vasoconstriction owing to the predominance of direct effects on smooth muscle cells. Thrombin is another mediator that causes constriction of stenotic epicardial arteries. This happens because of the poorly functioning endothelium-dependent vasodilation. Normally, thrombin increases coronary blood flow in resistance vessels by exploiting endothelium-dependent vasodilation. Finally, thromboxane A2 and ADP are platelet-derived factors: the former induces strong vasoconstriction of conduit arteries and the latter dilation of coronary microvessels and conduit arteries.

2.7.3 Fractional Flow Reserve

Myocardial perfusion is closely linked to myocardial ischemia and is directly dependent on the coronary driving pressure associated with three major coronary vascular resistances. The myocardial perfusion pressure

(AoP minus LV pressure or RA pressure) is reduced when an epicardial stenosis causes pressure loss distal to the stenosis. If the coronary vessels are stimulated to maximal hyperemia and resistances remain constant, the post-stenotic hyperemic coronary artery pressure is the maximal achievable perfusion available in that vessel and can be used to produce an estimate of normal coronary blood flow and an ischemic threshold. Using coronary pressure measured at constant and minimal myocardial resistances (i.e. maximal hyperemia), Pijls et al. [31] and De Bruyne et al. [32] derived an estimate of the percentage of normal coronary blood flow expected to go through a stenotic artery. This pressure-derived ratio is called the fractional flow reserve (FFR). FFRcor is defined as the maximum coronary flow in the presence of a stenosis divided by the normal maximum flow of the artery (i.e. the maximum flow in that artery if no stenosis were present) [33]. Similarly, FFRmyo is defined as maximum myocardial blood flow distal to an epicardial stenosis divided by its value if no epicardial stenosis were present. Hence, FFR represents that fraction of normal maximum flow that remains despite the presence of an epicardial lesion. FFR can be derived separately for the myocardium, epicardial coronary artery, and collateral supply. FFR has a normal value of 1.0 for every patient and every coronary artery. It is independent of gender or coronary artery disease risk factors such as hypertension and diabetes. Because of the need to know Pw, FFRcor can be calculated only during percutaneous transluminal coronary angioplasty (PTCA) and during diagnostic procedures. FFR reflects both antegrade and collateral myocardial perfusion rather than merely trans-stenotic pressure loss (i.e. a stenosis pressure gradient). Because it is calculated only at peak hyperemia, FFR is also differentiated from CVR by being largely independent of basal flow, driving pressure, heart rate, systemic blood pressure, or status of the microcirculation. Absolute CVR did not correlate with percent area stenosis or FFR. In patients with a nonuniform microcirculation, such as those with myocardial infarction, neither absolute CVR nor rCVR can be used for assessment of lesion severity. Even in patients with potential microcirculatory impairment, an epicardial narrowing is best assessed by FFR. In patients with an abnormal microcirculation, it can be argued that a normal FFR indicates the conduit resistance is not a major contributing factor to perfusion impairment, and that focal conduit enlargement (e.g. stenting) would not restore normal perfusion. As a conclusion, we can say that assessing qualitative perfusion differences is useful because relative perfusion deficit size is an important determinant of prognosis and post-procedural outcomes.

2.8 Nonobstructive Coronary Artery Disease

2.8.1 Endothelial Dysfunction

Endothelial dysfunction is the first pathophysiologic step of clinical atherosclerosis. Therefore, it is undetectable on angiography and intravascular ultrasonography, although microscopic abnormalities are likely present in the endothelial cells.

Hyperlipidemia, cigarette smoking, uncontrolled hypertension, diabetes mellitus and post-menopausal condition seem to degrade endothelial function. Recently, some evidence suggests that infectious pathogens and environmental pollution may lead to endothelial injury. When endothelial dysfunction occurs, some pathophysiologic mechanisms lead to an alteration in the normal equilibrium between vasoconstriction and vasodilation. Moreover, some structural changes of the vessel wall can hesitate in classical manifestation of coronary artery disease. Therefore, the expression of adhesion molecules on the cell surface, the leukocyte recruitment by increased oxidative stress, and the entry and oxidation of low-density lipoprotein into the intima induce the formation of foam cells and atherosclerotic plaques. Endothelial dysfunction also leads to reduced bioavailability of nitric oxide through multiple deleterious mechanisms, and stimulates the formation of endothelin which impairs vasomotion. Sometimes the altered vasomotion results in coronary spasm that can cause transient functional occlusion of a coronary artery. In the setting of endothelial disruption the normal vasodilation from autacoids and sympathetic stimulation is deficient and coronary constriction predominates. The presence of a superimposed element, such as thrombus formation or sympathetic stimulation, has consequences not counterbalanced owing to the lack of endothelium-dependent vasodilation.

Acetylcholine can be selectively infused into the coronary arteries to test for the presence of endothelial dysfunction. In normal individuals, acetylcholine stimulates the production and release of nitric oxide from the endothelium, which results in vasodilatation and increased coronary blood flow. In patients with endothelial dysfunction, acetylcholine is ineffective in releasing nitric oxide and, with the effect on smooth muscle cells predominating, causes vasoconstriction.

References

1. Saltin B, Astrand PO (1967) Maximal oxygen uptake in athletes. J Appl Physiol 23:353-358
2. Klocke FJ (1976) Coronary blood flow in man. Prog Cardiovasc Dis 19:117
3. Canty Jr JM (1988) Coronary pressure-function and steady-state pressure-flow relations during autoregulation in the unanesthetized dog. Circ Res 63:821-836
4. Shaw RF, Mosher P, Ross J Jr et al (1962) Physiologic principles of coronary perfusion. J Thorac Cardiovasc Surg 44:608-616
5. Feigl EO (1983) Coronary physiology. Physiol Rev 63:1-205
6. Kuo L, Davis MJ, Chilian WM (1995) Longitudinal gradients for endothelium-dependent and -independent vascular responses in the coronary microcirculation. Circulation 92:518-525
7. Miller FJ, Dellsperger KC, Gutterman DD (1997) Myogenic constriction of human coronaryarterioles. Am J Physiol Heart Circ Physiol 273:H257-264
8. Kuo L, Davis MJ, Chilian WM (1990) Endothelium-dependent, flow-induced dilation of isolated coronary arterioles. Am J Physiol 259:H1063-1070
9. Liu Y, Gutterman DD (2009) Vascular control in humans: Focus on the coronary microcirculation. Basic Res Cardiol 104:211-227
10. Miura H, Wachtel RE, Liu Y et al (2001) Flow-induced dilation of human coronary arterioles: Important role of Ca2+-activated K+ channels. Circulation 103:1992-1998
11. Dube S, Canty Jr JM (2001) Shear-stress induced vasodilation in porcine coronary conduit arteries is independent of nitric oxide release. Am J Physiol 280:H2581-2590
12. Niebauer J, Cooke JP (1996) Cardiovascular effects of exercise: role of endothelial shear stress. J Am Coll Cardiol 28:1652-1660
13. Duncker DJ, Bache RJ (2008) Regulation of coronary blood flow during exercise. Physiol Rev 88:1009-1086
14. Duncker DJ, Bache RJ (2000) Regulation of coronary vasomotor tone under normal conditions and during acute myocardial hypoperfusion. Pharmacol Ther 86:87-110
15. Daggett WM, Nugent GC, Carr PW et al (1967) Influence of vagal stimulation on ventricular contractility, O2 consumption, and coronary flow. Am J Physiol 212:8-18
16. Heusch G, Baumgart D, Camici P et al (2000) α-Adrenergic coronary vasoconstriction and myocardial ischemia in humans. Circulation 101:689-694
17. Eckstein RW, Stroud M 3rd, Eckel R et al (1950) Effects of control of cardiac work upon coronary flow and O2 consumption after sympathetic nerve stimulation. Am J Physiol 163:539-544
18. Mudge GH Jr, Grossman W, Mills RM Jr et al (1976) Reflex increase in coronary vascular resistance in patients with ischemic heart disease. N Engl J Med 295:1333-1337
19. Vatner SF, Hintze TH, Macho P (1982) Regulation of large coronary arteries by beta-adrenergic mechanisms in the conscious dog. Circ Res 51:56-66
20. Ross G, Jorgensen CR (1970) Effects of a cardio-selective beta-adrenergic blocking agent on the heart and coronary circulation. Cardiovasc Res 4:148-153
21. Roberts WC, Dicicco BS, Waller BF et al (1982) Origin of the left main from the right coronary artery or from the right aortic sinus with intramyocardial tunneling to the left side of the heart via the ventricular septum: the case against clinical significance of myocardial bridge or coronary tunnel. Am Heart J 104:303-305
22. McGinn AL, White CW, Wilson RF (1990) Interstudy variability of coronary flow reserve: Influence of heart rate, arterial pressure, and ventricular preload. Circulation 81:1319-1330
23. Marcus ML, Mueller TM, Gascho JA, Kerber RE (1979) Effects of cardiac hypertrophy secondary to hypertension on the coronary circulation. Am J Cardiol 44:1023-1031
24. Marcus ML, Doty DB, Hiratzka LF et al (1982) Decreased coronary flow reserve: a mechanism for angina pectoris in patients with aortic stenosis and normal coronary arteries. N Engl J Med 307:1362-1367
25. Wieneke H, Haude M, Ge J et al (2000) Corrected coronary flow velocity reserve: a new concept for assessing coronary perfusion. J Am Coll Cardiol 35:1713-1720
26. Akasaka T, Yoshida K, Hozumi T et al (1997) Retinopathy identifies marked restriction of coronary flow reserve in patients with diabetes mellitus. J Am Coll Cardiol 30:935-941
27. Baumgart D, Haude M, Liu F et al (1998) Current concepts of coronary flow reserve for clinical decision making during cardiac catheterization. Am Heart J 136:136-149
28. Gould KL, Lipscomb K (1974) Effects of coronary stenoses on coronary flow reserve and resistance. Am J Cardiol 34:48-55
29. White F, Carroll S, Magnet A et al (1992) Coronary collateral development in swine after coronary artery occlusion. Circ Res 71:1490-1500
30. Miwa K, Fujita M, Kameyama T et al (1999) Absence of myocardial ischemia during sudden controlled occlusion of coronary arteries in patients with well-developed collateral vessels. Coron Artery Dis 10:459-463
31. Pijls NH, De Bruyne B, Peels K et al (1996) Measurement of fractional flow reserve to assess the functional severity of coronary-artery stenoses. N Engl J Med 334:1703-1708
32. De Bruyne B, Bartunek J, Sys SU et al (1996) Simultaneous coronary pressure and flow velocity measurements in humans: feasibility, reproducibility, and hemodynamic dependence of coronary flow velocity reserve, hyperemic flow versus pressure slope index, and fractional flow reserve. Circulation 94:1842-1849
33. Pijls NH, Van Gelder B, Van der Voort P et al (1995) Fractional flow reserve: a useful index to evaluate the influence of an epicardial coronary stenosis on myocardial blood flow. Circulation 92:3183-3193

Subclinical Atherosclerosis and Primary Prevention

3

Giuseppe Tarantini, Paolo Buja, and Michela Facchin

3.1 Introduction

During the past four decades, there has been a dramatic decline in the age-adjusted rate of death from cardiac disease in the United States and many other developed countries [1-3]. This reduction is attributed in large part to primary and secondary prevention strategies that target modifiable risk factors [2, 4]. Despite these advances, cardiovascular disease remains the leading cause of death in developed countries as well as in most developing countries, [1, 3, 5] and there is concern that the growing prevalence of obesity and type 2 diabetes will reverse the gains of the past 40 years. Therefore, prevention of atherosclerotic cardiovascular events (myocardial infarction, sudden death, and stroke) remains a major imperative for health care professionals. The process of atherosclerosis, now considered to be a chronic immunoinflammatory disease of medium- and large-sized arteries, often begins in childhood and adolescence and frequently remains clinically dormant until plaque rupture or plaque erosion leads to abrupt thrombosis triggering acute clinical events [6]. Approximately 40% to 60% of major occlusive atherosclerotic cardiovascular events (myocardial infarction, sudden death) occur as the first manifestation (unheralded events), accounting for >700,000 such events annually in the U.S. [7]. The identification of subjects at risk of such events is obviously important, if identification leads to implementation of and compliance with effective preventive measures that reduce such risk. Stress testing to detect a flow-limiting coronary stenosis among asymptomatic subjects is unlikely to identify a significant majority of at-risk individuals because nearly 70% of acute coronary events result from coronary lesions that are not hemodynamically significant or flow limiting before the event [8].

Moreover, the risk factors for cardiovascular disease are present and poorly controlled in the majority of persons who have no symptoms [3-9]. Adult Treatment Panel III (ATP III) of the National Cholesterol Education Program [10] based its 2001 recommendations for the treatment of hypercholesterolemia for primary prevention of cardiovascular disease on the assessment of individual risk factors and global risk as indicated by the Framingham risk score, which is determined on the basis of age, blood pressure, levels of total cholesterol and HDL cholesterol, and smoking status. With the use of these criteria, persons without established coronary heart disease are considered to be at high risk if they have either a condition that is equivalent to coronary heart disease with respect to the risk of a coronary event (e.g. peripheral-artery atherosclerotic disease or diabetes) or more than a 20% estimated likelihood of a coronary event over the next 10 years; they are considered to be at low risk if the estimate is less than 10%. Although at the time of their first acute coronary event more than 85% of patients have at least one of the major established risk factors for heart disease [11, 12], the presence of only a single risk factor would place most people in the low-risk category according to the ATP III criteria — meaning that intensive measures to reduce risk factors would not be considered necessary. The 2004 ATP III update [13] also defined patients at *moderate risk* for a coronary event as those having two or more risk factors and a 10-year risk of less than 10% and patients at *moderately high* risk (previously termed *intermediate risk*) as those with a 10 to 20% likelihood of having a coronary event during the next 10 years. Neither patients at moderate risk nor those at moderately high risk would be considered candidates for the aggressive treatment of risk factors that is recommended for patients at high risk. The observation that a person classified as being at low, moderate, or moderately high risk for a coronary event according to the updated ATP III criteria [13] may nonetheless have a coronary event has spurred interest in new markers of such risk that might identify those who would benefit from more rigorous attention to risk-fac-

G. Tarantini (✉)
Interventional Cardiology Division,
Department of Cardiac, Thoracic and Vascular Sciences,
University of Padua,
Padua, Italy

F. Cademartiri, G. Casolo, M. Midiri (eds.), *Clinical Applications of Cardiac CT*,
© Springer-Verlag Italia 2012

tor modification [14-16]. In this regard, the potential role for imaging of subclinical atherosclerosis — in particular, the use of electron-beam computed tomography (EBCT) or multidetector computed tomography (MDCT) to detect CAC — has generated considerable attention and debate.

3.2 Risk-Estimation Systems and Primary Prevention

The atherosclerosis underlying most cardiovascular disease is rarely the result of a single risk factor, such as familial hyperlipidemia, but more usually the end result of the combined effect of several factors. Different risk scores have been proposed as potential means for quantifying the assessment of cardiovascular risk in asymptomatic patients as shown in Table 3.1.

3.2.1 Framingham Risk Score

The Framingham Heart Study is a landmark achievement [17], well known for its 10-year risk score for prediction of CHD events in asymptomatic patients [18]. Risk factors used in the Framingham risk score (FRS) include age, sex, total cholesterol, high-density lipoprotein cholesterol (HDL-C), blood pressure and cigarette smoking. Importantly, the FRS is easy to apply and clinically relevant. The FRS for hard CHD events has been incorporated into several guidelines for CVD prevention [19-22] and been used to guide treatment of risk factors (Table 3.1).

The FRS was adapted and then incorporated into the National Cholesterol Education Program Expert Panel on Detection, Evaluation, and Treatment of High Blood Cholesterol in Adults (Adult Treatment Panel III [ATP III]) for use in their recommendations for screening for and treatment of dyslipidemia [19]. Although the FRS has been validated in many populations, including Caucasian Americans and African Americans [23] its accuracy is somewhat limited among some European and Asian populations, and some risk markers are not incorporated. In a systematic review of 27 studies using the Framingham scoring system, the predicted-to-observed ratios ranged from an underprediction of 0.43 in a high-risk population to an overprediction of 2.87 in a low-risk population [24]. The FRS has been evaluated in the largest number of diverse settings, and many of these problems are likely to be relevant to the other risk scores.

In addition to the coronary event risk score, the FRS has been developed for a composite of all atherosclerotic CVD (CHD composite including angina, cerebrovascular

events, peripheral artery disease, and heart failure) [23] as well as individual risk scores for each specific components, including peripheral artery disease [25], stroke [26], and heart failure [27]. Risk scores have also been developed for lifetime risk [28-29] and 30-year risk [30] as opposed to 10-year risk. These latter scores require further validation.

3.2.2 ATP III

The ATP III document updated clinical guidelines for cholesterol testing and management [19]. The ATP III identified 3 categories of risk that modify the goals and modalities of low-density lipoprotein cholesterol (LDL-C) lowering therapy on the basis of CHD as an end point. The category of highest risk (>20% per 10 years) consists of CHD and CHD risk equivalents (atherosclerotic disease of other arterial beds and diabetes mellitus). The LDL-C goal is <100 mg/dL. The second category consists of multiple [23] risk factors and the LDL-C goal is <130 mg/dL. The major risk factors include cigarette smoking, blood pressure 140/90 mm Hg or receiving antihypertensive medication, low HDL-C, family history of premature CHD, and age 45 years in men or 55 years in women. The ATP III risk algorithm stratifies these persons into those with 10-year risk for CHD of >20%, 10% to 20%, and <10%. The third category consists of persons with 0 to 1 risk factor and the LDL-C goal of <160 mg/dL. In 2004, a modification of the risk categories was proposed [13]; the multiple risk factor category was divided into a moderately high risk group (2 risk factors and 10-year CHD risk 10% to 20%), and a moderate risk group (2 risk factors and 10-year CHD risk <10%). For the moderately high risk group, there is an optional LDL-C goal of <100 mg/dL largely based on the ASCOT (Anglo-Scandinavian Cardiac Outcomes Trial) of lipid lowering in adults with treated hypertension [31].

3.2.3 The SCORE Project

The SCORE (Systematic Coronary Risk Evaluation) project intended to provide better predictive accuracy for European patients. The SCORE system was derived from data from >200,000 patients pooled from 12 European cohort studies [32]. The SCORE system estimates the 10-year risk of a first fatal atherosclerotic event including heart attack, stroke, or aortic aneurysm. This is significant because it estimates the risk for any fatal atherosclerotic event, but is limited in that it does not consider nonfatal events.

Table 3.1 Characteristics of the cardiovascular risk. (Adapted from [22], with permission from Elsevier)

Study	Variables Included	Outcomes	Population Derived	Population Validated	ROC	Limitations
FRS	Age, sex, BP, smoking, use of HTN medications, TC, and HDL	CHD (angina, MI, sudden death)	U.S. white men and women, ages 30-62 yrs	Men, women, blacks, Europe, Mediterranean, and Asia	0.7744 (w) 0.7598 (m)	Age _30 yrs, _65 yrs, Japanese- American men, Hispanic men, Native-American women, LVH, DM, and severe HTN
Global cardiovascular	Age, sex, SBP, smoking, TC, HDL, DM, and use of HTN medications	CHD, stroke, CHF, or PVD	U.S. white men and women, ages 30-74 yrs	Framingham offspring 0.763 (m)	0.793 (w)	Mainly white
SCORE	Age, sex, smoking, either TC or TC/HDL ratio, broken up into areas of high and low CVD risk	Fatal CV events	European men and women, ages 45–64 yrs	Europe	0.71-0.84	No nonfatal events, "single" risk factor measurements made, rather than "usual"
ASSIGN	Age, sex, SBP, TC, HDL, family history, social deprivation	CV death, CHD admission, CABG, or PTCA	Scotland men and women, ages 30–74 yrs	Scotland 0.7644 (m)	0.7841 (w)	Marginally better than Framingham, still overestimated risk
Reynolds	Age, SBP, smoking, total cholesterol, HDL, hsCRP, family history, hgbAIc if DM	MI, stroke, coronary revascularization, or CV death	U.S. women, age 45 yrs	U.S. women	0.808 (w)	Mainly white, all women, socioeconomic status not generalizable, BP, weight, and family history, all taken by self-report
QRISK	Age, sex, SBP, smoking, ratio of TC/HDL, family history, use of HTN medications, BMI, social deprivation	MI, CHD, stroke, TIA	United Kingdom men and women, ages 35–74 yrs	United Kingdom 0.7674 (m)	0.7879 (w)	"Home advantage," data validated from same population from which it was originally derived

ASSIGN, Assessing Cardiovascular Risk to Scottish Intercollegiate Guidelines Network/SIGN to Assign Preventative Treatment; *BMI*, body mass index; *BP*, blood pressure; *CABG*, coronary artery by-pass graft surgery; *CHD*, coronary heart disease; *CVD*, cardiovascular disease; *DM*, diabetes mellitus; *FRS*, Framingham risk score; *HDL*, high-density lipoprotein; *hgb*, hemoglobin; *hsCRP*, high-sensitivity C-reactive protein; *HTN*, hypertension; *LVH*, left ventricular hypertrophy; *m*, men; *MI*, myocardial infarction; *PTCA*, percutaneous transluminal coronary angiography; *ROC*, receiver-operating characteristic; *QRISK*, QRESEARCH Cardiovascular Risk Algorithm; *SBP*, systolic blood pressure; *SCORE*, Systematic Coronary Risk Evaluation; *TC*, total cholesterol; *TIA*, transient ischemic attack; *w*, women.

Risk factors used in the SCORE system include age, sex, total cholesterol, total cholesterol to HDL-C ratio, systolic blood pressure and cigarette smoking. A unique aspect of the SCORE system is that it has separate risk scores for higher risk and lower risk regions of Europe. Nevertheless, the predictive value of the SCORE system was high in each component study cohort from Europe. There are now multiple country-specific versions of the SCORE system.

3.2.4 Reynolds Risk Score

The Reynolds risk score was initially designed to develop and validate an algorithm for global cardiovascular risk in healthy women [33]. Thirty-five factors were assessed among 25,000 initially healthy female health professionals enrolled in a clinical trial in the U.S. The Reynolds risk score estimates the 10-year risk of cardiovascular events, a composite of MI, ischemic stroke, coronary revascularization, and cardiovascular death. Of note, risk factors such as blood pressure and body weight were not directly measured but were self-reported in categories, which may have diminished some of their utility as predictive variables, allowing opportunities for other covariates to add predictive utility. Additionally, the risk score was validated from the same population it was derived. The authors provided 2 models: a best-fitting model and a clinically simplified model (the Reynolds risk score). The Reynolds risk score was composed of age, systolic blood pressure, hemoglobin A1c if diabetic, smoking, total and HDL-C, C-reactive protein measured by a high-sensitivity assay (hsCRP), and parental history of MI before age 60 years. In contrast to the FRS and SCORE system, the Reynolds score evaluated and incorporated the risk factors of parental history of premature CHD and hsCRP. Recently, the Reynolds risk score, using male-specific equations, was applied to healthy nondiabetic men with good results [34]. Similar to women, the authors showed that the addition of hsCRP and parental history of MI before age 60 years improved global cardiovascular risk prediction and reclassification of risk as compared with the traditional FRS employed in the ATP III in a population of male health professionals enrolled in a clinical trial. Despite improved risk assessment with RRS compared with the traditional FRS, neither scheme is sufficiently accurate for individual risk assessment and, unlike the FRS, the RRS has not yet been fully validated outside the Women's Health Study and Physicians Health Study participants.

3.2.5 The ASSIGN Risk Score

Using a representative database from Scotland, the ASSIGN (Assessing Cardiovascular Risk to Scottish Intercollegiate Guidelines Network/SIGN to Assign Preventative Treatment) risk score was developed [35]. This score was derived from men and women ages 30 to 74 years and free of symptomatic CVD. The ASSIGN score estimates the 10-year risk of CVD, including cardiovascular death or any hospital discharge diagnosis of CHD, cerebrovascular disease, or coronary artery intervention. Traditional risk factors, including number of cigarettes smoked, plus social deprivation and family history, but not obesity, were significant factors in this risk score. The ASSIGN scoring system was novel because the authors included an index of social status, which may account for social gradients in disease.

3.2.6 QRISK Risk Score

The QRISK (QRESEARCH cardiovascular risk algorithm) CVD risk score was derived from a large United Kingdom primary care population [36, 37]. The derivation cohort consisted of 1.3 million subjects ages 35 to 74 years free from diabetes and CVD. The QRISK score estimates the 10-year risk of CVD, including MI, CHD, stroke, and transient ischemic attack. Risk factors were age, sex, smoking status, systolic blood pressure, ratio of total to HDL-C, body mass index, family history of CHD, a measure of social deprivation, and treatment with antihypertensive agent. This was the first study to use data from a general practice population and not use an observational study in a predefined cohort. Both the QRISK and ASSIGN risk scores include social deprivation, an important step in acknowledging inequalities in cardiovascular risk. A major limitation of this risk score was that it was validated from the same population from which it was derived.

3.2.7 Example Risk Estimation

The following case vignette is an example of risk-estimation assessment. A 56-year-old woman without any cardiovascular symptoms comes to your office to establish care. She does not smoke currently, but she reports having smoked until 4 years ago when her sister at age 54 had an ischemic stroke. There is no family history of myocardial infarction (MI) or sudden cardiac death. Her resting blood pressure is 150/90 mmHg, fasting glucose is 135 mg/dL, total cholesterol is 240 mg/dL, high-den-

3 Subclinical Atherosclerosis and Primary Prevention

Table 3.2 Risk Score of the Patient Described in Case Vignette. (Adapted from [22], with permission from Elsevier)

Risk score	Estimated Risk
Framingham	
10-yr CHD risk score	2%
Global CVD score	10%
Heart age/vascular age	73%
Reynolds	6%
SCORE (fatal CVD)	1-2%
QRISK	11%
ASSIGN	14%
Lifetime risk for CVD	39%

Abbreviations as in Table 3.1.

Table 3.3 Standard risk factor-adjusted coronary event rates in 4 racial/ethnic groups of asymptomatic subjects based on coronary calcium score (multi-ethnic study of atherosclerosis). (Adapted from [54], with permission from Elsevier)

Calcium Score	Hazard Ratio	Annual Number and Rate of Coronary Events
0 (n=3409)	1	15 (0.1%)
1-100 (n=1728)	3.6	39 (0.6%)
101-300 (n=752)	7.73	41 (1.4%)
>300 (n=833)	9.67	67 (2.9%)

Note that 90% of all events occurred in subjects with coronary calcification, and nearly 50% of the subjects had no coronary calcification.

sity lipoprotein (HDL) is 35 mg/dL, and triglyceride level is 240 mg/dl. She is physically inactive, and her body mass index (the weight in kilograms divided by the square of the height in meters) is 31. She has never taken any medication. The cardiovascular risk of the reported patient, according to the risk score used, is shown in Table 3.2.

In conclusion, we recommend that heath care providers discuss the 10-year cardiac heart disease as well as global cardiovascular risk, and the lifetime cardiovascular risk score assessment with each patient to better explore each individual patient's future risk. However, it should be also acknowledged that risk-scoring models are derived from populations and applied to patients and thus, although they can improve the prediction of risk, their adoption into clinical practice is poor. In particular, for the purpose of deciding whether to start therapy, each risk score assessment should be evaluated in future studies and only adequately designed prospective trials will be able to evaluate whether the risk score improves important health outcomes and health care expenditures.

3.3 Noninvasive Imaging of Subclinical Atherosclerosis and Primary Prevention

There is considerable variation in the severity of atherosclerotic burden at any given level of risk factor exposure, presumably attributable to additional known or unknown genetic and environmental risk factors and risk modifiers. There are multiple noninvasive imaging techniques that can identify subclinical atherosclerosis in various vascular beds, including ultrasonography, coronary Ca^{2+} assessment by computed tomography (CT), noninvasive CT angiography, and magnetic resonance imaging. Although all of these methods have their rela-

tive advantages and drawbacks, imaging of coronary arteries to identify coronary calcium, a validated measure of atherosclerotic plaque, by computed tomography without contrast and use of B-mode ultrasonography to detect carotid intima-media thickness and carotid plaque have been most extensively studied and have the potential to be suitable screening tools for the detection of subclinical atherosclerosis.

3.3.1 Coronary Calcium Score

Coronary calcium detection by CT has been shown to identify atherosclerotic plaque and to quantitatively assess coronary calcium; using the Agatston coronary calcium score (CCS), a surrogate for plaque burden, has been shown to provide powerful prognostic information in multiple studies involving both sexes and multiple ethnic groups [38-54]. Furthermore, CCS has been shown to provide prognostic information that is independent of and substantially incremental to that provided by the FRS and hsCRP [38-54] (Table 3.3). The CCS can provide individual risk assessment and can reclassify the low and particularly intermediate Framingham risk cohort into lower- and higher-risk strata, as shown by Preis et al. [55] in a study involving 3,529 asymptomatic subjects from the Framingham Offspring Cohort (Table 3.4). Absence of coronary calcium (CCS=0), while not excluding the presence of noncalcified plaque, virtually excludes significant coronary atherosclerosis, but more importantly is associated, in an asymptomatic population, with an extremely low risk of cardiovascular events in the ensuing 5 to 10 years ranging from annual event rates of 0% to 0.6% [50]. The higher event rates reported in subjects with a 0 coronary calcium score by Greenland et al. [43] came from a study that used 6-mm thick slices, which is known to result in data loss compared with 3-mm slices. In an observational cohort of

Table 3.4 Reclassification of Framingham Risk by Coronary Calcium Score in the Framingham Offspring and Third-Generation Cohort. (Adapted from [54], with permission from Elsevier)

FRS	FRS + Coronary calcium Score		
	Low	Intermediate	High
Low (n=2410)	89% (92%)	11% (8%)	22% (39%)
Intermediate (n=595)	25% (25%)	53% (35%)	
High (n=245)			100% (100%)

Coronary calcium score criterion was either the 90th percentile value or absolute score 100; data using the absolute coronary calcium score is shown in parentheses. Note that in the FRS intermediate group, coronary calcium score reclassified 25% of subjects into a lower risk stratum and 22% to 39% into a higher risk stratum. Eight percent to 11% of those at low risk FRS level were upgraded to intermediate risk level with the addition of coronary calcium score. *FRS*, Framingham risk score.

35,765 asymptomatic subjects from published studies, 16,106 (45%) had zero coronary calcium; their annual event rate was only 0.027% [50]. Blaha et al. [56] reported from an asymptomatic cohort of 44,052 subjects referred for coronary calcium scanning that 19,898 of these subjects (45% of the total cohort) had a CCS of 0 and a 10-year all-cause mortality rate of 1%; the mortality rate was 2-fold higher in subjects with minimal coronary calcification with a CCS of 1 to 10 and nearly 9-fold higher with a CCS >10 [56]. In a systematic review of 13 published studies involving 64,873 asymptomatic subjects undergoing coronary calcium assessment and prognostic evaluation, 25,903 subjects (45% of cohort) with zero coronary calcium were identified whose cardiovascular event rate was 0.56% during a 4.25-year follow-up [57]. In another registry study involving >25,000 subjects, Budoff et al. [41], in a follow-up extending up to 12 years, demonstrated a mortality rate of 0.4%. These observations highlight the fact that asymptomatic subjects with a CCS of 0 have an extremely low 5- to 10-year risk of cardiovascular and all-cause mortality and that such patients are unlikely to benefit from lipid-lowering therapy and any additional downstream tests for vaso-occlusive disease. Interestingly, in a cohort of 900 subjects with diabetes, a CCS of 0 was associated with a 5-year survival rate of 98.8%, and the survival of diabetic and nondiabetic patients with a CCS of 0 was remarkably similar (98.8% vs. 99.4%) [48]. In another prospective study of patients with type 2 diabetes, a CCS <10 was associated with a zero event rate at 2 years of follow-up [58]. Such very low-risk individuals constitute 40% to 50% of asymptomatic cohorts [41], are unlikely to benefit from aggressive preventive interventions, and may be recommended only to follow a healthy lifestyle and could well be spared the cost and side effects of aggressive lipid-lowering therapy. It is, however, important to point out that in a symptomatic population with clinical evidence of myocardial ischemia, absence of coronary calcium is not totally reassuring and may be associated with a higher event rate (annual event rate of 3.6%) [59-61].

This is consistent with recent observations from noninvasive contrast CT coronary angiography revealing that 6% to 11.6% of subjects may have only noncalcified plaque, which would be missed on coronary calcium scoring [62, 63]. The major drawbacks of this CT-based technique include exposure to a small amount of radiation, which may be particularly undesirable in young subjects, especially women, and the very rare but definite instance in which a subject with only a noncalcified plaque is labeled as normal [62, 63]; such an eventuality is quite rare in asymptomatic subjects. When a coronary event occurs in a subject with a CCS of 0, besides a noncalcified culprit plaque, one must also consider other unpredictable reasons for cardiovascular events that have nothing to do with atherosclerosis such as acute myocarditis simulating myocardial infarction, coronary embolism, coronary dissection presenting as an acute coronary syndrome, and stress-induced acute myocardial syndrome in women. None of these relatively uncommon nonatherosclerotic events could be predicted by any known tests.

3.3.2 B-Mode Ultrasonography

B-mode ultrasound imaging of carotid arteries provides yet another noninvasive, simple, and relatively inexpensive modality for the detection of subclinical atherosclerosis or pre-atherosclerosis as measured by a thickened intima-media (carotid artery intima-media thickness [CIMT]); this technique is safe and, unlike coronary calcium scanning, carries no risk of radiation exposure [64, 65]. Several prospective studies, including the MESA (Multi-Ethnic Study of Atherosclerosis), of asymptomatic subjects demonstrated that increased CIMT over 75th percentile for a person's age, sex, and race (using nomograms from large population-based studies) is associated with future risk of myocardial infarction, stroke and death from coronary heart disease that in most studies was independent of traditional risk factors [64, 65].

Furthermore, several large studies have shown that the presence of carotid plaque on ultrasonography (defined as focal thickening of the carotid wall that is at least 50% greater than that of surrounding wall or as a focal region with CIMT >1.5 mm that is distinct from adjacent boundary and protrudes into the lumen) in asymptomatic subjects is associated with increased risk of cardiovascular events that is comparable to or better than that of increased CIMT [65]. A meta-analysis by Lorenz et al. [66] reported significant relative risks of coronary heart disease of 1.26 for myocardial infarction and 1.32 for stroke for each 1-SD increment of CIMT. More recently, it has been shown that the maximum internal and mean common carotid-artery intima–media thicknesses both predict cardiovascular outcomes, but only the maximum intima–media thickness of (and presence of plaque in) the internal carotid artery significantly (albeit modestly) improves the classification of risk of cardiovascular disease in the Framingham Offspring Study color [67].

3.3.3 Comparative Prognostic Value of Coronary Calcium Scanning Versus Carotid Ultrasonography

Although atherosclerosis is generally considered to be a diffuse or at least multifocal process and both carotid ultrasonography as well as coronary calcium scanning can detect subclinical atherosclerosis, CIMT and CCS are only modestly correlated in individual subjects, with some patients exhibiting a CCS of 0 in the context of abnormal CIMT or carotid plaque and some patients with an abnormal CCS exhibiting normal CIMT and no carotid plaque. Two recent prospective studies compared the incremental prognostic value of CIMT and coronary calcium scanning in initially asymptomatic subjects [68, 69]. Newman et al. [66] found that in adults older than 70 years, CIMT and CCS similarly predicted cardiovascular disease and coronary heart disease, but CIMT was a better predictor of stroke. However, Folsom et al. [69] reported the results of MESA and showed that the CCS was a stronger predictor of cardiovascular events than CIMT. For cardiovascular events, the traditional risk factor-adjusted hazard increased 2.1-fold for each SD greater level of log-transformed CCS versus 1.3-fold for each SD greater maximum CIMT; comparable differences in relative risk were noted for coronary heart disease [69]. That CIMT was modestly better than CCS in predicting stroke reflects a closer correlation between stroke and the relevant vascular territory. These results were further supported by receiver-operator characteristic analysis in which adding CCS to risk factor analysis significantly improved the area under the curve, whereas CIMT provided little additional value [69].

The CCS and CIMT fulfill many but not all of these requirements; in particular, the added value of imaging-guided management in improving patient outcomes has not yet been proven using randomized, controlled clinical trials, and therefore, in that sense, to a purist the "jury" is still out. However, we must acknowledge that FRS-based management using NCEP guidelines has also not been subjected to similar rigorous clinical trials and yet is accepted as a reasonable strategy for risk detection and modification based on purely observational data. Holding noninvasive imaging to a different standard even when its prognostic value has been unequivocally demonstrated to be significantly incremental to FRS, especially among low- and intermediate-risk categories, is indicative of a double standard [70]. Despite the lack of randomized clinical trial evidence, the totality of observational evidence supports imaging-guided management because: 1) detecting disease with its consequences we would like to prevent is no doubt better than simply identifying risk factors that have only a modest specificity and a highly variable relationship with the development of disease; 2) imaging can reclassify intermediate- and low-risk FRS subjects into higher-risk strata for which more aggressive medical therapy and lower cholesterol targets would be recommended, thereby tangibly altering therapy while at the same time identifying a very low-risk cohort that could avoid aggressive drug therapy given the lack of a likely near-term benefit; and 3) imaging-based identification of at-risk subjects may improve compliance and adherence to risk-modifying interventions; this is particularly germane because long-term compliance with effective preventive therapy results in better outcomes, making adherence a surrogate for outcomes. A random-effects meta-analysis of 5 recent trials involving 52,319 patients showed that adherence to statin therapy averaged only 65% [71]. In a study involving 505 subjects on statin therapy followed for 3 years, Kalia et al. [71] showed that the overall statin compliance was lowest (44%) among those with a CCS in the first quartile (0 to 30), whereas 91% of individuals with a baseline CCS in the fourth quartile adhered to statin therapy. Taylor et al. [72] reported on the association of the CCS detected on a screening examination with subsequent use of statins and aspirin in 1,640 asymptomatic men 40 to 50 years of age. In this prospective cohort followed for up to 6 years, the presence of coronary calcification was associated with a 3-fold greater likelihood of statin and aspirin use that was independent of NCEP risk variables and baseline medication use. These findings from a community-based nonreferred study population provide strong evidence of a significant and incremental impact of subclinical atherosclerosis detection, over and above FRS-NCEP risk assessment, on patient management, thus supporting the use of such an approach to refine cardiovascular risk assessment [72]. Therefore, the recommendations of the SHAPE (Screening for Heart Attack Prevention and Education) Task Force, although based on a wealth of published observational data but not randomized, controlled trials, represent a reasonable blueprint for an imaging-augmented strategy for risk assessment and management [73]. The SHAPE Task Force recommended noninvasive atherosclerosis imaging of all asymptomatic men (age 45 to 75 years) and women (age 55 to 75 years), except those at very low risk, to augment conventional cardiovascular risk assessment algorithms [73]. Recent observations from 2,611 participants 30 to 65 years of age from the Dallas Heart Study provided evidence in favor of the SHAPE algorithm because SHAPE recommendations resulted in bidirectional reclassification of eligibility for lipid-lowering therapy in the participants [74]. Application of imaging according to the SHAPE guidelines to the Dallas Heart Study Cohort reclassified 35% to 48% of the cohort into a higher-risk stratum, making them eligible for lipid-lowering therapy, and the number needed to reclassify 1 individual as newly eligible (or no longer eligible) for lipid-lowering therapy ranged from 4.1 to 7.8, depending on the coronary calcium score threshold used [74]. An important consideration in any recommendation for large-scale screening is the cost-effectiveness of such an approach. Diamond and Kaul [75] recently compared the costs and effectiveness of unconditional treatment of all risk factor–based treatment recommended by the NCEP and imaging-based treatment recommended by the SHAPE Task Force while making certain assumptions regarding costs of imaging and treatment with statins. The Diamond and Kaul [75] analysis supported cost-effectiveness of the SHAPE algorithm over the NCEP strategy, as also found by the SHAPE Task Force analysis [73], but suggested that unconditional treatment was most cost-effective. However, Diamond and Kaul [75] were quick to point out that if the SHAPE algorithm improves adherence to preventive therapy, its cost-effectiveness could surpass unconditional treatment. We must also be clear that although detecting subclinical atherosclerosis is a logical first step after Framingham risk assessment to improve prognostic value, the answer to the question "plaque present or absent?" cannot be the final solution because the amount/extent of plaque (plaque burden) and the composition of plaque are likely to contribute additional important prognostic information and can further improve the sensitivity and specificity of noninvasive imaging for risk prediction. Adding some measures beyond arterial structure, specifically addressing arterial function (arterial compliance and

vasodilator function) [76], plaque phenotype as an index of vulnerability to acute thrombotic events will likely further improve imaging-based risk prediction. Such approaches might include assessing plaque composition/configuration (inflammation, lipid core, thin cap, increased plaque neovascularity, outward remodeling, intraplaque hemorrhage), circulating biomarker reflective of biological processes relevant to plaque rupture (proteomics/metabolomics/circulating biomarkers), and genotypes that are predictive of risk. Such a comprehensive multimodality approach is currently under way in the High Risk Plaque Initiative, which is likely to provide valuable new information in the near future [77].

3.3.4 Cardiac Computed Tomography Angiography Assessment and Prognostic Implications

Cardiac CT angiography (CCT) permits visualization of the coronary artery lumen and detection of coronary artery stenoses [78]. In addition, nonstenotic coronary atherosclerotic plaques can be depicted. In contrast to *calcium screening*, CCT also allows visualization and, to some extent, quantification and characterization of noncalcified plaque deposits. However, all of this requires excellent image quality without artifacts. In addition, image acquisition for CCT is substantially more elaborate than coronary calcium imaging. Intravenous injection of contrast agent is required (60–100 mL). Data acquisition protocols as well as hardware must provide for extremely high spatial and temporal resolution (which may bring about a relatively high radiation exposure). In addition, image quality is strongly dependent on heart rate and it is usually required to lower the patients' heart rate to <65 bpm, preferably even <60 bpm [79]. This is usually achieved by administrating β-blockers. The need for strict heart rate control may not be as important for more recent scanner generations [80, 81]. CCT offers high accuracy for the detection and especially for ruling out coronary artery stenosis. However, as outlined above, to a certain extent patient selection is required. Sinus rhythm and the ability to follow breath-holding commands are a prerequisite and a low heart rate and the absence of severe obesity improve accuracy [82]. In two recent multicentre trials [83, 84], CCT was reported to have a sensitivity of 95–99%, specificity of 64–83% and negative predictive value of 97–99% to identify patients with at least one coronary artery stenosis among individuals at low to intermediate risk for coronary artery disease. Typically, the positive predictive value is lower (64 and 86% in the above-named trials), which is due to a tendency to overestimate stenosis degree in CCT as well as the fact that image artifacts often result in false-positive interpretations. CCT performs best in patient groups who are not at high likelihood of coronary artery disease [85]. A multicentre study of 291 patients with 56% prevalence of coronary artery stenoses, as well as 20% of patients with previous myocardial infarction and 10% with prior revascularization demonstrated a sensitivity of only 85% and specificity of 90% [86]. Ruling out obstructive coronary artery stenoses by CCT has prognostic value: several cohort studies have demonstrated extremely low rates of clinical events after CCT had ruled out coronary artery stenoses in patients with stable angina pectoris or acute chest pain [87-92]. Beyond the detection of coronary artery stenoses, CCT can demonstrate coronary atherosclerotic plaque. Calcified plaque can be detected just as in unenhanced scans, and more importantly, if image quality is high, noncalcified plaque components can also be visualized. To a certain degree, plaque characterization is possible. Obviously, CT is able to differentiate calcified, partly calcified, and noncalcified plaque (for noncalcified plaque, often the term *soft* plaque is used, but it lacks scientific justification). The aim of further characterization is to identify parameters that will be associated with increased plaque *vulnerability*. To a certain extent, the CT attenuation of noncalcified plaques may contribute towards plaque characterization. Computed tomography density within *fibrous* plaques is usually higher than within *lipid-rich* plaques - mean attenuation values have been reported in a range between 11 and 99 Hounsfield units (HU) for *lipid-rich* plaque vs. 77–121 HU for *fibrous* plaque [93-101]. However, the variability of density measurements within plaque types is large [98] and some studies did not even find any significant difference in CT attenuation between plaque types [93]. Furthermore, density measurements within coronary plaques are heavily influenced by the contrast attenuation in the adjacent lumen [101] and by image reconstruction parameters such as slice thickness and reconstruction kernel [102]. Therefore, accurate classification of plaque composition by measuring the CT attenuation is currently not reliable. However, based on studies performed in patients after acute coronary syndromes [103-105], it has been speculated that the identification of very low CT densities (below 30 HU) within a plaque may be associated with a higher predisposition towards rupture. Other plaque features which were demonstrated in patients who underwent CT imaging of the coronary arteries after acute coronary syndromes included a predominance of noncalcified plaque as well as pronounced positive remodeling, the assessment of which by CCT seems to correlate well with IVUS [106, 107]. Similar to the detection and quantification of coronary calcium, one

would expect that the detection and further characterization of noncalcified plaque should provide prognostic information concerning the occurrence of future acute coronary syndromes. Indeed, surrogate markers of plaque burden have been shown to be predictive of overall mortality in two other large trials. Ostrom et al. [108] demonstrated that the presence of nonobstructive plaque in all three coronary arteries was associated with increased mortality (risk ratio 1.77 when compared with individuals without any detectable plaque). The presence of non-obstructive plaque in only one or two coronary vessels was not associated with an increased risk. Min et al. [109] demonstrated that the presence of coronary atherosclerotic plaque in at least five coronary artery segments in symptomatic patients was associated with increased mortality when compared with patients with detectable plaque in less than five segments. In a landmark study, Motoyama et al. [110] demonstrated that beyond the mere assessment of plaque burden, specific plaque parameters may be associated with a particularly high risk. In 1059 patients who were followed over a mean period of 2.3 years after having undergone CCT, they clearly showed that plaques with positive remodeling and low CT attenuation were at particularly high risk for causing future cardiovascular events.

However, it should be acknowledged that the actual clinical utility of CCT for risk stratification purposes is very uncertain, especially when considering extending the currently available findings to a *screening* situation. The above-named trials which demonstrated a prognostic value of CCT were all retrospective analyses of individuals in whom CT was performed for a clinical reason, so most likely the populations mainly consisted of symptomatic patients. Because of the low overall event rate, predicting acute coronary syndromes in *asymptomatic* individuals is substantially more difficult. A further concern is the fact that CCT, as opposed to coronary calcium, requires the injection of contrast agent and is usually associated with substantially higher radiation exposure than calcium scans. Average effective doses for CCT are 12 mSv, but they can easily reach 20 mSv or more unless special measures to minimize the dose are implemented [111, 112]. Recently, numerous approaches to reduce the dose of CCT have been proposed and evaluated, and estimated effective doses <3 mSv [113-117], in selected cases even <1 mSv [118], can be achieved. However, such data sets will often have relatively high noise levels, and while they may be appropriate to detect or rule out coronary artery stenoses, the quality may not be sufficient for accurate plaque detection and characterization. While of intense scientific interest, the clinical use of CCT to detect plaque in asymptomatic individuals for purposes of risk stratification is therefore currently not considered an *appropriate* indication [119] and is uniformly discouraged [120, 121].

3.4 Clinical Implications and Future Perspectives

The modern integration of these risk factors together with age and gender into the Framingham risk score allows classification of patients into low-, intermediate-, and high-risk categories for the likelihood of development of acute coronary events Individuals with a risk of developing an acute coronary event over the next decade of up to approximately 5%, or <0.5% per year, are arbitrarily considered to be at low risk. Those who carry a risk of 5% to 20% over a 10-year period (0.5% to 2% per year) are at intermediate risk, while those with an acute coronary event rate of more than 20% over a decade (>2% per year) are generally considered to be at high risk. Approximately 40% of the population is at intermediate risk. A typical individual in this category would be a 55-year-old man with hypertension who is a nonsmoker and does not have hypercholesterolemia, diabetes, or a family history of coronary disease. In such individuals, additional testing may be helpful to aid in further risk stratification. For example, determining the CCS is recommended in the recent position statement of the European Society of Cardiology [122]. Such additional testing may allow reclassification of intermediate-risk patients into either low- or high-risk categories. For instance, if the hypertensive man described above exhibits a low CCS he may be reclassified as low risk and be a candidate for control of hypertension and follow-up, whereas if his CCS is elevated, this would place him into a higher risk category mandating for aggressive risk factor modification which include lipid lowering therapy and further assessment by myocardial perfusion scintigraphy. The high-risk category includes the remaining one-sixth of the adult population. Such individuals are known to have coronary, cerebral, or peripheral vascular disease or to suffer from diabetes mellitus or renal dysfunction. This category may also include patients upgraded from intermediate risk by additional testing. Patients identified as being at high risk should receive intense global risk factor reduction. In addition, these patients need further stratification to identify those with vulnerable plaques who are at very high risk (>15% acute coronary events per year). Identification of these *accidents waiting to happen* is a key goal for coronary artery imaging. Considering that the clinicians' expectations of the imagers are very high indeed, close collaboration of these two groups to reach this important goal is of the utmost importance.

References

1. National Heart, Lung, and Blood Institute (2009) Morbidity and mortality: 2007chartbook on cardiovascular, lung, and blood diseases. Washington, DC: Department of Health and Human Services, 2007. (Accessed July 21, 2009, at http:// www.nhlbi.nih.gov/resources/docs/ 07-chtbk.pdf.).
2. Ford ES, Ajani UA, Croft JB et al (2007) Explaining the decrease in U.S. deaths from coronary disease. N Engl J Med 356:2388-2398
3. Lloyd-Jones D, Adams R, Carnethon M et al (2009) Heart disease and stroke statistics – 2009 update: A report from the American Heart Association Statistics Committee and Stroke Statistics Subcommittee. Circulation 119:21-181
4. Hardoon SL, Whincup PH, Lennon LT et al (2008) How much of the recent decline in the incidence of myocardial infarction in British men can be explained by changes in cardiovascular risk factors? Evidence from a prospective population-based study. Circulation 117:598-604
5. Murray CJL, Lopez AD (1997) Mortality by cause for eight regions of the world: Global Burden of Disease Study. Lancet 349:1269-1276
6. Shah PK (2007) Molecular mechanisms of plaque instability. Curr Opin Lipidol 18:492-499
7. Gibbons RJ, Jones DW, Gardner TJ et al (2008) The American Heart Association's 2008 statement of principles for healthcare reform. Circulation 118:2209-2218
8. Falk E, Shah PK, Fuster V (1995) Coronary plaque disruption. Circulation 92:657-671
9. Stamler J, Stamler R, Neaton JD et al (1999) Low risk-factor profile and long-term cardiovascular and non cardiovascular mortality and life expectancy: findings for 5 large cohorts of young adult and middle-aged men and women. JAMA 282:2012-2018
10. Expert Panel on Detection, Evaluation, and Treatment of High Blood Cholesterol in Adults (2001) Executive summary of the Third Report of the National Cholesterol Education Program (NCEP) Expert Panel on Detection, Evaluation, and Treatment of High Blood Cholesterol in Adults (Adult Treatment Panel III). JAMA 285:2486-2497 (Also available at Http://www.nhlbi.nih.gov/guidelines/cholesterol/atp3full.pdf.)
11. Greenland P, Knoll MD, Stamler J et al (2003) Major risk factors as antecedents of fatal and nonfatal coronary heart disease events. JAMA 290:891-897
12. Khot UN, Khot MB, Bajzer CT et al (2003) Prevalence of conventional risk factors in patients with coronary heart disease. JAMA 290:898-904
13. Grundy SM, Cleeman JI, Merz CN et al (2004) Implications of recent clinical trials for the National Cholesterol Education Program Adult Treatment Panel III guidelines. Circulation 110:227-239
14. Greenland P, Smith SC Jr, Grundy SM (2001) Improving coronary heart disease risk assessment in asymptomatic people: role of traditional risk factors and noninvasive cardiovascular tests. Circulation 104:1863-1867
15. Smith SC Jr, Greenland P, Grundy SM (2000) Prevention Conference V: beyond secondary prevention: identifying the high-risk patient for primary prevention: executive summary. Circulation 101:111-116
16. Hlatky MA, Greenland P, Arnett DK et al (2009) Criteria for evaluation of novel markers of cardiovascular risk: a scientific statement from the American Heart Association. Circulation 119:2408-2416
17. Kannel WB, McGee D, Gordon T (1976) A general cardiovascular risk profile: the Framingham Study. Am J Cardiol 38:46 –51
18. Wilson PW, D'Agostino RB, Levy D et al (1998) Prediction of coronary heart disease using risk factor categories. Circulation 97:1837-1847

19. National Cholesterol Education Program Expert Panel on Detection, Evaluation, and Treatment of High Blood Cholesterol in Adults (2001) Executive summary of the third report of the National Cholesterol Education Program (NCEP) Expert Panel on Detection, Evaluation, and Treatment of High Blood Cholesterol in Adults (Adult Treatment Panel III). JAMA 285:2486-2497
20. U.S. Preventive Services Task Force (2009) Aspirin for the prevention of cardiovascular disease: U.S. Preventive Services Task Force recommendation statement. Ann Intern Med 150:396-404
21. Pearson TA, Blair SN, Daniels SR et al (2002) AHA guidelines for primary prevention of cardiovascular disease and stroke: 2002 update: Consensus Panel guide to comprehensive risk reduction for adult patients without coronary or other atherosclerotic vascular diseases. American Heart Association Science Advisory and Coordinating Committee. Circulation 106:388-391
22. Berger JS, Jordan CO, Lloyd-Jones D et al (2010) Screening for cardiovascular risk in asymptomatic patients. J Am Coll Cardiol 55:1169-1777
23. D'Agostino RB Sr, Grundy S, Sullivan LM et al (2001) Validation of the Framingham coronary heart disease prediction scores: results of a multiple ethnic groups investigation. JAMA 286:180-187
24. Brindle P, Beswick A, Fahey T et al (2006) Accuracy and impact of risk assessment in the primary prevention of cardiovascular disease: a systematic review. Heart 92:1752-1759
25. Murabito JM, D'Agostino RB, Silbershatz H et al (1997) Intermittent claudication. A risk profile from the Framingham Heart Study. Circulation 96:44-49
26. Wolf PA, D'Agostino RB, Belanger AJ et al (1991) Probability of stroke: a risk profile from the Framingham study. Stroke 22:312-318
27. Kannel WB, D'Agostino RB, Silbershatz H et al (1999) Profile for estimating risk of heart failure. Arch Intern Med 159:1197-204
28. Lloyd-Jones DM, Larson MG, Beiser A et al (1999) Lifetime risk of developing coronary heart disease. Lancet 353:89-92
29. Lloyd-Jones DM, Leip EP, Larson MG et al (2006) Prediction of lifetime risk for cardiovascular disease by risk factor burden at 50 years of age. Circulation 113:791-798
30. Pencina MJ, D'Agostino RB Sr., Larson MG et al (2009) Predicting the 30-year risk of cardiovascular disease: the Framingham Heart Study. Circulation 119:3078-3084
31. Sever PS, Dahlof B, Poulter NR et al (2003) Prevention of coronary and stroke events with atorvastatin in hypertensive patients who have average or lower-than-average cholesterol concentrations, in the Anglo-Scandinavian Cardiac Outcomes Trial-Lipid Lowering Arm (ASCOT-LLA): a multicentre randomised controlled trial. Lancet 361:1149 -1158
32. Conroy RM, Pyorala K, Fitzgerald AP et al (2003) Estimation of ten-year risk of fatal cardiovascular disease in Europe: the SCORE project. Eur Heart J 24:987-1003
33. Ridker PM, Buring JE, Rifai N et al (2007) Development and validation of improved algorithms for the assessment of global cardiovascular risk in women: the Reynolds Risk Score. JAMA 297:611-619
34. Ridker PM, Paynter NP, Rifai N et al (2008) C-reactive protein and parental history improve global cardiovascular risk prediction: the Reynolds Risk Score for men. Circulation 118:2243-2251
35. Woodward M, Brindle P, Tunstall-Pedoe H (2007) Adding social deprivation and family history to cardiovascular risk assessment: the ASSIGN score from the Scottish Heart Health Extended Cohort (SHHEC). Heart 93:172-176
36. Hippisley-Cox J, Coupland C, Vinogradova Y et al (2007) Derivation and validation of QRISK, a new cardiovascular disease risk score for the United Kingdom: prospective open cohort study. BMJ 335:136
37. Hippisley-Cox J, Coupland C, Vinogradova Y et al (2008) Performance of the QRISK cardiovascular risk prediction algorithm in an independent UK sample of patients from general practice: a validation study. Heart 94:34-39
38. Arad Y, Goodman KJ, Roth M et al (2005) Coronary calcification, coronary disease risk factors, C-reactive protein, and atherosclerotic cardiovascular disease events: the St. Francis Heart Study. J Am Coll Cardiol 46:158-65
39. Ardehali R, Nasir K, Kolandaivelu A et al (2007) Screening patients for subclinical atherosclerosis with non-contrast cardiac CT. Atherosclerosis 192:235- 242
40. Budoff MJ, Gul KM (2008) Expert review on coronary calcium. Vasc Health Risk Manag 4:315-324
41. Budoff MJ, Shaw LJ, Liu ST et al (2007) Long-term prognosis associated with coronary calcification: observations from a registry of 25,253 patients. J Am Coll Cardiol 49:1860 -1870
42. Detrano R, Guerci AD, Carr JJ et al (2008) Coronary calcium as a predictor of coronary events in four racial or ethnic groups. N Engl J Med 358:1336-1345
43. Greenland P, LaBree L, Azen SP et al (2004) Coronary artery calcium score combined with Framingham score for risk prediction in asymptomatic individuals. JAMA 291:210-215
44. Grundy SM (2004) Atherosclerosis imaging and the future of lipid management. Circulation 110:3509 -3511
45. Lakoski SG, Greenland P, Wong ND et al (2007) Coronary artery calcium scores and risk for cardiovascular events in women classified as "low risk" based on Framingham risk score: the Multi-Ethnic Study of Atherosclerosis (MESA). Arch Intern Med 167:2437-2442
46. Pohle K, Ropers D, Maffert R et al (2003) Coronary calcifications in young patients with first, unheralded myocardial infarction: a risk factor matched analysis by electron beam tomography. Heart 89:625- 628
47. Raggi P, Gongora MC, Gopal A et al (2008) Coronary artery calcium to predict all-cause mortality in elderly men and women. J Am Coll Cardiol 52:17-23
48. Raggi P, Shaw LJ, Berman DS et al (2004) Prognostic value of coronary artery calcium screening in subjects with and without diabetes. J Am Coll Cardiol 43:1663-1669
49. Rumberger JA (2008) Coronary artery calcium scanning using computed tomography: clinical recommendations for cardiac risk assessment and treatment. Semin Ultrasound CT MR 29:223-229
50. Shareghi S, Ahmadi N, Young E et al (2007) Prognostic significance of zero coronary calcium scores on cardiac computed tomography. J Cardiovasc Comput Tomogr 1:155-159
51. Shaw LJ, Raggi P, Schisterman E et al (2003) Prognostic value of cardiac risk factors and coronary artery calcium screening for all-cause mortality. Radiology 228:826-833
52. Taylor AJ, Bindeman J, Feuerstein I et al (2005) Coronary calcium independently predicts incident premature coronary heart disease over measured cardiovascular risk factors: mean three-year outcomes in the Prospective Army Coronary Calcium (PACC) project. J Am Coll Cardiol 46:807-814
53. Wayhs R, Zelinger A, Raggi P (2002) High coronary artery calcium scores pose an extremely elevated risk for hard events. J Am Coll Cardiol 39:225-230
54. Shah PK (2010) Asymptomatic subjects for subclinical atherosclerosis. Can we, does it matter, ans should we? J Am Coll Cardiol 56:98-105
55. Preis SR, Hwang SJ, Fox CS et al (2009) Eligibility of individuals with subclinical coronary artery calcium and intermediate coronary heart disease risk for reclassification (from the Framingham Heart Study). Am J Cardiol 103:1710-1715
56. Blaha M, Budoff MJ, Shaw LJ et al (2009) Absence of coronary artery calcification and all-cause mortality. J Am Coll Cardiol Img 2: 692-700
57. Sarwar A, Shaw LJ, Shapiro MD et al (2009) Diagnostic and prognostic value of absence of coronary artery calcification. J Am Coll

Cardiol Img 2:675- 688

58. Anand DV, Lim E, Lahiri A et al (2006) The role of non-invasive imaging in the risk stratification of asymptomatic diabetic subjects. Eur Heart J 27:905-912

59. Schenker MP, Dorbala S, Hong EC et al (2008) Interrelation of coronary calcification, myocardial ischemia, and outcomes in patients with intermediate likelihood of coronary artery disease: a combined positron emission tomography/computed tomography study. Circulation 117:1693-1700

60. Greenland P, Bonow RO (2008) How low-risk is a coronary calcium score of zero? The importance of conditional probability. Circulation 117:1627-1629

61. Henneman MM, Schuijf JD, Pundziute G et al (2008) Noninvasive evaluation with multislice computed tomography in suspected acute coronary syndrome: plaque morphology on multislice computed tomography versus coronary calcium score. J Am Coll Cardiol 52:216-222

62. Cheng VY, Lepor NE, Madyoon H et al (2007) Presence and severity of noncalcified coronary plaque on 64-slice computed tomographic coronary angiography in patients with zero and low coronary artery calcium. Am J Cardiol 99:1183-1186

63. Johnson KM, Dowe DA, Brink JA (2009) Traditional clinical risk assessment tools do not accurately predict coronary atherosclerotic plaque burden: a CT angiography study. AJR Am J Roentgenol 192:235-243.

64. de Groot E, van Leuven SI, Duivenvoorden R et al (2008) Measurement of carotid intima-media thickness to assess progression and regression of atherosclerosis. Nat Clin Pract Cardiovasc Med 5:280-288

65. Stein JH, Korcarz CE, Hurst RT et al (2008) Use of carotid ultrasound to identify subclinical vascular disease and evaluate cardiovascular disease risk: a consensus statement from the American Society of Echocardiography Carotid Intima-Media Thickness Task Force. Endorsed by the Society for Vascular Medicine. J Am Soc Echocardiogr 21:93-111, quiz 189-190

66. Lorenz MW, Markus HS, Bots ML et al (2007) Prediction of clinical cardiovascular events with carotid intima-media thickness: a systematic review and meta-analysis. Circulation 115:459-467

67. Polak JF, Pencina MJ, Pencina KM et al (2011) Carotid-Wall Intima-Media Thickness and Cardiovascular Events. N Engl J Med 365:213-222

68. Newman AB, Naydeck BL, Sutton-Tyrrell K et al (2002) Relationshipbetween coronary artery calcification and other measures of subclinical cardiovascular disease in older adults. Arterioscler Thromb Vasc Biol 22:1674-1679

69. Folsom AR, Kronmal RA, Detrano RC et al (2008) Coronary artery calcification compared with carotid intima-media thickness in the prediction of cardiovascular disease incidence: the Multi-Ethnic Study of Atherosclerosis (MESA). Arch Intern Med 168:1333-1339

70. Hecht HS (2008) The deadly double standard (the saga of screening for subclinical atherosclerosis). Am J Cardiol 101:1805-1807

71. Kalia NK, Miller LG, Nasir K et al (2006) Visualizing coronary calcium is associated with improvements in adherence to statin therapy. Atherosclerosis 185:394-399

72. Taylor AJ, Bindeman J, Feuerstein I et al (2008) Community-based provision of statin and aspirin after the detection of coronary artery calcium within a community-based screening cohort. J Am Coll Cardiol 51:1337-1341

73. Naghavi M, Falk E, Hecht HS et al (2006) The first SHAPE (Screening for Heart Attack Prevention and Education) guideline. Crit Pathw Cardiol 5:187-190

74. See R, Lindsey JB, Patel MJ et al (2008) Application of the Screening for Heart Attack Prevention and Education Task Force recommendations to an urban population: observations from the Dallas Heart Study. Arch Intern Med 168:1055-1062

75. Diamond GA, Kaul S (2007) The things to come of SHAPE: cost and effectiveness of cardiovascular prevention. Am J Cardiol 99:1013-1015

76. Cohn JN, Duprez DA (2008) Time to foster a rational approach to preventing cardiovascular morbid events. J Am Coll Cardiol 52:327-329

77. The HRP Initiative. Available at: http://www.hrpinitiative.com. Accessed May 12, 2010

78. Achenbach S (2007) Cardiac CT: state of the art for the detection of coronary arterial stenosis. J Cardiovasc Comput Tomogr 1:3-20

79. Abbara S, Arbab-Zadeh A, Callister TQ et al (2009) SCCT guidelines for performance of coronary computed tomographic angiography: a report of the Society of Cardiovascular Computed Tomography Guidelines Committee. J Cardiovasc Comput Tomogr 3:190-204

80. Achenbach S, Ropers U, Kuettner A, Anders K et al (2008) Randomized comparison of 64-slice singleand dual-source computed tomography for the detection of coronary artery disease. J Am Coll Cardiol Img 1:177-186

81. Alkadhi H, Scheffel H, Desbiolles L et al (2008) Dual-source computed tomography coronary angiography: influence of obesity, calcium load, and heart rate on diagnostic accuracy. Eur Heart J 29:766-776

82. Dewey M, Vavere AL, Arbab-Zadeh A et al (2010) Patient characteristics as predictors of image quality and diagnostic accuracy of MDCT compared with conventional coronary angiography for detecting coronary artery stenoses: CORE-64 Multicenter International Trial. Am J Roentgenol 194:93-102

83. Budoff MJ, Dowe D, Jollis JG et al (2008) Diagnostic performance of 64-multidetector-row coronary computed tomographic angiography for evaluation of coronary artery stenosis in individuals without known coronary artery disease. J Am Coll Cardiol 52:1724-1732

84. Meijboom WB, Meijs MF, Schuijf JD et al (2008) Diagnostic accuracy of 64-slice computed tomography coronary angiography: a prospective, multicenter, multivendor study. J Am Coll Cardiol 52:2135-2144

85. Meijboom WB, van Mieghem CA, Mollet NR et al (2007) 64-slice computed tomography coronary angiography in patients with high, intermediate, or low pretest probability of significant coronary artery disease. J Am Coll Cardiol 50:1469-1475

86. Miller JM, Rochitte CE, Dewey M et al (2008) Diagnostic performance of coronary angiography by 64-row CT. N Engl J Med 359:2324-2336

87. Danciu SC, Herrera CJ, Stecy PJ et al (2007) Usefulness of multislice computed tomographic coronary angiography to identify patients with abnormal myocardial perfusion stress in whom diagnostic catheterization may be safely avoided. Am J Cardiol 100:1605-1608

87. Gilard M, Le Gal G, Cornily JC et al (2007) Midterm prognosis of patients with suspected coronary artery disease and normal multislice computed tomography findings. A prospective management outcome study. Arch Intern Med 165:1686-1689

88. Hadamitzky M, Freissmuth B, Meyer T et al (2009) Prognostic value of coronary computed tomographic angiography for prediction of cardiac events in patients with suspected coronary artery disease. JACC Cardiovasc Imaging 2:404-411

90. Hollander JE, Chang AM, Shofer FS et al (2009) One-year outcomes following coronary computerized tomographic angiography for evaluation of emergency department patients with potential acute coronary syndrome. Acad Emerg Med 16:693-698

91. Rubinshtein R, Halon DA, Gaspar T et al (2007) Usefulness of 64-slice cardiac computed tomographic angiography for diagnosing acute coronary syndromes and predicting clinical outcome in emergency department patients with chest pain of uncertain origin. Circulation 115:1762-1768

92. Chow BJ, Wells GA, Chen L et al (2010) Prognostic value of 64-slice cardiac computed tomography severity of coronary artery disease, coronary atherosclerosis, and left ventricular ejection fraction. J Am Coll Cardiol 55:1017-1028

93. Petranovic M, Soni A, Bezzera H et al (2009) Assessment of nonstenotic coronary lesions by 64-slice multidetector computed tomography in comparison to intravascular ultrasound: evaluation of nonculprit coronary lesions. J Cardiovasc Comput Tomogr 3:24-31

94. Sun J, Zhang Z, Lu B et al (2008) Identification and quantification of coronary atherosclerotic plaques: a comparison of 64-MDCT and intravascular ultrasound. Am J Roentgenol 190:748-754

95. Schroeder S, Kopp AF, Baumbach A et al (2001) Noninvasive detection and evaluation of atherosclerotic coronary plaques with multislice computed tomography. J Am Coll Cardiol 37:1430-1435

96. Caussin C, Ohanessian A, Ghostine S et al (2004) Characterization of vulnerable nonstenotic plaque with 16-slice computed tomography compared with intravascular ultrasound. Am J Cardiol 94:99-100

97. Carrascosa PM, Capunay CM, Garcia-Merletti P et al (2006) Characterization of coronary atherosclerotic plaques by multidetector computed tomography. Am J Cardiol 97:598-602

98. Pohle K, Achenbach S, MacNeill B et al (2007) Characterization of non-calcified coronary atherosclerotic plaque by multi-detector row CT: comparison to IVUS. Atherosclerosis 190:174-180

99. Motoyama S, Kondo T, Anno H et al (2007) Atherosclerotic plaque characterization by 0.5-mm-slice multislice computed tomographic imaging. Circ J 71:363-366

100. Becker CR, Nikolaou K, Muders M et al (2003) Ex vivo coronary atherosclerotic plaque characterization with multi-detector-row CT. Eur Radiol 13:2094-2098

101. Cademartiri F, Mollet NR, Runza G et al (2005) Influence of intracoronary attenuation on coronary plaque measurements using multislice computed tomography: observations in an ex vivo model of coronary computed tomography angiography. Eur Radiol 15:1426-1431

102. Achenbach S, Boehmer K, Pflederer T et al (2010) Influence of slice thickness and reconstruction kernel on the computed tomographic attenuation of coronary atherosclerotic plaque. J Cardiovasc Comput Tomogr 4:110-115

103. Motoyama S, Kondo T, Sarai M et al (2007) Multislice computed tomographic characteristics of coronary lesions in acute coronary syndromes. J Am Coll Cardiol 50:319-326

104. Kitagawa T, Yamamoto H, Horiguchi J et al (2009) Characterization of noncalcified coronary plaques and identification of culprit lesions in patients with acute coronary syndrome by 64-slice computed tomography. JACC Cardiovasc Imaging 2:153-160

105. Hoffmann U, Moselewski F, Nieman K et al (2006) Noninvasive assessment of plaque morphology and composition in culprit and stable lesions in acute coronary syndrome and stable lesions in stable angina by multidetector computed tomography. J Am Coll Cardiol 47:1655-1662

106. Achenbach S, Ropers D, Hoffmann U et al (2004) Assessment of coronary remodeling in stenotic and nonstenotic coronary atherosclerotic lesions by multidetector spiral computed tomography. J Am Coll Cardiol 43:842-847

107. Kitagawa T, Yamamoto H, Ohhashi N et al (2007) Comprehensive evaluation of noncalcified coronary plaque characteristics detected using 64-slice computed tomography in patients with proven or suspected coronary artery disease. Am Heart J 154:1191-1198

108. Ostrom MP, Gopal A, Ahmadi N et al (2008) Mortality incidence and the severity of coronary atherosclerosis assessed by computed tomography angiography. J Am Coll Cardiol 52:1335-1343

109. Min JK, Shaw LJ, Devereux RB et al (2007) Prognostic value of multidetector coronary computed tomographic angiography for prediction of all-cause mortality. J Am Coll Cardiol 50:1161-1170

110. Motoyama S, Sarai M, Harigaya H et al (2009) Computed tomographic angiography characteristics of atherosclerotic plaques subsequently resulting in acute coronary syndrome. J Am Coll Cardiol 54:49-57

111. Hausleiter J, Meyer T, Hermann F et al (2009) Estimated radiation dose associated with cardiac CT angiography. JAMA 301:500-507

112. Raff GL, Chinnaiyan KM, Share DA et al (2009) Radiation dose from cardiac computed tomography before and after implementationof radiation dose-reduction techniques. JAMA 301:2340-2348

113. Bischoff B, Hein F, Meyer T et al (2009) Impact of a reduced tube voltage on CT angiography and radiation dose: results of the PROTECTION I study. JACC Cardiovasc Imaging 2:940-946

114. Earls JP, Berman EL, Urban BA et al (2008) Prospectively gated transverse coronary CT angiography versus retrospectively gated helical technique: improved image quality and reduced radiation dose. Radiology 246:742-753

115. Hirai N, Horiguchi J, Fujioka C et al (2008) Prospective versus retrospective ECGgated 64-detector coronary CT angiography: assessment of image quality, stenosis, and radiation dose. Radiology 248:424-430

116. Scheffel H, Alkadhi H, Leschka S et al (2008) Low-dose CT coronary angiography in the step-and-shoot mode: diagnostic performance. Heart 94:1132-1137

117. Husmann L, Valenta I, Gaemperli O et al (2008) Feasibility of low-dose coronary CT angiography: first experience with prospective ECGgating. Eur Heart J 29:191-197

118. Achenbach S, Marwan M, Ropers D et al (2010) Coronary computed tomography angiography with a consistent dose below 1 mSv using prospectively electrocardiogram-triggered high-pitch spiral acquisition. Eur Heart J 31:340-346

119. Hendel RC, Patel MR, Kramer CM et al (2006) American College of Cardiology Foundation Quality Strategic Directions Committee Appropriateness Criteria Working Group; American College of Radiology; Society of Cardiovascular Computed Tomography; Society for Cardiovascular Magnetic Resonance; American Society of Nuclear Cardiology; North American Society for Cardiac Imaging; Society for Cardiovascular Angiography, Interventions; Society of Interventional Radiology. ACCF/ACR/SC-CT/ SCMR/ASNC/NASCI/SCAI/SIR 2006 appropriateness criteria for cardiac computed tomography and cardiac magnetic resonance imaging: a report of the American College of Cardiology Foundation Quality Strategic Directions Committee Appropriateness Criteria Working Group, American College of Radiology, Society of Cardiovascular Computed Tomography, Society for Cardiovascular Magnetic Resonance, American Society of Nuclear Cardiology, North American Society for Cardiac Imaging, Society for Cardiovascular Angiography and Interventions, and Society of Interventional Radiology. J Am Coll Cardiol 48:1475-1497

120. Schroeder S, Achenbach S, Bengel F et al (2008) Cardiac computed tomography: indications, applications, limitations, and training requirements: report of a Writing Group deployed by the Working Group Nuclear Cardiology and Cardiac CT of the European Society of Cardiology and the European Council of Nuclear Cardiology. Eur Heart J 29:531-556

121. Bluemke DA, Achenbach S, Budoff M et al (2008). Noninvasive coronary artery imaging: magnetic resonance angiography and multidetector computed tomography angiography: a scientific statement from the American Heart Association Committee on cardiovascular imaging and intervention of the council on cardiovascular radiology and intervention, and the councils on clinical cardiology and cardiovascular disease in the young. Circulation 118:586-606

122. Perrone-Filiardi P, Achenbach S, Molenkamp S et al (2011) Cardiac Computed Tomography and Myocardial Perfusion Scintigra-

phy for risk stratification in asymptomatic individuals without known cardiovascular disease: a position statement of the working group of nuclear cardiology and cardiac CT of the European Society of Cardiology. Eur Heart J 32:1986-1993

Chronic (Stable) Coronary Artery Disease

4

Giancarlo Casolo

4.1 Introduction

Coronary Artery Disease (CAD) can be considered stable or chronic when obstructive atherosclerosis of the coronary vessels develops slowly and progressively without sudden and unexpected pathologic and clinical manifestations. This definition is somewhat arbitrary and includes all those clinical presentations of CAD that are not included in the chapter of acute coronary syndrome (ACS). It therefore describes a spectrum of conditions that do not require emergency hospital admission. These conditions, other than ACS, do not present any immediate danger for the patient and can be managed, at least initially, noninvasively and by clinical means. Chronic CAD conditions include, among others, post myocardial infarction patients, patients with chronic angina pectoris and patients who have been revascularized. A list of clinical conditions that may be part of this chapter is shown in Table 4.1.

4.2 Pathology

Coronary atherosclerosis is nowadays considered a chronic immune-inflammatory, fibro-proliferative dis-

Table 4.1 Clinical Conditions associated with the definition of Chronic CAD

Chronic stable angina
Post-myocardial infarction
Post-revascularization CAD
Obstructive CAD
CAD with demonstration of ischemia
CAD with demonstration of viability
Left ventricular dysfunction and CAD

G. Casolo (✉)
Cardiology Unit,
Versilia Hospital,
Lido di Camaiore (LU), Italy

ease of large and medium-sized arteries fuelled by lipid. Endothelial cells, leukocytes and intimal smooth muscle cells are the major players in the development of this disease [1, 2]. Long considered a disease of the aged vessels, coronary artery disease can be documented in young asymptomatic adults although obstructive lesions are rare in this population [3]. There is now wide evidence supporting the progression of coronary atherosclerosis over time [4] and studies show that obstructive lesions (>75%) can be documented in as many as 2% of asymptomatic individuals [5]. The spatial distribution of coronary stenosis along the vessels is not homogeneous, being more common in the proximal arteries, the first portion of the LAD and second portion of the RCA [6]. Factors such as shear stress, coronary anatomy and hereditary factors may all play a role in this spatial distribution. While the composition of the plaques causing an acute coronary syndrome more frequently show a thin-cap fibroatheroma and/or a large necrotic core, those belonging to patients with chronic angina usually show larger amount of fibrous tissue and calcium deposits.

4.3 Physiopathology

Whereas the presence of coronary atherosclerosis is the hallmark of a disease which does not necessarily promote clinical symptoms, it does trigger some changes in the vessel wall which may ultimately cause an imbalance between oxygen supply and metabolic needs under some circumstances. An atherosclerotic lesion may cause some degree of flow disturbance by decreasing the coronary arterial lumen. Under physiologic conditions coronary flow is not altered in a coronary bed served by an epicardial coronary artery with stenosis of the vessel lumen up to 65-70% [1, 7]. A reduction in flow reserve is observed beyond this narrowing of the epicardial arteries and an increase in metabolic needs of the myocardium in this condition results in ischemia. This imbalance is thought to take place in a sequence of

F. Cademartiri, G. Casolo, M. Midiri (eds.), *Clinical Applications of Cardiac CT*,
© Springer-Verlag Italia 2012

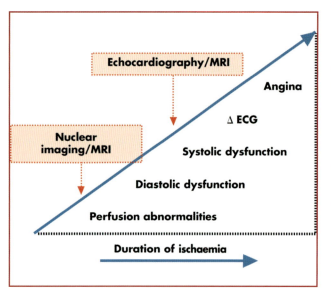

Fig. 4.1 The ischaemic cascade represents the sequence of pathophysiological ischaemia. (Reproduced from [9], with permission)

events which can be termed the ischemic cascade [8]. In this model, several phenomena take place which can be detected by appropriate diagnostic means before the appearance of chest pain or even without the patient suffering pain (Fig. 4.1).

4.4 Clinical Manifestations

Coronary atherosclerosis, even when characterized by obstructive lesions, may not be clinically manifest. It is usually recognized when anginal symptoms are present. Diabetic patients frequently do not experience chest pain and may be totally asymptomatic. Chest pain occurs as the ultimate manifestation of the ischemic cascade and it may be accompanied by dyspnea. This latter symptom may represent an angina-equivalent symptom.

The clinical assessment of a patient with suspected or known CAD includes a careful physical examination, recording of an ECG, and may be completed by imaging the left ventricle at rest by echocardiography [10].

Simple clinical information can be used to suspect CAD. The probability of disease increases significantly based upon the presence or absence of typical chest pain, age, and gender. Anginal symptoms can be either suggestive or not of CAD. Based upon this simple clinical information several tools have been developed to aid in evaluating the probability of CAD; one of the most known is the Duke probability risk score (Table 4.2) [11-13].

The Canadian Cardiovascular Society classification of angina pectoris is one of the most common systems for characterizing the severity of symptoms. The classification uses the extent of limitation on daily activities and the kind of physical activity which precipitates the anginal episode (Table 4.3) [14].

4.5 Diagnostic Tests

Between attacks, the ECG (and usually LV function) at rest is normal in about 30% of patients with a typical history of angina pectoris, even those with extensive 3-vessel disease. In the remaining 70%, the ECG shows several kinds of abnormalities. However, an abnormal resting ECG alone does not establish or refute the diagnosis.

Several noninvasive diagnostic tools can be used to increase the ability of recognizing CAD (Table 4.4). The most common tool is stress testing. This widely used test possesses a reasonable specificity and a low sensitivity in diagnosing CAD, particularly in females. The reported mean sensitivity is around 68%; mean specificity is 77% [15, 16].

Table 4.2 The Duke probability risk score. (Adapted from [12])

Age, years	Gender	Typical or definite angina pectoris	Atypical or probable angina pectoris	Nonanginal chest pain	No symptoms
30-39	Male	Intermediate	Intermediate	Low	Very low
	Female	Intermediate	Very low	Very low	Very low
40-49	Male	High	Intermediate	Intermediate	Low
	Female	Intermediate	Low	Very low	Very low
50-59	Male	High	Intermediate	Intermediate	Low
	Female	Intermediate	Intermediate	Low	Very low
60-69	Male	High	Intermediate	Intermediate	Low
	Female	High	Intermediate	Intermediate	Low

Table 4.3 The Canadian Cardiovascular Society classification of angina pectoris. (Adapted from [12])

Class	Definition	Specific Activity Scale
I	Ordinary physical activity (e.g. walking and climbing stairs) does not cause angina; angina occurs with strenuous, rapid, or prolonged exertion at work or recreation.	Ability to ski, play basketball, jog at 5 mph, or shovel snow without angina
II	Slight limitation of ordinary activity. Angina occurs on walking or climbing stairs rapidly, walking uphill, walking or stair climbing after meals, in cold, in wind, or under emotional stress, or only during the few hours after awakening, when walking more than two blocks on level ground, or when climbing more than one flight of stairs at a normal pace and in normal conditions.	Ability to garden, rake, roller skate, walk at 4 mph on level ground, have sexual intercourse without stopping
III	Marked limitation of ordinary physical activity. Angina occurs on walking one to two blocks on level ground or climbing one flight of stairs at a normal pace in normal conditions.	Ability to shower or dress without stopping, walk 2.5 mph, bowl, make a bed, play golf
IV	Inability to perform any physical activity without discomfort.	Anginal symptoms may be present at rest. Inability to perform activities requiring 2 or fewer metabolic equivalents without angina

Table 4.4 Summary of test characteristics for investigations used in the diagnosis of stable angina. (Adapted from [16], with permission)

Diagnosis of CAD	Sensitivity %	Specificity %
Exercise ECG	68	77
Exercise echo	80–85	84–86
Exercise myocardial perfusion	85–90	70–75
Dobutamine stress echo	40–100	62–100
Vasodilator stress echo	56–92	87–100
Vasodilator stress myocardial perfusion	83–94	64–90

In order to improve the accuracy in detecting CAD other common diagnostic tools used in clinical practice are myocardial perfusion scintigraphy, stress-echocardiography, stress-CMR, MDCT and diagnostic invasive coronary angiography.

The presence and severity of ischemia (spatial extent and temporal time of onset), and the angiographic severity of disease negatively and independently affect prognosis. By using stress testing either with or without associated imaging, it is possible to derive prognostic information that may help in deciding whether or not an invasive approach is advisable. The mortality risk that can be expected based upon a score calculated from variables collected during exercise stress testing.

A comprehensive summary of the appropriate indications for each test and invasive angiography in patients with suspected or ascertained CAD for diagnosis and prognostic assessment is shown in Table 4.5.

4.6 Medical vs. Invasive Management

Medical therapy of CAD has greatly improved symptoms and survival of CAD patients in the past few years. The control of the modifiable Framingham risk factors (smoke cessation, control of hypertension), as well as the use of statins, ACEi, beta blockers and ASA, have positively modified the prognosis.

The aim of therapy in patients with stable CAD has two main objectives: relief of symptoms when present, and improvement of survival. Symptom relief may not have relevant benefits in terms of survival, the latter depending on the severity of ischemia. Most meta-analyses report no mortality benefit, increased nonfatal periprocedural MI, and reduced need for repeat revascularization by choosing a systematic invasive strategy [18]. The COURAGE trial showed that the routine use of PCI with or without stenting in CAD patients with objective documentation of ischemia and optimal therapy is not superior to medical therapy alone in the composite of death, MI, stroke, or hospitalization for unstable angina [19]. Recent data show that a long-term survival benefit may be expected when using PCI in CAD patients with an ischemic area >10% of the left ventricle [20].

CABG shows a survival benefit over medical therapy in patients with LM or three-vessel disease, particularly when the proximal LAD coronary artery is involved. Greater benefits can be expected in those with severe symptoms, early positive exercise tests, and impaired LV function [21].

The ESC/EACTS have recently jointly released the guidelines for revascularization in CAD patients (Table 4.6) [18].

Table 4.5 Indications for noninvasive tests and invasive angiography in CAD patients. (Reproduced from [18], with permission)

	Asymptomatic (screening)	Symptomatic			Prognostic value of positive result[a]	Prognostic value of negative result[a]
		Pretest likelihood[b] of obstructive disease				
		Low	Intermediate	High		
Anatomical test						
Invasive angiography	III A	III A	IIb A	I A	I A	I A
MDCT angiography	III B[c]	IIb B	IIa B	III B	IIb B	IIa B
MRI angiography	III B	III B	III B	III B	III C	III C
Functional test						
Stress echo	III A	III A	I A	III A[d]	I A	I A
Nuclear imaging	III A	III A	I A	III A[d]	I A	I A
Stress MRI	III B	III C	IIa B	III B[d]	IIa B	IIa B
PET perfusion	III B	III C	IIa B	III B[d]	IIa B	IIa B

[a]For the prognostic assessment of known coronary stenosis, functional imaging is similarly indicated.
[b]The pretest likelihood of disease is calculated based on symptoms, sex and risk factors.
[c]This refers to MDCT angiography, not calcium scoring.
[d]In patients with obstructive CAD documented by angiography, functional testing may be useful in guiding the revascularization strategy based on the extent, severity and location of ischemia.
CAD, coronary artery disease; *MDCT*, multidetector computed tomography; *MRI*, magnetic resonance imaging; *PET*, positron emission tomography.

Table 4.6 Indications for revascularization in stable angina or silent ischaemia. (Reproduced from [18], with permission)

	Subset of CAD by anatomy	Class[a]	Level[b]
For prognosis	Left main >50%	I	A
	Any proximal LAD>50%	I	A
	2VD or 3VD with impaired LV function[c]	I	B
	Proven large area of ischemia (>10% LV)	I	B
	Single remaining patent vessel >50% stenosis[c]	I	C
	IVD without proximal LAD and without >10% ischemia	III	A
For symptoms	Any stenosis >50% with limiting angina or angina equivalent, unresponsive to OMT	I	A
	Dyspnea/CHF and >10% LV ischemia/viability supplied by >50% stenotic artery	IIa	B
	No limiting symptoms with OMT	III	C

[a]Class of recommendation.
[b]Level of evidence.
[c]With documented ischemia or FFR <0.80 for angiographic diameter stenoses 50-90%
CAD, coronary artery disease; *CHF*, chronic heart failure; *FFR*, fractional flow reserves; *LAD*, left anterior descending; *LV*, left ventricle; *OMT*, optimal medical therapy; *VD*, vessel disease.

4.7 Conclusions

- Stable coronary artery disease refers to patients with obstructive CAD both asymptomatic or with angina but without the features of an acute coronary syndrome (ACS).
- CAD is a common manifestation of coronary atherosclerosis and can be documented from an early age in otherwise normal subjects.
- Symptoms of CAD are related to an imbalance between metabolic needs of the myocardium and the ability of the coronary circulation to adapt. Significant stenosis limits the flow reserve causing ischemia when the narrowing exceeds 70-75% of the luminal area.
- Only about 2% of the population show at least one significant (>75%) stenosis of a major epicardial vessel
- Angina or dyspnea are relatively late phenomena of the ischemic cascade.
- The diagnosis of stable CAD relies upon a thorough clinical assessment and some tests, either functional or anatomical.
- Prognosis is affected by the extent of CAD and presence and severity of inducible ischemia. Only patients with severe ischemia show benefit over medical therapy alone from revascularization.
- Medical therapy improves symptoms and survival. PCI and CABG have a positive impact on both in some well characterized patients.

References

1. Hansson GK (2005) Inflammation, atherosclerosis, and coronary artery disease. N Engl J Med 352:1685-1695
2. Falk E (2006) Pathogenesis of atherosclerosis. J Am Coll Cardiol 47:7-12
3. Tuzcu EM, Kapadia SR, Tutar E et al (2001) High prevalence of coronary atherosclerosis in asymptomatic teenagers and young adults: evidence from intravascular ultrasound. Circulation 103:2705-2710
4. Lavoie AJ, Bayturan O, Uno K et al (2010) Plaque Progression in Coronary Arteries With Minimal Luminal Obstruction in Intravascular Ultrasound Atherosclerosis Trials. Am J Cardiol 105:1679-1683
5. Choi EK, Choi SI, Rivera JJ et al (2008) Coronary computed tomography angiography as a screening tool for the detection of occult coronary artery disease in asymptomatic individuals. JACC 52:357-365
6. Cheruvu PK, Finn AV, Gardner C et al (2007) Frequency and distribution of thin-cap fibroatheroma and ruptured plaques in human coronary arteries: a pathologic study. J Am Coll Cardiol 50:940-949
7. Gould KL, Kirkeeide RL, Buchi M (1990) Coronary flow reserve as a physiologic measure of stenosis severity. J Am Coll Cardiol 15:459-474
8. Nesto RW, Kowalchuk GJ (1987) The ischemic cascade: temporal sequence of hemodynamic, electrocardiographic and symptomatic expressions of ischemia. Am J Cardiol 59:23C-30C
9. Schuijf JD, Shaw LJ, Wijns W et al (2005) Cardiac imaging in coronary artery disease: differing modalities. Heart 91:1110-1117
10. Pryor DB, Linda S, McCants CB et al (1993) Value of the history and physical in identifying patients at increased risk for CAD. Ann Int Med 118:81-90
11. Diamond GA, Forrester JS (1979) Analysis of probability as an aid in the clinical diagnosis of coronary-artery disease. N Engl J Med 300:1350-1358
12. Gibbons RJ, Balady GJ, Beasley JW, et al (1997) ACC/AHA guidelines for exercise testing: Executive summary. A report of the American College of Cardiology/American Heart Association Task Force on Practice Guidelines (Committee on Exercise Testing). Circulation 96:345-354
13. http://www.westhertshospitals.nhs.uk/WHC/risk-duke.html. Accessed 7 September 2011
14. Goldman L, Hashimoto B, Cook EF, Loscalzo A (1981) Comparative reproducibility and validity of systems for assessing cardiovascular functional class: advantages of a new specific activity scale. Circulation 64:1227-1234
15. Okin PM, Klingfield P (1995) Gender-specific criteria and performance of the exercise electrocardiogram. Circulation 92:1209-1216
16. Fox K, Garcia MA, Ardissino D et al (2006) Guidelines on the management of stable angina pectoris: executive summary: the task force on the management of stable angina pectoris of the European society of cardiology. Eur Heart J 27:1341-1381
17. Mark DB, Shaw L, Harrell FE Jr et al (1991) Prognostic value of a treadmill exercise score in outpatients with suspected coronary artery disease. N Engl J Med 325:849-853
18. Wijns W, Kolh P, Danchin N et al (2010) Guidelines on myocardial revascularization: The Task Force on Myocardial Revascularization of the European Society of Cardiology (ESC) and the European Association for Cardio-Thoracic Surgery (EACTS). Eur Heart J 31:2501-2555
19. Boden WE, O'Rourke RA, Teo KK et al (2007) Optimal medical therapy with or without PCI for stable coronary disease. N Engl J Med 356:1503-1516
20. Shaw LJ, Berman DS, Maron DJ et al (2008) Optimal medical therapy with or without percutaneous coronary intervention to reduce ischemic burden: results from the Clinical Outcomes Utilizing Revascularization and Aggressive Drug Evaluation (COURAGE) trial nuclear substudy. Circulation 117:1283-1291
21. Yusuf S, Zucker D, Peduzzi P et al (1994) Effect of coronary artery bypass graft surgery on survival: overview of 10-year results from randomised trials by the Coronary Artery Bypass Graft Surgery Trialists Collaboration. Lancet 344:563-570

Acute Coronary Syndrome: Clinical Assessment

5

Paolo Buja and Giuseppe Tarantini

5.1 Introduction

The term acute coronary syndrome (ACS) refers to any group of clinical symptoms compatible with acute myocardial ischemia and covers the spectrum of clinical conditions ranging from unstable angina (UA) to non ST-segment elevation (NSTE) myocardial infarction (MI) to ST-segment elevation (STE) MI. UA and NSTE-MI are closely related conditions, in fact their pathophysiologic origins and clinical presentations are similar, but they differ in severity. The pathogenesis of ACS involves a complex interplay among the endothelium, the inflammatory cells, and the thrombogenicity of the blood. Autopsy studies have shown that plaque rupture causes approximately 75% of fatal MIs, whereas superficial endothelial erosion accounts for the remaining 20-25% [1-5].

Indeed, the clinical manifestation may vary widely from asymptomatic patients to sudden cardiac death. In clinical practice, the correct diagnosis and risk stratification of this life-threatening condition is based mainly on clinical, electrocardiographic (ECG) and laboratory data. All patients presenting at the emergency department (ED) with chest discomfort or other symptoms suggestive of ACS should be considered high-priority triage cases [1, 2].

The general clinical approach to the patient with suspected ACS includes [1, 2]:

1) establishing the likelihood that clinical findings are secondary to ACS and coronary artery disease (CAD);
2) categorizing operatively the type of ACS;
3) stratifying the risk of patients to define the most appropriate treatment and prognosis.

G. Tarantini (✉)
Interventional Cardiology Division,
Department of Cardiac, Thoracic and Vascular Sciences,
University of Padua,
Padua, Italy

5.2 Likelihood that Clinical Findings Are Due to ACS and CAD

Different clues to establish the likelihood of ACS are reported in Table 5.1. They include clinical history and physical examination, ECG analysis and cardiac biomarkers count. It is noteworthy that in up to 25% of cases this early evaluation might be inconclusive and thus, the diagnosis remains unclear. A longer ED observation period and the use of other noninvasive tests (e.g. stress tests) should be considered before discharge to improve the accuracy of the diagnosis as well as the risk stratification of these patients (Fig. 5.1) [1, 2, 5].

5.2.1 Clinical History and Physical Examination

Medical history and physical examination play a major role in defining the early likelihood that the clinical scenario is due to an ACS. Family history, the presence of co-morbidities (i.e. diabetes), age, gender, the history of a previous CAD or MI, type, time-course and characteristics of the symptoms and drug abuse (e.g. cocaine) are all related to the likelihood of an ACS being caused by CAD or not [5, 6].

Chest pain is the main symptom of myocardial ischemia. Typical angina is characterized by heavy chest pressure or squeezing, a burning feeling. Although its predominant location is the retrosternal region, sometimes it can be referred to the epigastric area or to the back. It frequently radiates to the left arm or shoulder, and more rarely it may radiate to the neck, the jaw, the right (or both) arm/shoulder or to other regions [1, 2, 5, 6].

Pulmonary edema, dyspnea, rales, nausea and vomiting, diaphoresis, pale and cool skin, and unexplained fatigue can often be associated with angina. Nevertheless, they might be present alone as angina "equivalent" or "atypical" and might challenge the diag-

---

F. Cademartiri, G. Casolo, M. Midiri (eds.), *Clinical Applications of Cardiac CT*,
© Springer-Verlag Italia 2012

Table 5.1 Likelihood that signs and symptoms indicate an acute coronary syndrome secondary to CAD. (Adapted from [6], with permission)

Feature	HIGH likelihood Any of the following	INTERMEDIATE likelihood No high-likelihood and any of the following	LOW likelihood No high/intermediate-likelihood but may have any of the following
History	Chest/left arm pain or discomfort reproducing previously documented angina. Known history of CAD/MI.	Chest/left arm pain or discomfort. Age ≥70 years old Male sex. Diabetes mellitus.	Probable ischemic symptoms without any intermediate-likelihood features. Recent cocaine use.
Examination	Transient MR murmur, hypotension, diaphoresis, pulmonary edema, rales	Extra-cardiac vascular disease.	Chest discomfort reproduced by palpation.
ECG	New or presumably new, transient ST-segment deviation (≥1 mm) or T-wave inversion in multiple precordial leads.	Fixed Q waves. ST-segment depression 0.5-1 mm or T-wave inversion >1 mm.	T-wave flattening or inversion <1 mm in leads with dominant R waves. Normal.
Cardiac markers	Elevated Tn I or T or CK-MB.	Normal.	Normal.

CAD, coronary artery disease; *CK-MB*, MB fraction of creatine-kinase; *ECG*, electrocardiogram; *MI*, myocardial infarction; *MR*, mitral regurgitation; *Tn*, troponin.

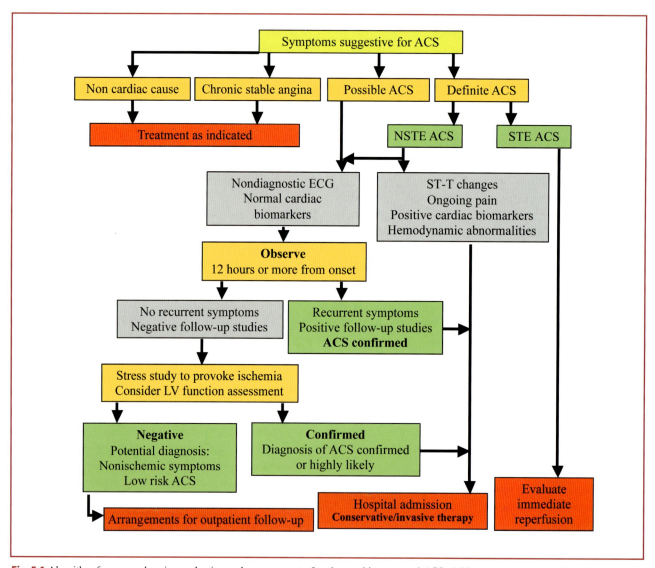

Fig. 5.1 Algorithm for comprehensive evaluation and management of patients with suspected ACS. *ACS*, acute coronary syndrome; *ECG*, electrocardiogram; *LV*, left ventricular; *NSTE*, non ST-segment elevation; *STE*, ST-segment elevation. (Adapted from [2], with permission)

nosis of ACS. This presentation is frequently observed in women, elderly or diabetics patients [1, 2, 5, 6].

The symptoms appear generally at rest and their relief after nitroglycerin administration may be suggestive of angina. Their duration can vary from a few minutes to hours and can occur as single or multiple episodes [1, 2, 5, 6].

Other kinds of pain that are not characteristic but that do not exclude myocardial ischemia include [2]:
- Pleuritic pain, i.e. sharp or knifelike pain brought on by respiratory movements or cough.
- Primary or sole location of discomfort in the middle or lower abdominal region.
- Pain that may be localized at the tip of one finger, particularly over the left ventricular apex or a costochondral junction.
- Pain reproduced with palpation or movement of the chest wall or arms.
- Very briefs episodes of pain that last few seconds or less.
- Pain that radiates into the lower extremities.

The most frequent presentations of ACS are [1, 2]: a) Angina at rest: prolonged pain at rest (usually >20 minutes); b) New onset angina: new onset severe angina of at least Canadian Cardiovascular Society (CCS) class III (i.e. marked limitations of ordinary physical activity) [7]; c) Increasing angina: recent destabilization of previously stable angina with at least CCS class III [7] angina characteristics, angina that has become distinctly more frequent, longer in duration, or lower in threshold; d) Post-MI angina. A more detailed scheme for classifying UA is [8]:
Severity
I. New onset of severe or accelerated angina, no pain at rest.
II. Angina at rest <1 month but not within preceding 48 hours (sub-acute).
II. Angina at rest <48 hours.
Clinical circumstances
A. Angina develops in the presence of an extra-cardiac condition which intensifies myocardial ischemia (e.g. secondary).
B. Angina develops in the absence of extra-cardiac conditions (e.g. primary).
C. Angina develops within 2 weeks after acute MI (e.g. post-MI).
Intensity of anti-ischemic treatment
1. Angina occurs in the absence of treatment.
2. Angina occurs during usual treatment.
3. Angina occurs despite maximal treatment.

5.2.2 ECG

The analysis of the ST segment and T wave helps to confirm the diagnosis of ACS, especially when a previous ECG is available for comparison. Nevertheless, it should be emphasized that a normal ECG does not rule out an ACS, although it is frequently observed in low risk patients. Nevertheless, in the presence of a reasonable clinical likelihood of ACS, serial or continuous ECG monitoring are recommended [1, 2] because myocardial ischemia is a dynamic process and ECG provides only a snapshot view. Lastly, the presence of ST-T segment changes at baseline, as observed in bundle branch blocks or ventricle hypertrophy, may hide the classic ECG signs and challenge the diagnosis of acute ischemia. New ST-segment depression of ≥0.05 mV is a specific sign of ongoing ischemia, whereas T-wave inversion is a less specific finding compared to ST-depression. In contrast, an STE of ≥0.1 mV in at least 2 contiguous leads indicates STEMI in most cases [9-11].

The leads in which ST-T changes are present can easily identify the extent and the location of ischemia: roughly, anterior and septal (V1-V4), lateral (V4-V6, D1, aVL), inferior (D2, D3, aVF). This can also suggests the culprit vessel because the anterior/lateral wall is generally supplied by the left anterior descending artery and the inferior/lateral wall by the left circumflex or the right coronary arteries.

5.2.3 Biomarkers of Cardiac Necrosis

All patients who present with a confirmed or suspected ACS should have multiple and consecutive repeated measures of cardiac biomarkers, such as myoglobin, troponins T or I and CK-MB [1, 2]. The main features of these biomarkers are reported in Table 5.2. The most accurate, sensitive, and specific biomarker used in clinical practice is troponin T or I. However, the troponin count also has some drawbacks. To be detected at least 3-12 hours need to have passed since the onset of symptoms. Therefore, a negative result obtained within this period should prompt a repetition of the assay 8 to 12 hours after the onset of symptoms. Because troponin levels remain elevated for a prolonged period (up to 14 days) after MI, their usefulness in detecting recurrent myocardial damage is limited. However, they are helpful in detecting myocardial injury several days after the onset of symptoms. Because of the shorter half-life of myoglobin and CK-MB, their levels are useful for diagnosing re-MI and periprocedural MI [1, 2]. A universal definition of MI has recently been proposed to standardize the criteria for its diagnosis in different clinical subsets which also include those observed after myocardial revascularization [12]:
A) Criteria for acute MI. The term MI should be used when there is evidence of myocardial necrosis in a

Table 5.2 Characteristics of cardiac biomarkers of necrosis. (Adapted from [2], with permission)

Marker	Advantages	Disadvantages	POC test?	Comment	Recommendation
Cardiac troponins	- Powerful toot for risk stratification. - Greater sensitivity and specificity than CK-MB. - Detection of recent - MI up to 2 wk after onset. - Useful for therapy selection.	- Low sensitivity in very early phase of MI (<6 h after onset) and requires repeated measurement at 8-12 h, if results are negative. - Limited ability to detect late minor re-MI.	Yes	Data on diagnostic performance and potential therapeutic implications increasingly available from clinical trials.	Useful as a single test for efficiently diagnosing NSTEMI (including minor myocardial damage), with serial measurements. Clinician should familiarize themselves with cutoffs used in their local hospital laboratory.
CK-MD	- Rapid, cost-efficient, accurate assays. - Ability to detect early re-MI.	- Loss of specificity in setting of skeletal muscle disease or injury, including surgery. - Low sensitivity during very early MI (<6 h after onset) or later after onset (>36 h) and for minor myocardial damage (detectable with troponins).	Yes	Familiar with most clinicians.	Previous standard and still acceptable diagnostic test in most clinical circumstances.
Myoglobin	- High sensitivity. - Useful in early detection of MI. - Detection of reperfusion. - Most useful in ruling out MI.	- Very low specificity in setting of skeletal muscle injury or disease. - Rapid return to normal range limits sensitivity for later presentations.	Yes	More convenient early marker than CK-MB isoforms because of greater availability of assays for myoglobin; rapid-release kinetics make myoglobin useful for noninvasive monitoring of reperfusion in patients with established MI.	

ACS, acute coronary syndrome; *CK-MB*, MB fraction of creatine-kinase; *MI*, myocardial infarction; *NSTEMI* non ST-elevation myocardial infarction; *POC*, point-of-care.

clinical setting consistent with myocardial ischemia; under these conditions any one of the following criteria meets the diagnosis:

- Detection of rise and/or fall of biomarkers (preferably troponins) with at least one value above the 99th percentile of the URL together with evidence of myocardial ischemia with at least one of the following: symptoms of ischemia; ECG changes indicative of new ischemia, i.e. new ST-T changes/left bundle branch block (LBBB); development of pathologic Q waves; imaging evidence of new loss of viable myocardium or new regional wall motion abnormality.
- Sudden, unexpected cardiac death, involving cardiac arrest, often with symptoms suggestive of myocardial ischemia, and accompanied by presumably new ST elevation/LBBB, and/or evidence of fresh thrombus at coronary angiography and/or at autopsy, but death occurring before blood samples could be obtained, or at a time before the appearance of cardiac biomarkers in the blood.
- For percutaneous coronary intervention (PCI) in patients with normal baseline troponin values, elevations of cardiac biomarkers above the 99th percentile URL are indicative of periprocedural myocardial necrosis. By convention, increases of biomarkers >3 x 99th percentile URL have been designated as defining PCI-related MI. A subtype related to a documented stent thrombosis is recognized.
- For coronary artery by-pass graft (CABG) in patients with normal baseline troponin values, elevated cardiac biomarkers above the 99th percentile URL are indicative of periprocedural myocardial necrosis. By convention, increases of biomarkers >5 x 99th percentile URL plus either new pathologic Q waves or new LBBB, or angiographically documented new graft or native coronary artery occlusion, or imaging evidence of new loss of viable myocardium have been designated as defining CABG-related myocardial.
- Pathologic findings of an acute MI.

B) Criteria for prior MI. Any one of the following criteria meets the diagnosis:

- Development of new pathologic Q waves with or without symptoms.
- Imaging evidence of a region of loss of viable myocardium that is thinned and fails to contract, in the absence of a non-ischemic cause.
- Pathologic findings of a healed or healing MI.

C) Clinical classification of the types of MI.

1) Spontaneous MI related to ischemia due to a primary coronary event such as plaque erosion and/or rupture, fissuring, or dissection.

2) MI secondary to ischemia due to either increased O2 demand or decreased supply, e.g. coronary artery spasm, coronary embolism, anemia, arrhythmias, hypertension, or hypotension.

3) Sudden unexpected cardiac death, including cardiac arrest, often with symptoms suggestive of myocardial ischemia, accompanied be presumably new ST elevation, or new LBBB, or evidence of fresh thrombus in a coronary angiography and/or at autopsy, but death occurring before blood samples could be obtained, or at a time before the appearance of cardiac biomarkers in the blood.

4a) MI associated with PCI.

4b) MI associated with stent thrombosis at angiography/autopsy.

5) MI associated with CABG.

5.2.4 Other Tests

A chest radiograph is usually performed at the time of admission so that the patient can be evaluated for other causes of chest pain and screened for pulmonary congestion, which implies a higher risk and an adverse prognosis [1, 2]. A transthoracic echocardiogram and a lipid profile should be obtained early after admission when available [1, 2]. Other blood samples should be considered for the diagnosis in selected cases: for example, thyroid function should be evaluated when a patient presents with symptoms of ACS and has persistent tachycardia. Also the contribution of cardiovascular imaging (e.g. multidetector CT scan) may be important in this setting to identify unstable plaques at high-risk of rupture, to contribute to the diagnosis in patients with equivocal signs and symptoms, and to simultaneously evaluate other potentially life-threatening conditions in the differential diagnosis of acute chest pain [13].

5.3 Operative Classification of ACS

The classification of ACS is usually obtained by integrating both ECG patterns and cardiac biomarkers of myocardial injury as shown in Fig. 5.2:

- NSTE ACS, e.g. absence of STE or transient (less than 30 minutes) STE, can be further classified in UA and NSTEMI, when cardiac biomarkers are negative or positive, respectively. The diagnostic patterns at ECG might be the depression or the transient, less than 30 minutes, STE and/or the inversion of the T wave. The ECG may be normal as well [1, 2].
- STE MI, which is characterized from STE ≥ 0.1 mV in

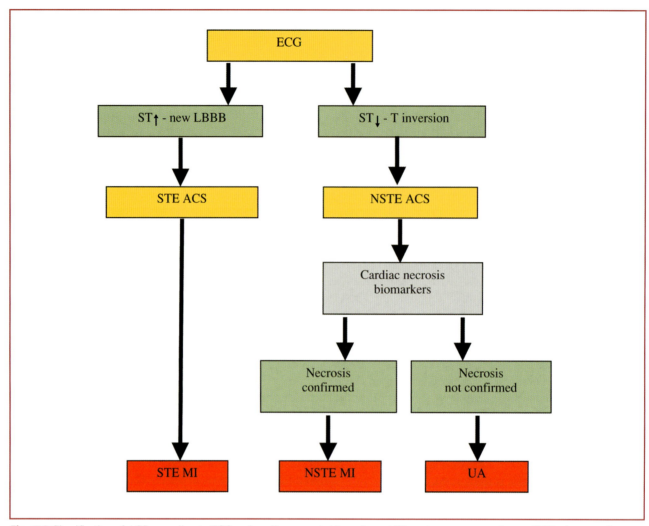

Fig. 5.2 Classification of ACS according to ECG and cardiac necrosis biomarkers. *ACS*, acute coronary syndrome; *ECG*, electrocardiogram; *LBBB*, left bundle branch block; *MI*, myocardial infarction; *NSTE*, non ST-segment elevation; *STE*, ST-segment elevation; *UA*, unstable angina

at least two contiguous leads or new onset of LBBB and increase of cardiac markers of necrosis [3, 4]. The associated symptoms are similar to those of classic angina but the chest discomfort usually appears suddenly at rest and it is more intense, longer, continuous or intermittent, and less responsive to nitrates compared to NSTE ACS [5].

Although this classification does not allow for discerning between different causes of ACS (e.g. caused by atherothrombosis or not), it is clinically useful to activate different pathways for the correct assessment and prompt management of patients with ACS. The cases with a definite diagnosis of ACS with a high likelihood of CAD should be hospitalized and evaluated for coronary angiography. However, when a cause other than coronary atherothrombosis is suspected, clinicians should consider that ACS can occur even in the absence of CAD with an onset similar to NSTE ACS and more rarely to STE ACS. The conditions which may require additional tests to be ruled out are:

- Coronary artery narrowing not due to atherosclerosis: coronary spasm, dissection or anomalous origin, dissection of the aorta with coronary ostium compression.
- Emboli: thromboembolism from atria (such as atrial fibrillation), left ventricle or prosthetic valves (especially mechanical), endocarditis, cardiac myxoma.
- Inadequate myocardial oxygen demand/supply: tachyarrhythmias, aortic stenosis or insufficiency, hypertrophic cardiomyopathy, high output states or low output states with sustained and severe hypotension, malignant hypertension, aortovenous shunts, fever, thyrotoxicosis or pheochromocytoma, cocaine or amphetamine use, anemia or polycythemia, hypoxemia.
- Others: apical ballooning syndrome, myocarditis, pericarditis, arteritis, chest wall trauma with myocardium involvement, tumors.

5.4 Risk Stratification

Choices among alternative strategies regarding ACS are based on an early assessment of the patient's risk. In this scenario, multiple clinical variables (Tables 5.3 and 5.4) at admission are useful for achieving the correct risk stratification and, among them, the most important are age, the pattern and location of ST-segment changes, and the hemodynamic status (heart rate, blood pressure, and Killip class). Other variables, such as the type of treatment, diabetes mellitus, extra-cardiac vascular disease, ongoing use

Table 5.3 Short-term risk of death of non-fatal MI in patients with UA/NSTEMI. (Adapted from [6], with permission)

Feature	HIGH likelihood Any of the following	INTERMEDIATE likelihood No high-likelihood and any of the following	LOW likelihood No high/intermediate-likelihood but may have any of the following
History	Accelerating tempo of ischemic symptoms in preceding 48 h.	Prior MI, peripheral or cerebrovascular disease or CABG; prior aspirin use.	
Character of pain	Prolonged ongoing (>20 min) pain at rest.	Prolonged (>20 min) rest angina, now resolved, with moderate or high likelihood of CAD. Rest angina (>20 min) or relieved with rest or sublingual NTG. Nocturnal angina. New onset or progressive CCS class III or IV angina in the past 2 weeks without prolonged (>20 min) rest pain but with intermediate or high likelihood of CAD	Increased angina frequency, severity or duration. Angina provoked at a lower threshold. New onset angina with onset 2 weeks to 2 months prior to presentation.
Clinical findings	Pulmonary edema, most likely due to ischemia. S3 or new/worsening rales. Hypotension, brady- or tachycardia. Age >75 years.	Age >75 years.	Chest discomfort reproduced by palpation.
ECG	Angina at rest with transient ST-segment changes (>0.5 mm). New or presumably new bundle branch block.	T-wave changes. Pathologic Q waves or resting ST-depression <1 mm in multiple lead groups (anterior, inferior, lateral). ST-segment depression 0.5-1 mm or T-wave inversion >1 mm.	Normal or unchanged.
Cardiac markers	Elevated Tn I or T (>0.1 ng/ml) or CK-MB.	Slightly elevated Tn I or T (>0.001 but <0.1 ng/ml) or CK-MB.	Normal.

CABG, coronary artery bypass graft surgery; *CAD*, coronary artery disease; *CCS*, Canadian Cardiovascular Society; *CK-MB*, MB fraction of creatine kinase; *ECG*, electrocardiogram; *MI*, myocardial infarction; *MR*, mitral regurgitation; *NSTEMI*, non–ST-elevation myocardial infarction; *NTG*, nitroglycerin; *Tn*, troponin; *UA*, unstable angina.

Table 5.4 Panel A) Risk scores to predict outcome in acute coronary syndromes: the higher the score, the higher the risk

	Risk Factor	Points
TIMI score for STEMI (0-14) [14]	Age 65-74 / ≥75 years	3
	Systolic blood pressure <100 mmHg	2
	Heart rate >100 bpm	2
	Killip class II-IV	1
	Anterior STEMI or left bundle branch block	1
	Diabetes mellitus, hypertension or angina pectoris	1
	Weight <67 Kg	1
	Time to treatment >4 hours	1
TIMI score for NSTE ACS (0-7) [15]	Age >65 years	1
	At least 3 risk factors for CAD	1
	Prior coronary stenosis >50 %	1
	ST-segment deviation	1
	At least 2 anginal events <24 hours	1
	Aspirin use <7 days	1
	Increased cardiac biomarkers	1

(cont.) →

Table 5.4 (*continued*)

GRACE score (0-372) [16-18]	Age, years	
	<30	0
	30-39	8
	40-49	25
	50-59	41
	60-69	58
	70-79	75
	80-89	91
	≥90	100
	Heart rate, beats/min	
	<50	0
	50-69	3
	70-89	9
	90-109	15
	110-149	24
	150-199	38
	>200	46
	Systolic blood pressure, mmHg	
	<80	58
	80-99	53
	100-119	43
	120-139	34
	140-159	24
	160-199	10
	>200	0
	Creatinine, mg/dl	
	0-0.39	1
	0.4-0.79	4
	0.8-1.19	7
	1.2-1.59	10
	1.6-1.99	13
	2-3.99	21
	>4	28
	Killip class	
	I	0
	II	20
	III	39
	IV	59
	Cardiac arrest at admission	39
	Increased cardiac markers	14
	ST-segment deviation	28

Table 5.4 Panel B) In-hospital and 6-month mortality according to GRACE score [16-18]

Risk category(tertiles)	Score	In-hospital death (%)
Low	≤108	<1
Intermediate	109-140	1-3
High	>140	>3
	Score	6-months death (%)
Low	≤88	<3
Intermediate	89-118	3-8
High	>118	>8

Killip class, I) absence of congestive heart failure, II) presence of rales and/or jugular venous distention, III) presence of pulmonary edema, IV) cardiogenic shock; *NSTE ACS*, non ST-elevation acute coronary syndrome; *Risk factors for CAD (coronary artery disease)*, family history hypertension, hypercholesterolemia, diabetes, smoke; *STEMI*, ST-elevation myocardial infarction.

of aspirin, prior CABG or MI, and others are of lesser but nonetheless modifiable importance [1-4, 6, 14-17].

Several scores for ACS have been developed to provide an accurate stratification of the risk and the most used at the moment are reported in Tables 5.3 and 5.4. One of the first validated scores was the Thrombolysis In Myocardial Infarction (TIMI) score, addressed to STEMI [14] and NSTE ACS [15]. Subsequently, the Global Registry for Acute Coronary Events (GRACE) score [16, 17], based on a large registry and applicable to all ACS, was developed and seems to be the best risk score for prediction of death and MI at the moment (Table 5.4).

The treatment of ACS depends firstly on the ECG pattern, but the other main factor which drives the decision strategy is once again the patient's risk [1-4]. In fact, the higher the risk the more aggressive will be the treatment, lasting from conservative to invasive treatment. Patients who present with UA seem to show a decreasing risk of adverse events compared to NSTEMI and STEMI respectively [18], and usually they are not candidates for immediate reperfusion. Two different arms are possible for the treatment (Fig. 5.1 and Table 5.5) [1, 2, 19]:

Table 5.5 Panel A) Selection of the initial treatment strategy in non ST-segment elevation acute coronary syndromes according to ACC-AHA Guidelines. (Adapted from [2], with permission)

Invasive strategy	Conservative strategy
Recurrent angina/ischemia at rest or with low-level activities despite intensive medical therapy	Low risk score (e.g. TIMI, GRACE). Patient or physician preference in the absence of high-risk conditions..
Elevated cardiac biomarkers (troponins).	
New/presumably new ST-depression.	
Signs/symptoms of heart failure.	
New/worsening mitral regurgitation.	
High-risk findings from non-invasive tests.	
Hemodynamic instability.	
Sustained ventricular tachycardia.	
Percutaneous coronary interventions <6 months.	
Prior coronary artery by-pass grafts.	
High risk score (e.g. TIMI, GRACE).	
Reduced left ventricular ejection fraction (<40%).	

Table 5.5 Panel B) Selection of the initial treatment strategy in non ST-segment elevation acute coronary syndromes according to ESC Guidelines. (Adapted from [19], with permission)

Features	Class of recommendation	Level of evidence
An invasive strategy is indicated in patients with: - GRACE risk score >140 or at least 1 high-risk criterion - Recurrent symptoms - Inducible ischemia at stress tests	I	A
An early (<24h) invasive strategy is indicated in patients with GRACE risk score >140 or multiple other high-risk criteria	I	A
A late (<72 h) invasive strategy is indicated in patients with GRACE risk score <140 in absence of multiple other high-risk criteria but with recurrent symptoms or stress-inducible ischemia	I	A
Patients at very high ischemic risk (refractory angina, associated heart failure, arrhythmias, hemodynamic instability) should be considered for emergent (<2 h) coronary angiography	IIa	C
An invasive strategy should not be performed in patients: - At low overall risk - At particular high-risk for invasive procedures	III	A

- Invasive strategy (e.g. coronary angiography within 24-72 hours from admission). This approach is reserved to patients with high risk features and scores, in case of recurrent symptoms or positive non-invasive test. On the basis of CAD and anatomy, revascularization with PCI or CABG is performed as appropriate.
- Conservative strategy (optimal medical therapy). This approach is reserved for patients at low overall risk or at high-risk of complications at coronary angiography or interventions.

Patients who present with STE ACS are at higher risk compared to NSTE ACS and they need an immediate reperfusion of the culprit vessel which can be obtained by either thrombolysis or primary percutaneous intervention (Fig. 5.1). This goal must be achieved as soon as possible because time is of the essence and every delay is related to an increased rate of death [3, 4].

References

1. Bassand JP, Hamm CW, Ardissino D et al (2007) Guidelines for the diagnosis and treatment of non-ST-segment elevation acute coronary syndromes. The Task Force for the Diagnosis and Treatment of Non-ST-Segment Elevation Acute Coronary Syndromes of the European Society of Cardiology. Eur Heart J 28:1598-1660
2. Anderson JL, Adams CD, Antman EM et al (2007) Writing Committee to Revise the 2002 Guidelines for the Management of Patients With Unstable Angina / Non-ST-Elevation Myocardial Infarction. ACC/AHA 2007 guidelines for the management of patients with unstable angina/non-ST-elevation myocardial infarction. J Am Coll Cardiol 50:1-157
3. Van de Werf F, Bax J, Betriu A et al (2008) Management of acute myocardial infarction in patients presenting with persistent ST-segment elevation The Task Force on the management of ST-segment elevation acute myocardial infarction of the European Society of Cardiology. Eur Heart J 29:2909-2945
4. Antman EM, Anbe DT, Armstrong PW et al (2004) Writing Committee to Revise the 1999 Guidelines for the Management of Patients With Acute Myocardial Infarction. ACC/AHA Guidelines for the Management of Patients With ST-Elevation Myocardial Infarction. J Am Coll Cardiol 44:671-719
5. Zipes DP, Libby P, Bonow RO, Braunwald E (2005) Part II (Examination of the Patient) and Part IV (Atheroslcerotic Cardiovascular Disease). In: Braunwlad's Heart Disease: a Textbook of Cardiovascular Medicine, 7th edn. Elsevier Saunders, Philadelphia, USA
6. Braunwald E, Jones RH, Mark DB et al (1994) Diagnosing and managing unstable angina. Agency for Health Care Policy Research. Circulation 90:613-622
7. Campeau L (1976) Letter: Grading of angina pectoris. Circulation 54:522-523
8. Braunwald E (1989) Unstable angina: a classification. Circulation 80:410-414
9. Platelet Receptor Inhibition for Ischemic Syndrome Management in Patients Limited by Unstable Signs and Symptoms (PRISM-PLUS) Trial Investigators (1998) Inhibition of the platelet glycoprotein IIb/IIIa receptor with tirofiban in unstable angina and non-Q-wave myocardial infarction [published correction appears in N Engl J Med 1998; 339:415]. N Engl J Med 338:1488-1497
10. Cannon CP, McCabe CH, Stone PH et al (1997) The electrocardiogram predicts one-year outcome of patients with unstable angina and non-Q wave myocardial infarction: results of the TIMI III Registry ECG Ancillary Study. J Am Coll Cardiol 30:133-140
11. Savonitto S, Ardissino D, Granger CB et al (1999) Prognostic value of the admission electrocardiogram in acute coronary syndromes. JAMA 281:707-713
12. Thygesen K, Alpert JS, White HD (2007) Universal definition of myocardial infarction. Eur Heart J 28:2525-2538
13. Giugliano RP, Braunwald E (2010) The year in non ST-segment elevation acute coronary syndromes. J Am Coll Cardiol 25:2126-2138
14. Morrow DA, Antman EM, Charlesworth A et al (2000) TIMI risk score for ST-elevation myocardial infarction: a convenient, bedside, clinical score for risk assessment at presentation: an Intravenous nPA for Treatment of Infarcting Myocardium Early II trial substudy. Circulation 102:2031-2037
15. Antman EA, Cohen M, Bernink PJLM et al (2000) The TIMI risk score for unstable angina/non–ST elevation MI: a method for prognostication and therapeutic decision making. JAMA 284:835-842
16. Granger CB, Goldberg RJ, Dabbous OH et al for the GRACE Investigators(2003) Predictors of hospital mortality in the global registry of acute coronary events. Arch Intern Med 163:2345-2353
17. Eagle KA, Lim MJ, Dabbous OH et al for the GRACE investigators (2004). A validated prediction model for all forms of acute coronary syndrome. Estimating the risk of 6-month postdischarge death in an international registry. JAMA 291:2727-2733
18. Fox KAA, Dabbous OH, Goldberg RJ et al (2006) Prediction of risk of death and myocardial infarction in the six months after presentation with acute coronary syndrome: prospective multinational observational study – GRACE. BMJ 333:1091-1094
19. Wijns W, Kolh P, Danchin N et al (2010) Guidelines on myocardial revascularization. The Task Force on Myocardial Revascularization of the European Society of Cardiology (ESC) and the European Association for Cardio-Thoracic Surgery (EACTS) with the special contribution of the European Association for Percutaneous Cardiovascular Interventions (EAPCI). Eur Heart J 3:2501-2555

Section II

Targets of Coronary and non Coronary Imaging

Coronary Plaques

6

Antonio L'Abbate, Massimo Lombardi, and Gualtiero Pelosi

6.1 Introduction

Noninvasive imaging of the coronary arteries has without doubt been a decisive step forward in cardiologic diagnostic procedures. However, we feel it is worth discussing, particularly with the operators of the new imaging modalities, the advantages and limitations of the noninvasive detection of coronary artery disease (CAD), in the light of its clinical and pathophysiologic significance.

6.2 Relationship between Coronary Atherosclerotic Disease and Coronary Heart Disease

Since the introduction of angiography in the 1960s it has been known that in patients with coronary heart disease (CHD), which is still the leading cause of death in Industrialized countries, the prevalence of CAD is about 90%. Many still attribute to this strong correlation between CHD and CAD a pathophysiologic and causal significance which on the one hand suggests CAD is a prerequisite of CHD, and on the other, that CHD is the natural progression of CAD. A natural consequence of this conviction is the accepted equivalence between CAD and CHD and the increasingly widespread use of coronary revascularization, particularly angioplasty, as a definitive solution to the real or potential effects of coronary stenosis [1-3].

However, the hard scientific facts tell a different story and they can be summarized as follows. Since the 1950s postmortem studies performed on subjects who died accidentally or on patients who died for non-cardiovascular causes have shown that CAD affects most people in

industrialized countries whereas CHD affects only a small fraction (2-3%) of CAD patients.

Clearly, the invasive nature of coronary angiography has impeded its use to date on the general population. Nonetheless, while awaiting confirmation from hypothetical epidemiologic studies, the postmortem data suggest that CHD is an exceptional event rather than the rule in the progression of CAD. The postmortem studies also demonstrate that with age and gender being equal, coronary atherosclerosis is neither more severe nor more extensive in patients with CHD than in others.

Since the beginning of the 1980s the large-scale application of coronary angiography has clearly demonstrated, in contrast to what was believed until then, that disease of the large coronary vessels in patients with CHD is different neither in severity nor in extension and that paradoxically myocardial infarction or sudden death are not consequences of the most severe forms of CAD. The logical conclusion of these observations and of the direct measurements of perfusion and ventricular function performed on individual patients is that the presence of stenosis, even severe, does not necessarily lead to a reduction in blood flow in the corresponding myocardial region, let alone ischemia. Even the finding of the complete occlusion of a large coronary branch does not necessarily imply the presence of infarction distally. This justifies the limited diagnostic and predictive value of coronary stenosis in itself, both in terms of perfusion and ventricular function and the implicit need for additional information to establish for each stenosis what is usually called "hemodynamic" or "pathophysiologic significance" or in more practical terms its "ischemic power".

In recent years, the disappointing conclusion of the absence of an association between degree of coronary stenosis, intended as the degree of the reduction of the coronary lumen, and the presence of severity of ischemia, has been obviated by the replacement with the quality evaluation of stenosis and the introduction of the concept of plaque instability or vulnerability. In other words, several characteristics of the composition of ath-

M. Lombardi (✉)
Cardiovascular MR Unit,
Fondazione CNR/Regione Toscana "G. Monasterio",
Pisa, Italy

F. Cademartiri, G. Casolo, M. Midiri (eds.), *Clinical Applications of Cardiac CT*,
© Springer-Verlag Italia 2012

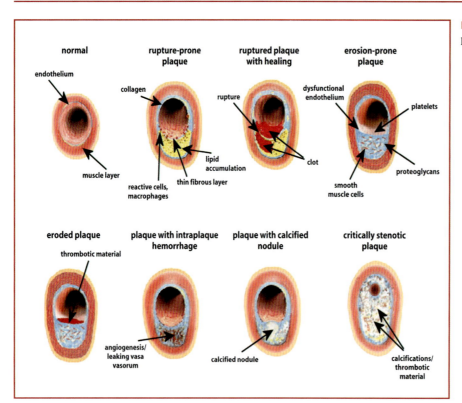

Fig. 6.1 Different types of vulnerable plaques. (Modified from [1])

erosclerotic plaque have been attributed with the potential of triggering local phenomena capable of acutely occluding the vessel, regardless of the initial degree of its obstruction, with the exception of the particular case of non collateralized severe stenosis which per se represents a vulnerable status. The phenomena proposed, which to date have only in part been documented, include plaque rupture, ulceration, intramural hemorrhage, thrombosis and embolization of the downstream microcirculation.

About 10% of patients with CHD, including cases of acute myocardial infarction, have a negative coronary angiography. This is further evidence of the non-equivalence between ischemia and coronary atherosclerosis. Similarly, despite the absence of coronary stenosis at angiography, a significant number of patients with cardiovascular risk factors (e.g. arterial hypertension, hyperlipidemia, smoking, diabetes, etc.) are affected by regional alterations of myocardial perfusion. These changes appear to be the same as those found in patients with CHD and CAD in terms of extent and severity. By exclusion, the alterations can be attributed to microvascular coronary disease.

The benefits of statin therapy or physical training in preventing major cardiac events in patients with CHD appear totally independent of their effect on coronary stenosis [4, 5].

In conclusion, on the basis of this brief summary of clinical and postmortem findings on the pathophysiology of CHD over the past 50 years, the equation CAD = CHD is unfounded.

6.3 Current View

Under the pathophysiologic profile, the prevailing unifying theory of CHD encapsulates all the problems of the disease into different moments of a single phenomenon: the development of an atherosclerotic plaque and its progression towards the occlusion of the vessel in a more or less discontinuous and more or less rapid process. The stages of this process, which are dictated by both local and general factors, condition and characterize the clinical manifestations.

The individual plaques therefore have different fates and only some of the plaques present in an individual will progress and produce clinical events. This is the underlying concept of the *vulnerable* plaque, a distinctive quality identifying it as a plaque destined to cause complications, as opposed to other quiescent plaques defined as *stable*. The study of the atherosclerotic plaque in its vulnerable variant (Fig. 6.1) should therefore be the rational approach of a pathophysiologic diagnosis. For this to occur the new imaging modalities

Table 6.1 Major and minor criteria for the definition of vulnerable plaque. (Modified from [3])

Major criteria	Minor criteria
Presence of active inflammatory process	Superficial calcified nodule
(infiltration of macrophages, monocytes, T-cells)	Glistening yellow appearance
Thin fibrous cap in the presence of a large lipid core	Intraplaque hemorrhage
Endothelial erosion with deposit of fibrin	Endothelial dysfunction
Plaque fissure	Expansive remodeling
Stenosis >90%	

(intravascular ultrasound, multidetector computed tomography, magnetic resonance imaging) need to reach a level of accuracy and reliability to enable the detailed description of the plaque and scientific validation of the techniques needs to be performed. These features are however currently lacking.

Despite the extraordinary technologic progress achieved to date, we are still a long way from identifying the real morphology and composition of individual plaques in the individual patient. The situation is further complicated by the fact that although the lesion held responsible for an acute event in 70% of postmortem cases is plaque rupture [1], only in 20% of cases does this involve a severely stenotic plaque. In addition, in 30% of cases thrombosis occurs in the absence of a ruptured plaque and in the presence of superficial erosion or a calcified nodule only. Lastly, retrospective studies in patients affected by unstable angina have demonstrated that about 70% of symptomatic lesions (culprit lesions) at initial angiography occupy <50% of the vascular lumen [6, 7]. These data clearly show that the challenge for the new imaging modalities goes beyond the simple detection of critical stenoses, or calcified or high-lipid-content stenoses.

6.4 Culprit Plaque and Vulnerable Plaque

The two terms *culprit plaque* and *vulnerable plaque* refer to two different concepts. The culprit plaque is the lesion identified at primary angioplasty by the cardiologist/interventional radiologist, or at postmortem by the pathologist, as being responsible for the ischemic event, provided the existence of an anatomic correspondence between the vessel and the ischemic territory. In contrast, the vulnerable plaque is the lesion the cardiologist and imaging expert would like to be able to attribute with an unfavorable prognostic value and thus preventively treat.

The term culprit lesion dates back to the first histopathologic studies conducted in the 1930s, and then broadened in the 1960s and 1970s [6, 8]. The link between the two types of lesions still remains elusive and

the choice of invasive treatment of one plaque rather than another is a process lacking scientific proof of its effectiveness. Our changing understanding of the vulnerable plaque is an excellent example of how difficult it is to establish the link between a lesion and its clinical progression (i.e. establish a link between a vulnerable plaque and the consequent cardiac event). In 1994 a vulnerable plaque was thought to be lipid-laden with a thin fibrous cap and an inflammatory component rich in macrophages at the level of or immediately below the surface [9]. Today we know that the plaque which produces an ischemic event can have decidedly different characteristics or not be part of such a clearly defined class.

A possible simplification has been proposed with the identification of major and minor criteria for defining a vulnerable plaque (Table 6.1). On the other hand, the awareness of the existence of different types of vulnerable plaques is not associated with an understanding of the prevalence of each type nor of the effective prognostic relevance (which plaques will become culprit lesions?).

6.5 Natural History of Atherosclerotic Plaque and its Classification

The available data on the very early stages of plaque formation (atherogenesis) derive mainly from experimental studies: plasma LDL accumulate in the intimal space at dysfunctional endothelial sites and are modified (ox-LDL), triggering the accumulation, proliferation and phagocytosis of blood-borne (monocytes) and resident (dendritic) phagocytic cells, which transform into foam cells.

In human pathology, these changes are more marked in arteries which at the same time show thickening of the intima, such as commonly found at bifurcations. This type of lesion is identified as Type I in the American Heart Association (AHA) classification. These phenomena are practically present in all humans – they do not reduce the vascular lumen and can be interpreted as adaptations to local mechanical forces.

Type II atherosclerotic plaque consists of layers of foamy macrophages and lipid laden smooth muscle cells. This type of lesion is grossly designated as fatty streaks. Present in neonates, the lesion is associated with the level of maternal cholesterolemia, and easily regresses in humans and in experimental animal models of atherosclerosis. It probably has no relationship with the clinical manifestations of atherosclerosis nor with the natural history of the atherosclerotic plaque. In this respect it has a prognostic value similar to the diffuse intimal thickening described in Type I and which is normally present in human coronary arteries [10, 11].

Type III plaques contain isolated pools of extracellular lipids. These pools are thought to be part of the initial phase of more extensive and destructive lipid accumulations found in Type IV plaques.

Type V plaques are characterized by both the presence of lipid accumulations and a thick layer of fibrous tissue (Va) or ample calcified deposits (Vb) or fibrous tissue without significant accumulations of lipids or calcium (Vc). Lastly, in addition to the lipid accumulations Type VI is characterized by fissure, hematoma and thrombus.

Despite its schematic nature and the questionable inclusion of intimal thickening and fatty streaks in the natural history of coronary atherosclerosis, this morphologic classification contains the important concept that each plaque may reach the various stages in different times and that the progression to the most *advanced* stage is not compulsory, rather it requires an additional stimulus. The morphologic characteristics of the plaques and their incidence in subjects of different ages suggest that Type I, II and III are successive stages in the development of the atherosclerotic lesion. A common feature in these three types of plaques is absence of major alterations of the matrix and/or of the microscopic structures of the intima and media, which favour their potential regression. The more advanced lesions in contrast contain accumulations of extracellular lipids which end up destroying the structure of the intima and, in the most advanced cases, the media and adventitia too. In advanced lesions the thrombotic mechanisms become predominant. Type I, II and III lesions can therefore be interpreted as hypothetic silent precursors of a possible future atherosclerotic *disease*.

It should, however, be underlined once again that given the impossibility of following the natural progression of a single lesion in vivo, our current view on the natural history of the atherosclerotic plaque is derived from extrapolations of data from subgroups of individuals belonging to different age ranges.

6.6 Vulnerable Coronary Plaque: Morphologic Presentation and Clinical Significance

For a long time in the past there was the prevailing and rather simplistic belief that the atherosclerotic lesion was directly responsible for the clinical manifestations of CHD, which was however in contrast with the results of several studies which demonstrated the inconsistency of the cause-effect relationship between CAD and CHD [12, 13]. Over the last decade, thanks largely to the development of invasive and noninvasive cardiac imaging, the elusive nature of the relationship between the morphologic presentation of the so-called vulnerable or high-risk plaque and the acute coronary event has been made apparent.

It has been demonstrated that [14]: (1) the so-called morphologic progression of the coronary atherosclerotic plaque and the clinical manifestations are not directly correlated and both are not predictable on the basis of clinical and angiographic variables; (2) the *progression* of the plaque is in reality the sum of individual occlusive and nonocclusive thrombotic episodes, hemorrhages, and proliferative and inflammatory phenomena; and (3) in different patients, and even in the vascular district of the single patient, atherosclerotic plaques progress in a completely different manner, both due to the different predisposing genetic and environmental factors (risk factors) and the different weight of the hemodynamic factors to which they are exposed. It has also been clarified that most plaques associated with acute myocardial infarction produce a stenosis markedly below the level of hemodynamic significance.

About 60% of cases of infarction are associated with the rupture of a fibrolipid plaque with a thin cap, presence of foci of macrophages and T-cells, intraplaque hematoma and calcium deposits. In 30-40% of cases thrombosis alone overlies plaques denuded of endothelium with diffuse T-cell infiltrates, and both luminal and periadventitial infiltrates [14].

The inflammatory response holds the most currency as the cause of the transformation of a vulnerable plaque into the culprit of an acute coronary event such as myocardial infarction [15]. It has been demonstrated that C-reactive protein (CRP) is a better predictor of infarction and stroke than LDL cholesterol levels, even though the presence of a systemic inflammatory state is not peculiar to particular vascular districts (coronary, aortic, carotid or peripheral atherosclerosis). In addition, there are still serious uncertainties regarding the incidence of vulnerable plaques in patients with CAD. It is still uncertain whether vulnerable

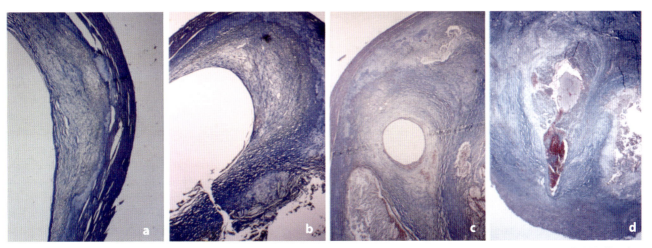

Fig. 6.2 Histologic sections of human atherosclerotic plaques (H&E stain 10x final magnification). From left to right: Type III lipid infiltration plaque (**a**), Type IV fibrolipid plaque (**b**), Type Va severely stenotic fibrolipid plaque (**c**) and Type VI complicated fibrous calcified plaque with fissure and thrombosis (**d**)

plaques are present in all cases of CAD or only in cases of high levels of CRP and unstable angina, whether they all undergo rupture, erosion and thrombosis, whether these events can occur silently with repeated episodes of inflammation and healing and consequent progression of the degree of stenosis, or whether they can stabilize and lose their characteristic vulnerability [14].

While the *hypercholesterolemia* hypothesis of plaque vulnerability sees the cause of the acute coronary event in the morphologic sequence transendothelial infiltration of lipoproteins → fatty streaks → macrophage infiltration → formation of atheroma with fibrous cap → rupture of the cap → thrombosis and embolization, other authors have proposed a *myohyperplasia* hypothesis, based on postmortem observations of human coronary arteries [11]. This theory sees the sequence of nodular hyperplasia of smooth muscle cells and elastic fibers → fibrous substitution → accumulation of glycoproteins below the fibrous cap between media and intima → passive deposit of lipoproteins and calcium in the glycoprotein matrix and appearance of foam cells → growth of plaque and late vascularization of the intima.

Supporting the latter theory is the fact that the natural history of human coronary atherosclerosis is not the same which is seen in the experimental models of hypercholesterolemia and in patients with familial hypercholesterolemia. Therefore, fatty streaks are not the initial lesions of human plaques. Furthermore, inflammation of the prevalently macrophagic plaque seems more likely to be due to healing, with the removal of foreign material, than to an active inflammatory process, rich in neutrophils and lymphocytes, typical of vasculitis. In this setting the infiltrate is not likely to be the cause of the rupture of the plaque. Plaque rupture and thrombosis may be secondary phenomena and therefore the onset, progression and complications of CAD may be unpredictable on the basis of the number and severity of the coronary atherosclerotic lesions.

6.7 Histologic Characteristics of Plaque in Relation to Vascular District

The main components of atherosclerotic plaque are: (1) an extracellular collagen matrix, i.e. collagen, proteoglycans and elastic fibers: (2) crystalline cholesterol, cholesteryl esters and phospholipids; (3) monocytes, macrophages, T-cells and smooth muscle cells. These components are present in varying proportions in the plaques of different arterial regions and in different stages, thus giving rise to a broad spectrum of lesions (Fig. 6.2). In particular, the plaque at high risk of rupture and successive thrombosis presents very different characteristics in relation to location (carotid arteries, coronary arteries, aorta).

With regard to the coronary arteries, the so-called vulnerable plaques have a thin fibrous cap (65/150 μm) and a large lipid core. According to the AHA classification described above, the most clinically relevant plaques are Type IV, Va and the complicated Type VI plaque, which is the result of the rupture of two previous types.

Type IV and Va are not generally stenotic, and therefore not detectable at angiography, while Type VI is generally associated with an occlusive thrombus. Type VI and Va plaques are thought to be responsible for 2/3 of acute coronary syndromes, whereas the coronary plaques responsible for angiographically visible stenosis and composed prevalently of smooth muscle cells, collagen and a minimal quantity of lipids are the least susceptible of all to rupture.

Unlike coronary plaques, high-risk carotid plaques are always severely stenotic and heterogeneous, being composed prevalently of fibrous tissue and calcium with a variable lipid component. These complex plaques often have internal hemorrhages with or without dissection and grow by a series of intraplaque circumscribed hematomas.

The morphologic appearance of atherosclerotic plaques in the peripheral arteries is not unlike that described in the carotid arteries.

In the thoracic aorta the morphology of vulnerable atherosclerotic plaques is essentially similar to Type IV and Va coronary plaques, such that postmortem and clinical studies with transesophageal echocardiography have provided evidence that the presence of this type of noncalcified plaque of the thoracic aorta is a predictor of CAD [15].

6.8 In Vivo Imaging of Atherosclerotic Plaque

The direct visualization of atherosclerotic plaques in vivo is the only way forward for studying the natural history of atherosclerotic disease. The invasive and noninvasive techniques currently being used are in general able to provide adequate information on the lumen diameter, the wall thickness and the plaque volume. However, sufficiently accurate techniques capable of performing a complete three-dimensional reconstruction of the histologic composition of the plaque are unavailable [16].

The development of new noninvasive coronary imaging modalities could open up new horizons in our understanding of the pathophysiology of atherosclerotic plaques.

Given the extremely complex histopathologic and pathophysiologic characteristics summarized in the previous paragraphs, reaching that goal appears a mighty challenge for the current diagnostic imaging techniques. Although highly sophisticated, the imaging modalities available today are only able to tell a part of the morphofunctional story. In theory, an imaging modality for this purpose would require the following features: be noninvasive and without risks for the patient and therefore repeatable, have submillimeter spatial resolution, enable the differentiation between the various histologic components of the plaque, and be able to give not only a morphologic but also a functional evaluation of stenosis. Although such a modality does not exist, it should not be forgotten that great leaps forward have been made in recent years.

Invasive angiography is the criterion standard for determining the degree of stenosis of coronary, carotid, peripheral and aortic plaques with sufficient resolution, even though it is unable to provide information regarding the intramural characteristics of the plaque. The major limitation is its underestimation or even failure to detect plaques eccentric to the vessel lumen or the atherosclerosis responsible for a uniform narrowing of the lumen along its entire length.

Intravascular ultrasonography (IVUS), which is performed with catheters and ultrasound, and angioscopy have made it possible to obtain more direct information regarding the vessel wall and plaque, including some characteristics of the content of the atheroma. With the use of an ultrasound catheter the technique is able to roughly distinguish between plaques with a prevalently fibrous, lipid or calcified component (Fig. 6.3), to recognize the presence of fissured or ulcerated plaque whereas angioscopy provides the possibility of visualizing the color of the plaque surface and the presence of thrombi, ulcerations or fissures with a higher degree of precision. The limitation to these techniques is their invasiveness and their use only in large-diameter vessels. More recently two new techniques have been proposed for characterizing the chemical composition of plaques: near infrared spectroscopy (NIRS) and optical coherence tomography (OCT). The in vitro and experimental findings are highly promising (Figs. 6.3-6.8).

At present, OCT is attracting the highest attention due to its capabilities in tissue characterization and to the very high spatial resolution. OCT measures the amplitude of backscattered light (optical echoes) from a sample as a function of time delay. Spatial resolution might reach 10 μm (10 times higher than IVUS) being able to resolve the thin fibrous caps (<65 μm) thought to be responsible for plaque vulnerability. Furthermore, the intrinsic optical properties of typical plaque constituents make OCT capable of differentiating between lipid, calcium and fibrous tissue. Also for limitations OCT seems to be the winning technique; in fact while the penetration capability cannot overcome the limit of 1.25 mm, it is even true that the most relevant morphologic findings are primarily localized within the first 500 μm under lumen surface [17-19]. Lastly, data acquired in patients affected by coronary artery disease have consistently shown that OCT is capable to provide microstructural images of atherosclerotic plaque (Figs. 6.4-6.8) [20].

The noninvasive modalities currently available offer unquestionable advantages for the study of the natural history of the plaque in the individual patient, even though their ability to discriminate the histologic characteristics of the plaque are still limited.

Surface or transesophageal ultrasonography, is wide-

6 Coronary Plaques 53

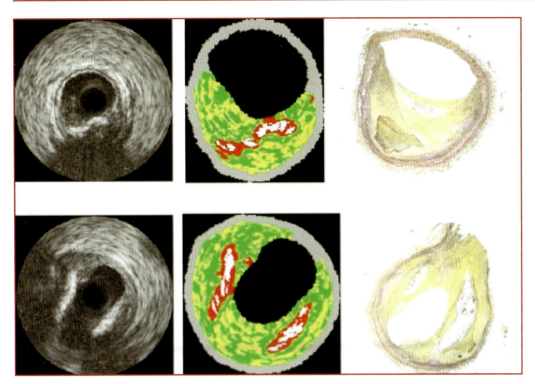

Fig. 6.3 The figure shows the correlation between histologic section (*right column*) and the corresponding images obtained with intravascular ultrasonography (IVUS – *left column*) and virtual histology (*central column*). The IVUS study enables the evaluation of the composition of the arterial wall, although the presence of calcium causes signal-loss artifacts. Although of lower resolution, the virtual histology images provide topographic and quantitative information of the various components of the plaque, regardless of the presence of calcifications (fibrosis in *green*, lipid components in *yellow*, necrosis in *red* and calcifications in *white*). Courtesy of Dr. Anuja Nair, Dr. Paulina Margolis and Goeffrey Vince, Volcano Corp

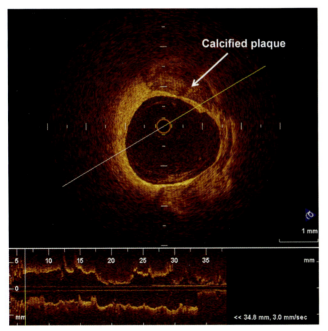

Fig. 6.4 Transversal section of human coronary artery obtained by Optical Coherence Tomography, OCT A calcified plaque is detectable as an area with low intensity signal, with sharp borders, surrounded by a thin fibrous cap. Fibrous tissue appears as a tissue with high intensity signal easily detected and measurable. (From OCT images archive of Cardiology Unit - Fondazione CNR/Regione Toscana "G. Monasterio")

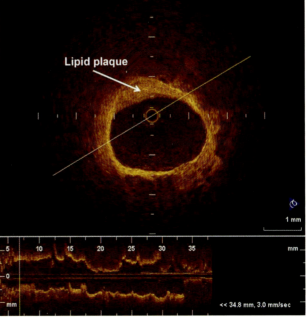

Fig. 6.5 Transversal section of human coronary artery obtained by Optical Coherence Tomography, OCT. The image shows a lipidic plaque which appears rich of low intensity signal tissue and with undefined borders. (From OCT images archive of Cardiology Unit - Fondazione CNR/Regione Toscana "G. Monasterio")

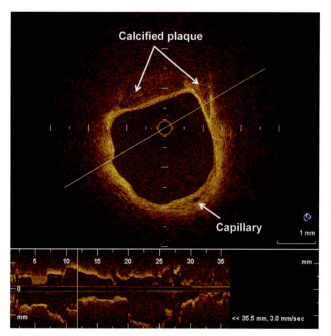

Fig. 6.6 Transversal section of human coronary artery obtained by Optical Coherence Tomography, OCT. The image shows a capillary structure within the calcified plaque (*dark structure*) The small vessel is of small dimension, well defined and with signal intensity comparable to the lumen. (From OCT images archive of Cardiology Unit - Fondazione CNR/Regione Toscana "G. Monasterio")

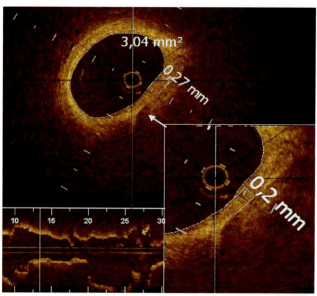

Fig. 6.7 Transversal section of human coronary artery obtained by Optical Coherence Tomography, OCT. Note how precise measurement of areas and thickness of the different components can be made. (From OCT images archive of Cardiology Unit - Fondazione CNR/Regione Toscana "G. Monasterio")

ly used in the diagnosis of carotid and aortic plaques respectively. Hypoechoic plaque suggests the presence of intraplaque hemorrhage or a prevalently lipid composition, whereas hyperechoic plaque is indicative of the fibrous and calcified component. The use of ultrasound contrast agents such as acoustic liposomes conjugated with monoclonal antibodies is a recent proposal for increasing the resolution and specificity of ultrasound examinations [21].

The techniques most likely to play a clinical role in the morphologic characterization of atherosclerotic plaque are multidetector computed tomography (MDCT), electron beam computed tomography (EBCT) and magnetic resonance imaging (MRI). The first two, and especially MDCT, currently appear the most advanced and provide a certain degree of accuracy in the study of the morphology and within certain limits the histopathologic composition [22] (Fig. 6.9) of the plaque. As described in other chapters, both the detection of coronary lumen narrowing and the differentiation

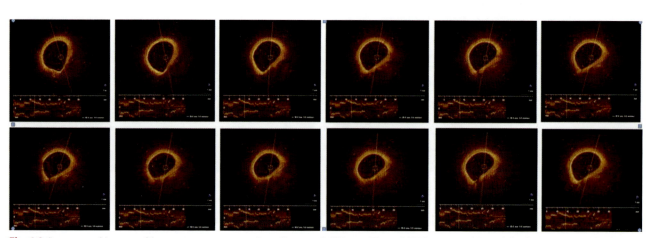

Fig. 6.8 Sequence of images of human coronary artery. Interslice gap 0.625mm. (From OCT images archive of Cardiology Unit - Fondazione CNR/Regione Toscana "G. Monasterio")

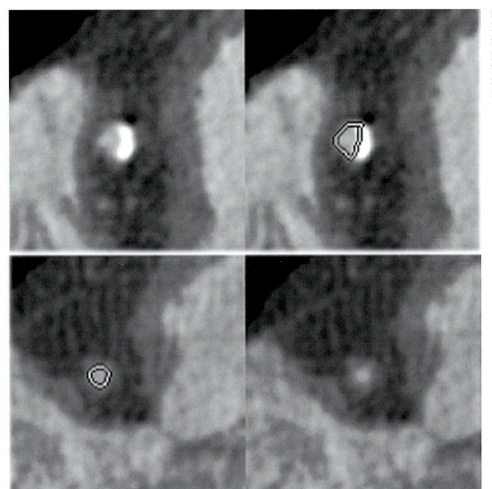

Fig. 6.9 Images obtained with MDCT. Cross-sections of coronary arteries. Images of calcified plaque (*above*) and diffuse wall thickening (*below*). Note the low resolution inherent in current imaging of the coronary arteries

between calcified and noncalcified (soft) plaque are possible in almost all coronary artery segments. In addition, the improved spatial resolution (about 0.4 mm) which can be obtained from 64-slice scanners offers the possibility of differentiating between the lipid and nonlipid components within the same plaque. The distinctive characteristic of the use of X-rays in this field is the ability to visualize and quantify the volume of calcium contained in the vascular wall [22-23]. This possibility is particularly significant for coronary plaques, given the demonstrated association between total amount of calcium and obstructive disease. However, it should be highlighted once again that the vulnerable plaques often present no calcium deposits and that the predictive value of coronary calcifications is not greater than that of common coronary risk factors. The use of appropriate acquisition and reconstruction algorithms is extending the possibilities of MDCT to visualizing all of the plaques with sufficient spatial resolution in various vascular regions, including those without calcium.

One of the current objective of methodological research is to identify the thin fibrous cap by noninvasive imaging techniques, such as MDCT, and eventually compare results with those obtained by OCT. Initial results appear promising; however, we are just at the beginning of the development process and much more data are needed before CT might be used for such purposes in real clinical life [24].

With regard to MRI, the reduced acquisition speed and the relatively low spatial resolution (about 1 mm) are severe limitations. In regions where these limitations can be overcome, e.g. the carotid arteries, very high resolution images can be obtained (0.35 mm) and the potential of the technique to characterize tissue can be exploited to the full (Fig. 6.10). In addition, much interest has been stimulated by the use of contrast agents such as USPIO (ultrasmall particles of iron oxide) which are actively taken up by macrophages present in the plaque [25]. Several clinical studies have also been performed using MRI to study the progression/regression of plaque in

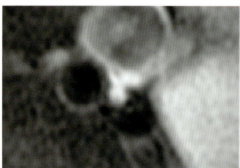
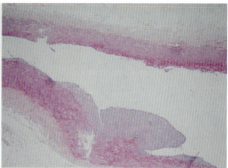

Fig. 6.10 Experimental model of aortic atherosclerosis. On the left, a magnetic resonance image of the abdominal aorta of a rabbit which reveals a marked thickening of the wall. SET1 image using high spatial resolution coil (350 micron). On the right, the corresponding histologic section

regions like the aorta and carotid arteries [26]. The visualization of coronary arteries is still a difficult objective which is pursued only in several specialized research centers [27]. New technologic developments and probably new contrast agents capable of marking particular cellular or molecular processes at the level of the plaque will be needed to make additional headway.

Tomographic scintigraphy has been used experimentally as a means for characterizing the presence of individual cellular or molecular components of atherosclerotic plaque. However, no tracer is currently available which is able to obtain clinically useful images of plaque, nor identify high-risk plaque [28].

6.9 Conclusions

Much is expected from the research and development into new contrast agents or innovative tracers capable, at least in theory, of identifying "active and vulnerable" plaque with a level of reliability much greater than is currently available. While invasive imaging of atherosclerotic plaque appears sufficiently advanced to consider realistic and reliable its information, noninvasive approaches are still under development and they have to be considered as research tools. Among noninvasive techniques, MDCT seems to have the highest possibility of fulfilling the expectations of researchers and clinicians.

However, the concept of unstable or vulnerable plaque is losing ground to the broader concept of *vulnerable patient*, i.e. the patient at high risk of developing a cardiac event in the short-to-medium term [1-3, 29]. This conceptual progression is fundamentally based on the recognition of the inability, if not impossibility, of identifying the distinctive characteristics of vulnerable plaque and moreover identifying the vulnerable plaque or plaques from among the many present in a single individual.

A further reason is the acceptance of the idea that the pathogenesis of acute coronary syndromes does not involve only factors operating at the level of the plaque, but rather there is the concurrence of local and extracoronary factors which involve coagulation, as well as the neuroendocrine and/or inflammatory and/or immune response of the vascular and myocardial tissue. In conclusion, the current and real opportunity of the noninvasive diagnosis of coronary stenosis should be framed in the correct pathophysiologic perspective if we are to avoid this major technologic progress being translated into an expensive instrument of confusion and alarm.

References

1. Naghavi M, Libby P, Falk E et al (2003) From vulnerable plaque to vulnerable patient: a call for new definitions and risk assessment strategies: Part I. Circulation 108:1664-1672
2. Naghavi M, Libby P, Falk E et al (2003) From vulnerable plaque to vulnerable patient: a call for new definitions and risk assessment strategies: Part II. Circulation 108:1772-1778
3. Naghavi M, Falk E, Hecht HS et al (2006) From vulnerable plaque to vulnerable patient. Part III. Executive Summary of the Screening for Heart Attack Prevention and Education (SHAPE) Task Force Report. Am J Cardiol 98:2-15
4. Pitt B, Waters D, Brown WV et al (1999) Aggressive lipid-lowering therapy compared with angioplasty in stable artery disease. N Engl J Med 341:70-76
5. Hambrecht R, Walther C, Mobius-Winkler S et al (2004) Percutaneous coronary angioplasty compared with exercise training patients with stable coronary artery disease: a randomised trial. Circulation 109:1371-1378
6. Stary HC, Chandler B, Dinsmore RE et al (1996) A definition of advanced types of atherosclerotic lesions and a histological classification of atherosclerosis. Circulation 92:1355-1374
7. Ambrose JA, Tannenbaum MA, Alexopoulos D et al (1988) Angiographic progression of coronary artery disease and the development of myocardial infarction J Am Coll Cardiol 12:56-62
8. Baroldi G, Silver MD, Mariani F et al (1988) Correlation of morphological variables in the coronary atherosclerotic plaque with the clinical patterns of ischemic heart disease. Am J Cardiovasc Pathol 2:159-172
9. Muller JE, Abela GS, Nesto RW et al (1994) Triggers, acute risk factors and vulnerable plaques: the lexicon of a new frontier. J Am Coll Cardiol 23:809-813

10. Stary HC, Chandler B, Glagov S et al (1994) A definition of initial, fatty streak, and intermediate lesions of atherosclerosis. Circulation 89:2462-2478
11. Baroldi G, Bigi R, Cortigiani L (2004) Ultrasound imaging versus morphopathology in cardiovascular diseases. Coronary atherosclerotic plaque. Cardiovascular Ultrasound 2:29
12. Baroldi G (1978) Coronary stenosis: ischemic or non-ischemic factor? Am Heart J 96:139-143
13. Maseri A, L'Abbate A, Baroldi G et al (1978) Coronary vasospasm as a possible cause of myocardial infarction. N Engl J Med 299:1271-1277
14. Casscells W, Naghavi M, Willerson JT (2003) Vulnerable atherosclerotic plaque: a multifocal disease: Circulation 107:2072-2075
15. Libby P, Okamoto Y, Rocha VZ, Folco E (2010) Inflammation in Atherosclerosis: Transition From Theory to Practice. Circ J 74:213-220
16. Fayad ZA, Fuster V (2001) Clinical imaging of the high-risk vulnerable atherosclerotic plaque. Circ Res 89:305-316
17. Davies MJ (1996) Detecting vulnerable coronary claque. Lancet 347:1422-1423
18. Lee RT, Libby P (1997) The unstable atheroma. Arterioscler Thromb Vasc Biol 17:1859-1867
19. Virmani R, Kolodgie FD, Burke AP et al (2000) Lesions from sudden coronary death: a comprehensive morphological classification scheme for atherosclerotic lesions. Arterioscler Thromb Vasc Biol 20:1262-1275
20. Jang IK, Bouma BE, Kang DH et al (2002) Visualization of coronary atherosclerotic claque in patients using optical coherence tomography: comparison with intravascular ultrasound. J Am Coll Cardiol 39:604-609
21. Lanza GM, Wallace KD, Scott MJ et al (1996) A novel site-targeted ultrasonic contrast agent with broad biomedical application. Circulation 94:3334-3340
22. Fayad ZA, Fuster V, Nikolaou K, Becker C (2002) Computed tomography and magnetic resonance imaging for noninvasive coronary angiography and plaque imaging: current and potential future concepts. Circulation 106:2026-2034
23. Clouse ME (2006) How useful is CT for screening for coronary artery disease? Circulation 113:125-146
24. Kashiwagi M, Tanaka A, Kitabata H et al (2009) Feasibility of non invasive assessment of thin-cap fibroatheroma by multi detector computer tomography. J Am Coll Cardiol Imaging 2:1412-1419
25. Ruehm SG, Corot C, Vogt P et al (2001) Magnetic resonance imaging of atherosclerotic plaque with ultrasmall superparamagnetic particles of iron oxide in hyperlipidemic rabbits. Circulation 103:415-422
26. Corti R, Fuster V, Fayad ZA et al (2005) Effects of aggressive versus conventional lipid-lowering therapy by simvastatin on human atherosclerotic lesions: a prospective, randomized, double-blind trial with high-resolution magnetic resonance imaging. J Am Coll Cardiol 46:106-112
27. Fayad ZA, Fuster V, Fallon JT et al (2000) Noninvasive in vivo human coronary artery lumen and wall imaging using black-blood magnetic resonance imaging. Circulation 102:506-511
28. Iuliano L, Mauriello A, Sbarigia E et al (2000) Radiolabeled native low-density lipoprotein injected into patients with carotid stenosis accumulates in macrophages of atherosclerotic plaque: effect of vitamin E supplementation. Circulation 101:1249-1254
29. Maseri A, Fuster V (2003) Is there a vulnerable plaque? Circulation 107:2068-2071

Myocardial Ischemia & Viability

7

Paolo G. Camici and Ornella Rimoldi

7.1 Introduction

The increasing use of thrombolytic therapy and primary percutaneous coronary interventions in association with optimized anti-thrombotic therapy has contributed to significantly reducing short-term mortality and morbidity in patients with acute coronary syndromes. The change of the epidemiology of myocardial infarction over the past 2 decades is due to the increase in NSTE-MI infarctions counterbalanced by a substantial reduction in ST-segment elevation [1]. Nevertheless, no further improvement in long term survival could be observed, probably due to the greater number of patients with residual left ventricular (LV) dysfunction undergoing progressive LV remodeling and congestive heart failure (CHF). A problem compounded by the rising age of the population and the higher prevalence of co-morbidities such as diabetes mellitus and hypertension which confer an increased risk of coronary artery disease (CAD) and CHF. Patients with CAD represent by far the most numerous cohort amongst those with CHF and their treatment remains a partial success [2]. Usually, these patients have multivessel disease, LV remodeling with increased LV volumes and variable degrees of regional and/or global systolic dysfunction, although recently more cases of isolated diastolic dysfunction have been reported [3, 4]. In these patients detection of myocardial viability followed by appropriate coronary revascularization may lead to symptomatic and prognostic improvement [5, 6] and these clinical benefits are accompanied by evidence of reverse LV remodeling [7].

7.2 Myocardial Ischemia and Function

The consequences of transient ischemia on myocardial contractile function were first described by Tennant and Wiggers in 1935 [8]. Subsequent observations in conscious dogs described the phenomenon of myocardial stunning: a regional dysfunction persisting for several hours after transient non-lethal occlusion of an epicardial coronary artery, which eventually results in full functional recovery [9].

In the mid eighties the term *myocardial hibernation* was introduced to the clinical community by Rahimtoola [10], who hypothesized that "hibernating myocardium refers to resting LV dysfunction due to reduced coronary blood flow that can be partially or completely reversed by myocardial revascularization and/or by reducing myocardial oxygen demand". However, this initial intuition was based mainly on qualitative studies with single photon emission computed tomography (SPECT). The assumption of a reduction in resting blood flow causing a decrease of contractile function has been debated at length and, more recently, a number of studies where absolute myocardial blood flow (MBF) was measured with positron emission tomography (PET) have demonstrated that baseline MBF is normal in most patients with hibernating myocardium whereas coronary flow reserve is severely reduced [6, 11].

A number of considerations need to be taken into account in order to have a comprehensive view of these issues.

7.2.1 The Technique

To date the criterion standard for the absolute quantitative measurement of MBF in humans is PET with $^{13}NH_3$ or $H_2^{15}O$ [12, 13]; the main factor limiting the widespread use of these tracers is the requirement of a cyclotron on site. Cardiac magnetic resonance (CMR) has the potential to provide quantitative measurements

P.G. Camici (✉)
Department of Cardiac, Thoracic and Vascular Sciences,
"San Raffaele" University Hospital,
Milano, Italy

F. Cademartiri, G. Casolo, M. Midiri (eds.), *Clinical Applications of Cardiac CT*,
© Springer-Verlag Italia 2012

7.2.2 The Tracer and the Amount of Scar

$^{13}NH_3$ is an extractable perfusion tracer and its transmembrane transport can occur by passive diffusion or can be active through the Na+K+ATPase pump. It has an 80% first pass extraction fraction and myocyte retention is energy-requiring and involves metabolic trapping. MBF measured using $^{13}NH_3$ is limited by high flow rate and energy dependent mechanisms [15, 16]. In patients with previous myocardial infarction the presence and amount of scar tissue within a dysfunctional region will affect the MBF estimates made with $^{13}NH_3$. The uptake in a given volume of interest reflects the average uptake and hence average flow in this mixture of viable and fibrotic tissue. On the other hand, since the uptake of $H_2^{15}O$ in scar tissue is negligible, washout of $H_2^{15}O$ will mainly reflect activity in perfused segments and the resulting flow can therefore be higher than that obtained with $^{13}NH_3$ in the same region [17]. $H_2^{15}O$ provides values of flow per gram of perfusable tissue and not per gram of volume of interest [18].

The awareness of the absolute value of flow in normal subjects of matched age and gender has important implications for the interpretation of myocardial perfusion studies in patients with hibernating myocardium. A large cohort of normal volunteers studied with PET and $H_2^{15}O$ has pointed out that: (1) in a population of normal subjects, baseline and hyperemic MBF are heterogeneous both within and between individuals; baseline and hyperemic MBF exhibit a similar degree of spatial heterogeneity which appears to be temporally stable; (2) baseline but not hyperemic MBF is significantly higher in females than in males; (3) there is a significant linear association between age and baseline MBF that is in part related to changes in external cardiac workload; (5) hyperemic MBF and hence coronary flow reserve (CFR - the ratio of myocardial blood flow during pharmacologically-induced hyperemia to baseline flow) declines over 55 years of age [19].

In addition, it has to be taken into consideration that chronically dysfunctional segments are generally thinner than remote normally contracting myocardium thus contributing to artificially increase the difference between hibernating and remote myocardium as a consequence of the partial volume effect [20]. This occurs whenever the dimension of the object to be imaged is comparable or smaller than the camera's spatial resolution. Although the detector will accurately record the total activity in the object, it will distribute it over an area larger than the actual size of the object. Hence, the detected radioactivity concentration per unit volume will be less than the actual value [21].

In a study with CMR, Selvanayagam et al. reported a transmural MBF of 0.8±0.2 mL/min/g in dysfunctional segments which is well within the range of normal values in humans [14].

In conclusion resting MBF in dysfunctional segments can be reduced in comparison with the remote myocardium in the same heart; however its absolute value can be below normal only if a consistent amount of scar or replacement fibrosis is present, but it is within normal limits in most patients.

In pathophysiologic terms, a unifying feature present in most of the available studies is the demonstration that a severe reduction in CFR is the *conditio sine qua non* for both stunning and hibernation (Fig. 7.1) [3]. Recovery of function in hibernating myocardium requires coronary revascularization which in turn restores an adequate CFR [22].

A wide spectrum of anatomic changes has been described in human hibernating myocardium [22-25], probably reflecting different stages of the condition.

A number of different techniques - dobutamine stress echocardiography, SPECT, CMR - have been used to investigate the presence of viable tissue or quantify the amount of scar before coronary revascularization. They have been described in detail and compared head-to-head in review articles and meta-analysis (Fig. 7.2) [6, 26].

According to the American College of Cardiology/American Heart Association/American Society of Nuclear Cardiology guidelines, FDG PET is considered a class I indication for assessment of viability in ischaemic cardiomyopathy [27].

7.3 The Concept of Myocardial Viability

In the setting of ischemic heart disease, the term *viability* describes dysfunctional myocardium subtended by diseased coronary arteries with limited or absent scarring which has the potential for functional recovery. Viability is a prospective definition, but it does not imply evidence of functional recovery following interventions. The term *hibernation*, which is often used as synonymous of tissue viability, is a retrospective definition based on evidence of functional recovery following interventions [6].

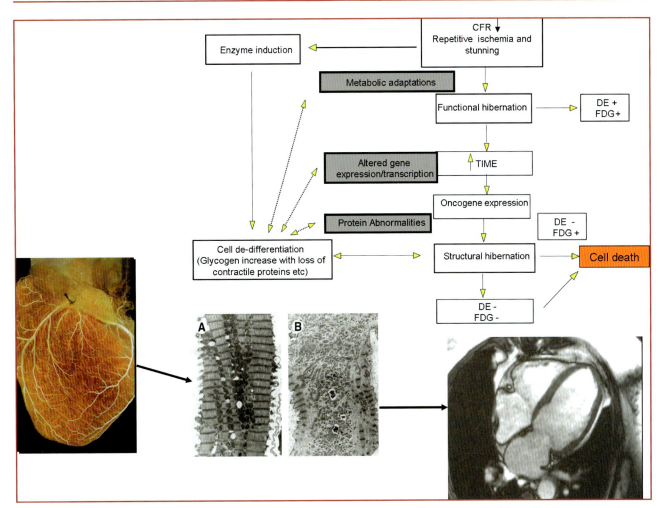

Fig. 7.1 Pathway leading from repetitive ischemia to irreversible cell death. *CFR*, coronary flow reserve; *DE*, dobutamine stress echocardiogram; *panel A*, EM of structurally altered cardiomyocytes showing glycogen increase and preserved sarcomeres; *panel B*, a more advanced stage of cell damage showing disrupted sarcomeres, glycogen accumulation, depletion of sarcoplasmic reticulum and numerous small mitochondria

7.4 Semiquantitative Viability Imaging Using Perfusion and 18FDG

Ischemic cardiomyopathy continues to be the most common etiology for myocardial dysfunction in developed countries [28]. The assessment of myocardial viability with ^{18}F-fluorodeoxyglucose (^{18}FDG) PET is based on its ability to distinguish between the two main pathogenic mechanisms for chronic myocardial dysfunction in ischemic cardiomyopathy (Fig. 7.1):

1. irreversible loss of myocardium due to prior myocardial infarction (scar);
2. at least partially reversible loss of contractility as a result of chronic or repetitive ischemia (hibernating myocardium).

The distinguishing feature of these two mechanisms is that revascularization has the potential to restore contractile function of hibernating myocardium but not scar. This distinction may be crucially important in clinical decision-making because of the upfront morbidity and mortality associated with revascularization procedures in patients with severe LV dysfunction.

Traditional ^{18}FDG-PET myocardial viability assessment requires integration of rest perfusion imaging with myocardial glucose metabolism imaging. PET MPI is preferable to SPECT for comparison with ^{18}FDG metabolism images because of limitations imposed by differences in attenuation correction algorithms [29-31]. PET MPI studies are acquired at rest with standard perfusion protocols and compared to ^{18}FDG [32-35]. For ^{18}FDG imaging, patients are generally studied after an oral glucose load. If the patient has glucose intolerance or diabetes, supplemental insulin will be required. Alternatively, some centers routinely employ the hyperinsulinemic euglycemic clamp or use it preferentially in patients with diabetes [29, 31, 36, 37].

Comparison of perfusion and metabolism images can

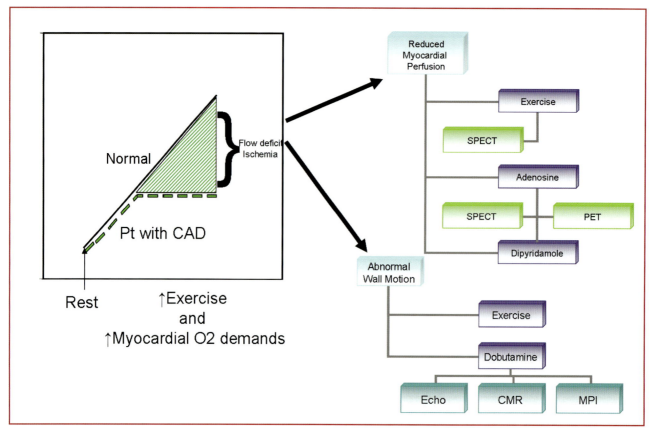

Fig. 7.2 The diagram summarizes the mechanism of the relation between myocardial oxygen demand and supply. In a patient with a fixed obstruction flow increases up to the ceiling of microvascular (arteriolar) vasodilatation. Flow can then no longer increase in spite of a persisting oxygen demand, the result will be ischemia and chest pain and contractile dysfunction. To assess the flow deficit we need to use standardized stressors

yield one of four common patterns:
1. *Viable* preserved perfusion and glucose metabolism;
2. *Viable-hibernation* reduced relative perfusion preserved glucose (mismatch);
3. *Non –viable* reduced perfusion and glucose metabolism (match);
4. *Viable* preserved perfusion reduced *glucose metabolism* (reverse mismatch).

Normal myocardium has preserved myocardial perfusion and metabolism.

In the perfusion-metabolism mismatch qualitative pattern, perfusion is relatively reduced whereas metabolism (^{18}FDG uptake) is preserved. This pattern has been traditionally considered the hallmark of myocardial hibernation [29, 31]. Higher degrees of mismatch have been shown to be associated with improved LV function with revascularization [35, 38]. Di Carli et al. demonstrated that when hibernation was present in as little as 5% of the myocardium, an outcome benefit from revascularization could be demonstrated [39]. This observation was recently supported in a post-hoc analysis of the prospective randomized trial, PET and Recovery Following Revascularization-2 (PARR-2) trial. D'Egidio et al. [40] identified a cutoff of >7% mismatch as an indicator that patients with ischemic cardiomyopathy would have outcome benefit from revascularization.

In a recent meta-analysis, the optimal threshold for the presence of viability required to improve *survival* with revascularization was estimated to be 25.8% (95% CI, 16.6-35.0%) by ^{18}FDG PET perfusion mismatch for the assessment of viability [41].

In the perfusion-metabolism match pattern, there is both reduced perfusion and reduced metabolism. This pattern is indicative of myocardium that is predominantly scarred. The extent of scar has also been shown to be important in the prediction of LV function recovery after revascularization [42]. Ottawa investigators showed that *quantification* of scar was an independent predictor of improvement of LV function following revascularization in a cohort of patients with severe LV dysfunction. Specifically, across tertiles of scar scores (small [0-16% scar]; moderate [16% to 27.5%]; large [27.5 – 45%]), changes in EF post-revascularization were 9%, 3.7%, and 1.3%, respectively [43].

Lastly, the reverse mismatch pattern denotes normal perfusion with relatively reduced metabolism. This pattern can be observed in several settings, including in patients with: nonischemic cardiomyopathy, left bundle branch block (LBBB), following revascularization early post-MI when the myocardium is stunned, and in some patients with diabetes. Reverse mismatch with LBBB has been suggested to be a consequence of altered septal glucose metabolism [44]. Recent evidence suggests that the presence of reverse mismatch (as well as the extent of lateral scar and the overall extent of viability), on perfusion/[18]FDG PET imaging can be used to predict outcome response in patients undergoing cardiac resynchronization therapy [45-47]. Nevertheless, the clinical significance of the reverse mismatch pattern itself warrants further investigation.

7.5 Quantitative Viability Imaging Using 18FDG Alone and Hyperinsulinemic Euglycemic Clamp

The semiquantitative and quantitative analyses of [18]FDG uptake may enhance detection of viable myocardium at the price of a rigorous standardization of the study conditions [48]. Many patients with CAD are insulin resistant, i.e. the amount of endogenous insulin released after feeding will not induce maximal stimulation due to partial resistance of the myocytes to the action of the hormone even if they are not diabetic [36]. This may often result in poor [18]FDG image quality after an oral glucose load. To circumvent the problem of insulin resistance, the hyperinsulinemic euglycemic clamp protocol has been applied to PET viability studies [11]. This protocol is based on the simultaneous infusion of insulin and glucose acting on the tissue as a metabolic challenge and stimulating maximal [18]FDG uptake. The use of the hyperinsulinemic euglycemic glucose clamp provides excellent image quality, usually demonstrates uniform tracer uptake and enables PET studies to be performed under steady and standardized metabolic conditions. If a fully quantitative analysis is carried out it is possible to compare absolute values of the metabolic rate of glucose uptake (μmol/g/min) between different subjects and centers.

A significant benefit of full quantification is its sensitivity in patients with CAD and poor LV function. Using this approach, Hammersmith Hospital investigators studied a large series of patients undergoing revascularization procedures and demonstrated good predictive accuracy of PET under different clinical conditions. A threshold value for the metabolic rate of glucose of 0.25 μmol/g/min corrected for perfusable tissue fraction, allowed the best prediction of improvement in functional class of at least one grade after revascularization [49,

50]. Lautamaki et al. [50] reported similar values in a population of patients with type 2 diabetes and CAD; during insulin stimulation they found myocardial glucose uptake in ischemic regions was similar to that of nonischemic regions.

While accuracy data have yielded results that are similar to perfusion/metabolism mismatch for predicting LV function recovery, most of the outcome data has applied perfusion/metabolism imaging approach. Currently the ASNC Guidelines recommend the use of perfusion with [18]FDG to assist in defining the perfusion/metabolism mismatch pattern, the hallmark of hibernation and the parameter most related to patient risk for adverse outcomes if they do not undergo revascularization [30].

7.6 Prospective Data on the Utility of 18FDG-PET on Assessment of Myocardial Viability

[18]FDG imaging is considered to be the most sensitive means of measuring myocardial viability. Several investigations have reported good accuracy of [18]FDG imaging in predicting improvement in LV function after revascularization [26, 30, 35, 38, 51-54]. A recent systematic review by Schinkel et al. [26] demonstrated that [18]FDG PET is more sensitive than any other viability imaging modality. A recent health technology assessment identified the pooled estimates of sensitivity and specificity of [18]FDG PET for predicting wall motion recovery to be 91.5% and 67.8% respectively [55].

Several observational studies have shown that [18]FDG PET is important for prognostication of patients with viable myocardium who do not undergo timely revascularization [5, 26, 39, 56-58]. However, only recently has the impact of [18]FDG viability imaging in clinical decision-making and its effect on patient outcome been evaluated. A patient-outcome oriented approach to imaging is particularly crucial in a contemporary era of rapidly proliferating imaging techniques and in the setting of resource limitations imposed by health care economic realities (Fig. 7.3).

Siebelink et al. [55] performed a randomized controlled trial comparing ^{99m}Tc-sestamibi SPECT to [13]NH3/[18]FDG PET in 103 patients. The PET arm had slightly fewer events but there was no significant difference in outcomes. However, only ~1/3 of these 103 patients had severe LV dysfunction (those most likely to benefit from revascularization). In addition there were long delays to revascularization which may limit the benefit of viability imaging in many patients and therefore may have made the study unable to detect differences. Prior studies have shown that benefits for revasculariza-

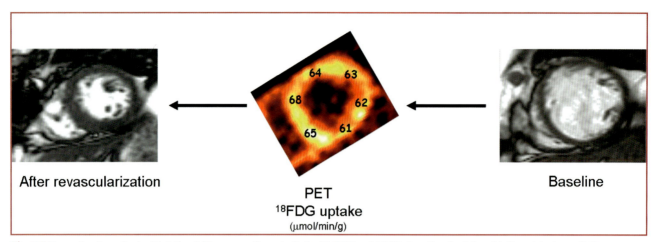

Fig. 7.3 Example of a patient with fully viable myocardium studied with PET and CMR. In spite of a thinned left ventricular wall there was no evidence of scar. The metabolic glucose rate measured with ^{18}FDG and PET during hyperinsulinemic euglycemic clamp was normal. After revascularization there was significant recovery of wall thickness and contractile function (CMR performed at Royal Brompton Hospital; courtesy of Prof. D.J. Pennell)

tion may be lost if there are excessive delays to revascularization [59, 60]. These limitations make it difficult to extrapolate data from this study regarding the viability detection in patients with severe LV dysfunction.

The PET and Recovery Following Revascularization-2 (PARR-2) study was a randomized controlled trial conducted to ascertain whether the use of ^{18}FDG PET in clinical decision-making resulted in better clinical outcome compared with standard care where PET was not available. This was a multicenter trial in patients with a LVEF ≤35% due to suspected coronary artery disease, who were being considered for revascularization, transplantation or heart failure work-up. In the PET arm, extent and severity of scar and mismatch were determined and considered in the context of a previously derived model to predict LV recovery after revascularization. Using the results of this model and the interpretation of PET images, the physician and surgeon would decide on whether or not to proceed with revascularization or revascularization work-up. Although there was a trend for better outcomes using the PET strategy compared to standard care, overall the trial was inconclusive as there was no statistically significant difference between the two groups. However, in a post hoc analysis that compared those that adhered to PET recommendations ("ADHERE" arm), there was a significant decrease in the hazard ratio for the primary outcome compared to standard care.

Taken together, the findings of the PARR-2 trial, its sub-studies and other outcome observational data, support that ^{18}FDG-PET viability imaging has clinical utility in identifying high risk patients who may benefit from revascularization and is a valuable tool in improving patient outcomes if ^{18}FDG based recommendations can be meaningfully incorporated into an overall management strategy. Further randomized trials incorporating viability imaging as part of the work up for management of ischemic cardiomyopathy which go beyond the observational studies that have populated much of the viability research to date, are still required to truly weigh the clinical value of these imaging techniques.

^{18}FDG-PET defines metabolic cell integrity and has the highest sensitivity compared to other methods for prediction of segmental contractile function recovery, whereas techniques challenging contractile reserve such as Dobutamine Stress with Echocardiogram (DSE) or Cardiac Magnetic Resonance (CMR) showed the highest specificity [26]. The ability of different imaging modalities to predict the recovery of LV function after revascularization in a population with a prevalence of viability assessed by the optimal cut-off (i.e. number of viable segments) identified by the Receiver Operating Curve (ROC) analysis confirm that SPECT and PET have higher sensitivity and DSE has superior specificity and lower PPV [6].

The importance of the cut-off value has been further highlighted in a recent paper by Inaba et al. [41]. The amount of myocardium deemed necessary for improvement of survival with revascularization was characteristic of each technique. PET requires the least amount of viable myocardium (25.8%) in comparison with DSE (35.9%) and SPECT (38.7%). Caution is of the essence when evaluating meta-analyses results and some limitations must be taken into consideration. The optimal cut-off for viability with different modalities was based on the assumption of a linear relationship between viability and survival. In more recent work by D'Egidio not included in this analysis, as little as 7% of the myocardium as mismatch may be needed to yield an outcome benefit from revascularization [40]. This cutoff is similar to early work by Di Carli et al. and Lee et al. who used 5% (1/20 segments) and 7.6% (1/13) respectively as the cutoff to define significant viability [39, 61]. Other limitations inherent to meta-analysis include the heterogeneity of the criteria used in different centers, the different duration of the follow up, the lag between viability assessment and revascularization, the extent of LV remodeling, co-morbidities preventing timely revascularization, failure of revascularization procedures, and adherence to current guidelines for medical therapy. Regarding CMR, a highly sensitive method to detect scarred myocardium, limited data are available so far on the prognostic value [6, 62].

Similarly to CMR MDCT has been proposed to evaluate myocardial viability by means of detection of scar after the administration of intravenous contrast agents [63]. Proof of principle studies have been carried out on acute infarcts in large animals [64]. However unresolved issues such as the required contrast dose, image quality and radiation exposure have hampered a clinical application.

7.7   Hybrid Imaging

Multimodality imaging offers unquestionable advantages through the routine availability of coregistered anatomical and functional images. Despite initial concerns relating to device running costs and the radiation dose this approach is being increasingly embraced by nuclear cardiologists. Nowadays, the major vendors no longer offer PET-only and combined PET/CT systems ensure state-of-the-art functionality for both modalities. Currently, a cardiac PET/CT configuration might comprise a 64-slice CT scanner and an LSO-based PET with 4-mm detector elements. These hybrid systems, use CT for attenuation correction of emission images, greatly accelerating acquisition protocols [65]. In three-vessel CAD measurement of coronary flow reserve and changes of LV ejection fraction during stress increase the diagnostic accuracy from 50% to 79% [39]. A further major advantage is the accurate assignment of perfusion data to a vascular territory assessed by means of CT coronary angiography, the merging of morphologic and functional data has a potential impact both on clinical decision making process and for monitoring of reperfusion procedures [66]. An ongoing limitation of CT angiography is that high-density objects, such as calcified coronary plaques [67], stent struts, and small vessels <1.5 mm in diameter, diminish the accuracy to delineate the degree of coronary luminal narrowing [68]. The European Association of Nuclear Medicine (EANM), the European Society of Cardiac Radiology (ESCR), and the European Council of Nuclear Cardiology (ECNC) in a joint position statement give recommendations on the appropriate use of cardiac hybrid imaging [69]. The statement supports the use of hybrid imaging in patients with an intermediate pre-test probability of CAD. At present hybrid imaging still needs evaluation in larger cohorts and multicentre investigations.

References

1. Roger VL, Go AS, Lloyd-Jones DM et al (2011) Heart disease and stroke statistics-2011 update: A report from the american heart association. Circulation. 123:18-209
2. Jessup M, Brozena S (2003) Heart failure. N Engl J Med 348:2007-2018
3. Wijns W, Vatner SF, Camici PG (1998) Hibernating myocardium. N Engl J Med 339:173-181
4. Bhatia RS, Tu JV, Lee DS et al (2006) Outcome of heart failure with preserved ejection fraction in a population-based study. N Engl J Med 355:260-269
5. Allman KC, Shaw LJ, Hachamovitch R, Udelson JE (2002) Myocardial viability testing and impact of revascularization on prognosis in patients with coronary artery disease and left ventricular dysfunction: A meta-analysis. J Am Coll Cardiol 39:1151-1158
6. Camici PG, Prasad SK, Rimoldi OE (2008) Stunning, hibernation, and assessment of myocardial viability. Circulation 117:103-114
7. Rizzello V, Poldermans D, Boersma E et al (2004) Opposite patterns of left ventricular remodeling after coronary revascularization in patients with ischemic cardiomyopathy: Role of myocardial viability. Circulation 110:2383-2388
8. Tennant R, Wiggers C (1935) Effect of coronary occlusion on myocardial contraction. Am J Physiol 112:351-361
9. Heyndrickx GR, Millard RW, McRitchie RJ et al (1975) Regional myocardial functional and electrophysiological alterations after brief coronary artery occlusion in conscious dogs. J Clin Invest 56:978-985
10. Rahimtoola SH (1989) The hibernating myocardium. Am Heart J 117:211-221
11. Marinho NV, Keogh BE, Costa DC et al (1996) Pathophysiology of chronic left ventricular dysfunction. New insights from the measurement of absolute myocardial blood flow and glucose utilization. Circulation 93:737-744
12. Ghosh N, Rimoldi OE, Beanlands RS, Camici PG (2010) Assessment of myocardial ischaemia and viability: Role of positron emission tomography. Eur Heart J 2984-2995
13. Camici PG, Rimoldi OE (2009) The clinical value of myocardial blood flow measurement. J Nucl Med 50:1076-1087
14. Selvanayagam JB, Jerosch-Herold M, Porto I et al (2005) Resting myocardial blood flow is impaired in hibernating myocardium: A magnetic resonance study of quantitative perfusion assessment. Circulation 112:3289-3296
15. Krivokapich J, Huang S-C, Phelps ME et al (1982) Dependence of 13-nh3 myocardial extraction and clearance on flow and metabolism. Am J Physiol 242:536-542
16. Bergmann SR, Hack S, Tewson T et al (1980) The dependence of accumulation of 13nh3 by myocardium on metabolic factors and its implications for quantitative assessment of perfusion. Circulation 61:34-43
17. Iida H, Kanno I, Takahashi A et al (1988) Measurement of absolute myocardial blood flow with h215o and dynamic positron-emission tomography. Strategy for quantification in relation to the partial-volume effect. Circulation 78:104-115

18. Schafers KP, Spinks TJ, Camici PG et al (2002)Absolute quantification of myocardial blood flow with h(2)(15)o and 3-dimensional pet: An experimental validation. J Nuc Med 43:1031-1040

19. Chareonthaitawee P, Kaufmann PA, Rimoldi O, Camici PG (2001) Heterogeneity of resting and hyperemic myocardial blood flow in healthy humans. Cardiovasc Res 50:151-161

20. Hoffman EJ, Huang SC, Phelps ME (1997) Quantitation in positron emission computed tomography: 1. Effect of object size. J Comput Assist Tomogr 3:299-308

21. Camici PG, Rosen SD, Spinks TJ (1998) Positron emission tomography. In: Murray IPC, Ell PJ, eds. Nuclear medicine in clinical diagnosis and treatment. London: Churchill-Livingstone pp 1353-1368

22. Pagano D, Fath-Ordoubadi F, Beatt KJ et al (2001) Effects of coronary revascularisation on myocardial blood flow and coronary vasodilator reserve in hibernating myocardium. Heart 85:208-212

23. Borgers M, Ausma J, Shivalkar B, Flameng W (1993) Structural correlates of regional myocardial dysfunction in patients with critical coronary artery stenosis: Chronic hibernation. Cardiovasc Pathol 2:237-245

24. Camici PG, Wijns W, Borgers M et al (1997) Pathophysiological mechanisms of chronic reversible left ventricular dysfunction due to coronary artery disease (hibernating myocardium). Circulation 96:3205-3214

25. Vanoverschelde JL, Depre C, Gerber BL et al (2000) Time course of functional recovery after coronary artery bypass graft surgery in patients with chronic left ventricular ischemic dysfunction. Am J Cardiol 85:1432-1439

26. Schinkel AF, Bax JJ, Poldermans D et al (2007) Hibernating myocardium: Diagnosis and patient outcomes. Curr Probl Cardiol 32:375-410

27. Klocke FJ, Baird MG, Lorell BH et al (2003)Acc/aha/asnc guidelines for the clinical use of cardiac radionuclide imaging–executive summary: A report of the american college of cardiology/american heart association task force on practice guidelines (acc/aha/asnc committee to revise the 1995 guidelines for the clinical use of cardiac radionuclide imaging). Circulation 108:1404-1418

28. He J, Ogden LG, Bazzano LA et al (2001) Risk factors for congestive heart failure in us men and women: Nhanes i epidemiologic follow-up study. Arch Intern Med 161:996-1002

29. Dilsizian V, Bacharach SL, Beanlands RS et al (2009) Pet myocardial perfusion and metabolism clinical imaging. J Nucl Cardiol 16:651

30. Beanlands RS, Chow BJ, Dick A et al (2007) Ccs/car/canm/cncs/canscmr joint position statement on advanced noninvasive cardiac imaging using positron emission tomography, magnetic resonance imaging and multidetector computed tomographic angiography in the diagnosis and evaluation of ischemic heart disease–executive summary. Can J Cardiol 23:107-119

31. Beanlands R, Thorn S, DaSilva J et al (2008) Myocardial viability. In: Wahl R, ed. Principles and practices of positron emission tomography. Philadelphia: Lippincott Williams and Wilkins

32. Tamaki N, Yonekura Y, Yamashita K et al (1989) Positron emission tomography using fluorine-18-deoxyglucose in evaluation of coronary artery bypass grafting. Am J Cardiol 64:860-865

33. Beanlands R, Ruddy T, deKemp R et al (2002) Positron emission tomography and recovery following revascularization (parr-1): The importance of scar and the development of a prediction rule for the degree of recovery of left ventricular function. J Am Coll Cardiol 40:1735-1743

34. Beanlands RS, Nichol G, Huszti E et al (2007) F-18-fluorodeoxyglucose positron emission tomography imaging-assisted management of patients with severe left ventricular dysfunction and suspected coronary disease: A randomized, controlled trial (parr-2). J Am Coll Cardiol 50:2002-2012

35. Tillisch J, Brunken R, Marshall R et al (1986) Reversibility of cardiac wall-motion abnormalities predicted by positron tomography. N Engl J Med 314:884-888

36. Paternostro G, Camici PG, Lammerstma AA et al (1996) Cardiac and skeletal muscle insulin resistance in patients with coronary heart disease. A study with positron emission tomography. J Clin Invest 98:2094-2099

37. Vitale G, deKemp R, Ruddy TD, Beanlands R (2001)Myocardial glucose utilization and the optimization of f-18-fdg pet imaging in patients with niddm, cad and lv dysfunction. J Nucl Med 42:1730-1736

38. vom Dahl J, Eitzman DT, Al-Aouar ZR et al (1994) Relation of regional function, perfusion, and metabolism in patients with advanced coronary artery disease undergoing surgical revascularization. Circulation 0:2356-2365

39. Di Carli MF, Davidson M, Little R et al (1994) Value of metabolic imaging with positron emission tomography for evaluating prognosis in patients with coronary artery disease and left ventricular dysfunction. Am J Cardiol 73:527-533

40. D'Egidio G, Nichol G, Williams K et al (2009) Identification of high-risk patients with increasing ischemic cardiomyopathy. JACC Cardiovasc Imaging 2:1060-1068

41. Inaba Y, Chen JA, Bergmann SR (2010) Quantity of viable myocardium required to improve survival with revascularization in patients with ischemic cardiomyopathy: A meta-analysis. J Nucl Cardiol 17:646-654

42. Kim RJ, Wu E, Rafael A et al (2000) The use of contrast-enhanced magnetic resonance imaging to identify reversible myocardial dysfunction. N Engl J Med 343:1445-1453

43. Advisory Secretariat, Medical (2010) Positron emission tomography (pet) for the assessment of myocardial viability: An evidence-based analysis

44. Thompson K, Saab G, Birnie D et al (2006) Is septal glucose metabolism altered in patients with left bundle branch block and ischemic cardiomyopathy? J Nucl Med 47:1763-1768

45. Inoue N, Takahashi N, Ishikawa T et al (2007) Reverse perfusion-metabolism mismatch predicts good prognosis in patients undergoing cardiac resynchronization therapy: A pilot study. Circ J 71:126-131

46. Birnie D, DeKemp RA, Ruddy TD et al (2009) Effect of lateral wall scar on reverse remodeling with cardiac resynchronization therapy. Heart Rhythm 6:1721-1726

47. Ypenburg C, Schalij MJ, Bleeker GB et al (2006) Extent of viability to predict response to cardiac resynchronization therapy in ischemic heart failure patients. J Nucl Med 47:1565-1570

48. DeFronzo R, Tobin J, Andres R (1979) Glucose clamp technique: A method for quantifying insulin secretion and resistance. Am J Physiol 273:E214-E223

49. Fath-Ordoubadi F, Beatt KJ, Spyrou N, Camici PG (1999) Efficacy of coronary angioplasty for the treatment of hibernating myocardium. Heart 82:210-216

50. Lautamaki R, Airaksinen KE, Seppanen M et al (2005) Rosiglitazone improves myocardial glucose uptake in patients with type 2 diabetes and coronary artery disease: A 16-week randomized, double-blind, placebo-controlled study. Diabetes 54:2787-2794

51. Knuuti J, Saraste M, Nuutila P et al (1994) Myocardial viability: Fluorine-18-deoxyglucose positron emission tomography in prediction of wall motion recovery after revascularization. Am Heart J 127:785-796

52. Marwick T, MacIntyre WJ, Lafant A et al (1992) Metabolic responses of hibernating and infarcted myocardium to revascularization. A follow-up study of regional perfusion, function, and metabolism. Circulation 85:1347-1353

53. Slart RH, Bax JJ, van Veldhuisen DJ et al (2006) Prediction of functional recovery after revascularization in patients with chronic ischaemic left ventricular dysfunction: Head-to-head comparison between 99mtc-sestamibi/18f-fdg disa spect and 13n-ammonia/ 18f-

fdg pet. Eur J Nucl Med Mol Imaging 33:716-723

54. Slart RH, Bax JJ, van Veldhuisen DJ et al (2006) Prediction of functional recovery after revascularization in patients with coronary artery disease and left ventricular dysfunction by gated fdg-pet. J Nucl Cardiol 13:210-219

55. Siebelink H-M, Blanksma PK, Crijns H et al (2001) No difference in cardiac event-free survival between positron emission tomography-guided and single-photon emission computed tomography-guided management. J Am Coll Cardiol 37:81-88

56. Eitzman D, Al-Aouar Z, Kanter HL et al (1992) Clinical outcome of patients with advanced coronary artery disease after viability studies with positron emission tomography. J Am Coll Cardiol 20:559-565

57. Lee KS, Marwick TH, Cook SA et al (1995) Prognosis of patients with left ventricular dysfunction, with and without viable myocardium after myocardial infarction: Relative efficacy of medical therapy and revascularization. Circulation 90:2687-2694

58. Desideri A, Cortigiani L, Christen AI et al (2005) The extent of perfusion-f18-fluorodeoxyglucose positron emission tomography mismatch determines mortality in medically treated patients with chronic ischemic left ventricular dysfunction. J Am Coll Cardiol 46:1264-1269

59. Pitt M, Dutka D, Pagano D et al (2004) The natural history of myocardium awaiting revascularisation in patients with impaired left ventricular function. Eur Heart J 25:500-507

60. Beanlands RS, Hendry P, Masters R et al (1998) Delay in revascularization is associated with increased mortality rate in patients with severe lv dysfunction and viable myocardium on fluorine-18-fluorodeoxyglucose positron emission tomography imaging. Circulation 98:51-56

61. Lee KS, Marwick TH, Cook SA et al (1994) Prognosis of patients with left ventricular dysfunction, with and without viable myocardium after myocardial infarction. Relative efficacy of medical

therapy and revascularization. Circulation 90:2687-2694

62. Steel K, Broderick R, Gandla V et al (2009) Complementary prognostic values of stress myocardial perfusion and late gadolinium enhancement imaging by cardiac magnetic resonance in patients with known or suspected coronary artery disease. Circulation 120:1390-1400

63. Schuleri KH, George RT, Lardo AC (2009) Applications of cardiac multidetector ct beyond coronary angiography. Nat Rev Cardiol 6:699-710

64. Lardo AC, Cordeiro MA, Silva C et al (2006) Contrast-enhanced multidetector computed tomography viability imaging after myocardial infarction: Characterization of myocyte death, microvascular obstruction, and chronic scar. Circulation 113:394-404

65. Di Carli MF, Dorbala S (2007) Cardiac pet-ct. J Thorac Imaging 22:101-106

66. Javadi MS, Lautamaki R, Merrill J et al (2010) Definition of vascular territories on myocardial perfusion images by integration with true coronary anatomy: A hybrid pet/ct analysis. J Nucl Med 51:198-203

67. Schenker MP, Dorbala S, Hong EC et al (2008) Interrelation of coronary calcification, myocardial ischemia, and outcomes in patients with intermediate likelihood of coronary artery disease: A combined positron emission tomography/computed tomography study. Circulation 117:1693-1700

68. Manghat N, Van Lingen R, Hewson P et al (2008) Usefulness of 64-detector row computed tomography for evaluation of intracoronary stents in symptomatic patients with suspected in-stent restenosis. Am J Cardiol 101:1567-1573

69. Flotats A, Knuuti J, Gutberlet M et al (2011) Hybrid cardiac imaging: Spect/ct and pet/ct. A joint position statement by the european association of nuclear medicine (eanm), the european society of cardiac radiology (escr) and the european council of nuclear cardiology (ecnc). Eur J Nucl Md Mol Imaging 38:201-212

Left and Right Ventricular Function, Contractility, Geometry, and Mass

8

Andrea I. Guaricci, Natale Daniele Brunetti, Roberta Romito, Giancarlo Casolo, and Matteo Di Biase

8.1 Introduction

The human heart lies within the central area of the thoracic cavity, in the mediastinal space. Its weight and size varies depending on age, sex, height, and nutritional status and it corresponds approximately to 300 grams in the adult male and 250 grams in the adult female [1, 2]. The heart has an inverted cone-shape, with the apex lying inferiorly and the great vessels entering the base superiorly.

The heart wall consists of three layers: the outermost, the epicardium, the innermost, the endocardium, and the middle, the muscular layer known as the myocardium, which is responsible for the major pumping action of the ventricles. The heart has four chambers, two atria and two ventricles.

8.2 Left and Right Hemodynamic

The right ventricle may be divided into the body of the right ventricle (i.e. an inflow region consisting of the tricuspid valve, the chordae tendineae, the papillary muscle, and a heavily trabeculated myocardium), and the infundibulum, a smooth outflow region. The inflow and outflow portions of the right ventricle are separated by four muscular bands: the infundibulum septum, the parietal band, the septal band, and the moderator band. The infundibulum septum and parietal band make up the crista supraventricularis [3]. Blood flows around the crista supraventricularis and is mixed by passing through the strands of the trabeculae carneae. The right ventricle receives blood from the right atrium through the tricuspid valve and ejects it through the pulmonary valve into the pulmonary artery where it travels to the lungs. Normal systolic pressure in the right ventricle ranges

A.I. Guaricci (✉)
Department of Cardiology,
University of Foggia,
Foggia, Italy

from 15 to 28 mmHg and end-diastolic pressure is 0 to 8 mmHg [4]. The right ventricle generates less than one fourth the stroke work of the left ventricle.

The left ventricle has a thick muscular wall. It receives blood from the left atrium through the mitral valve and ejects it through the aortic valve to the systemic circulation via the aorta. Pressure in the left ventricle is high. Normal systolic pressure is 90 to 140 mmHg and normal end-diastolic pressure is 4 to 12 mmHg. The ventricular septum, a thick muscular area that becomes membranous as it nears the atrio-ventricular valves, separates the right and left ventricles.

The heart consists of a right and left pump. The right pump is a low pressure system because, in a healthy person, the lungs offer little resistance to blood flow; the left pump is a high pressure system, because of higher systemic resistance to blood flow. Seventy percent of blood flows into both ventricles even before an atrial contraction occurs, while the atrial contraction contributes the remaining 25% to ventricular filling; thus, the atria function as primer pumps for the ventricles. The cardiac cycle is defined as the period from the beginning of one heartbeat to the beginning of the next beat. It includes systole (i.e. contraction), diastole (i.e. relaxation), and a short pause called the diastasis cordis (i.e. when both atria and ventricles relax). The duration of a cardiac cycle depends on the heart rate. During a mean cardiac cycle of 0.8 seconds, the atria are in systole for 0.1 seconds and in diastole 0.7 seconds; the ventricles are in systole 0.3 seconds and in diastole 0.5 seconds. The entire heart rests for about 0.4 seconds.

Ventricular systole is divided into three phases: isometric contraction, rapid ejection, and slow ejection [5]. The isometric contraction phase is the beginning of ventricular contraction. The resulting increase in pressure within the ventricle causes the atrioventricular valves to close. The isometric contraction phase is also called the isovolumetric contraction phase because all the valves are closed and there is no ejection of blood. The ventricular pressure rises above the aortic pressure curve. When left ventricular (LV) pressure exceeds aortic pressure

F. Cademartiri, G. Casolo, M. Midiri (eds.), *Clinical Applications of Cardiac CT*,
© Springer-Verlag Italia 2012

and right ventricular pressure pulmonary artery pressure, the aortic and pulmonary valves open and blood pours out of the ventricles. This is called the rapid ejection phase because 70% of the ventricular blood is emptied during the first third of the ejection period. The remaining 30% of ventricular blood is emptied during the latter two thirds of the ejection phase, and is called the slow ejection phase.

Ventricular diastole can be divided into four phases: isometric interval, rapid ventricular filling, slow ventricular filling, and atrial systole. The isometric or isovolumetric interval is a relaxation phase at the beginning of diastole. During diastole, ventricular pressure is lower than that in the aorta and the pulmonary artery and results in momentary backflow of blood. This backflow snaps the semilunar aortic and pulmonic valves shut. During this time, the ventricular pressure curve drops close to 0 mmHg. When ventricular pressure falls below atrial pressure, the atrioventricular (AV) valves open and blood rushes rapidly from the atria into the ventricles. The slow ventricular filling phase is also known as diastasis or the last part of diastole. The atrial contraction during the last phase of ventricular diastole contributes 25% more blood to the ventricles.

Toward the end of diastole, the blood volume in the ventricles (i.e. end-diastolic volume) is approximately 120 mL. At the end of systole, blood volume in the ventricles (i.e. end-systolic volume) is approximately 50 mL. The difference between the end-diastolic volume and the end-systolic volume (approximately 70 mL) is known as stroke volume (SV) and is the amount of blood ejected from the ventricles each time they contract. Cardiac output (CO) is the amount of blood in liters that is ejected from the heart per minute, and is equal to the SV multiplied by the heart rate. In normal conditions it is approximately 5 liters, but during heavy exercise this may increase to 35 liters a minute. The cardiac index (CI) is a measurement used by clinicians to adjust for individual differences in body size. It is the CO in terms of liters per/minute per square meter of body surface area. The CI gives a better indication of how well tissues are perfused than does CO alone because it addresses the actual size of the body and its blood supply needs. The normal CI is 2.5 to 4.0 liters/minute/m^2 of body surface. Both CO and CI are means of assessing the ability of a patient's heart to pump effectively.

There are four interrelated factors that govern cardiac output: preload (i.e. ventricular filling), afterload (i.e. resistance to ejection of blood), contractility, and heart rate. Preload refers to the volume of blood that fills the ventricles during diastole. It is influenced by the total volume of circulating blood. The greater the venous return to the heart, the more the myocardial fibers will stretch to accommodate that load. According to the Frank-Starling law, the greater the myocardial fiber stretch the greater the force of contraction will be. The increase in contractile force is related to an increase in sarcomere length that produces increased cross-bridge formation that regulates the amount of calcium released into the myocyte and thus regulates contraction. Clinically, preload can be determined by pulmonary capillary wedge pressure and pulmonary artery diastolic pressure.

Afterload is the amount of tension the ventricles must develop to eject the blood through the semilunar valves. In other words, afterload is the resistance against which the heart must pump the blood to all parts of the body. Many things can affect resistance. According to La Place's law, ventricular wall tension is a function of intraventricular systolic pressure, divided by ventricular wall thickness, and multiplied by intraventricular radius. An increase in chamber size (increased radius) necessitates more tension to eject the blood and raises resistance. These two factors (pressure and size) are offset by the thickness of the ventricular wall. The thicker the ventricular wall is, the less tension is needed to eject the blood and resistance is lowered.

8.3 Left Ventricular Contractility

The most commonly used tool to quantitatively evaluate global left ventricular contractility is ejection fraction (EF). To determine EF, stroke volume is divided by end-diastolic volume (EDV). Anomalies in these parameters reflect cardiac disorders. The EF indicates the pumping efficiency of the ventricle. It is reduced in patients with LV systolic dysfunction and is a good indicator of ventricular function.

The quantitation of left ventricle volumes and ejection fraction is an important aspect of cardiac evaluation in all cardiac disorders. Prognosis in many types of heart disease is closely related to global left ventricular ejection fraction (LVEF), falling off rapidly as the ejection fraction falls below 40%. However, although ejection fraction has the advantage of being a simple numerical parameter that reflects LV function, it is strongly influenced by loading conditions and does not correlate well with symptom status. Perhaps more importantly, although echocardiographic two dimensional ejection fraction is meaningful when applied across populations or to stratify risk in individuals, its value as a sequential test within individuals is constrained by limited test-retest reliability. Two dimensional echocardiography approaches for calculation of LV volumes have largely superseded M mode echocardiography techniques that used geometric assumptions based on the minor dimension of the ventricle to calculate fractional shortening.

Exercise 2D echocardiography may be useful for the identification of subclinical LV dysfunction - for example, in valvular heart disease. In this situation, standard measurements of ejection fraction have been used to measure the LV contractile reserve.

The qualitative, regional evaluation of LV systolic function is based on the division of the LV into a number of segments, after which each segment is scored as normal, hypokinetic, akinetic, or dyskinetic. The standard 16 segment model of the American Society of Echocardiography (septal, lateral, anterior, and inferior at the apex, with these segments as well as anteroseptal and posterior segments at the base and mid papillary muscle level), or 17 modified model (adding the "true apex") are the most commonly used.

LV global and segmental systolic dysfunction have been associated with myocardial ischemia and cardiovascular morbidity and mortality. Subclinical LV dilatation and LV systolic dysfunction, although uncommon in men free of overt cardiovascular disease, are associated with increased risk for new cardiovascular disease events [6]. In 1,493 men who were free of symptomatic cardiovascular disease underwent M-mode echocardiography, fractional shortening was a significant independent predictor of cardiovascular risk (relative risk 1.42 for decrease of fractional shortening by 4%). Increased risk was also associated with combinations of low fractional shortening and high end-diastolic internal dimension (RR 3.77) and with low percent fractional shortening with LV hypertrophy (RR 5.93).

Several treatment, both pharmacologic (Angiotensin Converting Enzyme-inhibitors, beta-blockers etc) and non pharmacologic, demonstrated to improve myocardial contractility, as expressed by increased ejection fraction and reduced ventricular volumes, and to proportionally improve prognosis. Results are obtained by cardiac resynchronization therapy (CRT). Compared with an Implantable Cardiovector Defibrillator (ICD) only strategy in patients with mildly symptomatic heart failure [7], the CRT-plus-ICD group had greater improvement in LV end-diastolic volume index, LV end-systolic volume index, LVEF (11% versus 3%), and right ventricular function. Moreover, improvement in end-diastolic volume at 1 year is predictive of a subsequent reduction in death or heart failure (each 10% decrease in end-diastolic volume is associated with a 40% reduction in risk).

8.4   Effect of Age and Gender

Aging and gender may affect LV mechanics [8]. The mean value of LV ejection fraction does not change with age. However, LV volumes, mass, sphericity index, and LV mass/volume ratio are altered by age. Sphericity index is highest in the first decade of age and then declines until the fifth decade; the LV mass/volume ratio significantly increases in older age, and it is significantly higher in aged women compared with age-matched men. Age has heterogeneous effects on LV shape and LV mass/volume ratio, potentially due to the growing process of myocardial fibers and the surrounding architecture in the younger population, as well as the aging process, with an increase in vascular stiffness and a loss of myocytes in older populations. Higher LV mass/volume ratios in older women might be a contributor to the preferential development of diastolic heart failure in this population.

Significant baseline relations are detectable between differences in sex, prevalent disease status, and echocardiographic measurements of LV mass and systolic function [9]. Age is weakly associated with LV mass measurements and LV ejection fraction abnormalities. These relations should be considered in evaluating the preclinical and clinical effects of cardiovascular risk factors in the elderly. M-mode LV mass adjusted for body weight increased modestly with age, increasing less than one gram per year increase in age for both men and women. After adjustment for weight, LV mass is significantly greater in men than in women and in subjects with clinical coronary heart disease (CHD) compared with those with neither clinical heart disease nor hypertension. Across all age subgroups, the difference in weight-adjusted LV mass by sex is greater in magnitude than the difference related to clinical CHD. In subjects with clinical CHD and with neither clinical heart disease nor hypertension, LV ejection fraction and segmental wall motion abnormalities are more prevalent in men than women. Of interest, 0.5% of men and 0.4% of women with neither clinical heart disease nor hypertension have LV segmental wall motion abnormalities, suggesting silent disease, compared with 26% of men and 10% of women in the clinical CHD group. Multivariate analyses revealed male sex and presence of clinical CHD to be independent predictors of LV akinesis or dyskinesis.

8.5   Diastolic Dysfunction

Abnormalities in LV diastolic function in the presence of normal LV systolic performance (isolated diastolic dysfunction) is one of the earliest cardiac manifestations of cardiovascular disease (i.e. systemic hypertension) [10]. Several studies indicate that abnormal diastolic function may be responsible, at least in part, for an impaired LV systolic response to isotonic or isometric exercise, even when systolic performance is normal at rest. Comprehensive Doppler echocardiography can now characterize diastolic function directly in addition to measurement of the EF. On the other hand, nearly all patients with systolic dysfunction have some degree of concomitant diastolic dysfunction, specifically, impaired relaxation and variable decreases in ventricular compliance which can contribute to symptoms.

Short and long term administration of some antihypertensive drugs, such as ACE-inhibitors and calcium antagonists may significantly improve diastolic function. Abnormal diastolic filling is significantly improved when LV mass is reduced by long term antihypertensive therapy [11]. Even when treatment is withdrawn and blood pressure increases again, LV mass remains reduced. These results suggest that regression of LV mass might improve LV diastolic function per se.

8.6 Right Ventricular Dysfunction

The right ventricle, unlike the left ventricle, is sensitive to acute increases in its afterload [12]. The right ventricle is usually dilated when its failure is the cause of shock. Three possible causes of right ventricular failure must be evaluated: decrease in contractility, pressure overload and volume overload. Many devices are available to assess right ventricular performance, but they are not equal in terms of accuracy and invasiveness. Compared with the left side, the assessment of right ventricular function remains fairly primitive. Standard two-dimensional echocardiographic views often are difficult to standardize to provide reproducible parameters, and the shape of the RV limits the use of simple geometric models to derive accurate volumetric data. As with the LV, RV pressures are not determined exclusively by the ventricle or vasculature but rather result from the dynamic interaction of the two. Pulmonary hypertension and accompanying right heart dysfunction is increasingly common in patients who have heart failure, regardless of EF, and potently affect exercise capacity and clinical outcome. With the wide use of echo-Doppler cardiography, pulmonary hypertension now is being increasingly recognized, particularly among older patients presenting with dyspnea.

Two main signs should be sought: right ventricular dilatation and paradoxical septal motion. Right ventricular failure may be responsible for, or participate in, shock in pulmonary embolism, acute respiratory distress syndrome and septic shock. A depression in right ventricular function that can be observed in many chronic heart diseases contributes to symptoms and leads to a worse prognosis.

Abnormal vasoconstriction of the lesser circulation characterizes a subset of patients with essential hyperten-

sion, a possible effect of mechanisms acting on both sides of the circulation or to backward transmission of increased pressure due to stiffer left ventricles with more advanced diastolic dysfunction. Elevated systemic pressure is also associated with thickening of the right ventricle. Right ventricular remodeling develops in parallel with a similar process occurring at the left side [13], likely as a result of ventricular interdependence under the influence of trophic factors targeting both ventricles, though other mechanisms, including increased pulmonary afterload, may also be operative [14]. By and large regardless of the extent of structural remodeling of both ventricles, systemic hypertension also conditions an impaired filling rate of the right ventricle that accompanies a similar phenomenon at the left side. Therefore, the right-sided cardiovascular system is not immune to the effect of systemic hypertension.

8.7 Determinants of Left Ventricular Mass

LV mass is affected by effects of obesity, hypertension, the level of cardiac volume load, and the level of LV myocardial contractility. Recently, additional independent associations of diabetes, arterial structure and function and as yet unknown genes to higher LV mass have been defined; angiotensin II and insulin have also been suggested to be additive stimuli to LV hypertrophy.

In patients with hypertension, LV hypertrophy and dysfunction is only modestly correlated with measurements of resting blood pressure [15]. LV performance declines when the pressure overload in hypertension is not offset by compensating hypertrophy, allowing wall stresses to increase. In 100 untreated patients with essential hypertension studied using cuff blood pressure and quantitative echocardiography to measure LV mass index and end-diastolic relative wall thickness (the ratio of wall thickness to chamber radius) as 2 indexes of LV hypertrophy, LV hypertrophy, as measured by both indexes, weakly correlated with all indexes of blood pressure including systolic, diastolic, and mean blood pressure. In contrast, end-diastolic relative wall thickness showed a closer direct relation with total peripheral resistance and a significant inverse relation with cardiac index. LV performance as assessed by fractional systolic shortening of LV internal dimensions is not significantly related to LV mass index, blood pressure, or peak systolic wall stress, but declines significantly with increasing mean systolic wall stress and even more with increasing end-systolic wall stress.

The weak relation of systolic blood pressure to LV mass in hypertensive patients is often interpreted as evidence of non-hemodynamic stimuli to muscle growth. To test the hypothesis that LV chamber size, which is indicative of hemodynamic volume load and myocardial contractility, influences the development of LV hypertrophy in hypertension, actual and theoretic relations of LV mass to LV diastolic chamber volume, pressure and volume load, and an index of contractility were studied. Two indices of overall LV load were assessed: total load (systolic blood pressure x LV endocardial surface area) and peak meridional force (systolic blood pressure x LV cross sectional area). A theoretically optimal LV mass, allowing each subject to achieve mean normal peak stress, was calculated as a function of systolic blood pressure and M-mode left ventricular end-diastolic diameter. LV mass measured by M-mode echo correlated better with two-dimensional echocardiogram derived LV end-diastolic volume than with systolic blood pressure and best with total load or peak meridional force [16]. In multivariate analysis both end-diastolic volume and blood pressure were independent predictors of systolic mass and explained most of its variability. Theoretically optimal LV mass was more closely related to end-diastolic volume than to systolic blood pressure; thus, the relatively weak correlation between blood pressure and optimal mass reflected the influence of LV cavity size, rather than a lack of proportionality between load and hypertrophy. Actual and theoretically optimal LV mass were closely related, indicating that LV hypertrophy in most cases paralleled hemodynamic load. LV mass is positively related to stroke index and inversely to contractility (as estimated by the end-systolic stress/volume index ratio), the main determinants of LV chamber volume. In multivariate analysis, systolic blood pressure, stroke index, and the end-systolic stress/volume index ratio are each independently related to LV mass index and accounted for 66% of its overall variability.

8.8 Left Ventricular Hypertrophy Clinical Implications

Numerous studies show that increased LV mass predicts cardiovascular events and death independently of all conventional risk factors; moreover, several studies strongly suggest that reversal of LV hypertrophy is associated with an improved prognosis.

LV hypertrophy as measured by M-mode echocardiography is an independent predictor of mortality and/or morbidity from CHD [17], behind other conventional risk factors. In a large prospective, multicenter, population-based study, the Cardiovascular Health Study, LV mass was significantly related to incident CHD, chronic heart failure (CHF), and stroke.

An increase in LV mass predicts a higher incidence of clinical events, including death, attributable to cardiovascular disease [18]. A pattern of LV hypertrophy evident on the electrocardiogram is a harbinger of morbidity and mortality from cardiovascular disease. In 3220 subjects enrolled in the Framingham Heart Study who were 40 years of age or older and free from clinically apparent cardiovascular disease, during a four-year follow-up period LV mass was determined echocardiographically and found to be associated with all outcome events. This relation persisted after adjustment for age, diastolic blood pressure, pulse pressure, treatment for hypertension, cigarette smoking, diabetes, obesity, the ratio of total cholesterol to high-density lipoprotein cholesterol, and electrocardiographic evidence of LV hypertrophy. In men, the risk factor-adjusted relative risk of cardiovascular disease was 1.49 for each increment of 50 g per meter in LV mass corrected for the subject's height; in women, it was 1.57. LV mass (corrected for height) was also associated with the incidence of death from cardiovascular disease and from all causes.

Echocardiographically determined LV hypertrophy maintains an important prognostic role regardless of the presence of coronary artery disease (CAD) [19]. Subjects with LV hypertrophy based on LV mass corrected for body surface area had worse survival than those without hypertrophy in both the group with CAD and the group without CAD. After adjustment was made for age at baseline, sex, and hypertension, the relative risk for death from any cause in patients with hypertrophy compared with patients without hypertrophy was 2.14 among those with CAD and 4.14 among those without.

Due to the different contribution of the myocardium layers to ejection, midwall left ventricular function (as expressed by midwall fractional shortening and by midwall-shortening/end-systolic stress relationship) better identifies early systolic depression, even in the presence of normal or supernormal ejection fraction, in an appreciable proportion of hypertensive patients with hypertrophied heart. Small studies have also identified adverse implications of low LV midwall function and high relative wall thickness (wall thickness/chamber radius ratio).

ACE-inhibition with ramipril is more effective than atenolol in reversing LV hypertrophy in essential hypertensive patients [20], but therapy with beta-blockers [21] or calcium channel blockers [22] may also efficiently reverse LV hypertrophy.

8.9 Left Ventricular Geometry

The adaptation of the cardiovascular system to various stimuli such as hypertension is structurally and functionally heterogeneous. By combining the level of LV mass and the relative wall thickness, four different geometric patterns can be identified: concentric LV hypertrophy (increased mass and wall thickness), eccentric hypertrophy (increased mass, normal relative wall thickness), concentric remodeling (increased relative wall thickness with normal mass) and normal LV geometry [23].

Among hypertensive patients, LV mass index and relative wall thickness is normal in 52%, whereas 13% have concentric remodeling, 27% have eccentric hypertrophy and only 8% have typical hypertensive concentric hypertrophy [24].

Concentric and eccentric hypertrophy, the two most common patterns of ventricular hypertrophy, are at the extremes of the geometric spectrum [25]. Concentric hypertrophy is characterized by an elliptic left ventricle, normal or supernormal stroke volume and high peripheral vascular resistance and elevated plasma renin. Conversely, most patients with eccentric hypertrophy have a spheric left ventricle, increased stroke volume and low peripheral vascular resistance. Its corresponding neurohormonal profile shows low serum renin and enhanced sympathetic nervous activity.

Plasma Atrial Natriuretic Peptide (ANP) and Brain Natriuretic Peptide (BNP) levels are increased in essential hypertensive patients with LV hypertrophy [26]. Furthermore, BNP secretion is augmented to a greater extent in concentric hypertrophy. Therefore, measurement of plasma ANP and BNP levels may be useful for the detection of concentric LV hypertrophy in patients with essential hypertension. Mean plasma ANP and BNP levels in all essential hypertensive patients were higher than those in age-matched normotensive control subjects. Plasma ANP levels in hypertensive patients with concentric remodeling, eccentric hypertrophy, and concentric hypertrophy were higher than in normotensive control subjects, although there were no differences between normotensive subjects and hypertensive patients with normal geometry. Plasma BNP levels tended to be higher in hypertensive patients with normal geometry, concentric remodeling, and eccentric hypertrophy than in normotensive control subjects; however, the differences were not significant. Plasma BNP levels and BNP/ANP ratio were specifically higher in concentric hypertrophy. There are significant correlations between ANP and left ventricular mass index, relative wall thickness, interventricular septal thickness, posterior wall thickness, and mean arterial pressure. Plasma BNP levels significantly correlated with relative wall thickness, interventricular septal thickness, posterior wall thickness, and left ventricular mass index but not with mean arterial pressure. In addition, plasma BNP levels are well correlated with ANP levels, and the slope for the linear regression model was steeper in concentric hypertrophy than in the other four groups.

8.10   Clinical Implications of Geometric Patterns

Each geometric pattern is associated with a distinct combination of pressure and volume stimuli (concentric hypertrophy is associated with especially high arterial pressure whereas eccentric hypertrophy is associated with obesity and elevated volume load), contractile efficiency (reduced in those with concentric left ventricular hypertrophy or remodeling) and prognosis (worst with concentric hypertrophy and best with normal left ventricular geometry) [27].

Among other hypertensive patients, even if endocardial and midwall shortening fraction were lower in concentric than in eccentric hypertrophy [28], only age >60 and LV mass above median were significant adverse prognostic predictors, while LV geometry (eccentric vs concentric hypertrophy) and ambulatory Blood Pressure (BP) were not.

Cardiac geometry and exercise capacity are strongly related [29]. In subjects with ejection fraction ≥50%, LV mass index and relative wall thickness were used to classify geometry into normal, concentric remodeling, eccentric hypertrophy and concentric hypertrophy. Geometry was related to exercise capacity in descending order: the maximum achieved metabolic equivalents were in normal, lesser in concentric remodeling, lesser in eccentric hypertrophy, and least in concentric hypertrophy. LV mass index and relative wall thickness were negatively correlated with exercise tolerance in metabolic equivalents. Augmentation of heart rate and EF with exercise were blunted in concentric hypertrophy compared with normal, even after adjusting for medications. The pattern of ventricular remodeling is related to exercise capacity. Subjects with concentric hypertrophy display the greatest limitation, and this is related to reduced systolic and chronotropic reserve (Fig. 8.1).

Concentric LV remodeling is an independent predictor of the coronary flow reserve in hypertensive patients with chest pain and normal coronary angiogram [30]. The impairment of coronary microcirculation probably contributes to the excess cardiovascular event rate associated with hypertensive concentric left ventricular remodeling.

A marked reduction in coronary flow reserve in all hypertensive groups was observed as compared with control values. Within the hypertensive subgroups, the coronary flow reserve was differentially reduced in the following rank order: concentric remodeling, approximately concentric hypertrophy, eccentric hypertrophy, normal geometry. Multifactorial regression analysis showed that the relative wall thickness but not LV mass was independently linked to the coronary flow reserve.

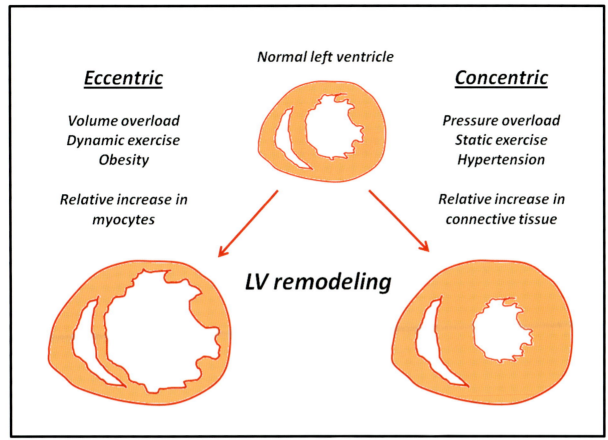

Fig. 8.1 Patterns of left ventricular hypertrophy and geometric remodeling

Several treatment regimens were shown to improve LV function and geometry; however, therapeutic response to angiotensin II antagonists and to beta-adrenergic blockers may be different among the four geometric patterns.

One year of anti-hypertensive treatment with angiotensin receptors blocker losartan is able to change LV geometric pattern [31]. A shift toward lower LV mass and relative wall thickness was found, as approximately 73% of those with concentric LV remodeling at baseline shifted to normal geometric pattern, whereas only 7% of those with normal pattern at baseline shifted to concentric LV remodeling. Of patients with concentric LV hypertrophy at baseline, 34% shifted to eccentric LV hypertrophy, whereas only 3% with eccentric LV hypertrophy at baseline had concentric LV hypertrophy. Furthermore, multiple regression analysis showed that Doppler stroke volume reduction was a significant correlate of LV mass reduction independent of BP, heart rate change, and assigned drug treatment.

A recent position statement introduced a different classification of left ventricular geometry, taking into account wall thickness and internal diameter. Indeed, among possibilities, wall thickness remains either normal, is reduced or increases, while internal diameter remains normal, increases or decreases. Therefore, nine possible combinations of altered cardiac structure may be defined. Changes in wall thickness or diameter can occur in the absence of any change in cardiac mass, but with evident alteration in cardiac structure, and obvious implications in cardiac function. An attempt to unify definitions and algorithms for the detection of abnormal ventricular phenotypes has also been proposed (Fig. 8.2) [32].

Using echocardiography and/or cardiac magnetic resonance the first step is the assessment of LV phenotypes that takes into account LV size and LV wall thickness and allows the discrimination between the different phenotypes; subsequent evaluation of resting LV function adds additional information. In the presence of normal ventricular function a noninvasive evaluation of the tolerance to stress, i.e. exercise test or catecholamines injection is proposed. Such functional assessment will more clearly locate the phenotype on the continuum of the natural history of the challenged heart.

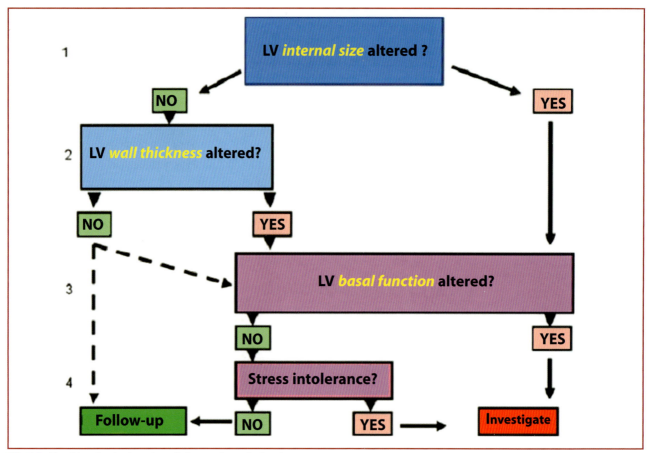

Fig. 8.2 Algorithm for the detection of abnormal ventricular phenotypes

References

1. Burrell LO (1992) Adult Nursing in Hospital and Community Settings. Norwalk, Conn: Appleton & Lange
2. Turner JR (1994) Cardiovascular Reactivity and Stress: Patterns of Physiological Response New York: Plenum Press
3. Farb A, Burke AP, Virmani R (1992) Anatomy and pathology of the right ventricle (including acquired tricuspid and pulmonic valve disease). Cardiol Clin 10:1-21
4. Lee FA (1992) Hemodynamics of the right ventricle in normal and disease states. Cardiol Clin 10:59-67
5. Gavaghan M (1998) Cardiac anatomy and physiology: A review. AORN J 67:802-822
6. Lauer MS, Evans JC, Levy D (1992) Prognostic implications of subclinical left ventricular dilatation and systolic dysfunction in men free of overt cardiovascular disease (the Framingham Heart Study). Am J Cardiol 70:1180-1184
7. Solomon SD, Foster E, Bourgoun M et al; MADIT-CRT Investigators (2010) Effect of cardiac resynchronization therapy on reverse remodeling and relation to outcome: multicenter automatic defibrillator implantation trial: cardiac resynchronization therapy. Circulation 122:985-992
8. Kaku K, Takeuchi M, Otani K et al (2011) Age- and gender-dependency of left ventricular geometry assessed with real-time three-dimensional transthoracic echocardiography. J Am Soc Echocardiogr 24:541-547
9. Gardin JM, Siscovick D, Anton-Culver H et al (1995) Sex, age, and disease affect echocardiographic left ventricular mass and systolic function in the free-living elderly. The Cardiovascular Health Study. Circulation 91:1739-1748
10. Agabiti-Rosei E, Muiesan ML (1993) Hypertension and diastolic function. Drugs 46:61-67
11. Wachtell K, Bella JN, Rokkedal J et al (2002) Change in diastolic left ventricular filling after one year of antihypertensive treatment: The Losartan Intervention For Endpoint Reduction in Hypertension (LIFE) Study. Circulation 105:1071-1076
12. Vieillard-Baron A (2009) Assessment of right ventricular function. Curr Opin Crit Care 15:254-260
13. Tumuklu MM, Erkorkmaz U, Ocal A (2007) The impact of hypertension and hypertension-related left ventricle hypertrophy on right ventricle function. Echocardiography 24:374-384
14. Pedrinelli R, Dell'Omo G, Talini E et al (2009) Systemic hypertension and the right-sided cardiovascular system: a review of the available evidence. J Cardiovasc Med 10:115-121
15. Devereux RB, Savage DD, Sachs I, Laragh JH (1983) Relation of hemodynamic load to left ventricular hypertrophy and performance in hypertension. Am J Cardiol 51:171-176
16. Ganau A, Devereux RB, Pickering TG et al (1990) Relation of left ventricular hemodynamic load and contractile performance to left ventricular mass in hypertension. Circulation 81:25-36
17. Gardin JM, McClelland R, Kitzman D et al (2001) M-mode echocardiographic predictors of six- to seven-year incidence of coronary heart disease, stroke, congestive heart failure, and mortality

in an elderly cohort (the Cardiovascular Health Study). Am J Cardiol 87:1051-1057

18. Levy D, Garrison RJ, Savage DD et al (1990) Prognostic implications of echocardiographically determined left ventricular mass in the Framingham Heart Study. N Engl J Med 322:1561-1566

19. Ghali JK, Liao Y, Simmons B et al (1992) The prognostic role of left ventricular hypertrophy in patients with or without coronary artery disease. Ann Intern Med 117:831-836

20. Agabiti-Rosei E, Ambrosioni E, Dal Palù C et al (1995) ACE inhibitor ramipril is more effective than the beta-blocker atenolol in reducing left ventricular mass in hypertension. Results of the RACE (ramipril cardio protective evaluation) study on behalf of the RACE study group. J Hypertens 13:1325-1334

21. Dunn FG, Ventura HO, Messerli FH et al (1987) Time course of regression of left ventricular hypertrophy in hypertensive patients treated with atenolol. Circulation 76:254-258

22. Fak AS, Okucu M, Tezcan H et al (1996) The Effects of Amlodipine on Left Ventricular Mass and Diastolic Function in Concentric and Eccentric Left Ventricular Hypertrophy. J Cardiovasc Pharmacol Ther 1:95-100

23. Devereux RB, Roman MJ (1999) Left ventricular hypertrophy in hypertension: stimuli, patterns, and consequences. Hypertens Res 22:1-9

24. Ganau A, Devereux RB, Roman MJ et al (1992) Patterns of left ventricular hypertrophy and geometric remodeling in essential hypertension. J Am Coll Cardiol 19:1550-1558

25. Dàvila DF, Donis JH, Odreman R et al (2008) Patterns of left ventricular hypertrophy in essential hypertension: should echocardiography guide the pharmacological treatment? Int J Cardiol 124:134-138

26. Nishikimi T, Yoshihara F, Morimoto A et al (1996) Relationship between left ventricular geometry and natriuretic peptide levels in essential hypertension. Hypertension 28:22-30

27. Devereux RB, de Simone G, Ganau A, Roman MJ (1994) Left ventricular hypertrophy and geometric remodeling in hypertension: stimuli, functional consequences and prognostic implications. J Hypertens 12:117-127

28. Verdecchia P, Schillaci G, Borgioni C et al (1996) Prognostic value of left ventricular mass and geometry in systemic hypertension with left ventricular hypertrophy. Am J Cardiol 78:197-202

29. Lam CS, Grewal J, Borlaug BA et al (2010) Size, shape, and stamina: the impact of left ventricular geometry on exercise capacity. Hypertension 55:1143-1149

30. Schäfer S, Kelm M, Mingers S, Strauer BE (2002) Left ventricular remodeling impairs coronary flow reserve in hypertensive patients. J Hypertens 20:1431-1437

31. Wachtell K, Dahlä B, Rokkedal J et al (2002) Change of left ventricular geometric pattern after 1 year of antihypertensive treatment: the Losartan Intervention For Endpoint reduction in hypertension (LIFE) study. Am Heart J 144:1057-1064

32. Knöll R, Iaccarino G, Tarone G et al (2011) Towards a re-definition of 'cardiac hypertrophy' through a rational characterization of left ventricular phenotypes: a position paper of the Working Group 'Myocardial Function' of the ESC. Eur J Heart Fail 13:811-819

Pulmonary Veins and Cardiac Veins

9

Maurizio Del Greco, Flavia Ravelli, and Massimiliano Marini

9.1 The Cardiac Veins

The cardiac veins offer the cardiologist-electrophysiologist relatively easy access to the epicardial surface of the left ventricle (LV) since they can be arrived at through the coronary sinus from the heart chamber easiest to reach with a catheter: the right atrium (RA). Although this approach has been little used in the past, and principally for the mapping of complex ventricular arrhythmias, in recent years it has become the foundation of a revolution in nonpharmacologic treatment for advanced heart failure (HF).

HF is a complex clinical syndrome which can arise from a variety of structural or functional cardiac disorders which limit the ability of the ventricle to fill with and eject blood. HF is a disease with a high social impact given its broad diffusion and associated morbidity and mortality. In Western populations the prevalence varies from 3 to 20% of individuals with the percentage increasing significantly among individuals older than 65 years. The incidence is 0.1-0.2%, and tends to double each decade after 50 years. Mortality is very high: 50% within the first 4 years from diagnosis [1]. Numerous large trials published in recent years [2-4] have highlighted the effectiveness of pharmacologic treatment in slowing the progression of HF, improving prognosis and reducing acute events (hospitalization). The recent American (ACC/AHA) [5] and European (ESC) [6] guidelines recommend the following drugs for the treatment of chronic HF: ACE inhibitors, diuretics, beta-blockers and aldosterone antagonists. In the advanced stages of the disease (classes III-IV NYHA), characterized by the worsening of quality of life and prognosis, heart transplant is the only real therapeutic solution. However, the limited number of organs available rules

out this treatment option for a significant number of patients.

In an attempt to find an alternative treatment for advanced HF, numerous studies were done throughout the 1990s to test the effect of cardiac resynchronization therapy (CRT) [7, 8]. Cardiac disorders which cause HF are often associated with damage to the myocardial conducting system. This produces dyssynchrony both in the contraction between the cardiac chambers and between the walls of individual chambers, which further aggravates the contractile ability of the heart. The understanding of the electroanatomic mechanisms of the heart coupled with materials development has in the last decade made selective pacing of any cardiac chamber possible. The development of increasingly complex pacemakers has made the selective programming of the pacing sequence possible.

Although CRT between atria and ventricles can produce beneficial hemodynamic effects in acute patients, clinical findings in chronic patients are conflicting [9, 10]. Greater benefit appears to be provided by biventricular pacing in patients with HF and electrical dyssynchrony at surface electrocardiogram (usually bundle-branch block) (Fig. 9.1a). In patients with left bundle-branch block the electrical impulse leaving the His bundle leads to delayed and nonuniform activation of the LV. This activation pattern not only produces the late contraction of the LV in respect to the right ventricle (RV) (interventricular dyssynchrony), but also nonuniform LV wall motion (intraventricular dyssynchrony) (Fig. 9.2a). This dysfunction of the conducting tissue can be of varying degrees and causes the late activation of the basal portions of the LV. This can lead to the contraction of the lateral and the posterior walls when the semilunar valves are already closed. In addition to a worsening of systolic function, the main hemodynamic consequence is a deterioration of mitral regurgitation produced by the asynchronous contraction of the papillary muscles.

CRT in patients with left bundle-branch block requires not only the traditional RV pacing, but also LV

M. Del Greco (✉)
Cardiology Unit, "Santa Chiara" Hospital,
Trento, Italy

F. Cademartiri, G. Casolo, M. Midiri (eds.), *Clinical Applications of Cardiac CT,*
© Springer-Verlag Italia 2012

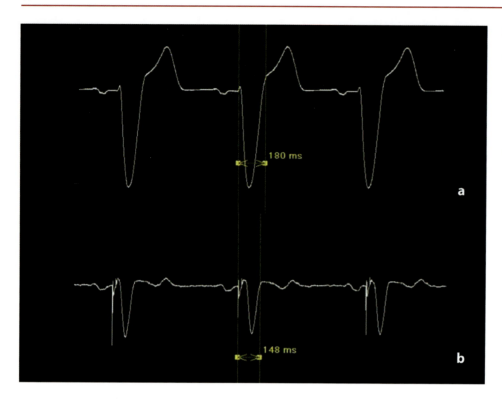

Fig. 9.1 The figure shows two electrocardiogram traces (single lead precordial V1) of a patient with refractory heart failure and left bundle-branch block, before (**a**) and after (**b**) cardiac resynchronization with biventricular pacing. A clear narrowing of the QRS complex during biventricular pacing can be appreciated

pacing. The LV is however an unsuitable chamber for permanent endocardial pacing, partly because the implantation of the pacing leads requires a retrograde (transaortic) arterial approach, and partly because of the elevated risk of thromboembolism associated with the presence of the leads in the chamber itself. In contrast, epicardial pacing is well tolerated over time (as cardiac surgeons are aware [11, 12]) and today can be done "non-invasively" with pacing leads capable of passing through the coronary sinus and along the cardiac venous system. The advantage of this approach is that even the LV lead can be inserted into the venous system (usually the left subclavian vein) like the leads for the right atrium and RV, thus simplifying the procedure. The difficulties associated with the transvenous approach are related to anatomic variability which can encumber the cannulation of the coronary sinus or the secondary branches proximal to the portion of the LV to be paced. Pacing lead placement is therefore usually preceded by selective venography of the coronary sinus to identify the target branch. This approach can however produce unsatisfactory visualization of complex venous anatomy, in part due to the limitations of the two-dimensional perspective offered by conventional angiography, and in part to insufficient perfusion of the retrograde-injected contrast material. In some centers venography is done several days before the procedure to allow planning of lead placement based on the anatomic findings. Where the anatomy precludes lead placement through a transvenous approach, thoracotomy is a second choice alternative for the placement of the epicardial lead. Despite the development of tools for catheter navigation in the cardiac veins, transvenous epicardial pacing is not possible in 5% to 11% of cases, not even in high-volume centers [13, 14]. Lastly, it should be recalled that general and specific risks need to be taken into account during pacemaker implantation. The general risks are those which are common to all pacemaker implantations (e.g. puncture of the subclavian artery, pneumothorax, bleeding, ventricular arrhythmias, infections, pressure sores, etc.). The specific risks include atrioventricular block, coronary sinus dissection (2.2%) and perforation of the coronary sinus complicated by pericardial effusion and/or cardiac tamponade [14].

The current configuration of CRT, therefore, sees a pacing lead on the endocardial surface of the RV (usually the apex), a pacing lead on the epicardial surface of the LV (preferably in a lateral or posterolateral vein through the coronary sinus) and in patients with a prevalently sinus rhythm a third pacing lead in the right atrium (usually the appendage) to optimize atrioventricular delay. Pacing is therefore "three chamber" and in the two ventricles it can occur simultaneously or be optimized with the delayed pacing of one of the two chambers according to electrocardiographic and echocardiographic parameters [15]. The result is a variable QRS narrowing at surface ECG (Fig. 9.1b) and even more importantly a resynchronization of LV contractility optimized at echocardiography [16] (Fig. 9.2b).

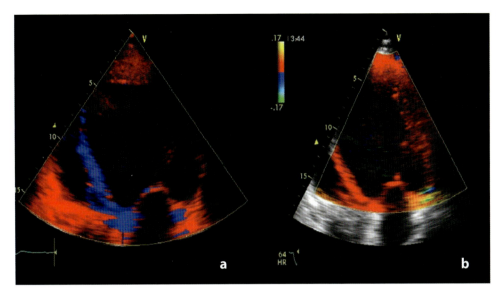

Fig. 9.2 The same patient as in Fig. 9.1. Echocardiography of the left ventricle (apical 4-chamber view) with tissue Doppler imaging showing delayed activation of the lateral wall represented by different color to interventricular septum (**a**); after biventricular pacing restored synchronization of the left ventricle can be appreciated (**b**), highlighted by the uniform color

The most important study to analyze the effects of pure CRT in a population with HF was the recent Care-HF [14]. The study compared the effect of CRT in addition to the optimal therapy for HF in NHYA class III-IV patients with depressed ventricular function (EF≤35%) and electrical dyssynchrony (QRS≥120 ms). The CRT group demonstrated not only a 40% reduction in mortality but also a drastic reduction in hospital stay and improvement of patient symptoms (improvement of NYHA class). The publication of the Care-HF study prompted the American, European and Italian societies to update their guidelines (ACC/AHA [5], ESC [6], and AIAC [17]), with the implantation of a biventricular pacemaker in patients with similar characteristics to those in the study becoming a Class I recommendation (Level of Evidence A).

9.2 The Pulmonary Veins

9.2.1 Introduction

The fact that the pulmonary veins are a *remote* part of the cardiovascular system and difficult to reach via catheterization is perhaps why they have been of no great interest to the medical community, except for some rare congenital malformations. Recent studies have however indicated their involvement in the genesis of atrial fibrillation (AF), sparking newfound interest in the pulmonary veins as a target for a new nonpharmacologic therapeutic approach to this arrhythmia.

AF is the most common clinically significant arrhythmia. The prevalence in the general population is about 0.95%, with a notably higher frequency among the elderly. The prevalence of 0.1% in the population below 55 years rises to 3.8% in patients above 60 years and reaches 9% in the population above 80 years [18]. The FIRE study (atrial Fibrillation/flutter Italian Registry) [19] gathered together data from 207 Italian centers and demonstrated that AF accounts for 1.5% of all emergency department admission diagnoses and that 61.9% of patients with AF are hospitalized, accounting for 3.3% of all hospital admissions. Subjects in the 65-74 years age range are a particular burden, with hospital expenses increasing by one third in comparison to the non AF population of the same age [20].

In addition to the economic burden of the condition, AF also has a high clinical cost, being associated with a mortality nearly twice that of non AF individuals [21], and a five-fold risk of stroke [22]. The quality of life of these patients is also significantly worse than that of the healthy population [23], being similar to that of patients affected by significant structural cardiac diseases, e.g. patients recovering from coronary angioplasty or myocardial infarction [24].

From the electrophysiologic point of view AF is characterized by highly disorganized electrical activity of the atria and by an irregular and often very rapid ventricular response (Fig. 9.3a). Although AF is very common, it does pose significant medical and economic problems for the cardiologist, probably due in part to an imperfect understanding of its pathogenetic mechanisms. AF is the end result of profoundly different electrophysiologic mechanisms and anatomic determinants [25]. Numerous experimental and clinical studies have in fact shown that all forms of arrhythmia mechanisms can be found in AF, including focal mechanisms and various forms of reentry (Fig. 9.3b).

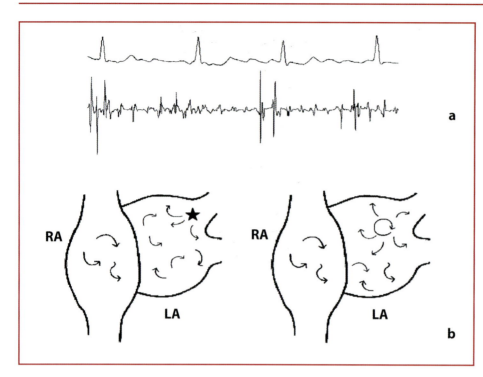

Fig. 9.3 Irregular electrical activity during atrial fibrillation and electrophysiologic mechanisms. **a** ECG and atrial electrogram recorded in the right atrium by bipolar electrodes. The atrial electrogram reveals elevated peak-to-peak variability both in the morphology of the depolarization waves and the frequency of activation. **b** The mechanisms of fibrillation include the presence of both focal activity, near the pulmonary veins (★), and a single reentry circuit. The electrical activity in the remaining part of the atria is made up of the random propagation of multiple wavefronts. *RA*, right atrium; *LA*, left atrium

9.2.2 The Mechanisms of Fibrillation: an Evolving Theory

The theoretical foundation for our understanding of the mechanisms of AF was laid at the beginning of the 20th century [26]. The main competing theories saw the underlying mechanisms of the fibrillation in ectopic discharges (Engelmann, Winterberg), single-circuit reentry (Lewis) and multiple-circuit reentry (Mines, Garrey). Over the past 50 years the multiple reentry notion has become the dominant conceptual model of AF. This has been largely due to the simulations of Moe [27] and the later experimental work of Allessie et al. [28]. Using a sophisticated mapping system Allessie was able to document the precise activation of the atria during the various stages of AF in canine hearts [28]. The study clearly demonstrates that the arrhythmia is maintained by the propagation of multiple wavefronts through both atria which interact with anatomic and/or functional obstacles, leading to fragmentation and wavelet formation. Though it has gained support as far as the propagation of electrical activity in a large part of the atrial mass is concerned, the theory of multiple wavelets has been revised by a number of clinical observations [29]. These demonstrate that focal and reentrant mechanisms prevalently situated in proximity to the pulmonary veins can coexist with a disordered propagation of wavefronts and prove crucial in triggering the arrhythmia. Haïaguerre et al. [30] were the first to observe that ectopic beats originating in the pulmonary veins can give rise to AF. Inside the pulmonary veins are present muscle fibers connected with the left atrium and potentially capable of arrhythmogenic activity. Other atrial regions which are possible trigger sites include the entrance of the coronary sinus, the superior vena cava and the ligament of Marshall [29].

Over the last decade a large part of our knowledge of the mechanisms of AF has been deduced during AF ablation procedures. As a result our understanding of the mechanisms of AF and catheter ablation strategies have evolved hand in hand [29]. The studies demonstrate that AF is the end result of diversified electrophysiologic mechanisms which can both trigger the arrhythmia and constitute the substrate which maintains it [31]. Trigger elements include ectopic foci or reentries which develop in sleeves of atrial tissue which extend into the cardiac veins. Elements constituting the electrophysiologic substrate include the dispersion of refractoriness, delayed conduction and short refractory periods. However, AF can only persist and not spontaneously cease after a couple of minutes in the presence of mechanisms which perpetuate the arrhythmia [32, 33]. The main mechanism responsible for maintaining the arrhythmia is electrical, contractile and structural remodeling of the atrium which results from repeated episodes of AF [32].

Alongside the revision to the theory of the mechanisms underlying AF, the concept of irregularity has also undergone some changes. In the wake of recent experimental observations regarding periodicity during fibrilla-

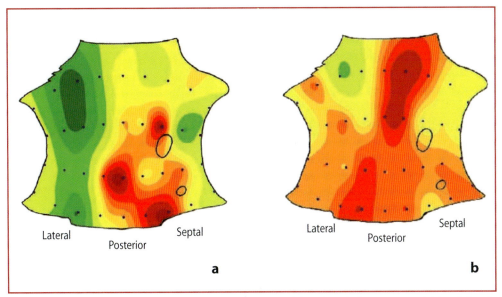

Fig. 9.4 Two-dimensional map of electrical organization in the right atrium during paroxysmal (**a**) and chronic (**b**) atrial fibrillation. The electrical signals used to build the activation maps were acquired with a basket catheter. The figure is a two dimensional depiction of the right atrium, opened along the anterior portion and shows the position of the electrodes on the endocardium. The colors indicate the degree of atrial activation (*green*: highly organized electrical activity; *red*: disorganized electrical activity). In patients with paroxysmal atrial fibrillation the lateral wall of the right atrium tends to have more organized electrical activity than the posterior wall and the interatrial septum. In chronic fibrillation the degree of disorganization increases. (Modified from [36])

tion [34], AF is no longer seen as disorganized or random electrical activity, but rather as an irregular process with transient periods of spatiotemporal organization. Recent studies [35, 36], some of which conducted with sophisticated mathematical models [37], have demonstrated how the complexity of atrial activation differs in different regions of the atria and varies according to the type of fibrillation (Fig. 9.4). The creation of activation maps has received considerable attention in clinical practice, with the proposal of using them to identify critical regions where different therapeutic approaches can be directed [38, 39]. In this setting, the integration of activation maps with anatomic images of the atria currently available thanks to the modern CT/MR imaging modalities will in the near future help to identify the exact critical region to be treated.

9.2.3 Treatment of Atrial Fibrillation

Given the complexity of the pathogenetic mechanisms of AF, therapy is neither simple nor immediate. Most antiarrhythmic drugs have a rate of relapse within 12-24 months of over 50% [40]. This rate can be lowered to 20% with electrical or pharmacologic conversion or a change in therapy should relapse occur [41]. A meta-analysis [42] examined all the randomized controlled trials on the prevention of AF relapse with antiarrhythmic drugs, for a total of 11,322 patients. The study reported the partial effectiveness of all antiarrhythmic drugs (percentage of relapse at 1 year varying between 44% and 77% vs. 71-84% in the control group) with side effects in 9-23% of cases (proarrhythmia in 1-7%) and an increase in mortality in the group of patients treated with class IA drugs ($p=0.04$). According to the AFFIRM study [43], not only was the strategy for controlling cardiac rhythm inferior to the one for controlling frequency (beta-blockers, calcium antagonists, digoxin), but also the risk of death among elderly patients, patients with coronary artery disease and patients with heart failure was greater. In the wake of these data a recent substudy [44] of the AFFIRM study confirmed that the presence of sinus rhythm is associated with a reduction in mortality and that while the use of antiarrhythmic drugs is effectively associated with an increase in mortality, they only have a negative effect on survival after the adjustment of therapy to restore sinus rhythm. Sinus rhythm proved to be the most important factor in improving quality of life [45]. As a result only highly effective therapy capable of maintaining sinus rhythm coupled with minimal side effects can lead to real benefits in patients with AF. Non pharmacologic therapy has played a particularly important role in this setting, with cardiac surgery historically leading the way. Cox [46] proposed the Maze technique which aimed to reduce the critical atrial mass in line with the multiple wavelet notion. Later, in addition to the variations on the initial technique proposed by Cox himself (Maze II and Maze III), many new approaches were used

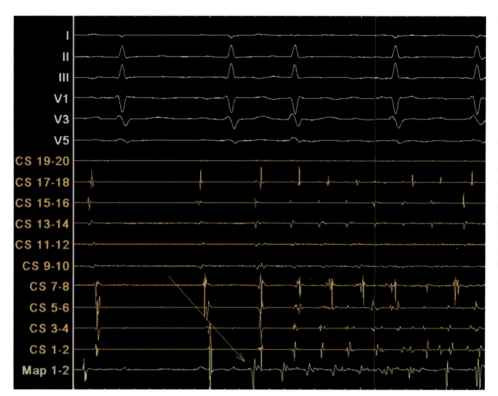

Fig. 9.5 Triggering of atrial fibrillation during electrophysiologic mapping. The following traces, from top to bottom, are depicted: six leads for the surface ECG, ten electrode catheters inserted in the coronary sinus and a combination monophasic action potential (MAP)/ablation catheter positioned in the right superior pulmonary vein. The *arrow* indicates the appearance of ectopic beats which trigger atrial fibrillation. The most premature electrogram at the level of the MAP catheter is compatible with the origin from the right superior pulmonary vein of the ectopic beats

[47], although the Maze technique still underlies surgical treatment of AF [48]. The results obtained with this technique were remarkable, with the abolition of arrhythmia in the absence of therapy in 93% of patients in the three months to eight and a half years after treatment [49]. The first attempts at catheter ablation of AF in fact attempted to emulate the Maze procedure [50]. At the beginning of the 1990s the Bordeaux group [51] concentrated on the possibility of AF ablation of the right atrium, but the results were disappointing. This was followed by catheter ablation of the left atrium [52] which shed light on the importance of this chamber in the genesis of AF. The real watershed, however, came at the end of the 1990s, when Haïsaguerre et al. [30, 53] discovered that AF can be triggered from a focal source located in the pulmonary veins (Fig. 9.5).

The atrial musculature extends for more or less lengthy tracts along the internal walls of the pulmonary veins to form myocardial sleeves [54]. The sleeves are composed of spiral, circular and longitudinal bundles of atrial myocytes like a network interspersed with areas of venous tissue and zones of fibrous degeneration. The venoatrial junction is also important for its abundance of nerve fibers and ganglia [55]. The Bordeaux group demonstrated that foci present in the pulmonary veins – multiple foci in the same vein or in several veins – can trigger arrhythmia. Instead of modifying the substrate responsible for maintaining AF, they proposed a therapeutic strategy capable of preventing AF through the elimination of the trigger. The Bordeaux group and then others developed a strategy aimed at eliminating the individual foci. This prompted pulmonary vein mapping to find the origin of the earliest electrical activity capable of triggering AF and enable it to be eliminated [53, 56, 57].

This first *focal* approach to AF was encumbered by important limitations (complexity of the procedure, relapse of AF caused by the appearance of other foci in other pulmonary veins, the possibility of pulmonary vein stenosis) and was quickly replaced by an approach aimed at the electrical disconnection of all the pulmonary veins from the atrial myocardial tissue. Although there are many variants, pulmonary vein ablation can be divided into two main approaches, both of which aim at the electrical disconnection of the pulmonary veins. These strategies are:
– segmental pulmonary vein ostial ablation. This uses predominantly electrophysiologic information and following the theory of the Bordeaux group aims at disconnecting the atrial myocardial tissue from the pulmonary veins through catheter ablation at the level of the pulmonary vein ostium. This technique uses a decapolar catheter with a circular tip to map the circumference of the pulmonary vein ostium (Fig. 9.6). Ablation is then performed along most of the ostium

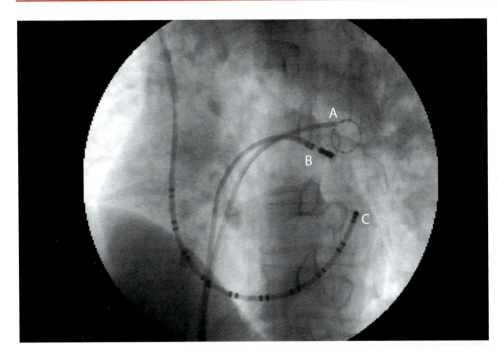

Fig. 9.6 Radiologic image in left anterior oblique view (40°) during mapping of the left superior pulmonary vein. Three catheters are visible: *A*, a circular decapolar catheter (Lasso, Cordis Webster) inserted in the left superior pulmonary vein (transeptal approach); *B*, a quadripolar catheter for mapping and ablation positioned at the level of the ostium of the same pulmonary vein (transeptal approach); *C*, a 20-pole catheter in the coronary sinus (the latter with right internal jugular vein access and the former two with right femoral vein access)

proximal to the mapping catheter, in the points of earliest activation until the pulmonary vein muscle potentials are eliminated (Fig. 9.7) [58];

– circumferential pulmonary vein ablation developed by Pappone et al. [59], despite recognizing the importance of the trigger provided by the pulmonary veins and the need for its disconnection, is aimed more at modifying the electroanatomic substrate as proposed by the compartmentalization concept of the Maze technique. This technique exploits the three-dimensional reconstruction of the atrium with non-fluoroscopic mapping systems (CARTO, Biosense Webster; EnSite Navx, St Jude Medical) which produces three-dimensional images of the atrium, the movements of the catheter and the ablation procedure by creating radiofrequency-induced contiguous linear lesions around the ostia of each vein, taken either individually or in pairs [60] (Fig. 9.8).

AF ablation procedures are long and complex still today. In both approaches one of the main obstacles to the electrical isolation of the pulmonary veins is anatomic variations and their relations to the adjacent structures [61-64]. Hand in hand with the progress made in catheter ablation has been the developing interest regarding cardiac anatomy and the imaging techniques for the heart, the left atrium and the pulmonary veins. Many modalities have been evaluated: transesophageal and intracardiac ultrasonography, computed tomography, magnetic resonance, etc. Regardless of the approach adopted, precise knowledge of the region to be treated is fundamental for the success of the procedure and for avoiding complications (including the much feared and not uncommon stenosis of the pulmonary veins). Studies have shown that as well as significant anatomic variability (38%) [61] the pulmonary veins are characterized by remarkable complexity of the form and variability in the diameter of the ostia, the morphology of the individual veins, the proximal and distal branches, the relations between the veins and the ostia, and the relations between the ostia and the cardiac structures (especially the appendage of the left atrium) [62, 63]. For example, holding the catheter stable for the ablation of the septum dividing the left pulmonary veins from the left appendage can be difficult, particularly due to the great anatomic variability in the septum itself. This thin structure is usually approached by the venous border rather than the left superior border, both for more effective ablation and to avoid the risk of perforating the thin wall of the appendage. Great care is required to not ablate too deep in the vein owing to the risk of stenosis. Detailed knowledge of cardiac anatomy which is today available thanks to CT/MR provides precious information, thus allowing the technician:

1. to avoid positioning errors of the ablation points due to *anatomic disorientation* or failure to recognize the structures during the procedure [65];
2. to design an ablation strategy *a priori* tailored to the anatomic variables of the individual;
3. to perform the ablation navigating directly in the 3D images of the cardiac chambers provided by CT/MR. This option (Carto Merge, Biosense Webster) enables CT data to be inserted directly into the system of

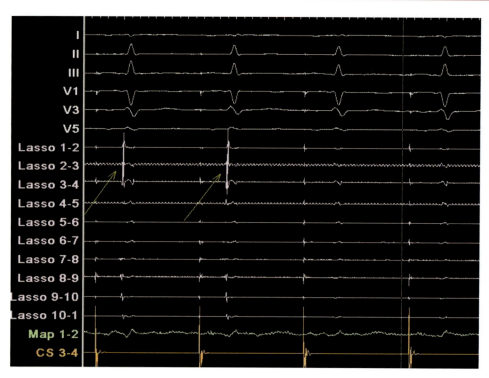

Fig. 9.7 Electrophysiologic mapping of the left superior pulmonary vein during ablation (and pacing of the coronary sinus). The following traces, from *top to bottom*, are depicted: six leads for the surface ECG, ten circular decapolar catheters (Lasso, Cordis Webster) inserted in the left superior pulmonary vein, a combination monophasic action potential (MAP)/ablation catheter positioned in the pulmonary vein and a catheter in the coronary sinus. The *arrows* indicate the presence of electrical activity within the pulmonary veins in the first two beats (clearly evident on Lasso 1-2, 2-3, 3-4), which disappears during ablation in the following two beats demonstrating the electrical disconnection of the vein

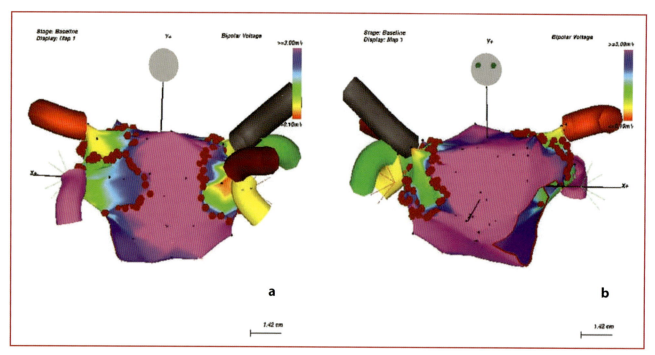

Fig. 9.8 Electroanatomic reconstruction (Carto, Cordis Webster) of the left atrium and the pulmonary veins after circumferential ablation (*see* text). The ablation points are depicted in dark red and their distribution follows the ostia of the pulmonary arteries. The atrium is depicted as a color-coded voltage map graded from *red* (lowest) to *purple* (greatest). Posteroanterior (**a**) and anteroposterior (**b**) views

electroanatomic mapping. Dedicated algorithms are then able to superimpose the electroanatomic images being created over the CT/MR images, thus informing the technician of the exact anatomic location of the radiofrequency catheter with a precision never seen before. All this opens up interesting scenarios in this field, especially with the advent of new technology which allows catheter movement through external magnetic fields (Stereotaxis, Inc., St. Louis, Missouri), thus paving the way for robotized procedures.

The incidence of significant peri- and postprocedural complications for AF catheter ablation is generally low and falling with the increasing experience of the technicians and the refinement of techniques (about 6% in the world survey and <3% in specialized centers) [66, 67].

The most significant nonfatal complications include transitory and nontransitory cerebral embolisms (0.4%-0.66% and 0.1%-0.28%, respectively), pericardial effusion and cardiac tamponade (0.5%-1.2%), and symptomatic or severe stenosis (>70%) of the pulmonary veins (0.3%-0.78%, requiring angioplasty in 0.71% of cases and surgery in 0.03% of cases) [66, 67]. A dangerous albeit rare complication of AF catheter ablation is atrialesophageal fistula secondary to radiofrequency ablation at the level of the posterior wall of the left atrium in proximity to the pulmonary vein ostia [68, 69]. Other possible complications of the procedure include severe vascular lesions at the catheter access site (arteriovenous fistulas, femoral pseudoaneurysm, inguinal hematoma requiring transfusion, etc.) (0.3%-0.95%) [66, 67]. Lastly, rare or minor complications include phrenic nerve paralysis [70], entrapment of the catheters in the mitral valves [71], acute coronary spasm and occlusion [72, 73], disseminated intravascular coagulation [74] and postprocedural increased resting heart rate [75], as well as the associated risks of radiation exposure [76].

The short- and medium- to long-term efficacy of radiofrequency catheter ablation for the cure of AF is still unknown. Overall, an analysis of the main data from the literature reveals an average success rate of 80% (3,062 out of 3,807 patients) at one year, with a range varying from 45% to 95% [77]. These data also reveal that 26% of patients without recurrence of AF in follow-up continue to take antiarrhythmic drugs which were generally ineffective prior to the procedure (9.7% of all patients who underwent catheter ablation). In the light of these data and the findings of several studies which compared the efficacy, safety and cost/benefit ratio of catheter ablation with traditional pharmacologic therapy [78-81], the AIAC Task Force [77] recommended left atrial catheter ablation for the treatment of AF as Class I (Level of Evidence B) for *non-elderly* patients with symptomatic paroxysmal/persistent AF refractory to drugs. A different stance was taken by the ESC/ACC/AHA Task Force [82] which recommended Class IIa for AF catheter ablation, stating that it can be considered a reasonable alternative to pharmacologic therapy in symptomatic patients.

References

1. Levy D, Kenchaiah S, Larson MG et al (2002) Long-term trends in the incidence of and survival with heart failure. N Engl J Med 347:1397-1402
2. The SOLVD Investigators (1991) Effect of Enalapril on survival in patients with reduced left ventricular ejection fractions and congestive heart failure. N Engl J Med 325:293-302
3. MERIT Investigators (1999) Effect of metoprolol CR/XL in chronic heart failure:Metoprolol CR/XL Randomised Intervention Trial in Congestive Heart Failure (Merit-HF). Lancet 353:2001-2007
4. Pitt B, Zannad F, Remme WJ et al (1999) The effect of spironolactone on morbidity and mortality in patients with severe heart failure. Randomised Aldactone Evaluation Study Investigators. N Engl J Med 341:709-717
5. Hunt SA, Abraham WT, Chin MH et al (2005) ACC/AHA 2005 Guideline Update for the Diagnosis and Management of Chronic Heart Failure in the Adult: a report of the American College of Cardiology/American Heart Association Task Force on Practice Guidelines (Writing Committee to Update the 2001 Guidelines for the Evaluation and Management of Heart Failure): developed in collaboration with the American College of Chest Physicians and the International Society for Heart and Lung Transplantation: endorsed by the Heart Rhythm Society. Circulation 112:e154-235
6. Swedberg K, Cleland J, Dargie H et al (2005) Guidelines for the diagnosis and treatment of chronic heart failure: executive summary (update 2005): The Task Force for the Diagnosis and Treatment of Chronic Heart Failure of the European Society of Cardiology. Eur Heart J 26:1115-1140
7. Cazeau S, Ritter P, Lazarus A et al (1996) Multisite pacing for end-stage heart failure: early experience. Pacing Clin Electrophysiol 19:1748-1757
8. Leclercq C, Cazeau S, Ritter P et al (2000) A pilot experience with permanent biventricular pacing to treat advanced heart failure. Am Heart J 140:862-870
9. Linde C, Gadler F, Edner M et al (1995) Results of atrioventricular synchronous pacing with optimized delay in patients with severe congestive heart failure. Am J Cardiol 75:919-923
10. Gold MR, Feliciano Z, Gottlieb SS et al (1995) Dual-chamber pacing with a short atrioventricular delay in congestive heart failure: a randomized study. J Am Coll Cardiol 26:967-973
11. Foster AH, Gold MR, McLaughlin JS (1995) Acute hemodynamic effects of atrio-biventricular pacing in humans. Ann Thorac Surg 59:294-300
12. Kleine P, Doss M, Aybek T et al (2000) Biventricular pacing for weaning from extracorporeal circulation in heart failure. Ann Thorac Surg 73:960-962
13. Bristow MR, Saxon LA, Boehmer J et al (2004) Cardiac-resynchronization therapy with or without an implantable defibrillator in advanced chronic heart failure. N Engl J Med 350:2140-2150
14. Cleland JG, Daubert JC, Erdmann E et al (2005) The effect of cardiac resynchronization on morbidity and mortality in heart failure. N Engl J Med 352:1539-1549
15. Bleeker GB, Bax JJ, Schalij MJ et al (2005) Tissue Doppler imaging to assess left ventricular dyssynchrony and resynchronization therapy. Eur J Echocardiogr 6:382-384
16. Yu CM, Bleeker GB, Fung JW et al (2005) Left ventricular reverse remodeling but non clinical improvement predicts long-term survival after cardiac resynchronization therapy. Circulation 112:1580-1586
17. Lunati M, Bongiorni MG, Boriani G et al (2005) Linee Guida AIAC 2006 all'impianto di pacemaker, dispositivi per la resincronizzazione cardiaca (CRT) e defibrillatori automatici impiantabili (ICD). GIAC 8:1-58
18. Go AS, Hylek EM, Phillips KA et al (2001) Prevalence of diag-

nosed atrial fibrillation in adults. JAMA 285:2370-2375

19. Santini M, De Ferrari GM, Pandozi C et al (2004) Atrial fibrillation requiring urgent medical care. Approach and outcome in the various departments of admission. Data from the atrial Fibrillation/flutter Italian Registry (FIRE). Ital Heart J 5:205-213

20. Wolf PA, Mitchell JB, Baker CS et al (1998) Impact of atrial fibrillation on mortality, stroke, and medical costs. Arch Intern Med 158:229-234

21. Benjamin EJ, Wolf PA, D'Agostino RB et al (1998) Impact of atrial fibrillation on the risk of death. The Framingham Heart Study. Circulation 98:946-952

22. Wolf PA, Abbott RD, Kannel WB (1991) Atrial fibrillation as an independent risk factor for stroke: the Framingham Study. Stroke 22:983-988

23. Luderitz B, Jung W (2000) Quality-of-life in patients with atrial fibrillation. Arch Intern Med 160:1749-1757

24. Dorian P, Jung W, Newman D et al (2000) The impairment of health-related quality of life in patients with intermittent atrial fibrillation: implications for the assessment of investigational therapy. J Am Coll Cardiol 36:1303-1309

25. Nattel S, Allessie M, Haissaguerre M (2002) Spotlight on atrial fibrillation -the 'complete arrhythmia'. Cardiovasc Res 54:197-203

26. Nattel S (2002) New ideas about atrial fibrillation 50 years on. Nature 415:219-226

27. Moe GK, Rheinboldt WC, Abildskov JA (1964) A computer model of atrial fibrillation. Am Heart J 67:200-220

28. Allessie MA, Lammers WEJEP, Bonke FIM et al (1985) Experimental evaluation of Moe's multiple wavelet hypothesis of atrial fibrillation. In: Cardiac electrophysiology and arrhythmias. Zipes DP, Jalife J (eds) Grune & Stratton Publ, Orlando, pp 265-275

29. Oral H (2005) Mechanisms of atrial fibrillation: lessons from studies in patients. Prog Cardiovasc Dis 48:29-40

30. Haissaguerre M, Jais P, Shah DC et al (1998) Spontaneous initiation of atrial fibrillation by ectopic beats originating in the pulmonary veins. N Engl J Med 339:659-666

31. Allessie MA, Boyden PA, Camm AJ et al (2001) Pathophysiology and prevention of atrial fibrillation. Circulation 103:769-777

32. Allessie M, Ausma J, Schotten U (2002) Electrical, contractile and structural remodeling during atrial fibrillation. Cardiovasc Res 54:230-246

33. Ravelli F (2003) Mechano-electric feedback and atrial fibrillation. Prog Biophys Mol Biol 82:137-149

34. Skanes AC, Mandapati R, Berenfeld O et al (1998) Spatiotemporal periodicity during atrial fibrillation in the isolated sheep heart. Circulation 98:1236-1248

35. Gaita F, Calo L, Riccardi R et al (2001) Different patterns of atrial activation in idiopathic atrial fibrillation: simultaneous multisite atrial mapping in patients with paroxysmal and chronic atrial fibrillation. J Am Coll Cardiol 37:534-541

36. Ravelli F, Faes L, Sandrini L et al (2005) Wave-similarity mapping shows the spatiotemporal distribution of fibrillatory wave complexity in the human right atrium during paroxysmal and chronic atrial fibrillation. J Cardiovasc Electrophysiol 16:1071-1076

37. Faes L, Nollo G, Antolini R et al (2002) A method for quantifying atrial fibrillation organization based on wave morphology similarity. IEEE Trans Biomed Eng 49:1504-1513

38. Nademanee K, McKenzie J, Kosar E et al (2004) A new approach for catheter ablation of atrial fibrillation: mapping of the electrophysiologic substrate. J Am Coll Cardiol 43:2044-2053

39. Sanders P, Berenfeld O, Hocini M et al (2005) Spectral analysis identifies sites of high-frequency activity maintaining atrial fibrillation in humans. Circulation 112:789-797

40. Delise P (2004) Fibrillazione atriale parossistica e persistente. Profilassi. In: Le aritmie: Diagnosi, prognosi e terapia. Delise P (ed) Casa Editrice Scientifica Internazionale Publ, Rome, pp 654-656

41. The AFFIRM Investigators (2003) Maintenance of sinus rhythm in patients with atrial fibrillation. An AFFIRM substudy of the first antiarrhythmic drug. J Am Coll Card 42:20-29

42. Lafuente-Lafuente C, Mouly S, Longas Tejero MA et al (2006) Antiarrhythmic drugs for maintaining sinus rhythm after cardioversion of atrial fibrillation. Arch Intern Med 166:719-728

43. The Atrial Fibrillation Follow-up Investigation of Rhythm Management (AFFIRM) Investigators (2002) A comparison of rate control and rhythm control in patients with atrial fibrillation. N Engl J Med 347:1825-1833

44. The AFFIRM Investigators (2004) Relationships between sinus rhythm, treatment, and survival in the Atrial Fibrillation Follow-up Investigation of Rhythm Management (AFFIRM) Study. Circulation 109:1509-1513

45. Hagens VE, Ranchor AV, Van Sonderen E et al (2004) Effect of rate or rhythm control on quality of life in persistent atrial fibrillation. Results from the rate control versus electrical cardioversion (RACE) study. J Am Coll Cardiol 43:241-247

46. Cox JL, Schuessler RB, D'Agostino Jr HJ et al (1991) The surgical treatment of atrial fibrillation. III. Development of a definitive surgical procedure. J Thorac Cardiovasc Surg 101:569-583

47. Jaïs P, Weerasooriya R, Shah DC et al (2002) Ablation therapy for atrial fibrillation: past, present and future. Cardiovasc Res 54:337-346

48. Gillinov AM, McCarthy PM, Marrouche N et al (2003) Contemporary surgical treatment for atrial fibrillation. Pacing Clin Electrophysiol 26:1641-1644

49. Cox JL, Schuessler RB, Lappas DG et al (1996) An 81/2-year clinical experience with surgery for atrial fibrillation.Ann Surg 224:267-275

50. Swartz JF, Pellersels G, Silvers J et al (1994) A catheter-based curative approach to atrial fibrillation in humans. Circulation 90(4 Part 2):I-335

51. Haïssaguerre M, Gencel L, Fischer B et al (1994) Successful catheter ablation of atrial fibrillation. J Cardiovasc Electrophysiol 5:1045-1052

52. Haïssaguerre M, Jaïs P, Shah DC et al (1996) Right and left atrial radiofrequency catheter therapy of paroxysmal atrial fibrillation. J Cardiovasc Electrophysiol 12:1132-1144

53. Jaïs P, Haïssaguerre M, Shah DC et al (1997) A focal source of atrial fibrillation treated by discrete radiofrequency ablation. Circulation 95:572-575

54. Saito T, Waki K, Becker AE (2000) Left atrial myocardial extension onto pulmonary veins in humans: anatomic observations relevant for atrial arrhythmias. J Cardiovasc Electrophysiol 11:888-894

55. Ho SY, Cabrera JA, Tran VH et al (2001) Architecture of the pulmonary veins: relevance to radiofrequency ablation. Heart 86:265-270

56. Haïssaguerre M, Jaïs P, Shah DC et al (2000) Electrophysiological end point for catheter ablation of atrial fibrillation initiated from multiple pulmonary venous foci. Circulation 101:1409-1417

57. Chen SA, Hsieh MH, Tai CT et al (1999) Initiation of atrial fibrillation by ectopic beats originating from the pulmonary veins. Circulation 100:1879-1886

58. Haïssaguerre M, Shah DC, Jaïs P et al (2000) Electrophysiological breakthroughs from the left atrium to the pulmonary veins. Circulation 102:2463-2465

59. Pappone C, Oreto G, Lamberti F et al (1999) Catheter ablation of paroxysmal atrial fibrillation using a 3D mapping system. Circulation 100:1203-1208

60. Pappone C, Oreto G, Rosanio S et al (2001) Atrial electroanatomical remodeling after circumferential radiofrequency pulmonary vein ablation. Circulation 104:2539-2544

61. Kato R, Lickfett L, Meininger G et al (2003) Pulmonary vein anatomy in patients undergoing catheter ablation of atrial fibrillation. Lessons learned by use of magnetic resonance imaging. Circulation 107:2004-2010

62. Scharf C, Sneider M, Case I et al (2003) Anatomy of the pulmonary veins in patients with atrial fibrillation and effects of segmental ostial ablation analyzed by computed tomography. J Cardiovasc Electrophysiol 14:150-155

63. Schwartzman D, Lacomis J, Wigginton WG (2003) Characterization of left atrium and distal pulmonary vein morphology using multidimensional computed tomography. J Am Coll Cardiol 41:1349-1357

64. Centonze M, Del Greco M, Nollo G et al (2005) The role of multidetector CT in the evaluation of the left atrium and pulmonary veins anatomy before and after radio-frequency catheter ablation for atrial fibrillation. Preliminary results and work in progress. Radiol Med 110:52-60

65. Del Greco M, Nollo G, Cristoforetti A et al (2005) Integration of electroanatomic mapping and multidetector computed tomography as a guide for atrial fibrillation catheter ablation. Europace 7(Suppl 1):941 P

66. Cappato R, Calkins H, Chen SA et al (2005) Worldwide survey on the methods, efficacy and safety of catheter ablation for human atrial fibrillation. Circulation 111:1100-1105

67. Verma A, Natale A (2005) Should atrial fibrillation ablation be considered first-line therapy for some patients? Circulation 112:1214-1231

68. Pappone C, Oral H, Santinelli V et al (2004) Atrio-esophageal fistula as a complication of percutaneous transcatheter ablation of atrial fibrillation. Circulation 109:2724-2726

69. Scanavacca MI, D'Avila A, Parga J, Sosa E (2004) Left atrial-esophageal fistula following radiofrequency catheter ablation of atrial fibrillation. J Cardiovasc Electrophysiol 15:960-962

70. Pai RK, Boyle NG, Child JS, Shivukmar K (2005) Transient left recurrent laryngeal nerve palsy following catheter ablation of atrial fibrillation. Heart Rhythm 2:182-184

71. Mansour M, Mela T, Ruskin J, Keane D (2004) Successful release of entrapped circumferential mapping catheters in patients undergoing pulmonary vein isolation for atrial fibrillation. Heart Rhythm 1:558-561

72. Tada H, Naito S, Oshima S, Taniguchi K (2005) Vasospastic angina shortly after left atrial catheter ablation for atrial fibrillation.Heart Rhythm 2:867-870

73. Takahashi Y, Jaïs P, Hocini M et al (2005) Acute occlusion of the left circumflex coronary artery during mitral isthmus linear ablation. J Cardiovasc Electrophysiol 16:1104-1107

74. Park H, Cho S, Kim K, Cho J (2005) Disseminated intravascular coagulation as a complication of radiofrequency catheter ablation of atrial fibrillation. J Cardiovasc Electrophysiol 16:1011-1013

75. Nilsson B, Chen X, Pehrson S et al (2005) Increased resting heart rate following radiofrequency catheter ablation for atrial fibrillation. Europace 7:415-420

76. Lickfett L, Mahesh M, Vasamreddy C et al (2004) Radiation exposure during catheter ablation of atrial fibrillation. Circulation 110:3003-3010

77. Disertori M, Alboni P, Botto G et al (2006) Linee Guida AIAC 2006 sul trattamento della fibrillazione atriale. GIAC 9:1-71

78. Pappone C, Rosanio S, Augello G et al (2003) Mortality, morbidity, and quality of life after circumferential pulmonary vein ablation for atrial fibrillation: outcomes from a controlled nonrandomized long-term study. J Am Coll Cardiol 42:185-197

79. Wazni OM, Marrouche N, Martin DO et al (2005) Radiofrequency ablation vs antiarrhythmic drugs as first-line treatment of symptomatic atrial fibrillation. JAMA 293:2634-2640

80. Stabile G, Bertaglia E, Senatore G et al (2006) Catheter ablation treatment in patients with drugrefractory atrial fibrillation: a prospective,multi-centre, randomized, controlled study (Catheter Ablation for the Cure of Atrial Fibrillation Study). Eur Heart J 27:216-221

81. Oral H, Pappone C, Chugh A et al (2006) Circumferential pulmonary-vein ablation for chronic atrial fibrillation. N Engl J Med 354:934-941

82. Fuster V, Ryden LE, Cannom DS et al (2006) ACC/AHA/ESC 2006 Guidelines for the Management of Patients with Atrial Fibrillation: a report of the American College of Cardiology/American Heart Association Task Force on Practice Guidelines and the European Society of Cardiology Committee for Practice Guidelines (Writing Committee to Revise the 2001 Guidelines for the Management of Patients With Atrial Fibrillation): developed in collaboration with the European Heart Rhythm Association and the Heart Rhythm Society. Circulation 114:e257-354

Section III

CT Semeiology

Heart Anatomy

10

Ludovico La Grutta, Giovanni Gentile, Giuseppe Runza, Massimo Galia, Filippo Cademartiri, and Massimo Midiri

10.1 Introduction

The anatomy of the heart and the coronary arteries should be nowadays a part of the standard cultural background of the radiologist. Nonetheless, the use of increasingly advanced imaging modalities has brought cardiac imaging into routine clinical practice.

The introduction of multidetector computed tomography (MDCT) scanners with elevated spatial and temporal resolution has led to the addition of ECG-gated MDCT coronary angiography among the techniques for evaluating coronary arteries and heart anatomy in selected patient populations with appropriated clinical criteria of application [1-4]. The state of the art of cardiac CT angiography technology consists of 64-slice generation, characterized by spatial resolution tending to voxel isotropy (~0.4 mm^3) and a gantry rotation time of 0.33 s (the effective temporal resolution with a 180° acquisition is 165 ms). The image quality for the visualization of the entire coronary tree is excellent, with very high sensitivity (86-99%) and negative predictive value (98-99%) in detecting significant coronary stenosis [5-7]. However, technology developments such as increasing number of slices, dual source systems, novel detector technology associated with sophisticated reconstruction algorithms, has improved spatial and temporal resolution, with a significant radiation dose reduction [8-10].

This chapter provides the basis for the study of the heart and the coronary artery tree with MDCT coronary angiography.

10.2 Cardiac Anatomy

The heart is an organ prevalently made up of smooth muscle situated in the thoracic cage cavity between the two lungs (Fig. 10.1), in a compartment known as the mediastinum and contained in a fibrous sac called the pericardium. The pericardium is a double-walled sac, made up of two thin layers (parietal and visceral) delimiting a virtual cavity, lubricated with fluid (Figs. 10.2, 10.3). The heart is a hollow organ divided into four chambers, two atria and two ventricles, divided into two atrioventricular pumps independent of each other (right and left heart separated by interatrial and interventricular septa), but in communication by valves. Between the two atrioventricular pumps is the pulmonary and systemic circulation.

The surface anatomy of the heart is described by an anterior or sternocostal surface, a posterior or diaphragmatic surface, a base which faces posteriorly and is in relation to the large vessels of the pulmonary and systemic circulation, an apex formed by the left inferolateral part of the left ventricle, and two borders, an acute right border and an oblique left border. An atrioventricular groove running transversally separates the atrial from the ventricular portion. The groove is visible on the posteroinferior surface for its entire length, whereas on the anterior surface it is partly hidden by the origin of the pulmonary artery and the aortic root. Two complete interventricular grooves (anterior and posterior) running longitudinally on the sternocostal and diaphragmatic surfaces mark the margins of the two ventricles (Fig. 10.4).

The heart is a pump which circulates the blood in the vessels by the pulmonary and systemic circulations. Systemic venous blood arrives at the heart from the superior and inferior vena cava which terminate respectively on the superior and inferior wall of the right atrium, and from here via the tricuspid valve the blood reaches the right ventricle. During systole the blood is pumped through the pulmonary valve into the pulmonary artery which conveys it to the pulmonary circu-

L. La Grutta (✉)
DIBIMEF, Department of Radiology,
"P. Giaccone" University Hospital,
Palermo, Italy

F. Cademartiri, G. Casolo, M. Midiri (eds.), *Clinical Applications of Cardiac CT*,
© Springer-Verlag Italia 2012

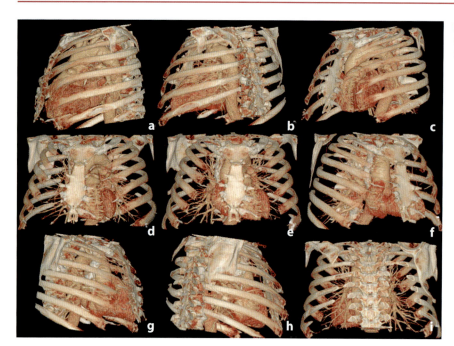

Fig. 10.1 Volume rendering images from different views (**a-i**) of the heart, located in the middle of the thorax

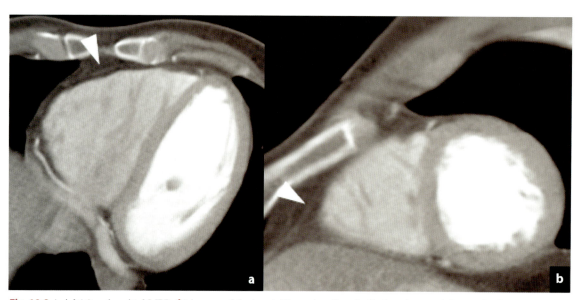

Fig. 10.2 Axial (**a**) and sagittal MPR (**b**) images of the heart. The pericardium is displayed as a subtle anterior layer (*arrowhead*)

lation (Fig. 10.5). Oxygenated blood then returns from the pulmonary circulation to the heart by the pulmonary veins (normally 4, but variable from 3 to 5), which drain into the left atrium (Figs. 10.5, 10.6), and from here through the mitral valve (Fig. 10.7) the blood reaches the left ventricle [11].

During systole the blood is pumped again through the aortic valve (Fig. 10.8) into the systemic circulation (Figs. 10.9, 10.10). The aortic valve is normally tricuspid (with three leaflets), although in 1% of the population it is found to be congenitally bicuspid (with two leaflets) (Fig. 10.11) [12]. The papillary muscles are located in the ventricles. They attach to the leaflets of the atrioventricular valves via the tendinous cords and contract to prevent inversion or prolapse of valves (Fig. 10.12).

The ascending aorta gives rise to two collateral branches, the coronary arteries, which supply the heart (Figs. 10.13, 10.14). The cardiac veins in contrast are tributaries of the coronary sinus (CS) which drains into the right atrium (Fig. 10.15).

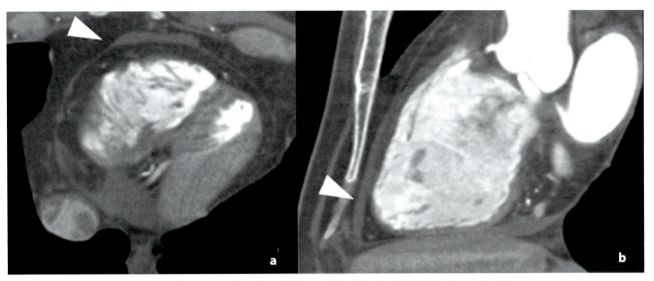

Fig. 10.3 Axial (**a**) and sagittal MPR (**b**) images of the heart display a minimal pericardial effusion (*arrowhead*)

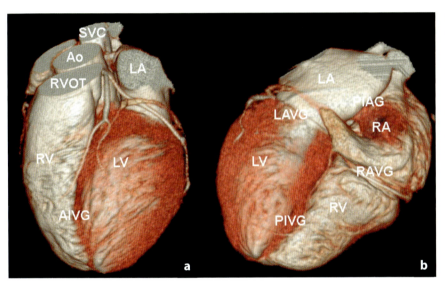

Fig. 10.4 Volume rendering images in anterior (**a**) and posterior (**b**) views depict the two complete longitudinal grooves: the anterior and posterior interventricular grooves, respectively. *SVC*, superior vena cava; *Ao*, ascending aorta; *RA*, right atrium; *RV*, right ventricle; *RVOT*, right ventricular outflow tract; *LA*, left atrium; *LV*, left ventricle; *AIVG*, anterior interventricular groove; *LAVG*, left atrioventricular groove; *PIAG*, posterior interatrial groove; *RAVG*, right atrioventricular groove; *PIVG*, posterior interventricular groove

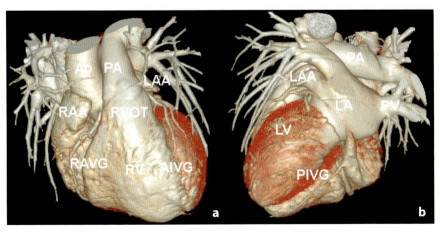

Fig. 10.5 Volume rendering images in anterior (**a**) and posterior (**b**) views display the pulmonary arterial and venous circulation. *Ao*, ascending aorta; *RAA*, right atrial appendage; *RV*, right ventricle; *RVOT*, right ventricular outflow tract; *LAA*, left atrial appendage; *LA*, left atrium; *LV*, left ventricle; *RAVG*, right atrioventricular groove; *AIVG*, anterior interventricular groove; *PIVG*, posterior interventricular groove; *PA*, pulmonary artery; *PV*, pulmonary vein

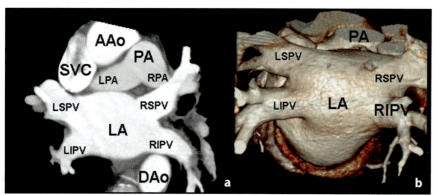

Fig. 10.6 MIP (**a**) and volume rendering images (**b**) display the left atrium and the pulmonary arterial and venous circulation. *SVC*, superior vena cava; *PA*, pulmonary artery; *AAo*, ascending aorta; *DAo*, descending aorta; *LA*, left atrium; *LPA*, left pulmonary artery; *RPA*, right pulmonary artery; *LSPV*, left superior pulmonary vein; *RSPV*, right superior pulmonary vein; *LIPV*, left inferior pulmonary vein; *RIPV*, right inferior pulmonary vein

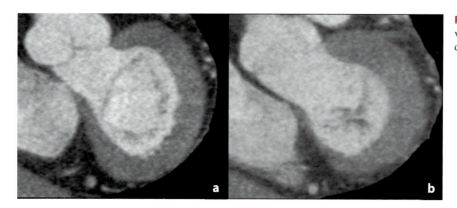

Fig. 10.7 MPR images depict the mitral valve, open during diastole (**a**) and closed during systole (**b**)

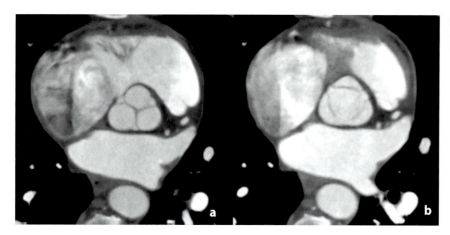

Fig. 10.8 MPR images depict the tricuspid aortic valve, closed during diastole (**a**) and open during systole (**b**)

10.3 Classification of Coronary Segments

The coronary segmentation classification recommended by the American Heart Association (AHA) can be used to create a MDCT reporting system as close as possible to that used in conventional coronary angiography, thus facilitating communication between the radiologist and the referring physicians (cardiologists or cardiac surgeons). The AHA classification divides the coronary arteries in to 15 or 16 segments (Figs. 10.13, 10.14, 10.16) [13-15].

The right coronary artery (RCA), which extends to the crux, is conventionally divided into three segments: the proximal (segment 1), the mid (segment 2), and the distal (segment 3), which runs in the posterior right atrioventricular groove from the acute margin of the heart to the origin of the posterior descending branch (PD). The PD runs in the posterior interventricular groove and is indicated as segment 4a; the posterolateral (PL) branch

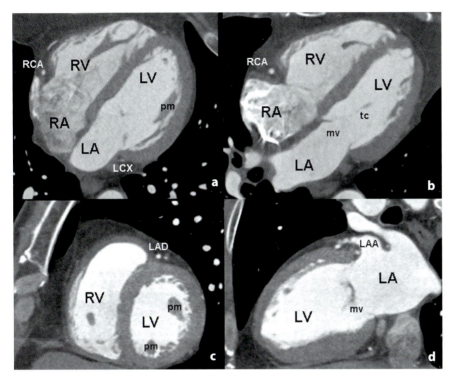

Fig. 10.9 Standard MPR images in different views: four-chamber-view (**a**, **b**), two-chamber-view short-axis (**c**) and long-axis view (**d**) images. *RCA*, right coronary artery; *RV*, right ventricle; *LV*, left ventricle; *pm*, papillary muscles; *RA*, right atrium; *LA*, left atrium; *LCX*, left circumflex coronary artery; *LAD*, left anterior descending coronary artery; *mv*, mitral valve; *tc*, tendinous cords; *LAA*, left atrial appendage

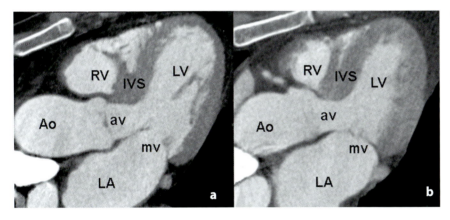

Fig. 10.10 MPR images in aortic and mitral valve plane of the heart during diastole (**a**) and systole (**b**). *Ao*, aorta; *LA*, left atrium; *LV*, left ventricle, *RV*, right ventricle; *IVS*, interventricular septum; *av*, aortic valve; *mv*, mitral valve

may be indicated as segment 4b.

The left main coronary artery (LM, segment 5) extends from the ostium of the left coronary artery (LCA) to the bifurcation in left anterior descending (LAD) and left circumflex (LCX) branches. The LAD, which runs in the anterior interventricular groove, is conventionally divided into: the proximal tract (segment 6), including the origin of the first diagonal branch (segment 9); the mid tract (segment 7), which extends to include the point where the LAD forms an angle and generally it coincides with the second diagonal branch (segment 10); the distal or apical tract (segment 8), which extends beyond the apex.

The LCX is divided into proximal (segment 11 including the origin of the first obtuse marginal branch) and distal tracts (segment 13 running in the left atrioventricular groove). The branches for the obtuse margin of the heart which supply the lateral wall of the left ventricle are called segment 12 (the first and the largest branch of the LCX) and segment 14 (the second marginal branch, which supplies the posterolateral face of the left ventricle). Segment 15, if present, identifies the PL branch which arises from the LCX. Segment 16 indicates a possible additional branch known as the "intermediate" (IM) which originates from the LM and runs along the anterolateral wall of the left ventricle.

The authors of the BARI trial (Bypass Angioplasty Revascularization Investigation) presented a different

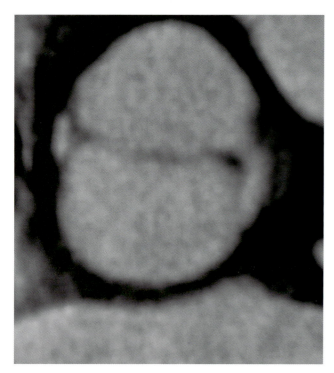

Fig. 10.11 MPR image of a bicuspid aortic valve

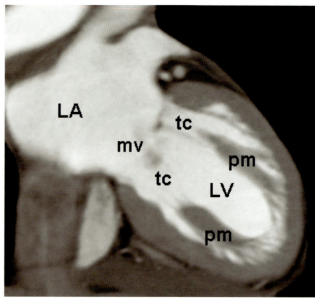

Fig. 10.12 Two-chambers long-axis view MIP image of the heart. *LA*, left atrium; *LV*, left ventricle; *mv*, mitral valve; *pm*, papillary muscles; *tc*, tendinous cords

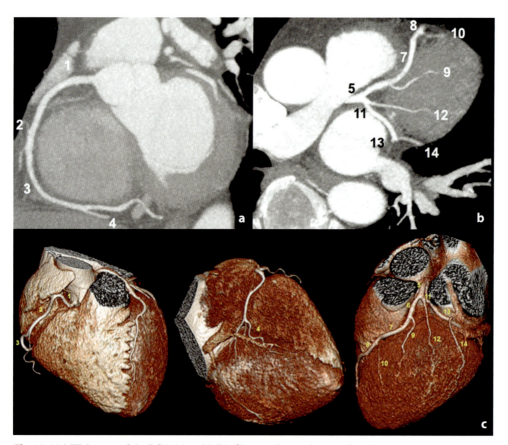

Fig. 10.13 MIP images of the RCA (**a**) and LCA (**b**) according to the American Heart Association classification [14]. Volume rendering images which more effectively depict the anatomy and the same classification of the RCA and LCA (**c**)

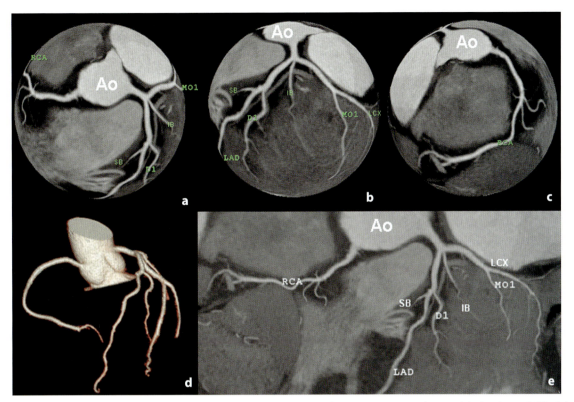

Fig. 10.14 Globe views (**a-c**), vessel-tree isolation volume rendering (**d**) and coronary map images (**e**). *Ao*, Aorta; *RCA*, right coronary artery; *LAD*, left anterior descending coronary artery; *D1*, first diagonal branch; *LCX*, left circumflex coronary artery; *MO1*, first marginal branch; *IB*, intermediate branch; *SB*, septal branch

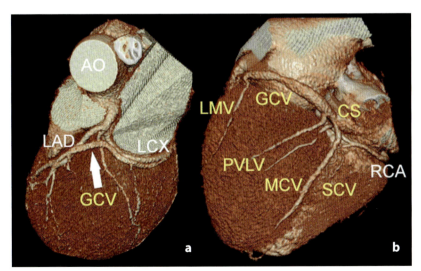

Fig. 10.15 Volume rendering images in anterior (**a**) and posterior (**b**) views of the heart depicting the cardiac vein anatomy. *Ao*, aorta; *LAD*, left anterior descending coronary artery; *LCX*, left circumflex coronary artery; *GCV*, great cardiac vein; *CS*, coronary sinus; *LMV*, left marginal vein; *PVLV*, posterior vein of left ventricle; *SCV*, small cardiac veins; *MCV*, middle cardiac vein; *RCA*, right coronary artery

and more detailed classification system of the coronary tree in 29 segments (Fig. 10.17; Table 10.1) [16]. The classification more analytically considers the different anatomy of the vessels according to the coronary dominance (right, left or mixed) [17-19].

10.4 MDCT Anatomy and Coronary Arteries

The major branches of the coronary arteries generally run on the surface of the epicardium. The septal branch-

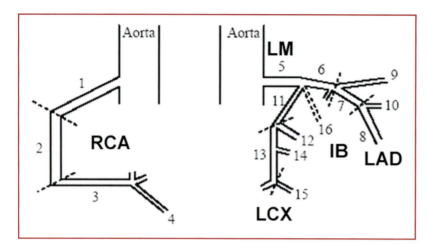

Fig. 10.16 Classification of coronary artery segments according to the American Heart Association [14]

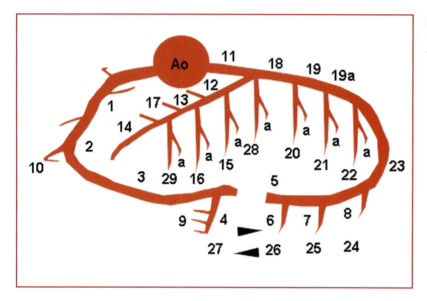

Fig. 10.17 Map of the coronary tree divided into 29 segments according to the BARI classification. *Ao*, aorta. (Adapted from [16], with permission)

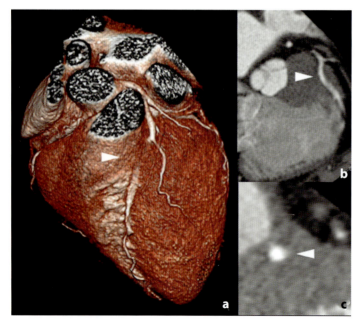

Fig. 10.18 Myocardial bridging (*arrowhead*) of the LAD depicted by volume rendering (**a**), MPR (**b**) and cross-sectional MPR images (**c**). *LAD*, left anterior descending coronary artery

Table 10.1 BARI Classification (Bypass Angioplasty Revascularization Investigation): table of coronary artery segments and corresponding map location. (Reproduced from [16], with permission)

Segment	Map location
1	Proximal RCA
2	Mid RCA
3	Distal RCA
4	Right PD
5	Right posterior AV
6	First right PL
7	Second right PL
8	Third right PL
9	PD septal perforators
10	Acute marginal segment(s)
11	LM
12	Proximal LAD
13	Mid LAD
14	Distal LAD
15	First diagonal branch
15a	Lateral diagonal branch
16	Second diagonal branch
16a	Lateral second diagonal branch
17	LAD septal perforators
18	Proximal LCX
19	Mid LCX
19a	Distal LCX
20	First OM
20a	Lateral first OM
21	Second OM
21a	Lateral second OM
22	Third OM
22a	Lateral third OM
23	LCX AV groove continuation segment
24	First left PL branch
25	Second left PL branch
26	Third left PL branch
27	Left PD segment
28	IM branch
28a	Lateral IM branch
29	Third diagonal branch
29a	Lateral third diagonal branch

RCA, right coronary artery; *PD*, posterior descending branch; *PL*, posterolateral branch; *LM*, left main coronary artery; *LAD*, left anterior descending artery; *LCX*, left circumflex coronary artery; *OM*, obtuse marginal branch; *AV*, atrioventricular; *IM*, intermediate branch.

es, which arise in a variable number from the LAD and PD, instead run along the inside of the myocardial muscle. Occasionally major coronary branches can also congenitally run intramurally through the myocardium (myocardial bridging, Fig. 10.18) [20, 21].

The measurement of the proximal diameters of the major coronary arteries in MDCT coronary angiography well correlates with measurements made with intravascular ultrasound and conventional angiography [22]. The LM measures 4.5±0.5 mm, the proximal LAD 3.7±0.4 mm, and the distal LAD 1.9±0.4 mm. The diameter of the LAD is not influenced by anatomic dominance, whereas the diameter of the RCA varies from 3.9±0.6 mm to 2.8±0.5 mm and the LCX varies from 3.4±0.5 mm to 4.2±0.6 mm according to right or left dominance. The diameter is not influenced by the age or the tortuosity of the vessel [23]. However, it may be affected by gender (female -9%) and myocardial diseases (left ventricular hypertrophy +17%; dilative cardiomyopathy +12%).

10.4.1 Right Coronary Artery

The RCA (Figs. 10.13a, 10.19) arises from the right coronary sinus (RCS). The RCA follows the atrioventricular groove, encircling the annulus of the tricuspid valve in a mirror image of the LCX to then reach the crux (segments 1, 2, and 3). Distally, the RCA (segment 3) continues towards the crux in the posterodorsal portion of the atrioventricular groove, in contact with the diaphragm. The PD is a branch of the RCA which runs from the base of the heart to the apex, in a mirror image of the LAD. Several septal branches arise from the PD and supply the posterior third of the interventricular septum.

10.4.2 Left Coronary Artery

Generally the LCA arises from the left coronary sinus (LCS) as the LM (segment 5) (Figs. 10.13b, 10.19) and in most cases bifurcates below the left appendage into the LAD and LCX.

The LAD passes to the left of the main pulmonary artery and continues anteriorly in the anterior interventricular groove to the apex of the heart. The LAD gives rise to two groups of branches: the diagonal (segments 9 and 10) and the septal branches. The diagonal branches generally supply the anterior wall of the left ventricle; the septal branches originate at right angles from the ventral portion of the LAD, are of smaller diameter than the diagonal branches, and supply the anterior two thirds of the interventricular septum. The terminal tract of the LAD (segment 8) encircles the apex of the heart and supplies the inferior portion of the left ventricle.

The LCX, which is usually of smaller diameter than the LAD, runs posteriorly shortly after its origin and follows the left atrioventricular groove, encircling the annulus of the mitral valve (segments 11 and 13). The LCX

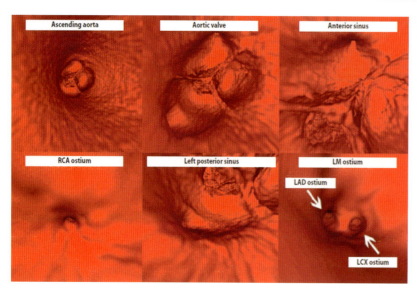

Fig. 10.19 Virtual angioscopy reconstructions from the ascending aorta up to the left posterior and anterior coronary sinuses of Valsalva. The ostia of the right coronary artery (*RCA*), the left main coronary artery (*LM*), the bifurcation of the left anterior descending coronary artery (*LAD*) and the left circumflex coronary artery (*LCX*) are depicted (*arrows*)

gives rise to several branches defined marginal (or branches for the obtuse cardiac margin; segments 12 and 14), which can have a considerable diameter and supply the lateral wall of the left ventricle.

10.5 Anatomic Variants of the Coronary Arteries

The anatomic variants of the coronary tree are extremely numerous and frequent. With the use of different postprocessing techniques (multiplanar reconstructions, curved multiplanar images, maximum intensity projections and volume rendering) MDCT coronary angiography is able to thoroughly visualize the complex and variable anatomy of the coronary arteries and provide valid support to the interventional cardiologist and cardiac surgeon [24]. Detailed knowledge of the normal coronary anatomy and its variants is therefore essential for the radiologist who is approaching MDCT cardiac imaging. The presence of coronary artery tree variants, which may be clinically significant, must be included in the report.

Angelini et al. [25] have developed a system for defining anatomic variability of the coronary tree. Any morphologic characteristic observed in more than 1% of a sample of randomly selected individuals is defined as normal, a normal variant is a relatively unusual morphologic feature encountered in more than 1% of the same sample, and anomaly is a condition observed in less than 1% of individuals [25].

Coronary dominance indicates which system of coronary vessels supplies the inferolateral wall of the left ventricle [17, 18]. In 80-90% of the population the PD is a branch of the RCA and runs from the base to the apex of the heart in a mirror image of the LAD. When coronary dominance is right-sided the RCA gives rise to a right posterolateral branch (RPL), which passing over the crux (the meeting point between the posterior interventricular groove and the posterior atrioventricular groove, i.e. the CS) continues on the left half of the heart following the homolateral atrioventricular groove and supplying the dorsal wall of the left ventricle (Fig. 10.20a). The RPL can be of considerable importance when the LCX is occluded, because it can uphold the supply to the posteroinferior wall of the left ventricle. When coronary dominance is left-sided, the LCX continues to the crux giving rise to the left posterolateral branch (LPL) and at times the PD (Fig. 10.20b).

The first branch of the RCA is the conus, which runs along the anterolateral surface of the right ventricular outflow tract. In a small percentage of cases this branch originates from the ostium of the RCA or separately from the aortic root (Fig. 10.21). The sinus node can have a variable vascularization: from the second branch which originates from the RCA, called the sinus node artery; from a proximal branch of the LCX; from both arteries (Fig. 10.22). Other branches for the right atrium and ventricle can be observed along the course of the RCA. In a small percentage of cases the RCA can give rise to a large branch which runs along the acute margin of the heart until continuing with the PD. Occasionally the RCA trifurcates at the crux giving rise to two branches (double PD) for the vascularization of the base of the heart and a RPL for the vascularization of the dorsal wall of the left ventricle.

The length of the LM in most cases is 1-2 cm, even though shorter segments are not uncommon, although longer ones are more rare (Fig. 10.23) [26]. In one third of cases the LM may divide into three or four branches with the presence of one or two additional intermediate

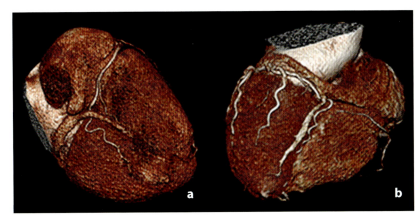

Fig. 10.20 Volume rendering images. In 90% of the population the RCA supplies the posterior wall of the left ventricle (right dominance, **a**), while in the remaining cases this wall is supplied by the LCX (left dominance, **b**). *RCA*, right coronary artery; *LCX*, left circumflex coronary artery

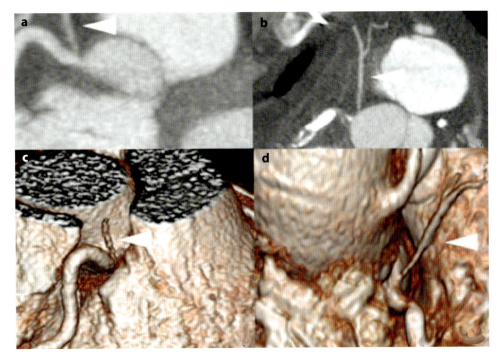

Fig. 10.21 The conus artery (*arrowhead*) is the first branch of the RCA (MIP reconstruction in **a** and volume rendering in **c**). Alternatively it can arise separately from the ascending aorta near the ostium of the RCA (MIP reconstruction in **b** and volume rendering in **d**). *RCA*, right coronary artery

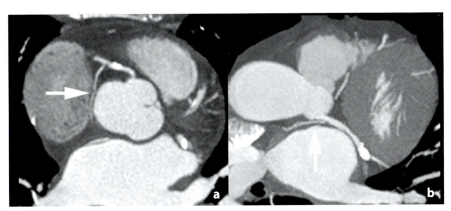

Fig. 10.22 MIP reconstruction. The sinus node artery (*arrow*) is the second branch of the RCA (**a**). In **b** the sinus node is supplied by a proximal branch of the LCX. *RCA*, right coronary artery; *LCX*, left circumflex coronary artery

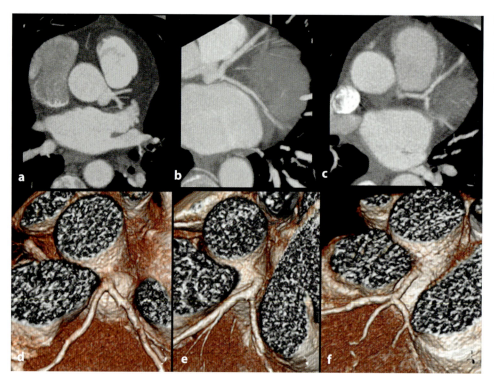

Fig. 10.23 MIP reconstructions (**a-c**) and corresponding volume rendering images (**d-f**) of the LM. The LM may vary in length from some millimeters to more than 2 cm. *LM*, left main coronary artery

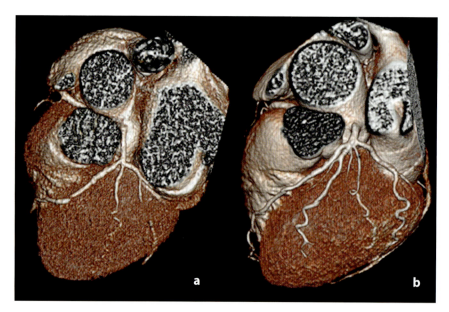

Fig. 10.24 Volume rendering image (**a, b**). In one third of cases the left main coronary artery trifurcates with variable arterial angulation and appearance: the intermediate branch (segment 16) runs along the anterolateral wall of the left ventricle

branches which run between the LAD and the LCX (Fig. 10.24) on the anterolateral wall of the left ventricle [27]. The diagonal branches of the LAD generally run towards the anterior wall of the left ventricle. Their number and course are variable, although at least one diagonal branch is usually present (Fig. 10.25). The marginal branches of the LCX can also vary in course and number (Fig. 10.26).

10.6 Coronary Artery Anomalies

According to literature, which is based on the findings of angiographies performed for suspected obstructive coronary artery disease, coronary artery anomalies (CAA) affect about 1.3% of the general population [28-30]. Many of these are clinically irrelevant and incidental

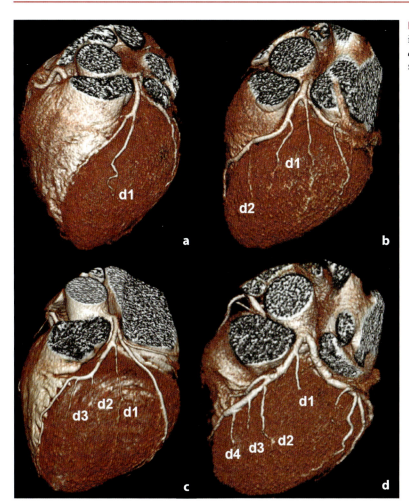

Fig. 10.25 Volume rendering images (**a-d**) depict increasing number of diagonal branches (*d1, d2, d3, d4*) with variable course. Absence of the LM with separate origin of LAD and LCX (**d**)

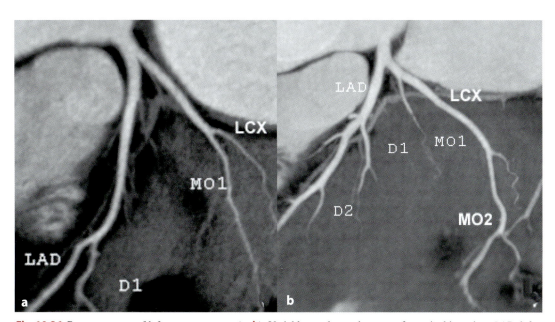

Fig. 10.26 Coronary maps of left coronary artery (**a**, **b**). Variable number and course of marginal branches. *LAD*, left anterior descending coronary artery; *LCX*, left circumflex coronary artery; *D*, diagonal branch; *MO*, marginal branch

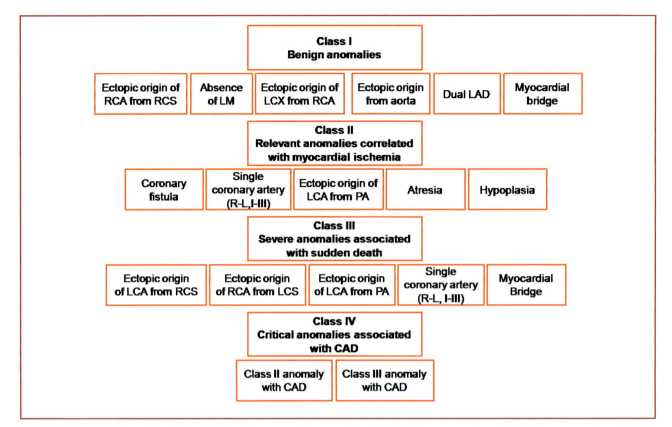

Fig. 10.27 Clinical relevance-based classification of coronary artery anomalies. *RCA*, right coronary artery; *RCS*, right coronary sinus; *LM*, left main coronary artery; *LCX*, left circumflex coronary artery; *LAD*, left anterior descending coronary artery; *LCA*, left coronary artery; *PA*, pulmonary artery; *LCS*, left sinus; *CAD*, coronary artery disease. (Modified from [31], with permission)

findings. However, those which are significant may induce angina pectoris, syncope, arrhythmias, myocardial infarction, sudden death and enhance the onset and progression of coronary atherosclerosis.

Several CAA are defined "malignant" due to their pathologic potential. Various anatomic and pathophysiologic classifications of CAA have been reported in the literature. The easiest classification used in clinical practice was proposed by Rigatelli et al. [31, 32]. To facilitate clinical management and follow-up, they divided CAA into four classes on the basis of clinical relevance (Fig. 10.27). The clinical classification is integrated with an anatomic classification (Tables 10.2, 10.3) which divides CAA on the basis of:
- origin (absence of the LM in Fig. 10.28, ectopic origin in Fig. 10.29);
- course (interarterial in Figs. 10.30, and 10.31, intraseptal in Fig. 10.32);
- intrinsic anatomy (aneurysm in Fig. 10.33, myocardial bridging in Fig. 10.18; dual LAD Fig. 10.34);
- anatomy of the termination (fistulas in Figs. 10.35-10.37) [31-33].

Interarterial course of a origin CAA is frequently associated with acute coronary syndromes and sudden death [34]. Patients with myocardial bridging may often develop coronary atherosclerosis in the segments proximal to the bridge [21].

With the integration of post-processing techniques, MDCT coronary angiography provides a much clearer visualization of CAA [35]. The radiologist therefore needs to be able to visualize and recognize the features which may have clinical relevance.

10.7 MDCT Angiography of the Cardiac Veins

During conventional coronary angiography the venous system can only be visualized in the late phase. Generally the venous system is not very evident unless its visualization is specifically desired. This can be achieved by optimizing the timing between contrast agent injection and the beginning of the angiographic scan. The visualization can be improved with delayed contrast administration by a variable period according to the scanner used. The great cardiac vein (GCV) may be

Table 10.2 Anomalies of origin and course. (Modified from [31], with permission)

Coronary artery anomaly	Anatomic finding		Clinical relevance
Absence of LM	LAD and LCX arise from two different ostia in LCS		Asymptomatic
Anomalous location of coronary ostium outside of normal coronary sinus	Origin from ascending Ao	Origin from proximal 2 cm of Ao	Possible iatrogenic complications
	Origin from non coronary sinus		Asymptomatic
	Origin from coronary sinuses	- LCA arising from RCS - LCX arising from RCS - LAD arising from RCS - RCA arising from LCS	Episodic myocardial ischemia Heart failure Sudden death
	Origin from PA (flow follows aortic -pulmonary pressure gradient)	Anomalous origin of the left coronary artery arising from the pulmonary artery (ALCAPA)	Episodic myocardial ischemia Congestive heart failure Sudden death
Ectopic origin of coronary ostium from opposite coronary sinus (either as main artery or with divided origin)	RCA arising from LCS with anomalous course: LCA arising from RCS with anomalous course	- Retrocardiac - Retroaortic - Interarterial (between Aorta and PA) - Intraseptal - Anterior to RVOT or precardiac	Potential compression of interarterial course may lead to episodic ischemia, myocardial infarction and sudden death
	Single coronary artery	R: ostium in RCS L: ostium in LCS I: Normal course of RCA or LCA II: Origin from proximal RCA or LCA III: LAD and LCX arise separately from proximal normal RCA	Episodic myocardial ischemia Sudden death
	LCX arising from RCS or from proximal RCA with anomalous course	- Posterior atrioventricular groove - Retroaortic	Asymptomatic. It may be incidentally compressed during valve substitution

RCA, right coronary artery; *LM*, left main coronary artery; *LCA*, left coronary artery; *LCX*, left circumflex artery; *LAD*, left anterior descending coronary artery; *LCS*, left coronary sinus; *RCS*, right coronary sinus; *Ao*, aorta; *PA*, pulmonary artery; *RVOT*, right ventricular outflow tract.

Table 10.3 Intrinsic anatomy and termination anomalies. (Modified from [31] with permission)

Coronary artery anomaly	Anatomic finding		Clinical relevance
Intrinsic anomaly	Stenosis or atresia of ostium (RCA, LCA, LAD, LCX)		Episodic myocardial ischemia at rest
	Hypoplasia		Episodic myocardial ischemia at rest
	Ectasia o aneurysm		Episodic myocardial ischemia
	Myocardial Bridge	Intramyocardial tunneling of epicardial coronary segments (proximal segments)	Episodic myocardial ischemia at-rest; increased risk of coronary artery disease
	Dual LAD (one short and another long artery)	- Type I: short LAD gives rise to septal branches; long LAD runs in AIVG and gives rise to diagonal branches - Type II: long LAD runs along the right ventricular surface before re-entering the AIVG - Type III: long LAD with intramyocardial course runs in the interventricular septum and gives rise to the septal branches; the diagonal branches arise from the short LAD - Type IV: long LAD arises from RCA; short LAD arises from the LM	Asymptomatic Misinterpretation during bypass grafting
Termination anomalies	Fistulas from RCA, LCA, or infundibular artery	Vessel arises from coronary artery branch and drains into a single chamber: right ventricle, right atrium, coronary sinus, superior vena cava, pulmonary artery, pulmonary vein, left atrium, left ventricle, multiple (right and/or left ventricle)	Episodic myocardial ischemia at-rest; right ventricular overload in the case of right ventricle fistula

RCA, right coronary artery; *LCA*, left coronary artery; *LCX*, left circumflex artery; *LAD*, left anterior descending coronary artery; *AIVG*, anterior interventricular groove.

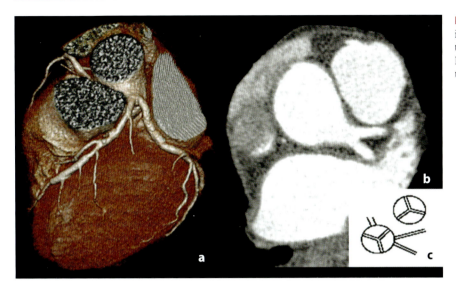

Fig. 10.28 Volume rendering (**a**) and MPR images (**b**) depicting the separate origin of the left anterior descending artery and the left circumflex artery. Schematic representation of the anomaly (**c**)

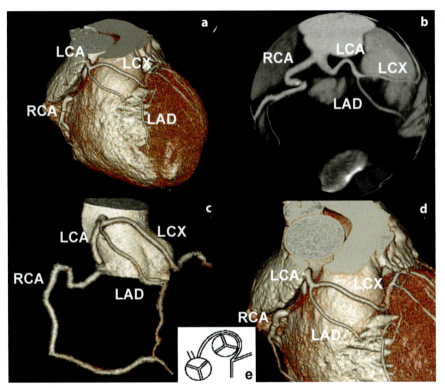

Fig. 10.29 Common origin of the entire coronary tree from the right coronary sinus of Valsalva. The LCA, which courses anteriorly, after a short tract bifurcates in LCX and LAD. The LAD reaches the anterior interventricular groove and runs along it to the apex of the heart. The LCX, which reaches and immediately terminates in the left atrioventricular groove, gives rise to several collateral branches which run along the lateral wall of the left ventricle. **a** Volume rendering image. **b** "Globe" view of the entire coronary tree. **c** Isolated coronary artery tree volume rendering. **d** Anomaly detail with volume rendering image. **e** Schematic representation of the anomaly. *RCA*, right coronary artery; *LCA*, left coronary artery; *LAD*, left anterior descending coronary artery; *LCX*, left circumflex coronary artery

visualized near the LCA bifurcation with a caudocranial scan (when the scan is performed in the craniocaudal direction the proximal venous tracts collect most of the contrast agent).

There are two main cardiac venous systems: the tributaries of the CS and the anterior cardiac veins. As in other regions of the human body, the veins tend to run parallel to the arteries [36]. The GCV drains the anterior two-thirds of the interventricular septum, arises from the apex of the heart and runs parallel to the LAD in the anterior interventricular groove up to the base of the heart. At the level of the origin of the LAD the GCV bends into the atrioventricular groove, where it runs parallel to the LCX, and from here drains into the CS. The CS continues parallel to the distal tract of the LCX and drains into the right atrium through the thebesian valve. The middle cardiac vein (MCV) arises in proximity to the apex of the heart, runs in the posterior interventricu-

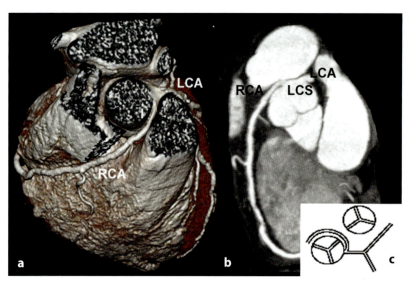

Fig. 10.30 Volume rendering (**a**) and MIP images (**b**) of the RCA with an anomalous origin from the left coronary sinus and interarterial course. This course is frequently associated with acute coronary syndromes. Schematic representation of the anomaly (**c**). *LCA*, left coronary artery; *RCA*, right coronary artery; *LCS*, left coronary sinus

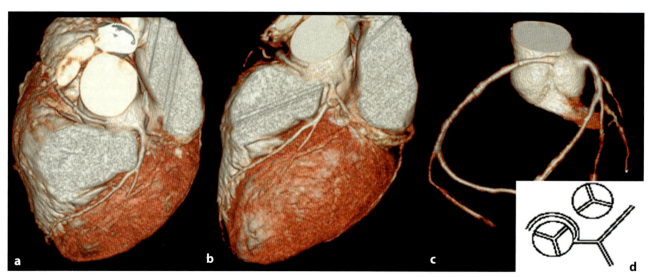

Fig. 10.31 Volume rendering (**a**, **b**), isolated tree (**c**), and schematic representation (**d**) of right coronary artery anomaly with origin from the left coronary sinus and interarterial course

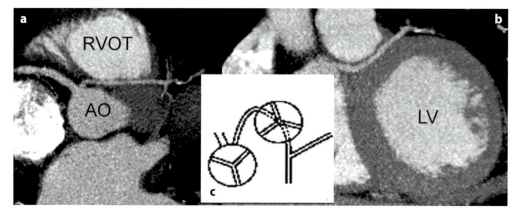

Fig. 10.32 Left coronary artery arising from the anterior coronary sinus of Valsalva and with intraseptal course. Curved MIP reconstructions of the anomalous left coronary artery in a para-axial (**a**) and oblique coronal (**c**) plane. Schematic representation of the anomaly (**b**). Upon reaching the anterior interventricular groove, it bifurcates in LAD and LCX. *RVOT*, right ventricular outflow tract; *Ao*, aorta; *LV*, left ventricle; *LAD*, left anterior descending coronary artery; *LCX*, left circumflex coronary artery

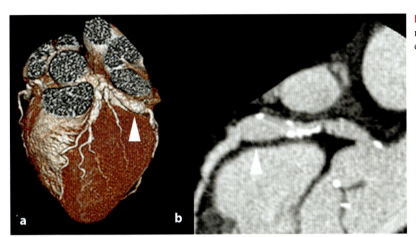

Fig. 10.33 Aneurysm of the left circumflex coronary artery (*arrowhead*) depicted with volume rendering (**a**) and MIP reconstructions (**b**), respectively

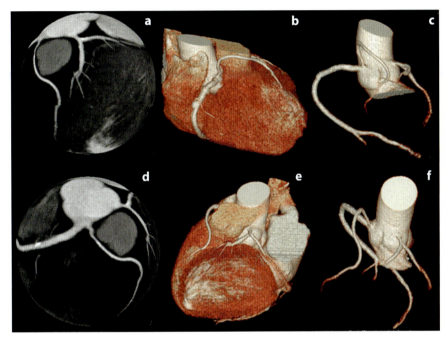

Fig. 10.34 Dual LAD depicted with globe view (**a**, **d**), volume rendering (**b**, **e**), and isolated coronary tree images (**c**, **f**). The short LAD arises from the LM; the long LAD arises from RCA and courses to the left side anterior to the right ventricular outflow tract (Type IV dual LAD). *LAD*, left anterior descending coronary artery; *LM*, left main coronary artery; *RCA*, right coronary artery

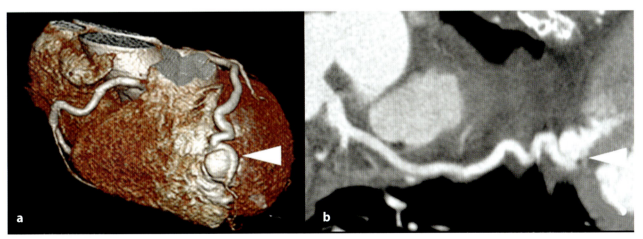

Fig. 10.35 Coronary fistula between the LAD and the right ventricle, depicted with volume rendering (**a**) and MIP reconstructions (**b**), respectively. *LAD*, left anterior descending coronary artery

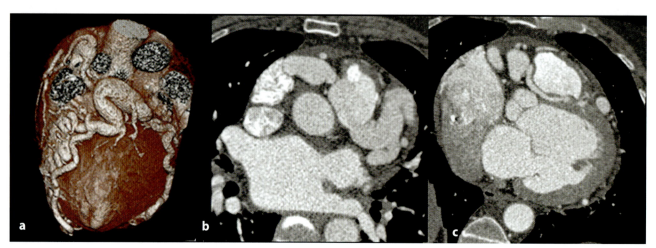

Fig. 10.36 Intrinsic anatomy and termination anomalies. Aneurysmal dilatation of the entire coronary artery tree visualized with volume rendering (**a**) and MPR reconstructions in different planes (**b**, **c**). LM is originating from the PA (**b**); an interarterial communication between the RCA and the LCA is observed (**c**). *LM*, left main coronary artery; *PA*, pulmonary artery; *RCA*, right coronary artery; *LCA*, left coronary artery

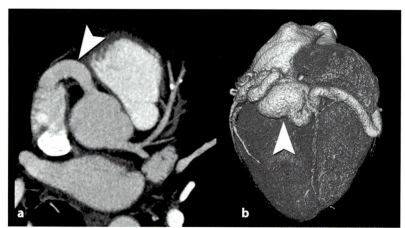

Fig. 10.37 Coronary fistula. MPR image in the oblique axial plane at the origin of the RCA and LCA from their respective coronary sinuses of Valsalva (**a**) and panoramic volume rendering image of the base of the heart (**b**). **a** depicts an anomalous ectasia of the proximal tract of the RCA (*arrowhead*). In **b**, the distal tract of the RCA with a tortuous course increases in diameter secondary to the communication with the cardiac venous circulation near the coronary sinus. *RCA*, right coronary artery; *LCA*, left coronary artery

lar groove and drains directly into the right atrium near the crux. In a minority of subjects it drains into the CS. Other small cardiac veins in variable number drain the lateral wall of the left ventricle and flow into the CS, between the GCV and the MCV. The anterior cardiac veins drain the circulation from the right ventricular wall to the right atrium via the atrial sinuses (Fig. 10.15).

10.8 Conclusions

MDCT provides detailed imaging of the heart anatomy and vessels thanks to its intrinsic ability to process volumetric data in an arbitrary number of planes in space. The consolidation of the technique and its widespread clinical application entail that the radiologist requires a thorough knowledge of cardiac and coronary artery anatomy.

References

1. Nieman K, Cademartiri F, Lemos PA et al (2002) Reliable noninvasive coronary angiography with fast submillimeter multislice spiral computed tomography. Circulation 106:2051-2054
2. Ropers D, Baum U, Pohle K et al (2003) Detection of coronary artery stenoses with thin-slice multidetector row spiral computed tomography and multiplanar reconstruction. Circulation 107:664-666
3. Schroeder S, Achenbach S, Bengel F et al (2008) Cardiac computed tomography: indications, applications, limitations, and training requirements: report of a Writing Group deployed by the Working Group Nuclear Cardiology and Cardiac CT of the European Society of Cardiology and the European Council of Nuclear Cardiology. Eur Heart J 29:531-556
4. Taylor AJ, Cerqueira M, Hodgson JM et al (2010) ACCF/SCCT/ACR/AHA/ASE/ASNC/NASCI/SCAI/SCMR 2010 Appropriate Use Criteria for Cardiac Computed Tomography: A Report of the American College of Cardiology Foundation Appropriate Use Criteria Task Force, the Society of Cardiovascular Computed Tomography, the American College of Radiology, the American Heart Association, the American Society of

Echocardiography, the American Society of Nuclear Cardiology, the North American Society for Cardiovascular Imaging, the Society for Cardiovascular Angiography and Interventions, and the Society for Cardiovascular Magnetic Resonance. Circulation. 122:e525-555

5. Mollet NR, Cademartiri F, van Mieghem CA et al (2005) High-resolution spiral computed tomography coronary angiography in patients referred for diagnostic conventional coronary angiography. Circulation 112:2318-2323

6. Leschka S, Alkadhi H, Plass A et al (2005) Accuracy of MSCT coronary angiography with 64-slice technology: first experience. Eur Heart J 26:1482-1487

7. Raff GL, Gallagher MJ, O'Neill WW, Goldstein JA (2005) Diagnostic accuracy of noninvasive coronary angiography using 64-slice spiral computed tomography. J Am Coll Cardiol 46:552-557

8. Korosoglou G, Mueller D, Lehrke S et al (2010) Quantitative assessment of stenosis severity and atherosclerotic plaque composition using 256-slice computed tomography. Eur Radiol. 20:1841-1850

9. Lell M, Marwan M, Schepis T et al (2009) Prospectively ECG-triggered high-pitch spiral acquisition for coronary CT angiography using dual source CT: technique and initial experience. Eur Radiol. 19:2576-2583

10. Einstein AJ, Elliston CD, Arai AE, et al (2010) Radiation dose from single-heartbeat coronary CT angiography performed with a 320-detector row volume scanner. Radiology 254:698-706

11. Centonze M, Del Greco M, Nollo G et al (2005) The role of multidetector CT in the evaluation of the left atrium and pulmonary veins anatomy before and after radio-frequency catheter ablation for atrial fibrillation. Preliminary results and work in progress. Technical note. Radiol Med. 110:52-60

12. Alkadhi H, Leschka S, Trindade PT et al (2010) Cardiac CT for the differentiation of bicuspid and tricuspid aortic valves: comparison with echocardiography and surgery. AJR Am J Roentgenol. 195:900-908

13. Luccichenti G, Cademartiri F, Pezzella FR et al (2005) 3D reconstruction techniques made easy: know-how and pictures. Eur Radiol 15:2146-2156

14. Austen WG, Edwards JE, Frye RL et al (1975) A reporting system on patients evaluated for coronary artery disease. Report of the Ad Hoc Committee for Grading of Coronary Artery Disease, Council on Cardiovascular Surgery, American Heart Association. Circulation 51:5-40

15. Detre KM, Wright E, Murphy ML, Takaro T (1975) Observer agreement in evaluating coronary angiograms. Circulation 52:979-986

16. Vander Salm TJ, Kip KE, Jones RH et al (2002) What constitutes optimal surgical revascularization? Answers from the Bypass Angioplasty Revascularization Investigation (BARI). J Am Coll Cardiol 39:565-572

17. Scanlon PJ, Faxon DP, Audet AM et al (1999) ACC/AHA guidelines for coronary angiography: executive summary and recommendations. A report of the American College of Cardiology/American Heart Association Task Force on Practice Guidelines (Committee on Coronary Angiography) developed in collaboration with the Society for Cardiac Angiography and Interventions. Circulation 99:2345-2357

18. Scanlon PJ, Faxon DP, Audet AM et al (1999) ACC/AHA guidelines for coronary angiography. A report of the Americ an College of Cardiology/American Heart Association Task Force on practice guidelines (Committee on Coronary Angiography). Developed in collaboration with the Society for Cardiac Angiography and Interventions. J Am Coll Cardiol 33:1756-1824

19. Pannu HK, Jacobs JE, Lai S, Fishman EK (2006) Coronary CT angiography with 64-MDCT: assessment of vessel visibility. AJR Am J Roentgenol 187:119-126

20. Alegria JR, Herrmann J, Holmes DR Jr (2005) Myocardial bridging. Eur Heart J 26:1159-1168

21. La Grutta L, Runza G, Lo Re G et al. (2009) Prevalence of myocardial bridging and correlation with coronary atherosclerosis studied with 64-slice CT coronary angiography. Radiol Med. 114:1024-1036

22. Sinha AM, Mahnken AH, Borghans A et al (2006) Multidetector-row computed tomography vs. angiography and intravascular ultrasound for the evaluation of the diameter of proximal coronary arteries. Int J Cardiol 110:40-45

23. Dodge JT Jr, Brown BG, Bolson EL, Dodge HT (1992) Lumen diameter of normal human coronary arteries. Influence of age, sex, anatomic variation, and left ventricular hypertrophy or dilation. Circulation 86:232-246

24. Cademartiri F, Malagò R, La Grutta L et al (2007) Coronary variants and anomalies: methodology of visualisation with 64-slice CT and prevalence in 202 consecutive patients. Radiol Med. 112:1117-1131

25. Angelini P, Velasco JA, Flamm S (2002) Coronary anomalies: incidence, pathophysiology, and clinical relevance. Circulation 105:2449-2454

26. James TN (1965) Anatomy of the coronary arteries in health and disease. Circulation 32:1020-1033

27. Levin DC, Fallon JT (1982) Significance of the angiographic morphology of localized coronary stenoses: histopathologic correlations. Circulation 66:316-320

28. Baltaxe HA, Wixson D (1977) The incidence of congenital anomalies of the coronary arteries in the adult population. Radiology 122:47-52

29. Click RL, Holmes DR Jr, Vlietstra RE et al (1989) Anomalous coronary arteries: location, degree of atherosclerosis and effect on survival–a report from the Coronary Artery Surgery Study. J Am Coll Cardiol 13:531-537

30. Yamanaka O, Hobbs RE (1990) Coronary artery anomalies in 126,595 patients undergoing coronary arteriography. Cathet Cardiovasc Diagn 21:28-40

31. Rigatelli G, Rigatelli G (2003) Coronary artery anomalies: what we know and what we have to learn. A proposal for a new clinical classification. Ital Heart J 4:305-310

32. Rigatelli G, Docali G, Rossi P et al (2003) Congenital coronary artery anomalies angiographic classification revisited. Int J Cardiovasc Imaging 19:361-366

33. Cademartiri F, Nieman K, Raaymakers RH et al (2003) Non-invasive demonstration of coronary artery anomaly performed using 16-slice multidetector spiral computed tomography. Ital Heart J 4:56-59

34. Cademartiri F, Runza G, Luccichenti G et al (2006) Coronary artery anomalies: incidence, pathophysiology, clinical relevance and role of diagnostic imaging. Radiol Med. 111:376-391

35. Cademartiri F, La Grutta L, Malagò R et al. (2008) Prevalence of anatomical variants and coronary anomalies in 543 consecutive patients studied with 64-slice CT coronary angiography. Eur Radiol. 18:781-791

36. Jongbloed MR, Lamb HJ, Bax JJ et al (2005) Noninvasive visualization of the cardiac venous system using multislice computed tomography. J Am Coll Cardiol 45:749-753

Calcium Score and Coronary Plaque

11

Sara Seitun, Erica Maffei, Chiara Martini, Margherita Castiglione Morelli, Anselmo A. Palumbo, and Filippo Cademartiri

11.1 Introduction

Noninvasive coronary imaging has for a number of years been a topic of great research interest with the involvement of researchers and clinicians from various specializations [1-5]. Different imaging modalities have been proposed as noninvasive alternatives to conventional angiography, which still today is the criterion standard for the evaluation of coronary arteries [1-5]. Until the advent of multidetector computed tomography (MDCT), the main obstacles hindering the noninvasive visualization of the coronary arteries were cardiac motion, the small size of the vessels and the need for elevated intravascular contrast resolution.

A precursor to the era of MDCT for the noninvasive imaging of the coronary arteries is electron beam computed tomography (EBCT), a technique with excellent temporal resolution but low spatial resolution [6]. EBCT has been used in the United States to quantitatively evaluate coronary artery disease [6].

Over the past years, several analyses have clearly demonstrated the superiority of 64-slice MDCT over previous technology due to the improved spatial resolution (more sensitive detectors, better performing X-ray tubes) and temporal resolution (increased gantry rotation speed) [7-10]. All of this has enabled acquisition of near isotropic volume data and excellent anatomic detail of the vascular structures with 64-slice MDCT, thus evaluation of main and side coronary artery branches is improved when compared to earlier types of MDCT scanners [7-10].

Several meta-analyses and large, multicenter trials reported high diagnostic accuracy with high sensitivity (range from 85% to 99%) and negative predictive value (range from 83% to 100%) by per-patient analysis for 64-slice MDCT (Table 11.1) [9-19]. Therefore, MDCT coronary angiography has become the noninvasive technique with the highest diagnostic accuracy compared with conventional angiography and is a reference standard for all other noninvasive imaging modalities [9-19].

Furthermore, MDCT with the use of emerging technology (dual-source MDCT; 256- or 320-slice MDCT; high definition MDCT) has the potential to significantly reduce the amount of contrast agent required and the radiation dose down to 1-5 mSv or less, depending on the technology applied (reduced tube voltage; prospective ECG-triggering protocol; high-pitch spiral acquisition; iterative reconstruction algorithms) while maintaining high diagnostic accuracy [20-24].

11.2 Atherosclerosis: Pathophysiology

Coronary stenosis is considered the major alteration linked to atherosclerosis, and by causing a reduction in blood supply to the heart is directly responsible for angina pectoris. However, the absence of hemodynamically significant coronary stenosis does not automatically exclude the advent of acute coronary events [25]. These events are the second significant feature of coronary artery disease (CAD), being linked to increased mortality and having a greater impact on the perception of CAD by the general population. Studies performed in the 1990s demonstrated a weak correlation between severity of stenosis and acute coronary events. Later, postmortem studies showed that the acute coronary event is linked less to severity of stenosis and more to instability or vulnerability of atherosclerotic plaque [26].

For several years now researchers have been focusing on the possibility of visualizing coronary atherosclerosis in the subclinical phase. In this setting the advantage of noninvasiveness, i.e. of the relative safety of MDCT and magnetic resonance imaging, has been one of the major points in favor of these two techniques. In particular, thanks to its elevated spatial and temporal resolution MDCT is becoming the method of choice for the noninvasive study of the coronary lumen and wall [27, 28].

S. Seitun (✉)
Department of Diagnostic and Interventional Radiology,
"San Martino" University Hospital – IST – IRCCS,
Genova, Italy

F. Cademartiri, G. Casolo, M. Midiri (eds.), *Clinical Applications of Cardiac CT,*
© Springer-Verlag Italia 2012

Table 11.1 Sensitivity, specificity, positive predictive value (PPV) and negative predictive value (NPV) of MDCT coronary angiography: comparison with conventional coronary angiography in the evaluation of hemodynamically significant coronary stenosis (stenosis ≥50%): data from meta-analysis and multicenter trials

S. Seitun et al.

116

Study	Study Type	Year	64-slice	MVD (%)	No. Studies	No. patients	Prevalence of obstructive CAD (%)	Inclusion criteria	Unassessable segments (%)	Sensitivity (%)	Specificity (%)	PPV (%)	NPV (%)
Hamon et al. [9]	Meta-analysis	2007	100	Yes	12	695	60	Suspected CAD	4	97	90	93	96
Vanhoenacker et al. [10]	Meta-analysis	2007	100	Yes	6	363	67[a]	Suspected CAD	2*	99	93	-	-
Abdulla et al. [11]	Meta-analysis	2007	100	Yes	13	875	58	Known and suspected CAD	-	98	91	94	97
Meijer et al. [12]	Meta-analysis	2008	85*[c]	Yes	20*	1331	50	Known[†] and suspected CAD	2[b]	98	91	91*	97*
Mowatt et al. [13]	Meta-analysis	2008	100	Yes	18	1286	58[b]	Known and suspected CAD	8	99	89	93[b]	100[b]
Schuetz et al. [14]	Meta-analysis	2010	87*[c]	Yes	49	4271*	-	Known and suspected CAD	-	98	89	-	-
Budoff et al. [15]	Multicenter	2008	100	No	-	230	25	Suspected CAD Age ≥ 18 y/o	0	95	83	64	99
Miller et al. [16, 17]	Multicenter	2008	100	No	-	291	56	Suspected CAD° AS ≤ 600 BMI ≤ 40; age ≥ 40 y/o	1	85	90	91	83
Meijboom et al. [18]	Multicenter	2008	100	Yes	-	360	68	Suspected CAD Age 50-70 y/o	0	99	64	86	97
Maffei et al. [19]	Multicenter	2010	100	Yes	-	1372	53	Suspected CAD	0	99	92	94	99

In most trials, unassessable segments were excluded from analysis. Data are expressed as number or percentage (%).

AS, Agatston Score; *64-slice*, prevalence of 64-slice MDCT scanner used; *MVD*, multivendor, i.e. whether MDCT systems from different manufacturers were used; *No. studies*, number of studies included in the meta-analysis; *No. patients*, number of patients enrolled in the study; *BMI*, body mass index; *CAD*, coronary artery disease; [a], pooled mean from all studies included in the meta-analysis (n=24); [b], expressed as median; [c], the remaining percentage was evaluated by 40-slice CT; *, estimated from text; [†], only studies with inclusion of less than 50% of patients with history of CAD were included; [°], patients with coronary artery stents were not excluded, but stented segments were excluded from the comparative analysis.

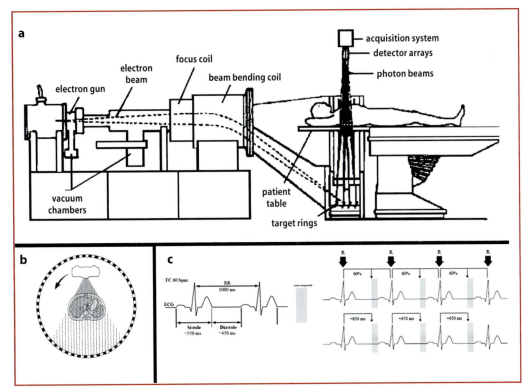

Fig. 11.1 Diagram of an electron beam computed tomography scanner (**a**). In contrast with traditional and spiral CT scanners, the anode and cathode are distant: in between is a beam bending coil which enables the photon beam to be swept around the patient, eliminating the need for a mechanically moving gantry. **b** Axial section of the gantry, the detector arrays are stationary and surround the patient at 360°. **c** Prospective modulation of the milliamperes. The maximum milliamperage is obtained in the cardiac mid-end diastole (about 60-65% of the RR interval) and the temporal reconstruction window (circa 100 ms) is positioned in the same interval

11.3 Electron Beam Computed Tomography

Prior to the advent of MDCT coronary angiography, noninvasive coronary artery imaging was performed with electron beam computed tomography (EBCT) [6]. For about a decade EBCT was the only tomographic scanner capable of noninvasively visualizing the coronary arteries [6]. This was possible because the technique requires no mechanical moving parts, which enables it to achieve a temporal resolution below 100 ms. The EBCT study is fast and relatively safe, in that it uses a low radiation dose and no contrast agents. The low radiation dose is made possible by a pulsed current acquisition in prospective ECG triggering. The main limitation of the technique lies in its poor spatial resolution (slice thickness of 3 mm) and the impossibility of performing angiographic scans, a not insignificant limitation when performing vascular studies [6].

The EBCT study is a safe examination due to the low radiation dose per patient and the absence of contrast agents. The only contraindication is pregnancy. Given the prospective nature of the acquisition, a minimum number of beats are required to perform the complete scan of the cardiac volume. In the event the heart rate is not high enough, positive chronotropic agents may be used (e.g. atropine). With a heart rate of 70-80 bpm the examination can be completed in a single breath-hold.

11.3.1 Scan Technique

The absence of moving scanner components is possible due to the deflection of the electron beam which strikes a tungsten ring surrounding the patient at 360°. The collision between electrons and tungsten produces a fan-shaped radiation beam which is made to rotate around the body of the patient (Fig. 11.1).

The radiation dose in this type of examination is contained because the acquisition is performed with prospective ECG triggering, and it is typically estimated to be approximately 1 mSv [29]. On the basis of the preset time interval a high-energy radiation beam is produced in the mid-end diastole, the phase of isovolumetric filling (60-80% of the interval between two QRS complexes) which is the phase less subject to cardiac motion.

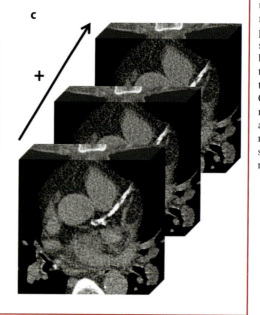

Fig. 11.2 The Agatston calcium score is calculated by multiplying the calcified plaque area (mm^2) by a density factor (between 1 and 4) based upon peak density of the plaque in each cross-sectional slice (**a**, **b**). The total CS of the patient is then automatically calculated by adding up the score for each region of calcification for all sequential slices in all coronary arteries (**c**)

11.4 Coronary Artery Calcium and Calcium Score

Agatston et al. in 1990 [30], supported by a method originally developed by David King (Imatron Inc), used the EBCT to detect and quantify baseline coronary artery calcium (CAC). The rationale for the detection of CAC was to identify those at risk for acute coronary event, since previous large angiographic studies have demonstrated that coronary calcium detected fluoroscopically is an independent predictor for future cardiac events when controlled for standard risk factors, in both symptomatic and asymptomatic, high risk subjects [31-34]. According to the scoring method introduced by Agatston [30], CAC is defined as a hyper-attenuating lesion with a density above a threshold of 130 Hounsfield units (HU) (a value which is at 3 standard deviations above the mean soft-tissue attenuation of the heart) with an area of ≥3 pixels (at least 1 mm^2). The method of calculation of the original Agatston calcium score (CS), obtained from 3-mm-thick nonoverlapping slices, is reported in Figure 11.2. The presence of CAC is sequentially quantified through all the major epicardial vessels. The total CS is then determined by adding up each lesion score for all sequential slices in all coronary arteries (Fig. 11.2).

Despite the limitations of spatial resolution, EBCT is able to make a very good evaluation of coronary calcifications by exploiting the elevated intrinsic contrast between the calcified component and the remaining cardiac tissue (Fig. 11.3). In the overall calculation of coronary atheromatous burden, the evaluation of the calcified component has high specificity (where there is a calcification there is definitely plaque), but low sensitivity (the noncalcified component is not calculated).

More recently, to improve interscan reproducibility of the CS, Callister et al. [35] introduced the volume score (isotropic interpolation) method. Volume score linearly interpolates the data set to isotropic volumes and computes the volume of the lesion above a 130 HU threshold. This measurement is considered the preferential method for the monitoring of regression or progression of atherosclerotic plaque [36]. However, the volume score is susceptible to partial volume artifacts that may impair its accuracy (overestimate volume), and may not be adequate to compare CS measurements obtained using different MDCT protocols [37].

Another scoring system, which is theoretically not dependent on slice thickness and spatial resolution of the acquisition, is the mass score that provides a quantitative assessment of the mineral content of a lesion. A threshold based on a fixed density or concentration of calcium hydroxyapatite (HA) (100 mg/cc of calcium HA) rather than the traditional fixed attenuation (130 HU) is applied. Several studies have demonstrated that the mass score is more accurate and less variable than the classic Agatston score or the volume score, but it requires scanner and scan protocol calibration to determine a specific calibrator factor [37-40].

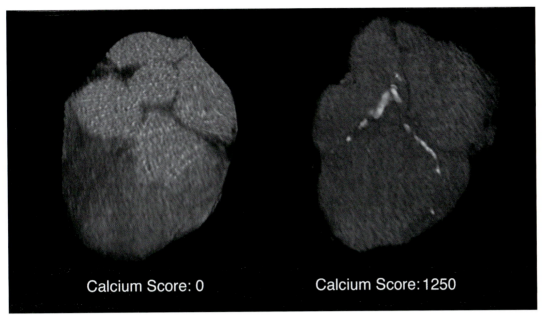

Fig. 11.3 Patients with different calcium scores. Coronary calcifications and the surrounding cardiac tissue intrinsically absorb photons differently. By exploiting this elevated contrast difference calcified components can be distinguished from all other structures

All these three types of measurements are repeatable and all have demonstrated the same accuracy in risk stratification [37, 38]. Standardization guidelines for CAC quantification have been recently proposed by a group of experts, which endorsed the mass score approach as the preferred method of quantifying CAC [41].

Although larger databases regarding CS are available for EBCT, numerous studies have suggested that MDCT is comparable to EBCT for coronary calcium scoring [42, 43]. Furthermore, the reproducibility of the CS has improved with newer-generation MDCT scanners, such that it is now similar to that with the EBCT scanner, which is approximately 15% [44].

MDCT not only enables EBCT-like acquisitions with prospective electrocardiographic (ECG) triggering (*step-and-shoot* technique, with radiation approximately equivalent to that delivered by EBCT), but also enables helical retrospectively ECG-gated acquisitions with reconstruction of partially overlapping sections. The latter has higher reproducibility due essentially to lower partial-volume effects, but it is still limited by the higher radiation dose compared with that of standard sequential acquisitions [45]. An example of a CS analysis using MDCT dedicated software is reported in Figure 11.4.

At present, the Agatston score is the scoring method widely used and largely accepted in the quantitative evaluation of calcified coronary atherosclerotic plaques, while the widespread use of the volume and mass scores is hindered by limited registry data for clinical decision-making [40].

11.5 Pathophysiology of Coronary Artery Calcium

Coronary artery calcium (CAC) is merely an epiphenomenon for the presence of atherosclerosis. Rumberger et al. have demonstrated that the total area of CAC, determined by EBCT, is correlated in a linear fashion with the histologically quantified coronary plaque area on a segmental, individual coronary artery and whole coronary artery system basis [46]. However, CAC amounts to only about 20% of the total plaque area determined at histologic examination, and the absence of detectable CAC cannot rule out the presence of atherosclerotic disease since not all plaques contain calcium [46].

The current evidence supports that CAC begins in the very early stages of atherosclerotic process via an active, complex process of mineralization with deposition of hydroxyapatite crystals (regulated by the expression of bone-related proteins) similar in many respects to bone formation and not only simple passive mineral precipitation [34]. Relatively consistent changes in calcium deposits parallel the natural history of atherosclerotic disease [47]. Calcium deposition begins in young people, just after fatty streak formation, as microscopic granules among the lipid droplets of lipid cores in atherosclerotic lesions defined histologically as type IV (see below) [47]. At this stage, extracellular small aggregates of crystalline calcium are, in part, granules that formed intracellularly (within some smooth muscle cells) and were

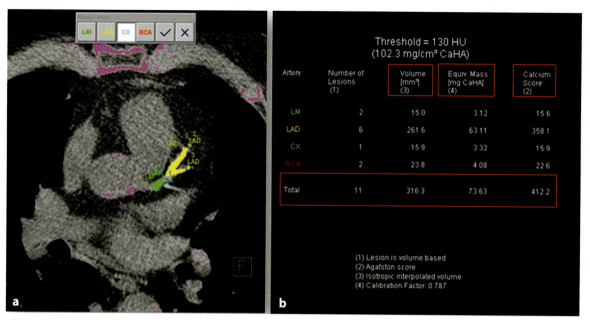

Fig. 11.4 Semi-automated quantification of coronary artery calcium (CAC) with multidetector computed tomography using dedicated software: quantification of the Agatston Score, calcium volume (Volume Score, VS) (mm^3) and calcium mass (Mass Score, MS) (mgCaHA). **a** CAC scores are typically calculated for each major coronary artery (*LM*, left main; *LAD*, left anterior descending; *CX*, circumflex; *RCA*, right coronary artery) separately. **b** For the purpose of outcomes data, risk stratification, or the serial assessment of patients over time the total CAC score is generally used, which is the sum of all vessels scores. The volume score tends to be similar in magnitude to the Agatston score except at very high and very low scores; the numeric value of the calcium mass is typically much lower than that of the Agatston score

released when cells died, and in part they represent extracellular calcification of cell remnants [47]. During the decade, the coalescence of microscopic extracellular calcium deposits form macro-aggregates (granules and plates which may measure hundreds of microns and even millimeters) until the greater part of a lesion core may be calcified (type VII lesion, see below) [47]. Lastly, organization of calcium deposits into bone (osseous metaplasia) may occur as a late step [47].

11.6 Role of Calcium Score

The evaluation of coronary calcium has proven feasible and the presence of calcification in addition to indicating the site of a plaque also suggests its extension [46]. Of course only a small percentage of patients with coronary calcifications also have a coronary stenosis. According to the Mayo Clinic guidelines, the probability of the presence of a hemodynamically significant stenosis is greater in patients with a calcium score (CS) >400, (Fig. 11.5) [48]. However, no correlation between the site of the calcification and the site of coronary stenosis has been demonstrated, even though there is a correlation between a CS>400 and the probability of an obstruction, i.e. an acute event [49].

On the basis of the above, the aim of the quantitative assessment of coronary calcium is to extrapolate the extent of atherosclerotic disease and to correlate this value with the possibility of an acute event occurring. Therefore, rather than having a role in the management of patients with CAD, the evaluation of CS is more an important element in the primary prevention of CAD.

The primary prevention population is made up of a very heterogeneous group of patients, whose risk of acute coronary events is estimated on the basis of the predictors of the Framingham Risk Score (FRS: age, gender, hypertension, dyslipidemia, diabetes, etc.) [50]. The score does however tend to underestimate risk and correctly classify only those patients with a low or high risk. There remains the problem of correctly classifying the majority of asymptomatic patients who on the basis of the FRS predictors have an intermediate risk of acute coronary events (risk of developing an acute coronary event between 10% and 20% over the next 10 years), which are approximately 40% of the population and for whom no consolidated treatment strategy has been established. Evidence suggests that the CS has a predictive value for mortality in asymptomatic patients, and if added to the FRS it significantly improves predictability (Fig. 11.6) [51, 52]. Therefore, considering that the CS is an independent risk factor, it could be used to more accurately stratify risk in this population [52].

The recent update of the Consensus Document of the

Agatston CS	CS Categories	Probability of significant CAD	Cardiovascular Risk	Recommendations
0	Absent	Very unlikely (<5%)	Vey low	Reassure patient. General guidelines for primary prevention of CV diseases
1-10	Minimal	Very unlikely (<10%)	Low	General guidelines for primary prevention of CV diseases
11-100	Mild	Mild or minimal coronary stenosis likely	Moderate	Counsel about risk factors modification, strict adherence with primary prevention goals Daily ASA.
101-400	Moderate	Nonobstructive CAD highly likely, obstructive CAD possible	Moderately high	Institute risk factor modification and secondary prevention goals. Consider exercise testing
>400	Extensive	High likelihood of significant coronary stenosis (>90%)	High	Institute very aggressive risk factors modification. Consider exercise or pharmacological nuclear stress testing for the detection of inducible ischemia

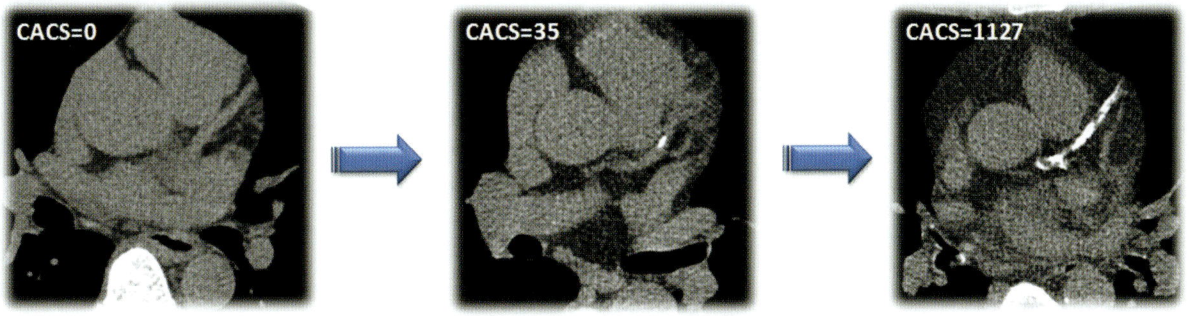

Fig. 11.5 Standardized categories for the calcium score (CS) have been developed to provide clinical guideline for interpretation of the CS values. *CV*, cardiovascular; *ASA*, acetilsalicylic acid. (Adapted from [48], with permission)

American College of Cardiology/American Heart Association (ACC/AHA) [53] and the more recent recommendation from the European Society of Cardiac Radiology and North American Society for Cardiovascular Imaging [40] provide support for the use of CS for risk stratification in asymptomatic populations with an intermediate FRS. In this clinical scenario, intermediate-risk FRS patients with a CS greater than or equal to 400 would be expected to have event rates that place them in the CAD risk equivalent status, with an event rate greater than or equal to 20% over 10 years (Fig. 11.7). Therefore in this high risk category, patient risk prediction and subsequent management may be modified.

Studies performed on the prognostic value of the CS have broadened our understanding of atherosclerosis and the progression of CAD. The absence of a technique capable of performing a direct angiographic evaluation of the coronary arteries has spurred the search for indirect markers of disease. The new concepts of the vulner-

ability of coronary plaque and more generally of the vulnerability of the patient with suspected CAD has reshaped the role of coronary calcium as a nonspecific predictor of disease. In the clinical setting of the near future, the use of MDCT for the noninvasive imaging of the coronary arteries will play a significant role in the global evaluation of the patient with suspected CAD, thanks to the possibility of integrating purely anatomic data with functional information and data on myocardial viability from challenge tests.

11.7 The Value of Zero Calcium Score

As discussed above, there is evidence of the increased risk of adverse events with increasing CS value. However, an even more clinically relevant finding may be the absence of CS. A systematic review of published studies using EBCT evaluating the outcome in both asymptomatic (n=71,595) and symptomatic (3,924)

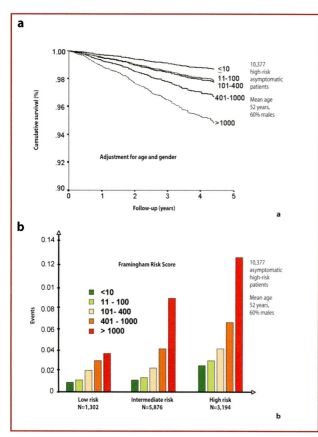

Fig. 11.6 Findings of the most important randomized studies on the prognostic value of the calcium score. Kaplan-Meier five-year survival curves of a high-risk asymptomatic patient population. **a** In patients with high calcium score (CS>1000) the incidence of major cardiac events is higher and survival is lower. **b** Cardiovascular risk stratification in asymptomatic patients using the Framingham risk score predictors. If the calcium score is added to the classic parameters a more accurate risk stratification of the population at intermediate risk is obtained. (Reproduced from [52])

patients with zero CS (CS=0), demonstrated a low risk for future events in both asymptomatic and symptomatic populations, but higher for the latter (mean cardiac event rate respectively: 0.47% vs. 1.8%) [54]. Furthermore, a distinction between zero CS (CS=0) and very low CS (CS=1-10) should be made. A recent large prospective study involving 44,052 patients followed over a 5-year period showed that in patients with low positive CS (CS=1-10) mortality was 1.06%, which was significantly higher than in patients with no coronary calcium (0.52%) and significantly lower than in patients with CAC >10 (3.96%) [55].

The exact prevalence of obstructive (noncalcified) plaque in the absence of any calcium remains to be fully elucidated; previous studies have shown a large variation, which may be explained by differences in study population [56]. Previous observations using 64-slice MDCT in patients with stable chest pain syndrome or with suspected acute coronary syndrome reported a prevalence of obstructive CAD with zero and low CS in the range of 6.2-10% [57-60]. A recent prospective multicenter trial including mainly intermediate-risk patients with suspected CAD and planned clinically-indicated conventional coronary angiography within 30-day from 64-slice MDCT examination reported a prevalence of 19% of obstructive CAD among patients with CS=0 [61]. Taken together these observations suggest that the absence of coronary calcium does not reliably exclude atherosclerosis or even obstructive CAD in patients at high cardiovascular risk and this may be especially true for high-risk subjects, such as diabetic patients [62].

Additionally, the current CS guideline does not provide support for the concept that high-risk asymptomatic

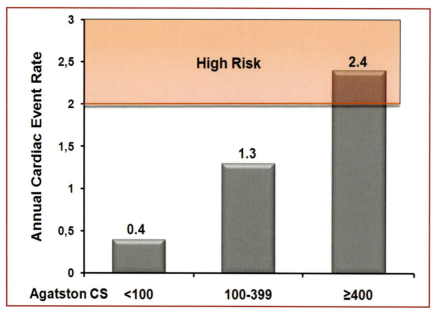

Fig. 11.7 Annual event rate (myocardial infarction or cardiac death) in different categories of CS among asymptomatic subjects at intermediate risk for cardiac event. In subjects with a high CS (≥400), the annual event rate exceeds the threshold for intensive risk factor modification (i.e. >2% per year, red line). A CS≥400 may therefore be considered as a risk equivalent. In patients with a low risk of coronary events (i.e. <1% risk per year), CS is not recommended, because even a high CS does not generally elevate the risk above the threshold to initiate therapy. Furthermore, even in patients at high risk (i.e. >2% risk per year) CS in not recommended because they are already candidates for intensive risk factor modification. (Modified from [53])

Table 11.2 American Heart Association histological classification of coronary atherosclerotic plaques. (Modified from [47])

Histological classification	Main histological characteristics
Type I	isolated macrophage foam cells appear
Type II	multiple layers of foam cells formed
Type III	small pools of extracellular lipid added
Type IV	confluent lipid core formed; calcium granules appear
Type V	fibrosis in addition to type IV changes; lumps or plates of calcium formed
Type VI	fissure, hematoma, thrombosis in addition to type IV or V changes
Type VII	predominantly calcified lesion; osseous metaplasia may appear
Type VIII	predominantly fibrotic lesion

individuals can be safely excluded from medical therapy for primary CAD prevention even if CS score is 0 [53].

11.8 Coronary Atherosclerotic Plaque

The most common classification of coronary atherosclerotic plaque is that provided by the American Heart Association, which distinguishes eight different types of lesions (Table 11.2) [47, 63-65]. This classification reflects the natural history of the disease, which is asymptomatic in the initial stages and has variable progression in more advanced stages. Advanced lesions may be quite heterogeneous and have different histologic features, giving rise to various clinical syndromes. Clinical manifestations and fatal outcomes are most often associated with processes included under the type VI (complicated) lesion, although even these processes may remain silent (Table 11.2).

In the initial stages atherosclerosis is characterized by histopathologic alterations without clinical signs. In particular, the fatty streak lesion may spontaneously disappear, although the natural history sees progressive involvement of the vascular wall up to the formation of prevalently fibrofatty atherosclerotic plaques. This transformation is particularly evident in areas with mechanical hemodynamic stimulation (vascular ostia and bifurcations) [66].

Smooth muscle cells migrate into the subendothelial space, divide and synthesize extracellular matrix. The result is the formation of a fibrous cap separating the lipid core of the lesion from the endothelial surface. This organization of the plaque is promoted by a series of inflammatory and immunoregulatory cytokines and growth factors. Due to hemodynamic stress, the chemical mediators facilitate the migration of the smooth muscle cells and the formation of the fibrous cap, which forms the barrier between the thrombogenic lipid core and the blood. The greater the thickness of the fibrous cap, the more stable the plaque and the lower the risk of acute vascular thrombosis [67, 68].The study of coronary arteries of patients deceased for sudden cardiac death has demonstrated that the fibrous cap thickness which guarantees an effective minimum barrier is about 65 micron [69].

The accumulation of lipid material is however a continuous process, and the growth of the plaque over time causes a reduction in vessel diameter which progressively reduces blood flow, thus causing exertional angina (Fig. 11.8).

Numerous studies have concluded that the acute coronary event is triggered by vascular thrombosis and that this is associated with the presence of nonocclusive plaques [70]. Histopathologic analysis of the coronary arteries has identified in these lesions the presence of surface fissures which pass through the endothelium reaching the lipid core. These fissures are considered the proof of plaque rupture [25]. The most recent discoveries have demonstrated that coronary plaque rupture is a complex process, linked to modifications related to inflammatory mechanisms. A number of phenomena have been highlighted which translate into typical morphologic alterations. The scale of these alterations is clearly extremely small and only with the advent of molecular imaging will it be possible to highlight these specific alterations and predict the outcome of coronary atherosclerotic plaque.

11.9 Evaluation of Coronary Plaque

11.9.1 Invasive Techniques

The technical and technologic instruments currently used in medicine are unable to identify with certainty the presence of coronary plaque prone to rupture in vivo. There are nonetheless a series of techniques capable of evaluating the vascular wall for which there are commonly accepted imaging characteristics of coronary plaque. The characterization of atheromatous coronary plaque is currently performed with intravascular ultrasound (IVUS), which is the only technique to receive Food and Drug Administration approval for the study of coronary ather-

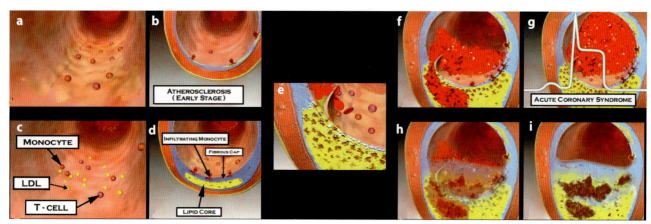

Fig. 11.8 Three dimensional reconstruction of the phases of coronary atherosclerosis. Initial modifications linked to the accumulation of lipid material at the level of the media (fatty streaks) (**a, b**). With the increasing accumulation of lipid material proinflammatory cells appear (monocytes/macrophages/T-cells) (**c**). The plaque core is separated from the lumen by a fibrous cap (**d**). Vulnerable atheromatous plaque characterized by large lipid core with inflammatory cellular infiltrates and thin fibrous cap. Fissuring of the fibrous cap places the highly thrombogenic lipid core in contact with the blood (**e**). Thrombus generated by plaque rupture causes acute coronary occlusion (myocardial infarction) (**f, g**). If the vascular thrombosis is followed by the rapid activation of thrombolysis, plaque rupture without painful symptoms occurs and the healing of the intraplaque hemorrhage leads to modifications of the composition of the plaque and a coronary stenosis (**h-i**)

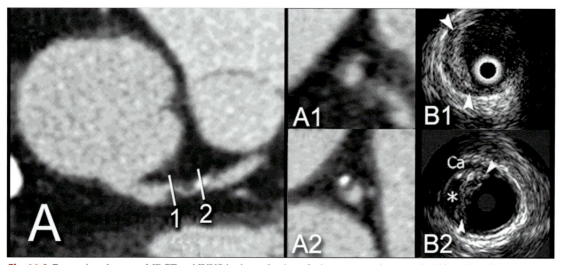

Fig. 11.9 Comparison between MDCT and IVUS in the evaluation of atheromatous plaque at the bifurcation of the left main coronary artery (**a**). MDCT axial images (**a1**) and IVUS (**b1**) of a fibrofatty atheromatous plaque: good correspondence in terms of imaging, with a tendency to volumetric underestimation by MDCT. MDCT axial images (**a2**) and IVUS (**b2**) of a mixed plaque. IVUS is the gold standard for the evaluation of the different plaque components: the fibrofatty tissue (asterisk) separating the lumen from the calcified component is also correctly visualized with MDCT as an area of low density which is underestimated due to artifacts linked to the presence of calcium

osclerosis. IVUS is able to visualize some of the main features of rupture-prone plaque [71]. There are nonetheless several findings with different interpretations and the spatial resolution of 100-200 micron does not enable to discriminate whether the fibrous cap is thick or thin. On the basis of current knowledge, IVUS is the reference technique for the evaluation of coronary plaque in vivo which has a clinical application with efficacy demonstrated and validated by an ACC/AHA consensus document [72] (Fig. 11.9).

Other invasive imaging modalities have been experimented in vivo, producing some very suggestive images of vulnerable plaque. Of particular note is elastography, which is able to characterize areas of plaque on the basis of deformability and therefore recognize the plaques with the largest lipid component and most prone to rupture [73]. Another recently introduced technique is virtual histology (VH-IVUS), which is able to obtain data on the microscopic structure of coronary plaque by processing the IVUS radiofrequency signal. With the application of mathematic models to the data obtained from IVUS, a spectral analysis of the radiofrequencies produced by IVUS can be performed and the data obtained can be correlated with different components of plaque in the form of a chromatic scale: the calcified component is visualized white, the fibrous component green, the fibrofatty component green-yellow and the necrotic core red [74-76]. Another technique is thermal imaging, which uses highly sensitive catheters (thermal sensitivity 0.05°C, spatial resolution 500 micron) capable of detecting the slightest variations in temperature which occur in the plaques where inflammatory processes are more marked and are therefore more prone to rupture [77].

Another technique is vascular angioscopy, which has the unique advantage of allowing direct visualization of the endothelium and superficial components of atherosclerotic plaque [78]. Compared with IVUS, angioscopy is more sensitive in evaluating the presence of the lipid core and thrombotic apposition in complicated plaque [28, 78]. The plaque in the coronary artery can be white or yellow angioscopically, depending on the histological presence of thick or thin fibrous cap, respectively [78]. Several studies have demonstrated that the risk of plaque rupture increases with the increase in the intensity of yellow color [78, 79]. However, major drawbacks of this technique are the need of a temporary occlusion of the vessel in order to view the lesion (as the light signal is heavily affected by the presence of blood), and the impossibility of providing a quantitative analysis [28].

Another optical method to detect vulnerable coronary plaque is the optical coherence tomography (OCT), which provides a spatial resolution of 10-20 micron, approximately ten times higher than that of IVUS [80]. OCT can clearly demarcate between tunica intima, media, and adventitia by differing level of reflecting signals. In contrast to IVUS, OCT is able to penetrate calcium and can image calcified plaques in the coronary vasculature. Currently, OCT is the only technique capable of accurately visualizing fibrous caps at risk of rupture (≤65 micron) and identifying a complicated lesion [81]. Furthermore, this technique may be able to image macrophage infiltration, which, in the clinical setting, was found to be greater in patients with acute coronary syndrome than in those with stable angina [82]. Its major limitation is signal attenuation, as electromagnetic waves are heavily attenuated by luminal blood, which reduces imaging time and complicates its use. Another limitation is its poor penetration depth (1–2 mm), which does not allow assessment of the entire thickness of the vessel [83].

Lastly, some investigators have tested the ability of intravascular spectroscopy for the identification of the composition of atherosclerotic plaques. The two most validated methods in this area are Raman spectroscopy (RS) and near-infrared spectroscopy (NIRS). RS is based on the phenomenon called Raman Effect whereby the inelastic collision of a photon (with λ between 750 and 850 nm) and a molecule generates light emissions with different frequencies [84]. A catheter (~1 mm) emits a laser beam focused on the tissue under examination, and the reflected beam contains the spectrum of the chemical structures present in the tissue. RS has been shown to be effective in detecting the molecular characteristics of the lipids and calcium in both ex-vivo and in-vivo studies [85-87]. RS has indisputable potential for the study of atherosclerosis in terms of chemical composition but provides no information on arterial morphology. NIRS, with λ between 750 and 2500 nm, has a penetration depth up to 2 mm. Most of the data available on the use of this technique are ex-vivo studies which demonstrated the presence of a characteristic spectrum for vulnerable plaque, reporting high sensitivity and specificity for lipid pool, thin-cap, and inflammatory cells in human atherosclerotic plaques [88, 89]. A catheter-based NIR spectroscopy device has now been developed and successfully tested in patients with stable angina and acute coronary syndromes [90]; however, its in-vivo use is limited to date.

The studies on the invasive characterization of coronary plaque have kindled great interest in recent years. The complexity of the equipment, the difficulty in performing the examinations, the cost and therefore the limited availability of these resources have however limited their application to ultraspecialized centers for the treatment of CAD. The exclusive nature of these techniques is poorly adapted to the type of disease and the impact it has on such a vast population. In contrast, the characteristics of the technique of choice for the study of CAD should not only be elevated sensitivity, but also availability in the clinical setting and safety of the technique, i.e. noninvasiveness.

11.9.2 Noninvasive Techniques: Multidetector Computed Tomography

It has been shown that during the progression of CAD the plaques responsible for acute coronary events are not hemodynamically significant, rather their degree of stenosis is <50% in almost 70% of cases [25]. This has been confirmed by the fact that a high percentage of subjects who die from acute myocardial infarction present no prior symptoms [70]. In this setting, where coronary stenosis is not the most important feature, conventional angiography appears not to be the diagnostic examination of choice, in that it significantly underestimates the degree of CAD in these patients. MDCT has the potential

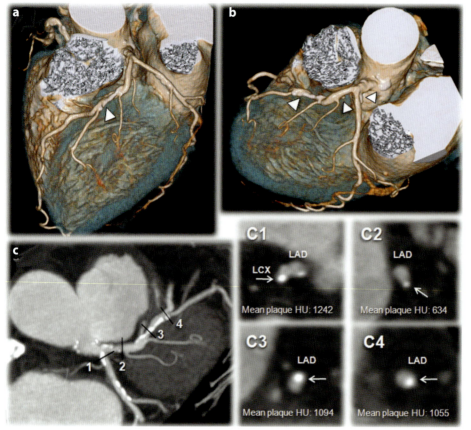

Fig. 11.10 Example of multiple calcified plaques with corresponding transversal sections. Calcified nodules and lamellar calcifications of left circumflex artery (LCX) and left descending anterior artery (LAD) are clearly depicted by volume rendering images (a and b, *arrowheads*) and maximum intensity projection reconstruction (MIP, c). Cross sectional views perpendicular to the axis of proximal LCX (c1), proximal LAD (c2) and distal LAD at two consecutive levels (c3, c4), showed calcified plaques without significant luminal obstruction and the corresponding HU values. Note the artifact of "blooming" due to partial volume averaging of dense calcium (which typically has an elevated atomic number), especially for the plaques with a high HU value (c1, c3 and c4)

to visualize the atherosclerotic lesions which present a series of typical morphologic characteristics and which seem to be linked to the predisposition of the plaque to rupture [91]. In view of its ability to assign density values (HU) to the structures being studied, MDCT appears to be the ideal imaging modality for visualizing and quantifying all plaque components, which angiography and EBCT are unable to detect [28].

MDCT classification of coronary plaques may be performed by using a qualitative [92] and a quantitative approach [93], or by both methods combined [94]. The former classifies coronary plaques as calcified (Fig. 11.10), mixed (Fig. 11.11), and noncalcified (Fig. 11.12) [92, 94], or as predominantly calcified, intermediate, or lipid-rich [95]. The quantitative approach assigns a specific density value to different plaque types [93].

Several in-vivo studies have investigated the ability of MDCT for plaque detection in comparison with IVUS, reporting high diagnostic accuracy (Table 11.3) [92, 96-100]. Of note, sensitivity, especially for noncalcified plaques and overall plaque burden, has increased parallel to the improvement of MDCT scanners in term of spatial and temporal resolution (Table 11.3). An underestimation of noncalcified and total plaque volumes and a trend to overestimate calcified plaque volume by quantitative MDCT analysis in comparison with IVUS have been reported [92, 98]; potential explanations are the lower spatial resolution of MDCT with respect to IVUS and the partial volume effects at MDCT.

Several in-vivo and ex-vivo studies have proved MDCT to be useful for distinction between lipid-rich, fibrous-rich, and calcified plaques based on HU values (Table 11.4) [93-96, 99-108]. MDCT plaque density values were systematically higher in plaques containing calcium as detected by grayscale IVUS, OCT or histopathology (Table 11.4). Furthermore, the majority of studies reported a statistically significant difference between the measured mean MDCT attenuations of plaques classified as lipid-rich and fibrous-rich; however, mean HU values vary widely from one study to the other (Table 11.4) According to the literature, specific MDCT density cut-off values have been proposed: lipid-rich plaque ≤60 HU, fibrous-rich plaque 61-119 HU, and calcified plaque ≥120 HU [95]. However, the HU score suggested for noncalcified plaques does not take into account the overlap in absolute density values between fibrous and lipid plaques, which may be substantial, as shown by ex-vivo and in-vivo studies, or the misdiagno-

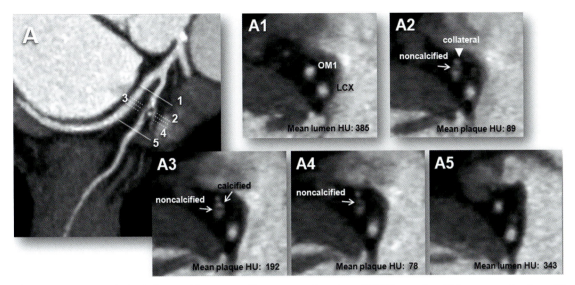

Fig. 11.11 Example of mixed plaque with corresponding transversal sections. MDCT curved multiplanar reconstruction of first obtuse marginal branch (OM1) showed a mixed plaque just distal to the origin of a small collateral vessel, associated with significant (>50%) obstruction of the lumen (**a**). MDCT axial images (**a1-a5**) display short axis views at the site of the coronary lesion (**a2-a4**) as well as proximal (**a1**) and distal (**a5**) short axis reference views. Note the small calcification embedded in the outer part of the noncalcified plaque material (**a3**); the mean MDCT density of the plaque at this level was 192 HU

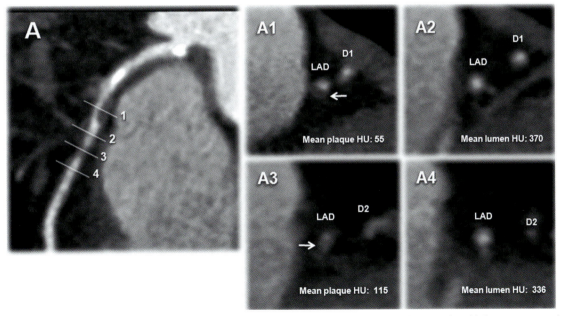

Fig. 11.12 Example of noncalcified plaques with corresponding transversal sections. MDCT curved multiplanar reconstruction of the left anterior descending artery (LAD) showed two noncalcified plaques associated with borderline (50%) and significant (>50%) obstruction of the lumen in the middle and distal segments, respectively (**a**). MDCT axial images (**a1-a4**) display short axis views at the site of the coronary lesions (**a1, a3**), between the two plaques (**a2**) and at the distal vessel reference view (**a4**). Note the different remodeling index of the proximal and distal noncalcified plaques (positive and negative remodeling, respectively); the mean MDCT densities of the plaques were 55 HU (**a1**) and 115 HU (**a3**), respectively. *D1* and *D2*, first and second diagonal branch, respectively

sis of thrombi, which have a similar attenuation value [28, 95].

Furthermore, previous phantom [109, 110], ex-vivo [111], and recent in-vivo [112, 113] studies have clearly demonstrated that intravascular attenuation significantly modifies the density values within plaque caused by partial volume effects, interpolation and, potentially, contrast enhancement of the atherosclerotic plaque. In particular, the density values of noncalcified components of the plaque (lipid-rich or fibrous-rich) increases nearly

Table 11.3 In vivo assessment of coronary atherosclerotic plaques: detection rate of noncalcified and calcified plaques by multidetector computed tomography (MDCT) vs. intravascular ultrasound (IVUS)

Study	N. patients	MDCT scanner	Sensitivity (%)			Total	Specificity
			Noncalcified		Calcified	(%)	(%)
			Soft	Fibrous			
Achenbach et al. [92]	22	420/16° x 0.75		53	94	82	88
Leber et al. [96]	37	420/16° x 0.75	78	78	95	85	92
Moselewski et al. [97]	26	420/16° x 0.75				91	94
Leber et al. [98]	19	330/64 x 0.6	83	94*	95	90	94
Sun et al. [99]	26	400/64 x 0.5		97	93	97	90
Petranovic et al. [100]	11	330/64 x 0.6		90	86	95	89

Data are expressed as number or percentage (%); *MDC scanner*, expressed as gantry rotation time (ms) / number of slices x slice thickness (mm); *, referred to mixed plaque; °, only the 12 inner detectors of the 16-detector scanner were used.

linearly to the intravascular attenuation; calcium attenuation and surrounding fat attenuation are, in contrast, not significantly affected [111]. The luminal density depends on several aspects, some related to the scanning procedure, and others related to the patients, e.g. the iodine concentration in the contrast agent, the volume administered, the flow rate of administration, the cardiac output and the body mass index of the patients. Therefore, the attenuation values measured inside the plaque should be calibrated on the basis of lumen density [28]. Density ranges defined for soft, fibrous and calcified plaque are therefore unlikely to have an absolute value [28].

In addition, previous phantom [114], ex-vivo [115] and recent in-vivo [116] studies have demonstrated that reconstruction parameters which influence the spatial resolution such as slice thickness and reconstruction kernel significantly affect the measured coronary plaque attenuation. "Sharper" convolution kernels, by increasing the spatial resolution (as well as image noise) and enhancing plaque structure boundaries, increase the attenuation of the calcium within the coronary plaques and reduce the attenuation of soft plaque tissues [115]. In contrast, thicker slices and "softer" reconstruction kernels, by reducing spatial resolution (as well as image noise), increase the MDCT attenuation values inside the noncalcified plaque due to partial volume effects [116].

Furthermore, as a decrease in tube voltage decreases the hardness of the X-ray beams and increases the absorbed portion of the radiation, a change in HU measurements would be theoretically expected using lower tube voltage setting (100 kV) in lower-weight patients. However, a phantom study [117] showed no difference in the HU densitometry of noncalcified plaque when comparing 100 kV and 120 kV MDCT protocols.

In summary, parameters such as lumen density, convolution filtering, slice thickness, and kV setting should be reported when attenuation values are shown in order to provide a standardization of the methodology.

In addition, some ex-vivo studies investigated the ability to identify and characterize coronary plaque composition according to the proposed classification of the American Heart Association (Tables 11.5 and 11.6) [93-95, 118-120]. The largest study to date by Leschka et al. [120] using a dual-source MDCT scanner reported high sensitivity with a detection rate of 79% (n= 245/322) for coronary artery plaques of any histopathologic type and of 100% for advanced-stage plaques (types IV-VIII) (Table 11.5). Furthermore, the average MDCT density of early-stage Stary type II-III plaques was significantly lower than that of advanced-stage Stary plaques (Table 11.6). Plaque classification as noncalcified was sensitive (100%) and specific (72%) for early, whereas classification as mixed/calcified was sensitive (92%, 89%) and specific (100%) for advanced plaques.

In conclusion, newer MDCT scanner generations (dual-source MDCT; 256- or 320-slice MDCT; high definition MDCT), which enable the acquisition of submillimeter isotropic volume data, have the potential to noninvasively evaluate the morphologic features of relevant coronary plaques associated with ACS and characterize subclinical coronary atherosclerosis. The association of this new information obtained in vivo with our post-mortem-derived knowledge of culprit lesions will in the future help reveal the mechanisms which lead to the transformation of unstable plaque and the generation of the acute event.

11.10 Vulnerable Plaque

The term vulnerable plaque was first introduced in the 1990s: the presentation of an angiographic series of culprit lesions before and after an acute coronary event prompted the reference to a rapidly evolving lesion associated with a high risk of thrombosis [121]. Since then this type of plaque has been studied ex vivo and in vivo

Table 11.4 Mean attenuation densities of coronary atherosclerotic plaques by MDCT: comparison with histology, intravascular ultrasound (IVUS) or optical coherence tomography (OCT)

Study	MDCT scanner	No. plaques	Comparison	Lumen attenuation (HU)	Plaque type Lipid-rich	Fibrous-rich	Calcified	p value*	p value**
Schroeder et al [101]	500/4 x 1	in vivo (34)[a]	IVUS	-	14 ± 26	91 ± 21	419 ± 194	<0.0001	<0.0001
Becker et al [94]	500/4 x 1	ex vivo (33)	Histology	~ 250	47 ± 9	104 ± 28	-	<0.01	-
Schroeder et al [95]	500/4 x 1	ex vivo (17)	Histology	182 ± 34	42 ± 22	71 ± 21	715 ± 328	<0.0001	<0.0001
Nikolau et al [93]	500/4 x 1	ex vivo (21)	Histology	242 ± 28	47 ± 13	87 ± 29	-	<0.01	-
Leber et al [96]	420/16 x 0.75	in vivo (299)	IVUS	-	49 ± 22	91 ± 22	391 ± 156	<0.02	<0.02
Ferencik et al [102]	420/16 x 0.75	ex vivo (164)[f]	OCT	~ 250	29 ± 43	101 ± 21	135 ± 199	<0.001	<0.001
Pohle et al [103]	420/16 x 0.75	in vivo (252)[b]	IVUS	-	58 ± 43	121 ± 34	-	<0.001	-
Sun et al [99]	400/64 x 0.5	in vivo (113)[g]	IVUS	398 ± 74	79 ± 34	90 ± 27	772 ± 251	n.s.	<0.01
Choi et al [104]	420/64x0.625	in vivo (80)[b]	VH-IVUS	-	41.3 ± 26.4	93.1 ± 37.5	-	<0.001	-
Kim et al [105]	350/64x0.625	in vivo (71)[b]	IVUS	-	52.9 ± 24.6	98.6 ± 34.9	-	<0.001	-
Petranovic et al [100]	330/64 x 0.6	in vivo (60)[g]	IVUS	275.3 ± 77.2	99.5 ± 28	77 ± 38.5	608.15 ± 216.9	n.s.	<0.05
Hur et al [106]	330/64 x 0.6	in vivo (61)[c]	IVUS	-	54 ± 13	82 ± 17	392 ± 155	n.s.	<0.01
Chopard et al [107]	420/64x0.625	ex vivo (83)	Histology	276 ± 42	70.9 ± 41	83 ± 35	966 ± 473	n.s.	<0.05
Soeda et al [108]	330/2x64 x 0.6[e]	in vivo (106)[d]	OCT	355.4 ± 64.6	28.9 ± 30.6	77.5 ± 25.7	515.9 ± 130.5	<0.0001	<0.0001

Data are expressed as number or mean ± standard deviation (SD); *No. plaques*, number of plaques identified by MDCT which could be compared; *MDCT scanner*, expressed as gantry rotation time (ms) / number of slices x slice thickness (mm); [a], only plaques narrowing the vessel lumen >40% were included; [b], calcified plaques were not included in the analysis; [c], only obstructive plaques were analyzed (coronary stenosis >50%); [d], non-stenotic coronary plaques within non-culprit coronary arteries in patients with acute coronary syndrome were analyzed; [e], dual-source MDCT scanner; [f], number of cross-sections analyzed by MDCT; [g], both MDCT and IVUS were performed in patients with significant CAD (>50% coronary stenosis); *, difference of the mean CT density values between lipid-rich and fibrous-rich plaques; **, difference of the mean CT density values between lipid-rich or fibrous-rich and calcified plaques.

Table 11.5 Ex-vivo assessment of coronary atherosclerotic plaques by MDCT: detection rate in comparison with histology according to the AHA classification

Study	MDCT scanner	No. plaques	Lumen attenuation (HU)	Sensitivity (%) Type II	Type III	Type IV	Type V	Type VI	Type VII	Type VIII
Becker et al [94]	500/4 x 1	50	~ 250	-	10	73	70	100	86	100
Nikolau et al [93]	500/4 x 1	28	242 ± 28	-		56	71	-	90	100
Galonska et al [118]	500/16 x 0.625	175	308 (93-625)*	0	0			94	100	88
Henzler et al [119]		58	~ 350							
	600/16 x0.6			14	100	100	100	-	100	-
	330/2x64 x0.6[a]			14	100	100	100	-	100	-
	330/2x64 x0.6[a] / DE[b]			14	100	100	100	-	100	-
Leschka et al [120]	330/2x64 x0.6[a]	322	~ 300	17	74	100	100	100	100	100

Data are expressed number, percentage (%) or mean ± standard deviation (SD); *No. plaques*, number of plaques identified by histology; *MDCT, scanner*, expressed as gantry rotation time (ms) / number of slices x slice thickness (mm); *, expressed as median (range); [a]: dual-source MDCT scanner; [b], DE: dual energy mode: 140 kV and 100 kV.

Table 11.6 Ex-vivo assessment of coronary atherosclerotic plaques by MDCT: CT density values of coronary plaques according to the AHA classification

Study	MDCT scanner	No. plaques	Lumen attenuation (HU)	Type II	Type III	Type IV	Type V	Type VI	Type VII	Type VIII	p value*	p value**
Becker et al. [94]	500/4 x 1	33	~ 250	-	-	-	47 ± 9[a]	-	104 ± 28[a]	-	<0.01	-
Schroeder et al. [95]	500/4 x 1	17	182 ± 34	-	46 ± 17	40 ± 24	71 ± 21	-	715 ± 328	-	<0.0001	<0.0001
Nikolau et al. [93]	500/4 x 1	21	242 ± 28	-	-	47 ± 13[a]	-	-	87 ± 29[a]	-	<0.01	-
Galonska et al. [118]	500/16 x 0.625	136	308 (93-625)	-	-	50 (33-59)	44 (26-63)	40 (36-67)	1089 (333-1944)	67 (37-124)	<0.001	<0.001
Henzler et al. [119]	600/16 x 0.6 330/2x64 x0.6[b] 330/2x64 x0.6[b] / DE[c]	52	~ 350	-	-	19[d] 11[d] 8[d]	52[d] 44[d] 45[d]	-	1079[d] 1088[d] 966[d]	-	≤0.05 ≤0.05 ≤0.05	≤0.05 ≤0.05 ≤0.05
Leschka et al [120]	330/2x64 x0.6[b]	245	~ 300	34 ± 17	48 ± 10	55 ± 12	34 ± 19	104 ± 84	501 ± 402	91 ± 16	<0.001[e]	<0.001

Data are expressed as number or mean ± standard deviation (SD); *No. plaques*, plaques identified by MDCT; *MDCT scanner*, expressed as gantry rotation time (ms) / number of slices x slice thickness (mm); *, difference of the mean CT density values between lipid-rich and fibrous-rich plaques; **, difference of the mean CT density values between lipid-rich or fibrous-rich and calcified plaques; [a] total CT density value for all lipid-rich or fibrous-rich plaques; [b], dual-source MDCT scanner; [c], DE: dual energy mode: 140 kV and 100 kV; [d]: standard deviation not reported; [e], difference between early-stage plaques (type II-III) and advanced-stage plaques (type IV-VIII).

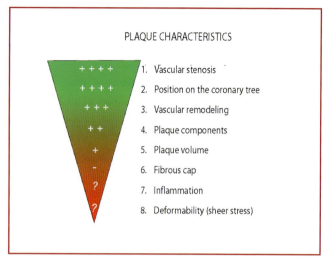

Fig. 11.13 Diagram of the characteristics of coronary plaque. Current MDCT scanners perform an excellent evaluation of most of the characteristics of instability, with greater accuracy in the evaluation of the morphologic features. The functional features cannot be evaluated with MDCT and the iodinated contrast agents currently used in clinical practice

and a number of highly characteristic anatomic and functional features have been identified which are considered predictors of an acute coronary event [122, 123]. In the past years there have been a number of Consensus Conferences which have established the morphologic and functional characteristics of unstable coronary plaque on the basis of current knowledge [1, 2, 5]. Several retrospective post-mortem studies reveal that different types of vulnerable plaque with various histopathology and biology exist [1]. Plaque rupture with superimposed acute coronary thrombosis is the most common type of plaque complication, accounting for approximately 70% of fatal myocardial infarctions and/or sudden coronary deaths [1]. Rupture-prone plaque has a specific morphology and has been termed *thin-cap fibroatheroma* (TCFA), characterized by a large, lipid-rich necrotic core, thin overlying fibrous cap (<65 micron) that contains few smooth muscle cells and many macrophages, angiogenesis, adventitial inflammation, and positive remodeling [1, 124, 125]. Other well-recognized underlying substrates of ACS are plaque erosion, calcified nodules, intraplaque hemorrhage secondary to leaking vasa vasorum and potentially other unknown, all of them lacking the distinct morphologic features of TCFA [1].

Given the extremely small dimensions of some of the characteristics of these plaques, very high spatial resolution is required to identify them, and the only noninvasive technique with the potential for this type of imaging is the latest generation MDCT scanners (Fig. 11.13).

11.10.1 Plaque Position and Area

The formation of atherosclerotic plaques prevalently occurs in areas where blood flow tends to be turbulent. The evaluation of coronary ostia and bifurcations can be very precisely performed with MDCT. Thanks to the three-dimensional imaging capabilities the best view can be created for evaluating the plaque/stenosis, a feature which is undoubtedly much more difficult with conventional angiography: in such situations there is the risk of underestimating the stenosis due to difficulties in obtaining the appropriate view [126]. Furthermore, plaques of potential clinical relevance such as the TCFAs - the precursors of acute plaque rupture - tend to be relatively large and have a sizeable necrotic core accounting for 10% to 25% of total plaque area, with a mean length of 8 mm (range: from 2 to 17 mm) and a mean area of 1.7 ± 1.1 mm^2 [125]. Furthermore, in plaque vulnerability the circumferential extent of the necrotic core may be important, since it has been demonstrated that approximately 75% of TCFAs have a necrotic core extending >120° in circumference of the intima affected by the necrosis [127]. In addition, TCFAs are often observed in the proximal-mid portion of the coronary arteries (approximately in 90% of cases), with the proximal left anterior descending coronary artery being the most common site (in over 50% of cases), and proximal right and left circumflex coronary arteries about half as common [125, 128]. All these characteristics make them potentially evaluable by MDCT.

11.10.2 Plaque Composition

A substantial difference in mean density (and therefore in composition) of plaques in patients with acute coronary syndromes and patients with stable angina has been demonstrated [129, 130]. However, the lipid component does not have a negative Hounsfield density as might be expected; instead it displays on average higher levels. This is linked to the micro-architecture composition of the plaque itself which in addition to triglycerides is also composed of cholesterol, necrotic material, smooth muscle cells and microscopic calcified components. Due to insufficient spatial resolution it has also been demonstrated that the levels of plaque density are influenced by many factors, mainly the elevated density of intravascular contrast agent (see above) [111, 112].

11.10.3 Vascular Remodeling

This is an early vascular adaptation in response to the accumulation of atheromatous material at the level of the media. Negative vascular remodeling is well known, consisting of the accumulation of large quantities of fibrocalcified material responsible for a reduction in vascular diameter with typical clinical signs of angina. Positive vascular remodeling is a more recent discovery and occurs in the initial phases of disease and tends to preserve coronary flow despite the increasing accumulation of atheromatous material (Fig. 11.14). This phenomenon was initially demonstrated by Glagov et al. [131] in a necropsy study and subsequently validated in vivo using IVUS imaging [132]. Glagov demonstrated that luminal area was unaffected by plaque growth until the lesion reached 40% area stenosis; above this threshold, luminal area diminished in a close relationship to the percentage of stenosis [131]. This type of remodeling is associated with relatively large plaque dimensions (plaque area or plaque volume) and it is more frequent in prevalently lipid-laden and more unstable plaques [133]. Retrospective post-mortem studies have demonstrated that TCFAs do not usually show severe narrowing but show positive remodeling, with an underlying cross-sectional area narrowing in over 75% of cases <75% (diameter stenosis <50%) [125]. Experimental studies indicate that processes in adventitia could play a decisive role in remodeling [124].

11.10.4 Calcified Nodules

There exists a growth pattern of these nodules, defined *superficial*, which is recognizable at the level of the coronary arteries most subject to the mechanical stress of the beating heart (right coronary artery). Their presence is correlated with plaque transformation, a precursor of the typical symptoms of acute coronary syndromes [63, 64]. Several researchers have used IVUS to demonstrate a relationship between calcification pattern, plaque morphology and type of vascular remodeling. The culprit lesions of patients with acute myocardial infarction, unstable angina and stable angina have been shown to have different calcification patterns. In particular, in acute myocardial infarction an association was observed between spotty calcified deposits within an arc of ≤90° with positive remodeling and large fibrofatty core (Fig. 11.15) [134]. On the basis of the good correlation between IVUS and MDCT in the evaluation of coronary plaques, and particularly the excellent sensitivity of MDCT in differentiating calcified and soft components, MDCT can be considered the noninvasive criterion standard to accompany the invasive imaging modalities.

Currently no definite relationship has been demonstrated between coronary stenosis and the predisposition of a plaque to rupture (vulnerability). It is nonetheless certain

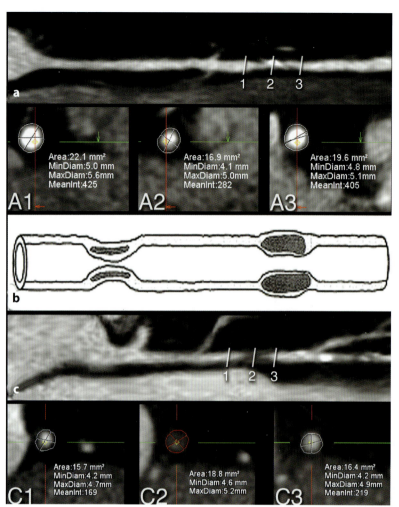

Fig. 11.14 Vascular remodeling. Negative remodeling (**a**): the ratio between the mean diameters of the vessel proximally and distally to the stenosis (**a1** and **a3**) and of the vessel at the level of maximum stenosis (**a2**) is <1. **b** Diagram of negative and positive vascular remodeling. Positive remodeling (**c**): the ratio between the mean diameters of the vessel proximally and distally to the stenosis (**c1** and **c3**) and of the vessel at the level of maximum stenosis (**c2**) is >1

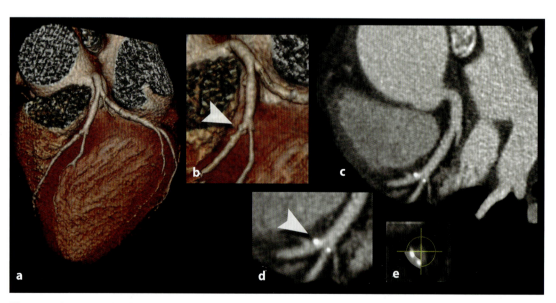

Fig. 11.15 Spotty calcification (**a**). Presence of calcified nodules at the level of the bifurcation of the left anterior descending coronary artery with the first diagonal branch (**b**, *arrowhead*). Multiplanar reconstructions provide a more accurate evaluation of the different components of the plaque (**c**) and the degree of stenosis it is causing in the vessel (**d**, *arrowhead*). The axial view enables the evaluation of the extent of the calcification: an angular involvement ≤90° was observed more frequently in the culprit lesions of patients with acute myocardial infarction

that over 50% of plaques which rupture are not hemodynamically significant and are therefore underestimated by conventional angiography. A new characterization of plaque is currently being formulated thanks to the knowledge acquired by postmortem and above all in vivo studies.

There is emerging clinical evidence which correlates the presence of some morphologic characteristics of coronary plaque visualized with MDCT with the occurrence of acute coronary syndrome (ACS). The largest prospective study to date evaluated plaque characteristics detected by 64-slice MDCT in a cohort of 1059 patients with suspected or known CAD, followed for 27 months for the development of ACS [135]. They found that patients with low-attenuation coronary plaques (density <30 HU) and associated positive remodeling (>10% diameter at the plaque site compared with the reference segment) showed a higher rate of ACS when compared with patients having lesions without these characteristics (respectively 22% vs. 0.5%) [135].

Furthermore, some recent studies conducted with MDCT in patients with ACS have demonstrated a higher prevalence of noncalcified plaques with vulnerable characteristics (low-attenuation plaques, positive remodeling and spotty calcifications) in patients with ACS as compared with stable clinical presentation [130, 136-140]. Interestingly, Pundziute et al. [137] performed 64-MDCT and VH-IVUS in patients with ACS or stable angina. They demonstrated that noncalcified plaque and mixed plaque were more prevalent in ACS patients, while calcified plaques were more prevalent in stable patients. They also found that VH-IVUS-defined TCFAs were more common in patients with ACS than stable angina, and that the TCFAs most frequently occurred in plaques classified as mixed by MDCT.

Recently, a new sign of plaque vulnerability has been proposed: a *contrast rim* around the plaque described as a ring-like contrast enhancement surrounding the coronary lesion. This imaging phenomenon possibly reflects vasa vasorum neovascularization of the plaque with active inflammation ring; other possible explanations are related to the presence of contrast surrounding thrombus material or of a large necrotic core separated by fibrous contents or native vessel wall [140, 141]. This sign, although insensitive, was shown to be the strongest MDCT feature associated with TCFA at the culprit site, with a reported specificity >95% [139-140].

11.11 Conclusions

In summary, the systematic evaluation of the parameters indicative of vulnerability and the improvement of protocols aimed at imaging plaque will help to define the individual degree of CAD and enable evidence-based risk stratification of major coronary events. This will have positive effects on the prevention of acute myocardial infarction and define the prognostic value of MDCT.

Ultimately, future developments other than increased spatial and temporal resolution may improve detection of vulnerable plaque by MDCT. These include the use of multiple energy data sets (80 kV and 140 kV) to reduce the overlap of the attenuation of plaque components, which would improve their classification [142] and the possibility of new nanoparticle contrast agents to target inflammatory components, such as macrophages, to highlight areas of potential vulnerability [143].

References

1. Naghavi M, Libby P, Falk E et al (2003) From vulnerable plaque to vulnerable patient: a call for new definitions and risk assessment strategies: Part I. Circulation 108:1664-1672
2. Naghavi M, Libby P, Falk E et al (2003) From vulnerable plaque to vulnerable patient: a call for new definitions and risk assessment strategies: Part II. Circulation 108:1772-1778
3. Cademartiri F, Malagutti P, Belgrano M et al (2005) Non-invasive coronary angiography with 64-slice computed tomography. Minerva Cardioangiol 53:465-472
4. Cademartiri F, Runza G, Belgrano M et al (2005) Introduction to coronary imaging with 64-slice computed tomography. Radiol Med (Torino) 110:16-41
5. Naghavi M, Falk E, Hecht HS et al (2006) From vulnerable plaque to vulnerable patient-Part III: Executive summary of the Screening for Heart Attack Prevention and Education (SHAPE) Task Force report. Am J Cardiol 98:2H-15H
6. Cademartiri F, Runza G, La Grutta L et al (2005) Non-invasive evaluation of coronary calcium. Radiol Med (Torino) 110:506-522
7. Achenbach S, Dilsizian V, Kramer CM, Zoghbi WA (2009) The year in coronary artery disease. JACC Cardiovasc Imaging 2:774-786
8. Pugliese F, Mollet NR, Hunink MG et al (2008) Diagnostic performance of coronary CT angiography by using different generations of multisection scanners: single-center experience. Radiology 246:384-393
9. Hamon M, Morello R, Riddell JW, Hamon M (2007) Coronary arteries: diagnostic performance of 16- versus 64-section spiral CT compared with invasive coronary angiography—meta-analysis. Radiology 245:720-731
10. Vanhoenacker PK, Heijenbrok-Kal MH, Van Heste R et al (2007) Diagnostic performance of multidetector CT angiography for assessment of coronary artery disease: meta-analysis. Radiology 244:419-428
11. Abdulla J, Abildstrom SZ, Gotzsche O et al (2007) 64-multislice detector computed tomography coronary angiography as potential alternative to conventional coronary angiography: a systematic review and meta-analysis. Eur Heart J 28:3042-3050
12. Meijer AB, O YL, Geleijns J, Kroft LJ (2008) Meta-analysis of 40- and 64-MDCT angiography for assessing coronary artery stenosis. AJR Am J Roentgenol 191:1667-1675
13. Mowatt G, Cook JA, Hillis GS et al (2008) 64-Slice computed tomography angiography in the diagnosis and assessment of coronary artery disease: systematic review and meta-analysis. Heart 94:1386-1393
14. Schuetz GM, Zacharopoulou NM, Schlattmann P, Dewey M (2010) Meta-analysis: noninvasive coronary angiography using comput-

ed tomography versus magnetic resonance imaging. Ann Intern Med 152:167-177

15. Budoff MJ, Dowe D, Jollis JG et al (2008) Diagnostic performance of 64-multidetector row coronary computed tomographic angiography for evaluation of coronary artery stenosis in individuals without known coronary artery disease: results from the prospective multi center ACCURACY (Assessment by Coronary Computed Tomographic Angiography of Individuals Undergoing Invasive Coronary Angiography) trial. J Am Coll Cardiol 52:1724-1732

16. Miller JM, Rochitte CE, Dewey M et al (2008) Diagnostic performance of coronary angiography by 64-row CT. N Engl J Med 359:2324-2336

17. Miller JM, Dewey M, Vavere AL et al (2009) Coronary CT angiography using 64 detector rows: methods and design of the multi-centre trial CORE-64. Eur Radiol 19:816-828

18. Meijboom WB, Meijs MF, Schuijf JD et al (2008) Diagnostic accuracy of 64-slice computed tomography coronary angiography: a prospective, multicenter, multivendor study. J Am Coll Cardiol 52:2135-2144

19. Maffei E, Palumbo A, Martini C et al (2010) Diagnostic accuracy of 64-slice computed tomography coronary angiography in a large population of patients without revascularisation: registry data and review of multicentre trials. Radiol Med 115:368-384

20. Earls JP, Berman EL, Urban BA et al (2008) Prospectively gated transverse coronary CT angiography versus retrospectively gated helical technique: improved image quality and reduced radiation dose. Radiology 246:742-753

21. Chao SP, Law WY, Kuo CJ et al (2010) The diagnostic accuracy of 256-row computed tomographic angiography compared with invasive coronary angiography in patients with suspected coronary artery disease. Eur Heart J 31:1916-1623

22. Dewey M, Zimmermann E, Deissenrieder F et al (2009) Noninvasive coronary angiography by 320-row computed tomography with lower radiation exposure and maintained diagnostic accuracy: comparison of results with cardiac catheterization in a head-to-head pilot investigation. Circulation 120:867-875

23. Min JK, Swaminathan RV, Vass M et al (2009) High-definition multidetector computed tomography for evaluation of coronary artery stents: comparison to standard-definition 64-detector row computed tomography. J Cardiovasc Comput Tomogr 3:246-251

24. Achenbach S, Marwan M, Ropers D et al (2010) Coronary computed tomography angiography with a consistent dose below 1 mSv using prospectively electrocardiogram-triggered high-pitch spiral acquisition. Eur Heart J 31:340-346

25. Falk E, Shah PK, Fuster V (1995) Coronary plaque disruption. Circulation 92:657-671

26. Topol EJ, Nissen SE (1995) Our preoccupation with coronary luminology. The dissociation between clinical and angiographic findings in ischemic heart disease. Circulation 92:2333-2342

27. Van Mieghem CA, McFadden EP, de Feyter PJ et al (2006) Noninvasive detection of subclinical coronary atherosclerosis coupled with assessment of changes in plaque characteristics using novel invasive imaging modalities: the Integrated Biomarker and Imaging Study (IBIS). J Am Coll Cardiol 47:1134-1142

28. Cademartiri F, La Grutta L, Palumbo A et al (2007) Imaging techniques for the vulnerable coronary plaque. Radiol Med 112:637-659

29. Hunold P, Vogt FM, Schmermund A et al (2003) Radiation exposure during cardiac CT: effective doses at multi-detector row CT and electron-beam CT. Radiology 226:145-152

30. Agatston AS, Janowitz WR, Hildner FJ et al (1990) Quantification of coronary artery calcium using ultrafast computed tomography. J Am Coll Cardiol 15:827-832

31. Margolis J, Chen J, Kong Y et al (1980) The diagnostic and prognostic significance of coronary artery calcification: a report of 800 cases. Radiology 137:609-616

32. Detrano RC, Wong ND, Tang W et al (1994) Prognostic significance of cardiac cinefluoroscopy for coronary calcific deposits in asymptomatic high risk subjects. J Am Coll Cardiol 24:354-358

33. Clouse ME (2006) How useful is computed tomography for screening for coronary artery disease? Noninvasive screening for coronary artery disease with computed tomography is useful. Circulation 113:125-146

34. Wexler L, Brundage B, Crouse J et al (1996) Coronary artery calcification: pathophysiology, epidemiology, imaging methods, and clinical implications. A statement for health professionals from the American Heart Association. Writing Group. Circulation 1996 94:1175-1192

35. Callister TQ, Cooil B, Raya SP et al (1998) Coronary artery disease: improved reproducibility of calcium scoring with an electron beam CT volumetric method. Radiology 208:807-814

36. McEvoy JW, Blaha MJ, Defilippis AP et al (2010) Coronary artery calcium progression: an important clinical measurement? A review of published reports. J Am Coll Cardiol 56:1613-1622

37. Rumberger JA, Kaufman L (2003) A Rosetta stone for coronary calcium risk stratification: Agatston, volume, and mass scores in 11,490 individuals. Am J Roentgenol 181:743-748

38. Hong C, Becker CR, Schoepf UJ Et al (2002) Coronary artery calcium: absolute quantification in nonenhanced and contrast-enhanced multi-detector row CT studies. Radiology 223:474-480

39. Hong C, Bae KT, Pilgram TK (2003) Coronary artery calcium: accuracy and reproducibility of measurements with multi-detector row CT—assessment of effects of different thresholds and quantification methods. Radiology 227:795-801

40. Oudkerk M, Stillman AE, Halliburton SS et al (2008) European Society of Cardiac Radiology; North American Society for Cardiovascular Imaging. Coronary artery calcium screening: current status and recommendations from the European Society of Cardiac Radiology and North American Society for Cardiovascular Imaging. Eur Radiol 18:2785-2807

41. McCollough CH, Ulzheimer S, Halliburton SS et al (2007) Coronary artery calcium: a multi-institutional, multimanufacturer international standard for quantification at cardiac CT. Radiology 243:527-538

42. Becker CR, Kleffel T, Crispin A et al (2001) Coronary artery calcium measurement: agreement of multirow detector and electron beam CT. AJR Am J Roentgenol 176:1295-1298

43. Stanford W, Thompson BH, Burns TL, Heery SD, Burr MC (2004) Coronary artery calcium quantification at multi-detector row helical CT versus electron-beam CT. Radiology 230:397-402

44. Budoff MJ, McClelland RL, Chung H et al (2009) Reproducibility of coronary artery calcified plaque with cardiac 64-MDCT: the Multi-Ethnic Study of Atherosclerosis. AJR Am J Roentgenol 192:613-617

45. Morin RL, Gerber TC, McCollough CH (2003) Radiation dose in computed tomography of the heart. Circulation 107:917-922

46. Rumberger JA, Simons DB, Fitzpatrick LA et al (1995) Coronary artery calcium area by electron-beam computed tomography and coronary atherosclerotic plaque area. A histopathologic correlative study. Circulation 92: 2157-2162

47. Stary HC (2000) Natural history of calcium deposits in atherosclerosis progression and regression. Z Kardiol 89 Suppl 2:28-35

48. Rumberger JA, Brundage BH, Rader DJ, Kondos G (1999) Electron beam computed tomography coronary calcium scanning: a review and guidelines for use in asymptomatic persons. Mayo Clin Proc 74:243-252

49. Kajinami K, Seki H, Takekoshi N, Mabuchi H (1997) Coronary calcification and coronary atherosclerosis: site by site comparative morphologic study of electron beam computed tomography and coronary angiography. J Am Coll Cardiol 29:1549-1556

50. Wilson PW, D'Agostino RB, Levy D et al (1998) Prediction of coronary heart disease using risk factor categories. Circulation 97:1837-1847

51. Greenland P, Abrams J, Aurigemma GP et al (2000) Prevention Conference V: Beyond secondary prevention: identifying the high-risk patient for primary prevention: noninvasive tests of atherosclerotic burden:Writing Group III. Circulation 101:E16-22

52. Shaw LJ, Raggi P, Schisterman E et al (2003) Prognostic value of cardiac risk factors and coronary artery calcium screening for all-cause mortality. Radiology 228:826-833

53. Greenland P, Bonow RO, Brundage BH et al (2007) ACCF/AHA 2007 clinical expert consensus document on coronary artery calcium scoring by computed tomography in global cardiovascular risk assessment and in evaluation of patients with chest pain: a report of the American College of Cardiology Foundation Clinical Expert Consensus Task Force (ACCF/AHA Writing Committee to Update the 2000 Expert Consensus Document on Electron Beam Computed Tomography). Circulation 115:402-426

54. Sarwar A, Shaw LJ, Shapiro MD et al (2009) Diagnostic and prognostic value of absence of coronary artery calcification. J Am Coll Cardiol Img 2:675-688

55. Blaha M, Budoff MJ, Shaw LJ et al (2009) Absence of coronary artery calcification and all-cause mortality. J Am Coll Cardiol Img 2:692-700

56. Schuijf JD, van der Wall EE, Bax JJ (2009) Lesions without calcium: lessons from CT angiography. Heart 95:1038-1040

57. Cheng VY, Lepor NE, Madyoon H et al (2007) Presence and severity of noncalcified coronary plaque on 64-slice computed tomographic coronary angiography in patients with zero and low coronary artery calcium. Am J Cardiol 99:1183-1186

58. Akram K, O'Donnell RE, King S et al (2009) Influence of symptomatic status on the prevalence of obstructive coronary artery disease in patients with zero calcium score. Atherosclerosis 203:533-537

59. Rubinshtein R, Gaspar T, Halon DA et al (2007) Prevalence and extent of obstructive coronary artery disease in patients with zero or low calcium score undergoing 64-slice cardiac multidetector computed tomography for evaluation of a chest pain syndrome. Am J Cardiol 99:472-475

60. Nieman K, Galema TW, Neefjes LA et al (2009) Comparison of the value of coronary calcium detection to computed tomographic angiography and exercise testing in patients with chest pain. Am J Cardiol 104:1499-1504

61. Gottlieb I, Miller JM, Arbab-Zadeh A et al (2010) The absence of coronary calcification does not exclude obstructive coronary artery disease or the need for revascularization in patients referred for conventional coronary angiography. J Am Coll Cardiol 55:627-634

62. Maffei E, Seitun S, Nieman K et al (2011) Assessment of coronary artery disease and calcified coronary plaque burden by computed tomography in patients with and without diabetes mellitus. Eur Radiol 21:944-953

63. Stary HC, Chandler AB, Glagov S Et al (1994) A definition of initial, fatty streak, and intermediate lesions of atherosclerosis. A report from the Committee on Vascular Lesions of the Council on Arteriosclerosis, American Heart Association. Circulation 89:2462-2478

64. Stary HC, Chandler AB, Dinsmore RE Et al (1995) A definition of advanced types of atherosclerotic lesions and a histological classification of atherosclerosis. A report from the Committee on Vascular Lesions of the Council on Arteriosclerosis, American Heart Association. Circulation 92:1355-1374

65. Stary HC (2000) Natural history and histological classification of atherosclerotic lesions: an update. Arterioscler Thromb Vasc Biol 20:1177-1178

66. Mann JM, Davies MJ (1996) Vulnerable plaque. Relation of characteristics to degree of stenosis in human coronary arteries. Circulation 94:928-931

67. Fuster V, Badimon L, Badimon JJ, Chesebro JH (1992) The pathogenesis of coronary artery disease and the acute coronary syndromes (1). N Engl J Med 326:242-250

68. Fuster V, Badimon L, Badimon JJ, Chesebro JH (1992) The pathogenesis of coronary artery disease and the acute coronary syndromes (2). N Engl J Med 326:310-318

69. Burke AP, Farb A, Malcom GT et al (1997) Coronary risk factors and plaque morphology in men with coronary disease who died suddenly. N Engl J Med 336:1276-1282

70. Fishbein MC, Siegel RJ (1996) How big are coronary atherosclerotic plaques that rupture? Circulation 94:2662-2666

71. Rioufol G, Finet G, Ginon I et al (2002) Multiple atherosclerotic plaque rupture in acute coronary syndrome: a three-vessel intravascular ultrasound study. Circulation 106:804-808

72. Mintz GS, Nissen SE, Anderson WD et al (2001) American College of Cardiology Clinical Expert Consensus Document on Standards for Acquisition, Measurement and Reporting of Intravascular Ultrasound Studies (IVUS). A report of the American College of Cardiology Task Force on Clinical Expert Consensus Documents. J Am Coll Cardiol 37:1478-1492

73. Schaar JA, Regar E, Mastik F et al (2004) Incidence of high-strain patterns in human coronary arteries: assessment with three-dimensional intravascular palpography and correlation with clinical presentation. Circulation 109:2716-2719

74. Rodriguez-Granillo GA, Bruining N, Mc Fadden E et al (2005) Geometrical validation of intravascular ultrasound radiofrequency data analysis (Virtual Histology) acquired with a 30 MHz boston scientific corporation imaging catheter. Catheter Cardiovasc Interv 66:514-518

75. Rodriguez-Granillo GA, Vaina S, Garcia-Garcia HM et al (2006) Reproducibility of intravascular ultrasound radiofrequency data analysis: implications for the design of longitudinal studies. Int J Cardiovasc Imaging 22:621-631

76. Rodriguez-Granillo GA, Garcia-Garcia HM, Valgimigli M et al (2006) In vivo relationship between compositional and mechanical imaging of coronary arteries. Insights from intravascular ultrasound radiofrequency data analysis. Am Heart J 151:1025 e1-6

77. Stefanadis C, Toutouzas K, Tsiamis E et al (2001) Increased local temperature in human coronary atherosclerotic plaques: an independent predictor of clinical outcome in patients undergoing a percutaneous coronary intervention. J Am Coll Cardiol 37:1277-1283

78. Mizuno K, Miyamoto A, Satomura K et al (1991) Angioscopic coronary macromorphology in patients with acute coronary disorders. Lancet 337:809-812

79. Uchida Y, Nakamura F, Tomaru T et al (1995) Prediction of acute coronary syndromes by percutaneous coronary angioscopy in patients with stable angina. Am Heart J 130:195-203

80. Patel NA, Stamper DL, Brezinski ME (2005) Review of the ability of optical coherence tomography to characterize plaque, including a comparison with intravascular ultrasound. Cardiovasc Intervent Radiol 28:1-9

81. Yabushita H, Bouma BE, Houser SL et al (2002) Characterization of human atherosclerosis by optical coherence tomography. Circulation 106:1640-1645

82. MacNeill BD, Jang IK, Bouma BE et al (2004) Focal and multifocal plaque macrophage distributions in patients with acute and stable presentations of coronary artery disease. J Am Coll Cardiol 44:972-979

83. Jang IK, Bouma BE, Kang DH et al (2002) Visualization of coronary atherosclerotic plaques in patients using optical coherence tomography: comparison with intravascular ultrasound. J Am Coll Cardiol 39:604-609

84. Raman C (1928) A new type of secondary radiation. Nature 121:501-502

85. Brennan JF III, Romer TJ, Lees RS et al (1997) Determination of human coronary artery composition by Raman spectroscopy. Circulation 96:99-105.

86. Buschman HP, Marple ET, Wach ML et al (2000) In vivo determination of the molecular composition of artery wall by intravascular Raman spectroscopy. Anal Chem 72:3771-3775

87. Romer TJ, Brennan JF III, Puppels GJ (2000) Intravascular ultrasound combined with Raman spectroscopy to localize and quantify cholesterol and calcium salts in atherosclerotic coronary arteries. Arterioscler Thromb Vasc Biol 20:478-483

88. Jaross W, Neumeister V, Lattke P, Schuh D (1999) Determination of cholesterol in atherosclerotic plaques using near infrared diffuse reflection spectroscopy. Atherosclerosis 147:327-337

89. Moreno PR, Lodder RA, Purushothaman KR et al (2002) Detection of lipid pool, thin fibrous cap, and inflammatory cells in human aortic atherosclerotic plaques by near-infrared spectroscopy. Circulation 105:923-927

90. Caplan JD, Waxman S, Nesto RW, Muller JE (2006) Near-infrared spectroscopy for the detection of vulnerable coronary artery plaques. J Am Coll Cardiol 47:C92-C96

91. Leber AW, Knez A, von Ziegler F et al (2005) Quantification of obstructive and nonobstructive coronary lesions by 64-slice computed tomography: a comparative study with quantitative coronary angiography and intravascular ultrasound. J Am Coll Cardiol 46:147-154

92. Achenbach S, Moselewski F, Ropers D et al (2004) Detection of calcified and noncalcified coronary atherosclerotic plaque by contrast-enhanced, submillimeter multidetector spiral computed tomography: a segment based comparison with intravascular ultrasound. Circulation 109:14-17

93. Nikolaou K, Becker CR, Muders M (2004) et al Multidetector-row-computed tomography and magnetic resonance imaging of atherosclerotic lesions in human ex vivo coronary arteries. Atherosclerosis 174:243-242

94. Becker CR, Nikolaou K, Muders M et al (2003) Ex vivo coronary atherosclerotic plaque characterization with multi-detector-row CT. Eur Radiol 13:2094-2098

95. Schroeder S, Kuettner A, Leitritz M et al (2004) Reliability of differentiating human coronary plaque morphology using contrast-enhanced multislice spiral computed tomography: a comparison with histology. J Comput Assist Tomogr 28:449-454

96. Leber AW, Knez A, Becker A et al (2004) Accuracy of multidetector spiral computed tomography in identifying and differentiating the composition of coronary atherosclerotic plaques: a comparative study with intracoronary ultrasound. J Am Coll Cardiol 43:1241-1247

97. Moselewski F, Ropers D, Pohle K et al (2004) Comparison of measurement of cross-sectional coronary atherosclerotic plaque and vessel areas by 16-slice multidetector computed tomography versus intravascular ultrasound. Am J Cardiol 94:1294-1297

98. Leber AW, Becker A, Knez A et al (2006) Accuracy of 64-slice computed tomography to classify and quantify plaque volumes in the proximal coronary system: a comparative study using intravascular ultrasound. J Am Coll Cardiol 47:672-677

99. Sun J, Zhang Z, Lu B et al (2008) Identification and quantification of coronary atherosclerotic plaques: a comparison of 64-MDCT and intravascular ultrasound. AJR Am J Roentgenol 190:748-754

100. Petranovic M, Soni A, Bezzera H et al (2009) Assessment of non-stenotic coronary lesions by 64-slice multidetector computed tomography in comparison to intravascular ultrasound: evaluation of nonculprit coronary lesions. J Cardiovasc Comput Tomogr 3:24-31

101. Schroeder S, Kopp AF, Baumbach A et al (2001) Noninvasive detection and evaluation of atherosclerotic coronary plaques with multislice computed tomography. J Am Coll Cardiol 37:1430-1435

102. Ferencik M, Chan RC, Achenbach S et al (2006) Arterial wall imaging: evaluation with 16-section multidetector CT in blood vessel phantoms and ex vivo coronary arteries. Radiology 240:708-716

103. Pohle K, Achenbach S, Macneill B et al (2007) Characterization of non-calcified coronary atherosclerotic plaque by multi-detector row CT: comparison to IVUS. Atherosclerosis 190:174-180

104. Choi BJ, Kang DK, Tahk SJ et al (2008) Comparison of 64-slice multidetector computed tomography with spectral analysis of intravascular ultrasound backscatter signals for characterizations of noncalcified coronary arterial plaques. Am J Cardiol 102:988-993

105. Kim SY, Kim KS, Lee YS et al (2009) Assessment of non-calcified coronary plaques using 64-slice computed tomography: comparison with intravascular ultrasound. Korean Circ J 39:95-99

106. Hur J, Kim YJ, Lee HJ et al (2009) Quantification and characterization of obstructive coronary plaques using 64-slice computed tomography: a comparison with intravascular ultrasound. J Comput Assist Tomogr 33:186-192

107. Chopard R, Boussel L, Motreff P (2010) et al How reliable are 40 MHz IVUS and 64-slice MDCT in characterizing coronary plaque composition? An ex vivo study with histopathological comparison. Int J Cardiovasc Imaging 26:373-383

108. Soeda T, Uemura S, Morikawa Y et al (2011) Diagnostic accuracy of dual-source computed tomography in the characterization of coronary atherosclerotic plaques: Comparison with intravascular optical coherence tomography. Int J Cardiol 148:313-318

109. Schroeder S, Flohr T, Kopp AF et al (2001) Accuracy of density measurements within plaques located in artificial coronary arteries by X-ray multislice CT: results of a phantom study. J Comput Assist Tomogr 25:900-906

110. Horiguchi J, Fujioka C, Kiguchi M et al (2007) Soft and intermediate plaques in coronary arteries: how accurately can we measure CT attenuation using 64-MDCT? AJR Am J Roentgenol 189:981-988

111. Cademartiri F, Mollet NR, Runza G et al (2005) Influence of intracoronary attenuation on coronary plaque measurements using multislice computed tomography: observations in an ex vivo model of coronary computed tomography angiography. Eur Radiol 15:1426-1431

112. Cademartiri F, Runza G, Palumbo A et al (2010) Lumen enhancement influences absolute noncalcific plaque density on multislice computed tomography coronary angiography: ex-vivo validation and in-vivo demonstration. J Cardiovasc Med (Hagerstown) 11:337-344

113. Dalager MG, Bøttcher M, Andersen G et al (2011) Impact of luminal density on plaque classification by CT coronary angiography. Int J Cardiovasc Imaging 27:593-600

114. Schroeder S, Flohr T, Kopp AF et al (2001) Accuracy of density measurements within plaques located in artificial coronary arteries by X-ray multislice CT: results of a phantom study. J Comput Assist Tomogr 25:900-906

115. Cademartiri F, La Grutta L, Runza G et al (2007) Influence of convolution filtering on coronary plaque attenuation values: observations in an ex vivo model of multislice computed tomography coronary angiography. Eur Radiol 17:1842-1849

116. Achenbach S, Boehmer K, Pflederer T et al (2010) Influence of slice thickness and reconstruction kernel on the computed tomographic attenuation of coronary atherosclerotic plaque. J Cardiovasc Comput Tomogr 4:110-115

117. Horiguchi J, Fujioka C, Kiguchi M et al (2011) In vitro measurement of CT density and estimation of stenosis related to coronary soft plaque at 100kV and 120kV on ECG-triggered scan. Eur J Radiol 77:296-298

118. Galonska M, Ducke F, Kertesz-Zborilova T et al (2008) Characterization of atherosclerotic plaques in human coronary arteries with 16-slice multidetector row computed tomography by analysis of attenuation profiles. Acad Radio 15:222-230

119. Henzler T, Porubsky S, Kayed H et al (2010) Attenuation-based characterization of coronary atherosclerotic plaque: Comparison of

dual source and dual energy CT with single-source CT and histopathology. Eur J Radiol 80:54-59

120. Leschka S, Seitun S, Dettmer M et al (2010) Ex vivo evaluation of coronary atherosclerotic plaques: characterization with dual-source CT in comparison with histopathology. J Cardiovasc Comput Tomogr 4:301-308

121. Little WC (1990) Angiographic assessment of the culprit coronary artery lesion before acute myocardial infarction.Am J Cardiol 66:44G-47G

122. Muller JE, Abela GS, Nesto RW, Tofler GH (1994) Triggers, acute risk factors and vulnerable plaques: the lexicon of a new frontier. J Am Coll Cardiol 23:809-813

123. Virmani R, Kolodgie FD, Burke AP et al (2000) Lessons from sudden coronary death: a comprehensive morphological classification scheme for atherosclerotic lesions. Arterioscler Thromb Vasc Biol 20:1262-1275

124. Falk E (2006) Pathogenesis of atherosclerosis. J Am Coll Cardiol 47(8 Suppl):C7-12

125. Virmani R, Burke AP, Farb A, Kolodgie FD (2006) Pathology of the vulnerable plaque. J Am Coll Cardiol 47(8 Suppl):C13-18

126. Galbraith JE, Murphy ML, de Soyza N (1978) Coronary angiogram interpretation. Interobserver variability. JAMA 240:2053-2056

127. Kolodgie FD, Virmani R, Burke AP et al (2004) Pathologic assessment of the vulnerable human coronary plaque. Heart 90:1385-1391

128. Kolodgie FD, Burke AP, Farb A et al (2001) The thin-cap fibroatheroma: a type of vulnerable plaque: the major precursor lesion to acute coronary syndromes. Curr Opin Cardiol 16:285-292

129. Leber AW, Knez A, White CW et al (2003) Composition of coronary atherosclerotic plaques in patients with acute myocardial infarction and stable angina pectoris determined by contrast enhanced multislice computed tomography. Am J Cardiol 91:714-718

130. Hoffmann U, Moselewski F, Nieman K et al (2006) Noninvasive assessment of plaque morphology and composition in culprit and stable lesions in acute coronary syndrome and stable lesions in stable angina by multidetector computed tomography. J Am Coll Cardiol 47:1655-1662

131. Glagov S, Weisenberg E, Zarins CK, Stankunavicius R, Kolettis GJ (1987) Compensatory enlargement of human atherosclerotic coronary arteries. N Engl J Med 316:1371-1375

132. Hermiller JB, Tenaglia AN, Kisslo KB et al (1993) In vivo valida-

tion of compensatory enlargement of atherosclerotic coronary arteries. Am J Cardiol 71:665-668

133. Rodriguez-Granillo GA, Garcia-Garcia HM,Wentzel J et al (2006) Plaque composition and its relationship with acknowledged shear stress patterns in coronary arteries. J Am Coll Cardiol 47:884-885

134. Ehara S, Kobayashi Y,Yoshiyama M et al (2004) Spotty calcification typifies the culprit plaque in patients with acute myocardial infarction: an intravascular ultrasound study. Circulation 110:3424-3429

135. Motoyama S, Sarai M, Harigaya H et al (2009) Computed tomographic angiography characteristics of atherosclerotic plaques subsequently resulting in acute coronary syndrome. J Am Coll Cardiol 54:49-57

136. Motoyama S, Kondo T, Sarai M et al (2007) Multislice computed tomographic characteristics of coronary lesions in acute coronary syndromes. J Am Coll Cardiol 50:319-326

137. Pundziute G, Schuijf JD, Jukema JW et al (2008) Head-to-head comparison of coronary plaque evaluation between multislice computed tomography and intravascular ultrasound radiofrequency data analysis. JACC Cardiovasc Interv 1:176-182

138. Kitagawa T, Yamamoto H, Horiguchi J et al (2009) Characterization of noncalcified coronary plaques and identification of culprit lesions in patients with acute coronary syndrome by 64-slice computed tomography. JACC Cardiovasc Imaging 2:153-160

139. Pflederer T, Marwan M, Schepis T et al (2010) Characterization of culprit lesions in acute coronary syndromes using coronary dual-source CT angiography. Atherosclerosis 211:437-444

140. Kashiwagi M, Tanaka A, Kitabata H et al (2009) Feasibility of noninvasive assessment of thin-cap fibroatheroma by multidetector computed tomography. JACC Cardiovasc Imaging 2:1412-1419

141. Maurovich-Horvat P, Hoffmann U, Vorpahl M et al (2010) The napkin-ring sign: CT signature of high-risk coronary plaques? JACC Cardiovasc Imaging 3:440-444

142. Tanami Y, Ikeda E, Jinzaki M et al (2010) Computed tomographic attenuation value of coronary atherosclerotic plaques with different tube voltage: an ex vivo study. J Comput Assist Tomogr 34:58-63

143. Hyafil F, Cornily JC, Feig JE et al (2007) Noninvasive detection of macrophages using a nanoparticulate contrast agent for computed tomography. Nat Med 13:636-641

Coronary Artery Stenosis on Cardiac CT

12

Sara Seitun, Erica Maffei, Chiara Martini, Margherita Castiglione Morelli, and Filippo Cademartiri

12.1 Invasive Coronary Angiography

Nearly 55 years after its invention, invasive coronary angiography is still considered to be the "gold standard" method for the assessment of coronary stenosis and for planning and guiding percutaneous coronary intervention (PCI) [1-3]. Angiography is a two-dimensional imaging modality that depicts coronary anatomy as a planar silhouette of the contrast-filled lumen. Modern angiographic equipment yields a spatial resolution approximately of 0.2 mm in the clinical setting [3]. The procedure is associated with a small but definable risk (<2%) and is relatively expensive [3].

In clinical practice, the most simple and frequently used method is subjective visual estimation of the percentage of stenosis. However, coronary angiography has major shortcomings. A high interobserver and intraobserver variability in the interpretation of coronary angiograms has been well documented [2, 3]. In the late 1970s, a quantitative coronary angiography (QCA) method was originally introduced as a computer-based system which can improve assessment of anatomic lesion characteristics and reduce the wide variability in readings of the angiogram [3]. However, QCA has not yet been used routinely in clinical practice.

Furthermore, comparative studies reported poor correlation between the severity of coronary stenosis as evaluated from coronary arteriogram and both intravascular ultrasound and postmortem histology, with angiography significantly underestimating the extent of atherosclerosis [2, 3]. Angiography consists of a *luminography* in which each stenosis can be evaluated only by comparison to an adjacent segment that is presumed to be free of disease. Therefore, it only visualizes the lumen and it cannot identify atherosclerotic plaque accumulation in the coronary wall. An adaptive phenomenon, positive coronary remodeling, contributes to the inability of coronary angiography to identify mild atherosclerosis. Coronary lesions are often geometrically complex, with an eccentric luminal shape such that, even with multiple projection angles, the degree of luminal narrowing may be underestimated (Fig. 12.1) [4]. Other factors such as tortuous vessels and overlapping of the multiple side branches may also interfere with the assessment of severity and extent of coronary artery lesions. In particular, evaluation of ostial lesions of the left main coronary artery is particularly troublesome for angiographic imaging [2].

12.2 Coronary Stenosis and Coronary Flow Reserve

The extent of coronary disease is usually defined as one-vessel, two-vessel, three-vessel, or left main disease, with a cut-off ≤ 50% of diameter reduction for significant stenosis, although many angiographers define a significant stenosis as being narrowed by 70% diameter reduction [3]. Both animal and human data showed that a stenosis that reduces lumen diameter by 50% (and hence cross-sectional area by 75%) is hemodynamically significant in that it reduces the coronary flow reserve (CFR) [2, 3]. This phenomenon is the ability to increase blood flow in response to metabolic demands. Determination of CFR requires measurement of blood flow at rest and after induction of reactive hyperemia, usually by administration of a coronary vasodilator [5]. The normal CFR of a coronary bed is typically a 5:1 to 7:1 ratio between hyperemic to basal flow. Several methods for measurement of CFR in patients have been developed, including intracoronary Doppler flow probes, digital angiography and quantitative PET [3]. For stenosis between 75% and 95% diameter narrowing, CFR falls progressively to reach values approaching a 1:1 ratio [2-4] (Fig. 12.2).

The anatomic severity of a coronary stenosis is, however, not always predictive of its physiologic effect. This

S. Seitun (✉)
Department of Diagnostic and Interventional Radiology,
"San Martino" University Hospital – IST – IRCCS,
Genova, Italy

F. Cademartiri, G. Casolo, M. Midiri (eds.), *Clinical Applications of Cardiac CT*,
© Springer-Verlag Italia 2012

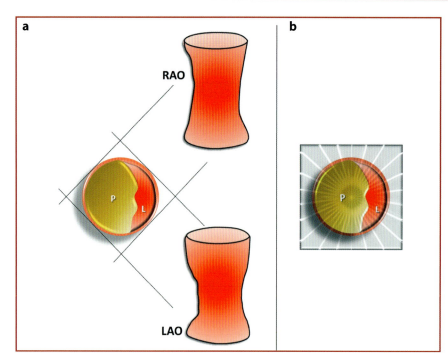

Fig. 12.1 a Conventional coronary angiograms yields two-dimensional (2D) images obtained at different angles for the evaluation of coronary stenosis. Therefore, the procedure may underestimate the degree of stenosis if the minimum luminal diameter is depicted at suboptimal projection angles. *RAO*, right anterior oblique projection; *LAO*, left anterior oblique projection. **b** Allows analysis of the coronary vessels in any desired spatial orientation; the cross-sectional image oriented perpendicular to the coronary vessel at the level of the stenosis clearly depicts both lumen and wall morphology allowing a better quantification of the degree of stenosis. *L*, lumen; *P*, plaque

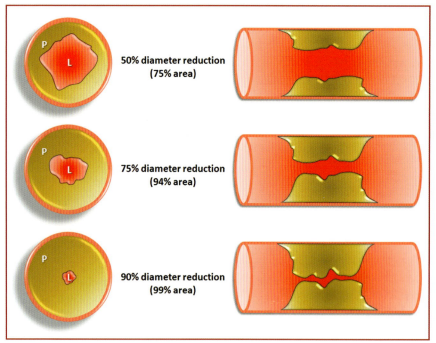

Fig. 12.2 Drawings illustrates cross-sectional and longitudinal views at different percentage of diameter and area reduction. The relationship between area reduction and diameter reduction in a completely concentric stenosis is described by the equation $A = D(2 - [D/100])$, where A= percentage of area reduction and D=percentage of diameter reduction. In the presence of eccentric stenosis, the relationship between area and diameter reduction is not constant [4]. *L*, lumen; *P*, plaque

is especially true in the case of an intermediate coronary lesion (40%-70% diameter stenosis), where angiography is very limited in distinguishing ischemia-producing intermediate coronary lesions from non-ischemia-producing ones [6, 7].

In 1995, fractional flow reserve (FFR) measurement was introduced to evaluate the clinical significance of a stenosis [8]. It can be measured during coronary angiography by calculating the ratio of the pressure after the stenosis measured with a pressure catheter to the aortic pressure measured simultaneously with the guiding catheter, at maximal coronary hyperemia induced by intravenous adenosine [8]. The established cut-off value for FFR is 0.75, which implies that the stenosis is considered significant when distal pressure during maximum hyperemia is <75% of aortic pressure and otherwise is not significant [3, 8, 9].

However, several anatomic variables of coronary stenosis other than reduction in lumen diameter affect the physiologic responses of the coronary circulation. These variables are: (a) stenosis geometry; (b) site of stenosis; (c) length of stenosis; and (d) number of stenoses in one vessel [10-14]. For example, previous works have shown that multiple stenoses have a cumulative hemodynamic effect even when none of the stenoses were critical. In particular, Feldaman et al. demonstrated that the hemodynamic responses observed with multiple 40% to 60% narrowings in series were comparable to effects observed with longer 40 to 60 % narrowings and with short narrowings of approximately an 80% reduction in diameter, although there seemed to be slightly more loss of pressure across the multiple stenosis [10].

Lastly, other factors including coronary collateral flow, ventricular hypertrophy, the metabolic state of the myocardium, and microvascular impairment may contribute to the hemodynamic effect of a stenosis [3].

12.3 Cardiac Computed Tomography

The high diagnostic accuracy of cardiac computed tomography angiography (CCT) in the noninvasive detection of significant coronary artery disease (CAD) ($\geq$50% luminal narrowing) is well established. Results from meta-analysis and multicenter trials are reported in Table 12.1 and Table 12.2 [15-25]. In general, CCT, after appropriate patient selection and with sufficient experience, demonstrates high accuracy particularly by its high sensitivity and negative predictive values, the latter implying that the symptoms leading to testing are very unlikely related to significant coronary stenosis. Several studies have demonstrated that at least three specific parameters capable of modulating accuracy can be identified in the literature: (a) body mass index (BMI); (b) heart rate, and (c) coronary artery calcium (i.e. Agatston calcium score). When high, these three parameters can negatively influence the diagnostic accuracy [26-28]. In particular, if extensive calcifications are present, CCT results tend to overestimate coronary stenosis as compared with conventional coronary angiography due to beam-hardening artifacts [25, 29, 30].

According to Bayes theorem, diagnostic accuracy is strictly dependent also on the disease prevalence of the study population, with an increased predictive accuracy of a positive CCT scan with increasing prevalence of dis-

ease in the population under study [25]. The clinical utility and diagnostic performance of CCT for detecting significant coronary disease in relation to the pre-test probability of CAD in patients with chest symptoms has been recently evaluated (Table 12.3) [31]. The study concluded that CCT seems to play a more important role in patients with an intermediate pre-test probability, in whom the test can distinguish which patients require invasive testing [31].

A further source of variability in CCT accuracy lies in the subjective interpretation strategy of the dataset. This is very particularly true in the presence of borderline lesions (around 50% luminal narrowing) and lesions that may be difficult to evaluate due to other limiting factors (e.g. calcium artifacts, residual motion, poor intraluminal contrast, arrhythmias, etc.).

Because CCT allows acquisition of volumetric data sets, coronary vessels can be visualized in any desired spatial orientation, (Fig. 12.1). With the use of dedicated 3D workstations, the images can be manipulated through a 360° perspective, offering distinct advantages compared to invasive coronary angiography.

Several studies have demonstrated that visual and quantitative assessments by CCT of stenosis severity are similar [22, 32]. In general, a quantitative assessment of stenosis severity by visual estimation is commonly used in clinical practice. Most previous studies on MDCT coronary angiography have used *binary* cut-off values, such as $\geq$50% diameter stenosis (more frequently) or $\geq$70% diameter stenosis, to define a clinically relevant coronary artery stenosis by CCT [33]. Table 12.4 reports the proposed quantitative stenosis systems most commonly adopted when reporting MDCT coronary angiography [25, 32, 34].

A schematic comparison in plaque imaging between CCT and conventional coronary angiography is illustrated in Table 12.5. From a purely diagnostic point of view, since invasive coronary angiography offers information on the intraluminal enhancement by direct injection of contrast material into the coronary artery after induction of a local vasodilatation, it is undoubtedly considered as the standard of reference for the assessment of the degree of stenosis. On the other hand, CCT has the potential to assess more accurately or even exclusively respect to standard angiography other major plaque characteristics:
- *site*: CCT provides a more detailed plaque identification and analysis of aorto-ostial lesions, which are challenging for invasive coronary angiography due to its intrinsic technical limits [35];
- *length of coronary plaque*: CCT in more detail may analyze the real extension of the atherosclerotic disease affecting the region of the stenosis, especially at the proximal and distal edge of the luminal narrow-

Table 12.1 Results of meta-analysis that have evaluated the diagnostic accuracy of CCT in comparison to conventional coronary angiography in the detection of significant coronary stenosis (stenosis ≥ 50%)

Study	Year	64-slice (%)	MVD	N. Studies	N. patients	Prevalence obstructive CAD (%)	Inclusion criteria	Unassessable segments (%)	Analysis	Sensitivity (%)	Specificity (%)	PPV (%)	NPV (%)
Hamon et al. [15]	2007	100	Yes	12	695	60	Suspected CAD	4	Per-patient	97	90	93	96
	2007	100	Yes	12	695	60	Suspected CAD	4	Per-segment	88	96	79	98
Vanhoenacker et al. [16]	2007	100	Yes	6	363	67[a]	Suspected CAD	2*	Per-patient	99	93	-	-
	2007	100	Yes	6	363	67[a]	Suspected CAD	2*	Per-segment	93	96	-	-
Abdulla et al. [17]	2007	100	Yes	13	875	58	Known and suspected CAD	-	Per-patient	98	91	94	97
	2007	100	Yes	19	1251	19	Known and suspected CAD	4	Per-segment	86	96	83	97
Meijer et al. [18]	2008	85*[c]	Yes	20*	1331	50	Known[†] and suspected CAD	2[b]	Per-patient	98	91	-	-
	2008	69*[c]	Yes	11*	765*	61*	Known[†] and suspected CAD	2[b]	Per-segment	91	96	-	-
Mowatt et al. [19]	2008	100	Yes	18	1286	58[b]	Known and suspected CAD	8	Per-patient	99	89	93[b]	100[b]
	2008	100	Yes	17	1078	-	Known and suspected CAD	8	Per-segment	90	97	76[b]	99[b]
Schuetz et al. [20]	2010	87*[c]	Yes	49	4271*	-	Known and suspected CAD	-	Per-patient	98	89	-	-

In most trials, unassessable patients or segments were excluded from analysis. Data are expressed as number or percentage (%). *PPV*, positive predictive value; *NPV*, negative predictive value; *64-slice*, prevalence of 64-slice CT scanner used; *MVD*, multivendor, i.e. whether CT systems from different manufacturers were used; *No. studies*, number of studies included in the meta-analysis; *No. patients*, number of patients enrolled in the study; *CAD*, coronary artery disease; [a], pooled mean from all studies included in the meta-analysis (n=24); [b], expressed as median; [c], the remaining percentage was evaluated by 40-slice CT; *, estimated from text; [†], only studies with inclusion of less than 50% of patients with history of CAD were included.

Table 12.2 Results of multicenter trials that have evaluated the diagnostic accuracy of CCT in comparison to conventional coronary angiography in the detection of significant coronary stenosis (stenosis ≥ 50%)

Study	Year	64-slice (%)	MVD	N. patients	Prevalence obstructive CAD (%)	Inclusion criteria	Analysis	Sensitivity (%)	Specificity (%)	PPV (%)	NPV (%)
Budoff et al. [21]	2008	100	No	230	25	Suspected CAD Age ≥ 18 y/o	Per-patient	95	83	64	99
	2008	100	No	229	10*	Suspected CAD Age ≥ 18 y/o	Per-vessel	84	90	51	99
Miller et al. [22, 23]	2008	100	No	291	56	Suspected CAD° AS ≤ 600 BMI ≤ 40; age ≥ 40 y/o	Per-patient	85	90	91	83
	2008	100	No	291	31*	Suspected CAD° AS ≤ 600 BMI ≤ 40; age ≥ 40 y/o	Per-vessel	75	93	82	89
Meijboom et al. [24]	2008	100	Yes	360	68	Suspected CAD Age 50-70 y/o	Per-patient	99	64	86	97
	2008	100	Yes	360	26*	Suspected CAD Age 50-70 y/o	Per-vessel	95	77	59	98
Maffei et al. [25]	2010	100	Yes	1372	53	Suspected CAD	Per-patient	99	92	94	99
	2010	100	Yes	1372	53	Suspected CAD	Per-segment	94	95	64	99

In most trials, unassessable patients or segments were excluded from analysis. Data are expressed as number or percentage (%). *PPV*, positive predictive value; *NPV*, negative predictive value; *AS*, Agatston Score; *64-slice*, prevalence of 64-slice CT scanner used; *MVD*, multivendor, i.e. whether CT systems from different manufacturers were used; *No. patients*, number of patients enrolled in the study; *BMI*, body mass index; *CAD*, coronary artery disease; *, vessel obstructive disease prevalence; °, patients with coronary artery stents were not excluded, but stented segments were excluded from the comparative analysis.

12 Coronary Artery Stenosis on Cardiac CT

Table 12.3 Diagnostic accuracy of CCT according to the pre-test probability of coronary artery disease (CAD). Estimated with the Duke Clinical Risk Score

Pre-test probability	Prevalence of CAD (%)	Sensitivity (%)	Specificity (%)	PPV (%)	NPV (%)
Low (<20%)	~ 15	100	89	69	100
Intermediate (20-80%)	~ 50	99	93	94	99
High (>80%)	~ 85	99	72	95	95

PPV, positive predictive value; *NPV*, negative predictive value.

Table 12.4 Proposed quantitative stenosis grading in CCT

Modified from Maffei et al. [25]		Cheng et al. [32]		Raff et al. [34]		Raff et al. [34]	
Grade	% stenosis	Grade	% stenosis	Grade	% stenosis	Grade	% stenosis
Normal	0%	0	0%	Normal	0%	Normal	0%
Non-significant/Non-obstructive	<50%	1	<25%	Minimal	<25%	Mild	<39%
Border-line	~50%	2	25%–49%	Mild	25%–49%	Moderate	40%–69%
Significant/Obstructive	>50%–100%	3	50%–69%	Moderate	50%–69%	Severe	70%–99%
		4	70%–89%	Severe	70%–99%	Occluded	100%
		5	≥90%	Occluded	100%		

Percentage stenosis refers to diameter stenosis usually extracted from two orthogonal projections.

Table 12.5 Summary of parameters in plaque imaging comparing CCT and conventional invasive coronary angiography (ICA)

	CCT	ICA
Plaque characteristics		
Site (aorto-ostial lesions)	+++	+
Grade of stenosis	++	+++
Morphology	+++	+
Length	+++	+
Remodeling	+++	-
Composition	++	-
Chronic total occlusion	+++	-
Overall plaque burden	+++	+

ing, providing potentially important information for the planning of percutaneous coronary intervention (PCI) [36];

- *morphology*: CCT shape analysis can accurately assess complex lesions (e.g. bifurcation lesions) and differentiate between concentric and eccentric plaques, the latter being lesions more frequently observed in acute coronary syndrome [37];
- *remodeling index*: CCT may identify areas of negative and positive remodeling, the latter being an adaptive phenomenon, correlated with acute aortic syndrome, for which the vessel wall may contain a large atheroma, despite an angiogram that shows little or no luminal narrowing [37, 38];
- *plaque composition*: CCT has the potential to detect different plaque components, such as calcium and noncalcified elements [39, 40];
- *chronic total occlusion*: CCT provides an accurate assessment of the length and composition of the occluded segment, which are important predictors of procedural success when attempting a PCI [41];
- *overall plaque burden*: CCT may evaluate the overall anatomic distribution and extent of coronary plaques and identify subclinical coronary atherosclerosis.

12.4 Anatomical vs. Functional Imaging

It is important to underlie that, as with standard coronary angiography, a significant discordance between visual estimates of luminal narrowing by CCT and the functional significance of stenosis may be observed. Therefore, both invasive and noninvasive coronary angiography need functional information in addition to the anatomic data to know which particular lesion is physiologically significant and responsible for reversible ischemia, (Fig. 12.3).

Revascularization of stenotic coronary lesions that induce ischemia can improve a patient's functional status and outcome [42, 43]. Conversely, for stenotic lesions not associated with ischemia, the benefit of revascularization is less clear, and medical therapy alone is likely to be equally effective [44, 45].

Previous studies comparing CCT with myocardial perfusion imaging have reported a positive predictive value of CCT for detecting hemodynamically significant stenosis on a vessel- and a patient-based level respectively at around 30% and 50%, (Fig. 12.4) [46-54]. Conversely, normal myocardial perfusion imaging cannot rule-out the presence of significant CAD or atherosclerosis in general.

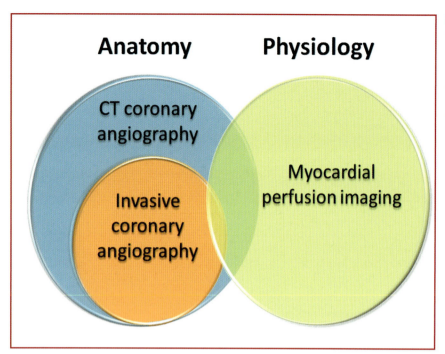

Fig. 12.3 CCT is an anatomic imaging method and as such shares the limitations of conventional invasive angiography: it cannot assess the hemodynamic consequences of the lesions it detects. Therefore, functional testing such as myocardial perfusion imaging is complementary in the work-up of patients with suspected CAD in order to demonstrate the presence of ischemia

With the advent of novel technologies such as dual-source CCT, 256- or 320-slice CCT, and high definition CCT, an improved spatial and/or temporal resolution is achieved, together with a higher volume coverage [55-58]. Furthermore, new radiation dose-saving techniques have recently become available. These have the potential to significantly reduce the radiation dose down to 1-5 mSv or less, depending on the technology applied (prospective ECG-triggering technique; reduced tube voltage; high-pitch spiral acquisition; iterative reconstruction algorithms) while maintaining high diagnostic accuracy [59]. For example, a recent meta-analysis evaluating 16 studies (comprising 960 patients) compared prospective electrocardiography-gated CCT with catheter coronary angiography (the criterion standard) in symptomatic patients with suspected CAD. The pooled patient-level sensitivity and specificity were high, respectively 100% and 89% [60].

References

1. Sones FM, Shirey EK (1962) Cine coronary arteriography. Mod Concepts Cardiovasc Dis 31:735-738
2. Topol EJ, Nissen SE (1995) Our preoccupation with coronary luminology. The dissociation between clinical and angiographic findings in ischemic heart disease. Circulation 92:2333-2342
3. Scanlon PJ, Faxon DP, Audet AM et al (1999) ACC/AHA guidelines for coronary angiography. A report of the American College of Cardiology/American Heart Association Task Force on practice guidelines (Committee on Coronary Angiography). Developed in collaboration with the Society for Cardiac Angiography and Interventions. J Am Coll Cardiol 33:1756-1824

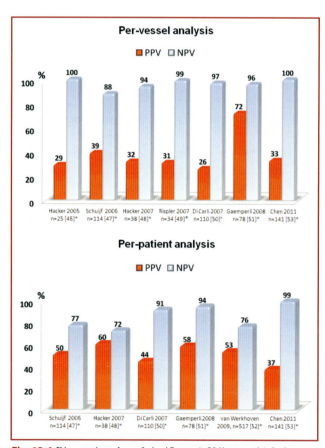

Fig. 12.4 Diagnostic value of significant (≥50% stenosis) lesions on CCT in predicting inducible ischemia on myocardial perfusion imaging. **a** Per-vessel analysis. **b** Per-patient analysis. *PPV*, positive predictive value; *NPV*, negative predictive value; *comparison between CCT and SPECT; #comparison between CCT and hybrid SPECT/CT; °comparison between CCT and hybrid PET/CT

4. Ota H, Takase K, Rikimaru H et al (2005) Quantitative vascular measurements in arterial occlusive disease. Radiographics 25:1141-1158

5. Gould KL, Lipscomb K, Hamilton GW (1974) Physiologic basis for assessing critical coronary stenosis: instantaneous flow response and regional distribution during coronary hyperemia as measures of coronary flow reserve. Am J Cardiol 33:87-94

6. Kern MJ, Donohue TJ, Aguirre FV et al (1993) Assessment of angiographically intermediate coronary artery stenosis using the Doppler flowire. Am J Cardiol 71:26D-33D

7. White CW, Wright CB, Doty DB et al (1984) Does visual interpretation of the coronary arteriogram predict the physiologic importance of a coronary stenosis? N Engl J Med 310:819-824

8. Pijls NH, Van Gelder B, Van der Voort P et al (1995) Fractional flow reserve. A useful index to evaluate the influence of an epicardial coronary stenosis on myocardial blood flow. Circulation 92:3183-3193

9. Pijls NHJ, De Bruyne B, Peels K et al (1996) Measurement of fractional flow reserve to assess the functional severity of coronary-artery stenoses. N Engl J Med 334:1703-1708

10. Feldman RL, Nichols WW, Pepine CJ, Conti CR (1978) Hemodynamic effects of long and multiple coronary artery narrowings. Chest 74:280-285

11. Feldman RL, Nichols WW, Pepine CJ, Conetta DA, Conti CR (1979) The coronary hemodynamics of left main and branch coronary stenoses. The effects of reduction in stenosis diameter, stenosis length, and number of stenoses. J Thorac Cardiovasc Surg 77:377-388

12. Harrison DG, White CW, Hiratzka LF et al (1984) The value of lesion cross-sectional area determined by quantitative coronary angiography in assessing the physiologic significance of proximal left anterior descending coronary arterial stenoses. Circulation 69:1111-1119

13. Kirkeeide RL, Gould KL, Parsel L (1986) Assessment of coronary stenoses by myocardial perfusion imaging during pharmacologic coronary vasodilation: VII. Validation of coronary flow reserve as a single integrated functional measure of stenosis severity reflecting all its geometric dimensions. J Am Coll Cardiol 7:103-111

14. Dodds SR, Phillips PS (2003) The haemodynamics of multiple sequential stenoses and the criteria for a critical stenosis. Eur J Vasc Endovasc Surg 26:348-353

15. Hamon M, Morello R, Riddell JW, Hamon M (2007) Coronary arteries: diagnostic performance of 16- versus 64-section spiral CT compared with invasive coronary angiography—meta-analysis. Radiology 245:720-731

16. Vanhoenacker PK, Heijenbrok-Kal MH, Van Heste R et al (2007) Diagnostic performance of multidetector CT angiography for assessment of coronary artery disease: meta-analysis. Radiology 244:419-428

17. Abdulla J, Abildstrom SZ, Gotzsche O et al (2007) 64-multislice detector computed tomography coronary angiography as potential alternative to conventional coronary angiography: a systematic review and meta-analysis. Eur Heart J 28:3042-3050

18. Meijer AB, O YL, Geleijns J, Kroft LJ (2008) Meta-analysis of 40- and 64-MDCT angiography for assessing coronary artery stenosis. AJR Am J Roentgenol 191:1667-1675

19. Mowatt G, Cook JA, Hillis GS et al (2008) 64-Slice computed tomography angiography in the diagnosis and assessment of coronary artery disease: systematic review and meta-analysis. Heart 94:1386-1393

20. Schuetz GM, Zacharopoulou NM, Schlattmann P, Dewey M (2010) Meta-analysis: noninvasive coronary angiography using computed tomography versus magnetic resonance imaging. Ann Intern Med 152:167-177

21. Budoff MJ, Dowe D, Jollis JG et al (2008) Diagnostic performance of 64-multidetector row coronary computed tomographic angiography for evaluation of coronary artery stenosis in individuals without known coronary artery disease: results from the prospective multi center ACCURACY (Assessment by Coronary Computed Tomographic Angiography of Individuals Undergoing Invasive Coronary Angiography trial). J Am Coll Cardiol 52:1724-1732

22. Miller JM, Rochitte CE, Dewey M et al (2008) Diagnostic performance of coronary angiography by 64-row CT. N Engl J Med 359:2324-2336

23. Miller JM, Dewey M, Vavere AL et al (2009) Coronary CT angiography using 64 detector rows: methods and design of the multi-centre trial CORE-64. Eur Radiol 19:816-828

24. Meijboom WB, Meijs MF, Schuijf JD et al (2008) Diagnostic accuracy of 64-slice computed tomography coronary angiography: a prospective, multicenter, multivendor study. J Am Coll Cardiol 52:2135-2144

25. Maffei E, Palumbo A, Martini C et al (2010) Diagnostic accuracy of 64-slice computed tomography coronary angiography in a large population of patients without revascularisation: registry data and review of multicentre trials. Radiol Med 115:368-384

26. Cademartiri F, Mollet NR, Lemos PA et al (2005) Impact of coronary calcium score on diagnostic accuracy for the detection of significant coronary stenosis with multislice computed tomography angiography. Am J Cardiol 95:1225-1227

27. Cademartiri F, Runza G, Mollet NR et al (2005) Impact of intravascular enhancement, heart rate, and calcium score on diagnostic accuracy in multislice computed tomography coronary angiography. Radiol Med 110:42-51

28. Mollet NR, Cademartiri F, van Mieghem CA et al (2005) High-resolution spiral computed tomography coronary angiography in patients referred for diagnostic conventional coronary angiography. Circulation 112: 2318-2323

29. Leschka S, Alkadhi H, Plass A et al (2005) Accuracy of MSCT coronary angiography with 64-slice technology: first experience. Eur Heart J 26:1482-1487

30. Leber AW, Knez A, von Ziegler F et al (2005) Quantification of obstructive and nonobstructive coronary lesions by 64-slice computed tomography: a comparative study with quantitative coronary angiography and intravascular ultrasound. J Am Coll Cardiol 46:147-154

31. Weustink AC, Mollet NR, Neefjes LA et al (2010) Diagnostic accuracy and clinical utility of noninvasive testing for coronary artery disease. Ann Intern Med 152:630-639

32. Cheng V, Gutstein A, Wolak A et al (2008) Moving beyond binary grading of coronary arterial stenoses on coronary computed tomographic angiography: insights for the imager and referring clinician. JACC Cardiovasc Imaging 1:460-471

33. Achenbach S (2008) Quantification of coronary artery stenoses by computed tomography. JACC Cardiovasc Imaging 1:472-474

34. Raff GL, Abidov A, Achenbach S et al (2009) Society of Cardiovascular Computed Tomography. SCCT guidelines for the interpretation and reporting of coronary computed tomographic angiography. J Cardiovasc Comput Tomogr 3:122-136

35. Kantarci M, Ceviz N, Sevimli S et al (2007) Diagnostic performance of multidetector computed tomography for detecting aorto-ostial lesions compared with catheter coronary angiography: multidetector computed tomography coronary angiography is superior to catheter angiography in detection of aorto-ostial lesions. J Comput Assist Tomogr 31:595-599

36. Hecht HS, Roubin G (2007) Usefulness of computed tomographic angiography guided percutaneous coronary intervention. Am J Cardiol 99:871-875

37. Virmani R, Burke AP, Farb A, Kolodgie FD (2006) Pathology of the vulnerable plaque. J Am Coll Cardiol 47(8 Suppl):C13-18

38. Achenbach S, Ropers D, Hoffmann U et al (2004) Assessment of coronary remodeling in stenotic and nonstenotic coronary atherosclerotic lesions by multidetector spiral computed tomography. J

Am Coll Cardiol 43:842-847

39. Schroeder S, Kuettner A, Leitritz M et al (2004) Reliability of differentiating human coronary plaque morphology using contrast-enhanced multislice spiral computed tomography: a comparison with histology. J Comput Assist Tomogr 28:449-454

40. Leschka S, Seitun S, Dettmer M et al (2010) Ex vivo evaluation of coronary atherosclerotic plaques: characterization with dual-source CT in comparison with histopathology. J Cardiovasc Comput Tomogr 4:301-308

41. Mollet NR, Hoye A, Lemos PA, et al (2005) Value of preprocedure multislice computed tomographic coronary angiography to predict the outcome of percutaneous recanalization of chronic total occlusions. Am J Cardiol 95:240-243

42. Shaw LJ, Berman DS, Maron DJ et al (2008) Optimal medical therapy with or without percutaneous coronary intervention to reduce ischemic burden: results from the Clinical Outcomes Utilizing Revascularization and Aggressive Drug Evaluation (COURAGE) trial nuclear substudy. Circulation 117:1283-1291

43. Erne P, Schoenenberger AW, Burckhardt D et al (2007) Effects of percutaneous coronary interventions in silent ischemia after myocardial infarction: the SWISSI II randomized controlled trial. JAMA 297:1985-1991

44. Boden WE, O'Rourke RA, Teo KK et al (2007) Optimal medical therapy with or without PCI for stable coronary disease. N Engl J Med 356:1503-1516

45. Pijls NH, van Schaardenburgh P, Manoharan G et al (2007) Percutaneous coronary intervention of functionally nonsignificant stenosis: 5-year follow-up of the DEFER Study. J Am Coll Cardiol 49:2105-2111

46. Hacker M, Jakobs T, Matthiesen F et al (2005) Comparison of spiral multidetector CT angiography and myocardial perfusion imaging in the noninvasive detection of functionally relevant coronary artery lesions: first clinical experiences. J Nucl Med 46:1294-1300

47. Schuijf JD, Wijns W, Jukema JW et al (2006) Relationship between noninvasive coronary angiography with multi-slice computed tomography and myocardial perfusion imaging. J Am Coll Cardiol 48: 2508-2514

48. Hacker M, Jakobs T, Hack N et al (2007) Sixty-four slice spiral CT angiography does not predict the functional relevance of coronary artery stenoses in patients with stable angina. Eur J Nucl Med Mol Imaging 34:4-10

49. Rispler S, Keidar Z, Ghersin E et al (2007) Integrated single-photon emission computed tomography and computed tomography coronary angiography for the assessment of hemodynamically significant coronary artery lesions. J Am Coll Cardiol 49:1059-1067

50. Di Carli MF, Dorbala S, Curillova Z et al (2007) Relationship between CT coronary angiography and stress perfusion imaging in patients with suspected ischemic heart disease assessed by integrated PET-CT imaging. J Nucl Cardiol 14:799-809

51. Gaemperli O, Schepis T, Valenta I et al (2008) Functionally relevant coronary artery disease: comparison of 64-section CT angiography with myocardial perfusion SPECT. Radiology 248:414-423

52. van Werkhoven JM, Schuijf JD, Gaemperli O et al (2009) Prognostic value of multislice computed tomography and gated single-photon emission computed tomography in patients with suspected coronary artery disease. J Am Coll Cardiol 53:623-632

53. Chen ML, Mo YH, Wang YC et al (2011) 64-slice CT angiography for the detection of functionally significant coronary stenoses: comparison with stress myocardial perfusion imaging. Br J Radiol [Epub ahead of print]

54. Di Carli MF, Dorbala S, Meserve J et al (2007) Clinical myocardial perfusion PET/CT. J Nucl Med 48:783-793

55. Chao SP, Law WY, Kuo CJ et al (2010) The diagnostic accuracy of 256-row computed tomographic angiography compared with invasive coronary angiography in patients with suspected coronary artery disease. Eur Heart J 31:1916-1623

56. Dewey M, Zimmermann E, Deissenrieder F et al (2009) Noninvasive coronary angiography by 320-row computed tomography with lower radiation exposure and maintained diagnostic accuracy: comparison of results with cardiac catheterization in a head-to-head pilot investigation. Circulation 120:867-875

57. Min JK, Swaminathan RV, Vass M et al (2009) High-definition multidetector computed tomography for evaluation of coronary artery stents: comparison to standard-definition 64-detector row computed tomography. J Cardiovasc Comput Tomogr 3:246-251

58. Achenbach S, Marwan M, Ropers D et al (2010) Coronary computed tomography angiography with a consistent dose below 1 mSv using prospectively electrocardiogram-triggered high-pitch spiral acquisition. Eur Heart J 31:340-346

59. Earls JP, Berman EL, Urban BA et al (2008) Prospectively gated transverse coronary CT angiography versus retrospectively gated helical technique: improved image quality and reduced radiation dose. Radiology 246:742-753

60. von Ballmoos MW, Haring B, Juillerat P, Alkadhi H (2011) Meta-analysis: diagnostic performance of low-radiation-dose coronary computed tomography angiography. Ann Intern Med 154:413-420. Erratum in: (2011) Ann Intern Med 154:848

Coronary Artery Stents

13

Francesca Pugliese, Katarzyna Gruszczynska, Ian Baron, Ceri L. Davies, and Steffen E. Petersen

13.1 Coronary Stent Assessment by MDCT

Percutaneous coronary intervention (PCI) with stent implantation is the primary form of coronary revascularization. Stents are positioned to resolve obstructing lesions by balloon inflation. Balloon inflation represents an injury for the vessel wall and leads to a healing response. An excessive healing response can cause narrowing of the stent lumen and be associated with recurrent chest pain. Recurrent chest pain however is not invariably secondary to stent occlusion or restenosis. The availability of a noninvasive technique able to diagnose and rule out the presence of restenosis would be very desirable.

Multidetector computed tomography (MDCT) is able to depict:

- stent patency (Fig. 13.1a);
- neo-intimal hyperplasia, defined as <50% diameter narrowing (Fig. 13.1b);
- in-stent restenosis, defined as diameter narrowing between 50% and 99% (Fig. 13.1c);
- stent occlusion, defined as total (100%) luminal obliteration (Fig. 13.1d).

In-stent restenosis and stent occlusion can be associated with recurrent chest pain.

13.2 The 'Blooming Effect'

Coronary stents can be difficult to assess by MDCT. Due to partial volume artifacts, stent struts are visualized larger than they actually are. When the smallest portion of a digital image, i.e. a pixel, contains tissues of different densities, the attenuation value to be assigned to that pixel will be obtained by averaging the attenuation values of the individual tissues. If the pixel is partially filled by a structure of very high attenuation (e.g. metal), a high attenuation value will be assigned to that pixel which will thus appear bright on the CT image. Structures with a very bright appearance (e.g. the stent struts) may obscure adjacent structures (e.g. the stent lumen). This phenomenon may hinder the ability to evaluate the in-stent lumen and is also referred to as the 'blooming effect'. The finding of contrast-enhancement distal to the stent is not sufficient to assume stent patency, because collateral pathways may provide retrograde filling of the vessel. Especially if the stent is being evaluated for the presence of nonocclusive in-stent restenosis, direct visualization of the in-stent lumen becomes mandatory.

The blooming effect (Fig. 13.2) is more disturbing:

- in smaller rather than larger stents, where the in-stent lumen might be completely obscured [1];
- in stents with thick struts (e.g. 0.15 mm and above) rather than in stents with thin struts (e.g. 0.14 mm) [2, 3];
- in steel, cobalt-chromium or tantalum stents rather than magnesium stents. Magnesium stents exhibit a lumen visibility of 90%, whereas the majority of the other stents exhibit a lumen visibility of 50–59% [4, 5];
- in overlapping (stent-in-stent) and bifurcation stenting rather than in simple stenting due to an excess of metal [6].

13.3 Technical Requirements

In order to compensate for the blooming effect, some technical features are required for coronary stent imaging:

- high spatial resolution, i.e. thin detectors as featured by 64-slice MDCT scanners or later systems;
- high temporal resolution is necessary because the

F. Pugliese (✉)
Centre for Advanced Cardiovascular Imaging,
Barts & The London NIHR Biomedical Research Unit,
The William Harvey Research Institute,
Queen Mary University of London,
The London Chest Hospital,
London, UK

F. Cademartiri, G. Casolo, M. Midiri (eds.), *Clinical Applications of Cardiac CT*,
© Springer-Verlag Italia 2012

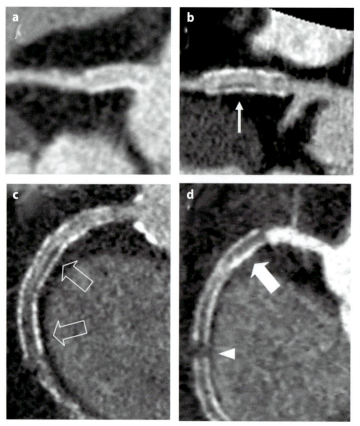

Fig. 13.1 MDCT appearance of a patent stent (**a**) implanted in the LM coronary artery. No filling defects are seen within the stent. Neo-intimal hyperplasia (**b**, *thin arrow*) is displayed as a dark rim of tissue within the stent implanted in the proximal LAD. This condition is mostly asymptomatic. In-stent restenosis (**c**, *hollow arrows*) is displayed as a thicker filling defect in a stent implanted in the RCA. This condition can be associated with recurrent chest pain. In stent occlusion (**d**, *thick arrow*) there is total obliteration of the in-stent lumen. Notice the gap (*arrowhead*) between 2 stents implanted in the RCA

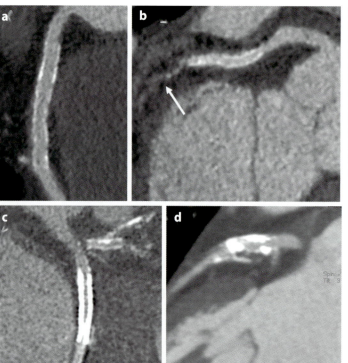

Fig. 13.2 In a 3 mm stent (**a**) implanted in the RCA the blooming effect is minimal and allows the exclusion of in-stent restenosis. In a 2.25 mm stent (**b**) implanted in the LCX the blooming effect is more detrimental and hinders the assessability of the in-stent lumen. In this case, the in-stent lumen may look erroneously patent in spite of the absence of distal runoff (*arrow*) which indicates restenosis.
The blooming effect from a 3 mm tantalum stent (**c**) implanted in the LCX is very marked and prevents from visualisation of the in-stent lumen. In the event of stent-in-stent configuration (**d**) or pre-existing heavy calcification of the vessel wall the blooming effect is secondary to multiple layers of metal and/or calcium

13 Coronary Artery Stents

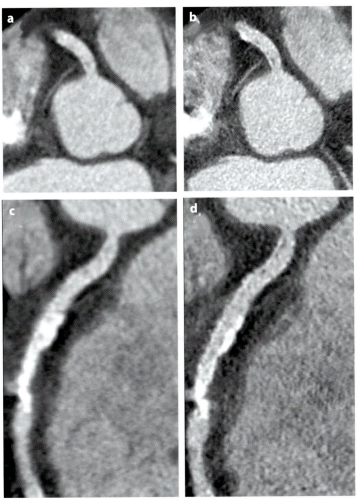

Fig. 13.3 MDCT angiograms obtained in a patient with multiple stents and heavy calcifications in the RCA. On the images reconstructed with a smooth convolution filter (**a** and **c**), the dark rim causing luminal defect in the proximal RCA is hardly visible. On the images reconstructed with a dedicated edge-enhancing kernel (**b** and **d**), visualization of in-stent neointimal hyperplasia in the proximal RCA is possible at the expense of a slight increase of image noise

blooming effect is exacerbated by motion artifacts (blurring) in the dataset;
- heart rate control through the administration of pre-scan beta-blockers can be advisable;
- dedicated (sharp) convolution kernels may decrease the degree of the blooming effect and are therefore recommendable (Fig. 13.3) [6];
- "dual energy" acquisition modes (application of 2 different kilovoltages, e.g. 80 and 140 kV) may improve the assessment of coronary stents in the near future [7] although the applicability of this technique is yet to be fully evaluated.

13.4 Diagnostic Usefulness

Several clinical studies [2, 3, 8-17] compared MDCT to conventional angiography for the detection of in-stent restenosis, defined as ≥50% luminal narrowing (Table 13.1).

These studies consistently demonstrated that:
- MDCT had a constantly high negative predictive value;
- stent diameter was the most important predictor of in-stent lumen visibility. Cut-off diameters of 2.75 mm or 3 mm were identified for patient selection.

In a study [18] including patients with stent diameters ≥3 mm, the sensitivity of dual source CT (98%) for the detection of in-stent restenosis was found to be significantly higher than that of a traditional diagnostic work-up (65%) based on the combination of exercise electrocardiography, myocardial perfusion imaging and dobutamine-stress echocardiography.

Stent implantation in the LM and proximal LAD/CX provides a suitable scenario for the use of MDCT to rule out in-stent restenosis (Fig. 13.4). This is due to the large size of stents implanted in the LM and proximal LAD/CX. Moreover, this part of the coronary tree is relatively protected from motion artifacts. Although coronary artery bypass graft surgery is still recommended in

Table 13.1 Detection of in-stent restenosis - diagnostic performance of MDCT versus conventional angiography in clinical studies

	Nonassessable stents (%)	Sensitivity (%)	Specificity (%)	PPV (%)	NPV (%)
64-MDCT					
Rixe [2]					
All diameters	42	86	98	86	98
>3mm	22	100	100	100	100
3mm	42	83	96	83	96
*<3mm**	92	.	100	.	100
Ehara [12]					
All diameters	12	92	81	54	98
Cademartiri [8]					
All diameters	7	90	86	44	98
Das [11]					
All diameters	3	97	88	78	99
Schuijf [3]					
All diameters	14	100	100	-	-
Carbone [9]					
All diameters	28	75	86	83	79
≥3mm	3	85	97	94	95
Hecht [13]					
All diameters	0	94	75	39	99
Carrabba [10]					
All diameters	0	84	97	92	97
Manghat [14]					
All diameters	10	85	86	61	96
≥3mm	0	100	94	81	100
DSCT					
Pugliese [16]					
All diameters	5	94	92	77	98
≥3.5mm	0	100	100	100	100
3mm	0	100	97	91	100
≤2.75mm	22	84	64	52	90
Oncel [15]					
All diameters	0	100	94	89	100
320-MDCT					
De Graaf [17]					
All diameters	8	92	91	65	98

*only 1 stent available, without in-stent restenosis.

patients with LM disease, PCI is increasingly performed on the unprotected LM coronary artery in the drug-eluting stent (DES) era. However, in-stent restenosis still occurs with DES and may cause fatal myocardial infarction or sudden death [19], therefore surveillance of asymptomatic patients with routine angiography 6 months after PCI for left main stem is highly recommended [20]. A study by Van Mieghem et al. [21] showed that MDCT is safe and reliable in excluding in-stent restenosis in patients with LM and proximal LAD/CX stents. This study suggested that MDCT might be a first-line alternative to conventional angiography for the follow-up of asymptomatic patients after unprotected LM stenting.

13.5 Conclusions

The available clinical data [2, 3, 8-16, 18, 21-24] suggest that MDCT could be used:
- in the follow-up of asymptomatic patients after unprotected LM stenting;

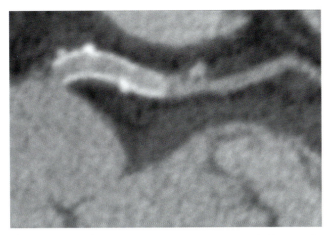

Fig. 13.4 The LM coronary artery represents a very suitable scenario for MDCT evaluation. The diameter of stents implanted in the LM is usually large. Moreover, the LM artery is relatively protected from motion artifacts

- in patients with symptoms but low clinical probability of in-stent retenosis.

The use of MDCT should be carefully weighed up in relation to the stent's characteristics which may predict inconclusive diagnostic findings. These include:
- diameter <2.75 mm;
- hyperdense metal, thick struts and/or under-deployed stent;
- stent-in-stent configuration;
- heavily calcified vessel wall.

Noninvasive assessment of disease progression in the native coronary tree is an appealing application of MDCT which raises however radiation dose concerns and warrants further research before routine clinical use can be implemented.

Tissue prolapses, stent malapposition and underdeployment are generally beyond the resolution of MDCT. It is conceivable that stents with thinner struts, absorbable and non-metallic stents [25] will be less susceptible to the blooming effect. The introduction of these new devices might increase the utility of MDCT in patients after PCI.

Disclosure:
This work forms part of the research themes contributing to the translational research portfolio of Barts and The London Cardiovascular Biomedical Research Unit which is supported and funded by the National Institute for Health Research.

References

1. Steen H, Andre F, Korosoglou G et al (2011) In vitro evaluation of 56 coronary artery stents by 256-slice multi-detector coronary CT. Eur J Radiol 80:143-150
2. Rixe J, Achenbach S, Ropers D, et al. Assessment of coronary artery stent restenosis by 64-slice multi-detector computed tomography. Eur Heart J 27:2567-2572
3. Schuijf JD, Pundziute G, Jukema JW et al (2007) Evaluation of patients with previous coronary stent implantation with 64-section CT. Radiology 245:416-423
4. Maintz D, Burg MC, Seifarth H et al (2009) Update on multidetector coronary CT angiography of coronary stents: in vitro evaluation of 29 different stent types with dual-source CT. Eur Radiol 19:42-49
5. Maintz D, Seifarth H, Raupach R et al (2006) 64-slice multidetector coronary CT angiography: in vitro evaluation of 68 different stents. Eur Radiol 16:818-826
6. Pugliese F, Cademartiri F, van Mieghem C et al (2006) Multidetector CT for visualization of coronary stents. Radiographics 26:887-904
7. Achenbach S, Anders K, Kalender WA (2008) Dual-source cardiac computed tomography: image quality and dose considerations. Eur Radiol 18:1188-1198
8. Cademartiri F, Schuijf JD, Pugliese F et al (2007) Usefulness of 64-slice multislice computed tomography coronary angiography to assess in-stent restenosis. J Am Coll Cardiol 49:2204-2210
9. Carbone I, Francone M, Algeri E et al (2008) Non-invasive evaluation of coronary artery stent patency with retrospectively ECG-gated 64-slice CT angiography. Eur Radiol 18:234-243
10. Carrabba N, Bamoshmoosh M, Carusi LM et al (2007) Usefulness of 64-slice multidetector computed tomography for detecting drug eluting in-stent restenosis. Am J Cardiol 100:1754-1758
11. Das KM, El-Menyar AA, Salam AM et al (2007) Contrast-enhanced 64-section coronary multidetector CT angiography versus conventional coronary angiography for stent assessment. Radiology 245:424-432
12. Ehara M, Kawai M, Surmely JF et al (2007) Diagnostic accuracy of coronary in-stent restenosis using 64-slice computed tomography: comparison with invasive coronary angiography. J Am Coll Cardiol 49:951-959
13. Hecht HS, Zaric M, Jelnin V et al (2008) Usefulness of 64-detector computed tomographic angiography for diagnosing in-stent restenosis in native coronary arteries. Am J Cardiol 101:820-824
14. Manghat N, Van Lingen R, Hewson P et al (2008) Usefulness of 64-detector row computed tomography for evaluation of intracoronary stents in symptomatic patients with suspected in-stent restenosis. Am J Cardiol 101:1567-1573
15. Oncel D, Oncel G, Tastan A et al (2008) Evaluation of coronary stent patency and in-stent restenosis with dual-source CT coronary angiography without heart rate control. AJR Am J Roentgenol 191:56-63
16. Pugliese F, Weustink AC, Van Mieghem C et al (2008) Dual source coronary computed tomography angiography for detecting in-stent restenosis. Heart 94:848-854
17. de Graaf FR, Schuijf JD, van Velzen JE et al (2010) Diagnostic accuracy of 320-row multidetector computed tomography coronary angiography to noninvasively assess in-stent restenosis. Investigative radiology 45:331-340
18. Van Mieghem CA WA, PuglieseF, Meijboom WB et al Clinical value of dual-source CT coronary angiography in symptomatic patients after previous percutaneous coronary stent implantation. Submitted for publication.
19. Takagi T, Stankovic G, Finci L et al (2002) Results and long-term predictors of adverse clinical events after elective percutaneous interventions on unprotected left main coronary artery. Circulation 106:698-702
20. Smith SC, Jr., Feldman TE, Hirshfeld JW, Jr. et al (2006) ACC/AHA/SCAI 2005 Guideline Update for Percutaneous Coronary Intervention—summary article: a report of the American College of Cardiology/American Heart Association Task Force on

Practice Guidelines (ACC/AHA/SCAI Writing Committee to Update the 2001 Guidelines for Percutaneous Coronary Intervention). Circulation 113:156-175

21. Van Mieghem CA, Cademartiri F, Mollet NR et al (2006) Multislice spiral computed tomography for the evaluation of stent patency after left main coronary artery stenting: a comparison with conventional coronary angiography and intravascular ultrasound. Circulation 114:645-653

22. Hamon M, Champ-Rigot L, Morello R et al (2008) Diagnostic accuracy of in-stent coronary restenosis detection with multislice spiral computed tomography: a meta-analysis. Eur Radiol 18:217-225

23. Sun Z, Almutairi AM (2010) Diagnostic accuracy of 64 multislice CT angiography in the assessment of coronary in-stent restenosis: A meta-analysis. Eur J Radiol 73:266-273

24. Vanhoenacker PK, Decramer I, Bladt O et al (2008) Multidetector computed tomography angiography for assessment of in-stent restenosis: meta-analysis of diagnostic performance. BMC Med Imaging 31:8-14

25. Ormiston JA, Webster MW, Armstrong G (2007) First-in-human implantation of a fully bioabsorbable drug-eluting stent: the BVS poly-L-lactic acid everolimus-eluting coronary stent. Catheter Cardiovasc Interv 69:128-131

Evaluation of Bypass Grafts

14

Riccardo Marano, Giancarlo Savino, Carlo Liguori, and Lorenzo Bonomo

14.1 Introduction

Surgical revascularization of the coronary arteries is one of the most frequent surgical procedures performed worldwide. The reduction or disappearance of angina, the improved tolerability of physical exercise and the overall improvement in quality of life and life expectancy have been the motivations underlying its use since the first procedures were performed in the 1950s. However, although the procedure is one of the major successes of modern medicine, it does not treat the disease underlying the symptoms (atherosclerosis) but only the clinical presentation of coronary artery disease (CAD).

The prognosis of patients who have undergone surgical revascularization depends not only on the outcome of the procedure but also on the progression of the disease in the native coronary arteries and in the conduits used to bypass the atherosclerotic lesions [1-4]. The large number of patients suffering a recurrence of angina after surgical revascularization represents a significant issue in clinical cardiology. Recurrence of angina can be present in association with myocardial ischemia both in previously reperfused and non reperfused regions. These patients should therefore undergo clinical and instrumental monitoring and in some cases a repeat procedure is required, which unfortunately is encumbered by a higher percentage of postprocedure complications.

14.2 Indications for Coronary Artery Bypass Grafting

The indications for coronary artery bypass grafting surgery (CABG) defined by the American College of Cardiology and the American Heart Association

R. Marano (✉)
Department of Bioimaging and Radiological Sciences,
Institute of Radiology, "A. Gemelli" Hospital,
Catholic University,
Rome, Italy

(ACC/AHA) [5] include three-vessel disease, two-vessel disease with the involvement of the proximal tract of the left anterior descending coronary artery (LAD) and/or in cases of altered left ventricular function. Stenosis of the left main coronary artery (LM), which is pathophysiologically comparable to two-vessel disease, is also an indication for surgical treatment, even though in some laboratories it is mechanically treated (percutaneous transluminal coronary angioplasty – PTCA – with stenting).

14.3 Imaging Techniques

Since its first specific application in the 1960s by Sones and Favaloro, conventional coronary angiography has been the criterion standard for the long-term evaluation of coronary revascularization procedures, whether CABG or PTCA. The limitations of angiography include invasiveness, high cost, the need for hospitalization, poor patient compliance, and although rare the risks correlated with the invasiveness of the procedure (hematomas, dissections, vascular rupture, arrhythmias, stroke and death), with morbidity and mortality of 1.5% and 0.05%, respectively [6, 7].

Conventional coronary angiography is a two-dimensional diagnostic technique which despite having high spatial resolution (50 lp/cm) and temporal resolution (<20 ms) is only able to visualize the vessel lumen, thus providing no direct information about the vessel wall. Since the technique is largely *luminographic* [8], coronary angiography can underestimate some severe vascular lesions, as in the case of diffuse CAD or lesions with a certain morphology, as well as overestimate the *gain* obtained with angioplasty, e.g. in the case of laceration of the atheromatous plaque. Another limitation, in the absence of continuous and widespread use of quantitative analysis of vessel diameter (quantitative coronary angiography – QCA), is low intra- and interobserver variability. Clearly then the use of alternative noninvasive imaging modalities can have a significant clinical and economic impact on the evaluation of post-CABG patients. In this setting, multidetector computed tomog-

F. Cademartiri, G. Casolo, M. Midiri (eds.), *Clinical Applications of Cardiac CT*,
© Springer-Verlag Italia 2012

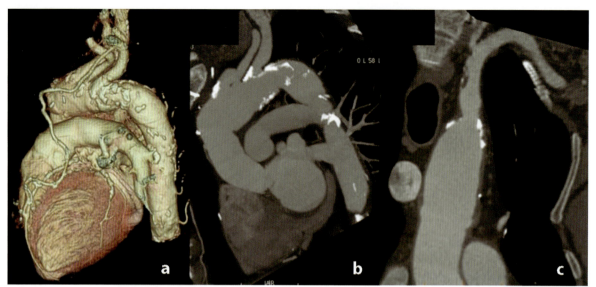

Fig. 14.1 The volume rendering (**a**), multiplanar reconstruction (**b**) and curved planar reconstruction (**c**) images clearly depict the diffuse aortic parietal calcifications at the level of the arch, the ostial calcifications at the origin of the left subclavian artery and a mixed plaque in the proximal tract of the vessel causing a nonsignificant stenosis. This information should be considered at examinations performed pre- or post-coronary revascularization with left internal thoracic artery (LITA)

raphy (MDCT) can play an important role, whether used with or without ECG gating. Without ECG gating MDCT can be useful in the preoperative phase for evaluating the course of arterial conduits to be used as grafts, such as the internal thoracic artery (ITA), or in the study of patients who have already been operated and need to undergo a redo-surgery due to the progression of CAD (evaluation of the course of previous grafts and their relations with the sternal plane, or in cases of dysmorphism of the thoracic cage). The use of ECG gating is mandatory for the evaluation of graft patency, and in preoperative planning for evaluating the wall, diameter and course of the target coronary artery, thus excluding possible anomalies such as myocardial bridging. In the evaluation of the characteristics of atherosclerotic disease, MDCT can easily identify calcifications and stenoses not only in the coronary arteries, but also on the aortic wall and the subclavian arteries (Fig. 14.1). Furthermore, the use of MDCT, with or without ECG gating (the choice depends on the specific problems), has particular clinical relevance in the detection of complications associated with grafting:

- *Pericardial effusion*: this occurs in 22-85% of cases [9] due to the antiplatelet therapy cardiac used in surgery patients; in a limited number of patients (0.8%-6%) [10] it can progress to cardiac tamponade;
- *Pleural effusion*: usually left unilateral; this occurs during the first week in 90% of cases [11] and clears up in a few weeks in most patients;
- *Sternal infection*: this is found in 2%-20% of cases [12] and can involve the presternal, sternal or retrosternal compartment, with a mortality of 4% in the latter case;
- *Pulmonary embolism*: this occurs in a relatively low number of cases (0.4%-9.5%) [13], although it can have fatal consequences precisely due to its unexpected nature.

14.4 Surgical Techniques

From the technical point of view, three main problem areas can be identified in the setting of CABG: the choice of surgical access, the choice of revascularization technique and the choice of conduits.

The surgical access can be distinguished in:
- sternotomy;
- complete median sternotomy
- T partial sternotomy
- reversed-J partial sternotomy
- minithoracotomy;
- left
- right
- left posterolateral thoracotomy.

Complete median sternotomy (Fig. 14.2a): the incision is typically made from the jugular notch to the xiphoid process. This is the most commonly performed access since it enables the control of all the cardiac structures and all the epicardial coronary branches, as well as the harvesting of both thoracic arteries.

T partial sternotomy (Fig. 14.2b): this spares the manubrium, thus maintaining the integrity of scapular

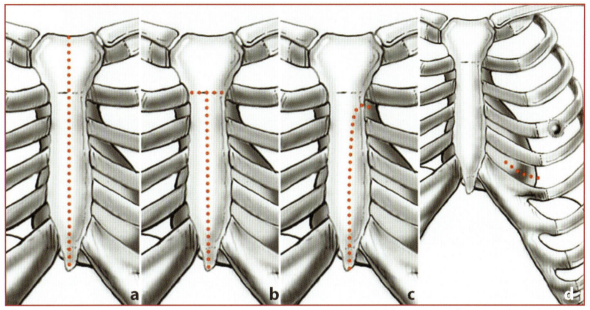

Fig. 14.2 Surgical access techniques: complete median sternotomy (**a**); mini-T partial sternotomy (**b**); reversed-J partial sternotomy (**c**); left minithoracotomy (**d**)

girdle mobility which is important for respiratory dynamics or in elderly patients at increased risk of sternal dehiscence.

Reversed-J partial sternotomy (Fig. 14.2c): alternative to the T sternotomy with few additional advantages.

Left minithoracotomy (Fig. 14.2d): performed with a minimally invasive incision (around 10 cm or even less if video-assisted techniques are used) at the level of the fourth-fifth left intercostal space. The technique is used for the revascularization of the LAD with the left ITA (LITA) in cases of single-vessel disease of the LAD or multivessel disease where the left circumflex coronary artery (LCX) and the right coronary artery (RCA) are chronically occluded or tributaries of a small necrotic myocardial area (<1.5 mm) or are extremely calcified.

Right minithoracotomy: performed at the level of the fifth right intercostal space and used to reperfuse the RCA with the right ITA (RITA) in situ. Since its introduction in 1995 and after an initial period of enthusiasm, right and left minithoracotomies have been used less frequently in light of the unjustifiably incomplete coronary revascularization, the technical difficulty of harvesting the LITA and last but not least the significantly increased use of PTCA for the treatment of single vessel disease of the LAD.

Left posterolateral thoracotomy: performed at the fourth-fifth left intercostal space, the technique provides a wide access which facilitates LITA harvesting right up to its origin with the consequent optimal mobilization and possible use for sequential anastomoses to diagonal branches. The technique enables an improved incision of the pericardium as well as greater control of the ascending aorta, thus offering a real alternative to off pump coronary artery bypass (OPCAB) with sternotomy. It should however be noted that the posterior access does not allow the control of the venae cavae, with the consequent cannulation of the pulmonary artery in case hemodynamic conditions of the patient requiring extracorporeal circulation.

14.5 Vascular Conduits

The development of surgical techniques and the introduction of new technologies (optical magnification and monofilament fine sutures) led to the shift from the initial venous revascularization of the 1960s and 1970s to mixed revascularization (arterial and venous). In light of the findings in terms of medium- and long-term patency, the use of the LITA began to be favored for the elective revascularization of the LAD, with use of the saphenous vein (SV) being limited to the revascularization of the other coronary branches.

The vascular conduits currently in use for coronary revascularization are: SV; ITA – both RITA and LITA; the radial artery (RA); the right gastroepiploic artery (RGEA); and the inferior epigastric artery (IEA).

These vessels differ from one another by distinctive anatomic and biologic characteristics which in most cases are the basis for their different use and different long-term patency [14].

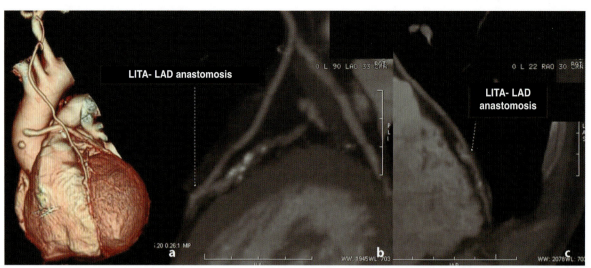

Fig. 14.3 Patient with triple coronary bypass: LITA to LAD, SVG to OM1, SVG to RCA. The volume rendering image (**a**) gives a panoramic view of the postsurgical vascular anatomy: the LITA graft, patent from its origin to the distal anastomosis, the graft to the obtuse marginal branch, patent from the proximal anastomosis to the mid-distal tract, and the venous graft for the right coronary artery, occluded at its origin. The multiplanar reconstructions provide a better evaluation of the distal anastomosis of the LITA with no signs of stenosis (**b**) and the distal tract of the LAD with regular contrast enhancement and diameter (**c**). *LITA*, left internal thoracic artery; *LAD*, left anterior descending coronary artery; *SVG*, saphenous vein graft; *OM1*, obtuse marginal branch; *RCA*, right coronary artery

14.5.1 Internal Thoracic Artery

The ITA is the vessel of choice for the surgical revascularization of the LAD, due to both its biologic and anatomic characteristics, being the vessel nearest the LAD and the most easily accessible surgically, both in terms of median sternotomy and left minithoracotomy [15]. It is used as an *in situ* bypass graft, i.e. with the anatomic origin conserved, for the revascularization of the anterior or anterolateral wall of the left ventricle with end-to-side distal anastomosis to the LAD (Fig. 14.3a-c) or to one of its diagonal branches. Multiple (sequential) anastomoses may also be done with an initial side-to-side anastomosis to the first diagonal branch and a successive end-to-side to the LAD. In the case of in situ use of both ITAs, the LITA is anastomosed to the LAD and the RITA to the RCA or to one of its collateral branches. In the event of revascularization of the left region with both ITAs in situ, two options are available. The first is performed with anastomosis of the RITA to the LAD and the LITA to the lateral superficial branches of the left ventricle (LCX and obtuse marginal branches, OM). The second option involves a retroaortic course of the RITA in situ to reperfuse the lateral wall of the left ventricle through the transverse sinus of the pericardium, whereas the LITA is anastomosed to the LAD.

The options available were later increased with the use of branching arterial conduits created from the in situ ITA with the addition of Y- or T-branching arterial segments in relation to the direction they were to take to reach the target coronary vessel. The RITA can also be used as a free graft, being anastomosed proximally to the ascending aorta and distally to the target vessel (generally the RCA).

ITA grafts are characterized by elevated long-term patency, low risk of occlusion with an incidence below 5% in the first year postprocedure and with a 10-year patency above 80% [4, 16]. The explanation for these positive data is found in the absence of vasa vasorum in the vessel wall, the presence of a fenestrated internal elastic lamina (factors which inhibit cellular migration and intimal hyperplasia), the absence of muscle cells in the media (poor vasoreactivity) and an endothelium capable of producing vasodilators.

With regard to MDCT evaluation, in situ ITA grafts have metal clips along their length, which are used in the process of skeletonization and harvesting. As a result, beam hardening artifacts and the blooming effect may compromise the evaluation of lumen patency.

14.5.2 Saphenous Vein

The advantages of using the SV are essentially due to the extreme ease of surgical access and harvesting and to the fact that the vessel is not subject to spasms during harvesting. Contraindications to its use include varicose and sclerotic disease: the incidence of atherosclerotic alterations after arterialization with consequent reduced long-term patency is its main limitation. Anatomically venous

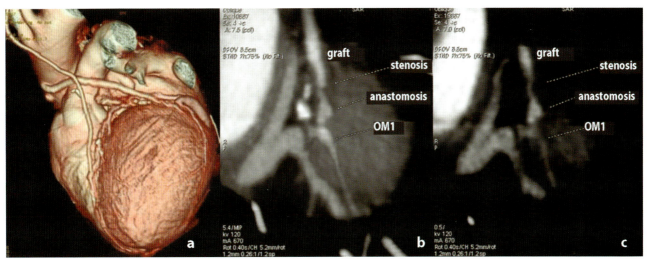

Fig. 14.4 The VR image of the lateral wall of the left ventricle shows the distal anastomosis of the venous graft to OM1 (**a**), while the MPR images (**b, c**) clearly depict the stenosis of the graft proximal to the distal anastomosis, with the distal coronary branch appearing thin and stenotic. *VR*, volume rendering; *OM1*, obtuse marginal branch; *MPR*, multiplanar reconstruction

grafts have larger diameters in comparison with arterial grafts, and combined with the fact that they have no surgical clips along their course they are easier to evaluate with noninvasive diagnostic imaging. A circumferential clip at the level of the proximal anastomosis may however be present in cases where the anastomosis was done by using a special metallic device (Bypass System Connector). While this may be helpful in angiographic procedures to recognize the anastomosis site, it may hamper MDCT evaluation.

The SV is prevalently used for the revascularization of the RCA, or by running posteriorly to the sternum and anteriorly to the right ventricular outflow tract (RVOT) it can be used for the revascularization of the vessels of the obtuse margin of the heart (LCX and OM) (Fig. 14.4) or the posterior descending artery (PDA) (Fig. 14.5). The frequency of disease in venous grafts is higher than in arterial grafts, with an incidence of occlusion at 10 years of 50%, with only 50% of patent grafts at 10 years (25%) free from disease [2, 3, 5] (Figs. 14.3, 14.4, 14.6).

14.5.3 Radial Artery

The RA is usually harvested from the nondominant arm and is occasionally used as a third arterial graft for the revascularization of the obtuse margin of the heart, or in the event the ITAs are not available when the use of venous grafts would rather be avoided [17-19]. Since it is a muscular artery the RA is characterized by elevated vasoreactivity with consequent reduced long-term patency, although its performance has been improved recently with the use of calcium antagonists. Another disadvantage is the large number of clips employed during skeletonization/harvesting, with a consequent increased incidence of beam hardening artifacts at MDCT.

14.5.4 Right Gastroepiploic Artery

Initially used for redo-surgery in the absence of other suitable conduits [20], the RGEA can be used as a second, third or fourth arterial conduit or used in situ to reperfuse the PDA. The absence of real advantages of a third or fourth arterial graft and the longer surgical procedure duration, related to the involvement of the abdominal cavity, have however limited its use.

14.5.5 Inferior Epigastric Artery

The IEA is an arterial branch of the abdominal wall arising from the external iliac artery and supplying the abdominal rectus muscle. Like the RA, it also has a prevalently muscular structure, but the short length of its tract with the largest diameter limit its use as the lateral branch of a sequential conduit [21].

14.6 MDCT Coronary Angiography: Study Technique and Postprocessing

The MDCT study of coronary artery bypass grafts is performed in the same way as in the study of the coronary

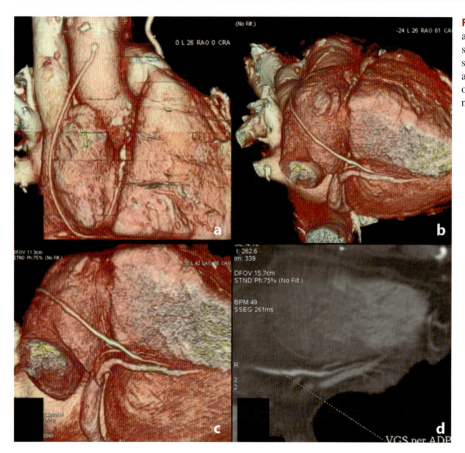

Fig. 14.5 Volume rendering images (**a-c**) and multiplanar reconstruction (**d**) of a saphenous vein graft: proximal anastomosis to the anterior wall of the ascending aorta (**a**), mid tract running posteroinferiorly to the right atrium (**b**), distal anastomosis to the PDA (**c,d**)

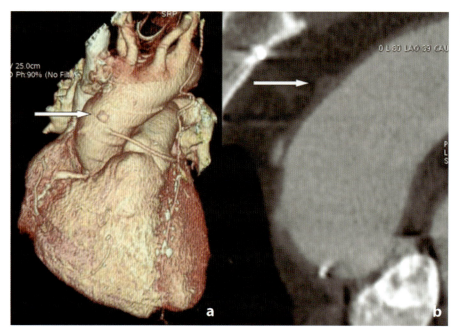

Fig. 14.6 Patient with triple coronary bypass: LITA to distal LAD, SVG to OM1, SVG to RCA. The volume rendering image (**a**) and the detailed multiplanar reconstruction (**b**) of the ascending aorta demonstrate the patency of the venous graft to OM1 and the occlusion at the origin of the graft to the LAD (*arrow*). *LITA*, left internal mammary artery; *LAD*, left anterior descending coronary artery; *SVG*, saphenous vein graft; *OM1*, obtuse marginal branch; *RCA*, right coronary artery

arteries, with the patient in the supine position and the acquisition being done in a single breath-hold. Once the ECG leads have been correctly positioned and an appropriate peripheral venous access has been prepared (18-20 Gauge) for the intravenous administration of contrast agent with automatic injector, usually in an antecubital vein of the right arm, the patient's heart rate needs to be monitored. Similar to the study of the coronary arteries,

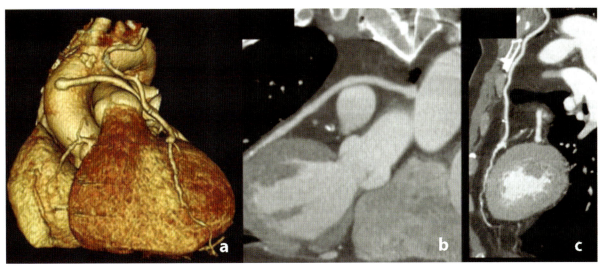

Fig. 14.7 Postprocessing techniques. The volume rendering image (**a**) provides a panoramic evaluation of the bypass graft anatomy and course. The curved multiplanar reconstructions enable the evaluation of the lumen of the grafts in a single image, with significant loss of anatomic orientation (**b**, **c**)

the heart rate should be lower than 65 bpm. In the event the heart rate is higher and in the absence of contraindications, negative chronotropic agents (beta-blockers) can be administered intravenously. Alternatively, the drugs can be administered orally, although this must be done at least one hour prior to the MDCT examination. Most CABG patients, however, are already following this line of pharmacologic treatment. After performing one or more scout-views (frontal and possibly lateral), a preliminary MDCT study of the chest should be done without contrast agent, not only to define the correct anatomic volume for the successive MDCT coronary angiography, but also to evaluate the presence of not rare incidental findings. In patients with a LITA graft, particularly with the most recent generation of scanners with 64 rows of detectors, the acquisition volume can depict the origin of the vessel from the subclavian artery and therefore detect the presence (in about 5% of cases) of non iatrogenic stenosis of the graft. Otherwise, in the presence of only venous grafts the acquisition volume need only include the proximal anastomosis of the most cranial graft. In the case of RGEA grafts to the PDA branch the study should be extended to the upper abdomen. The MDCT coronary angiography is performed with retrospective ECG gating and during intravenous contrast agent administration (120-130 mL; 370-400 mgI/mL; injection rate 3-5 mL/s). If dual-head automatic injectors are available, a bolus chaser following the contrast agent injection can serve several purposes: it consolidates the bolus of contrast agent, it acts as a further vis-a-tergo for the contrast agent administered and lastly it facilitates washout of the right cardiac sections.

An MDCT study with a 16-slice scanner of patients with LITA grafts requires an acquisition collimation of 1-1.5 mm depending on the scanner used to cover the entire anatomic volume of the graft (scan range 220-240 mm) during a single breath-hold (20-25 s). In the case of only venous grafts the acquisition volume (scan range 180 mm) can be covered with thinner collimations, between 0.5 mm and 0.75 mm according to the scanner used. The advantage a scanner with 64 rows of detectors has over a 16-slice system is its ability to acquire larger anatomic volumes with thinner collimations (0.4-0.625 mm vs. 0.5-0.75 mm) and more rapidly (20-24 s vs. 28-33 s).

Similar to the MDCT study of native coronary arteries, image reconstruction is performed in the mid-to-end-diastolic phase of the cardiac cycle. In choosing the most appropriate time window, which will vary according to the scanner type used, a fraction of the R-R interval (relative delay) or an absolute value (ms) in relation to the previous R wave (absolute delay) or the next R wave (inverse-absolute delay) is used. In this context it is worth noting that while with 16-MDCT optimal time windows vary between the right and left coronary arteries (even though in some cases a satisfactory result for the entire coronary tree can be achieved between 70% and 75% of the R-R interval), recent studies have shown that 64-MDCT with 330 ms gantry rotation speed achieves optimal image quality for all coronary segments with a reconstruction interval of 65% [22]. Once the phase of the cardiac cycle with the best diagnostic quality has been identified, the relative dataset of images is used for 2D and 3D post-processing on dedicated workstations. The 2D reconstructions (MPR, multiplanar

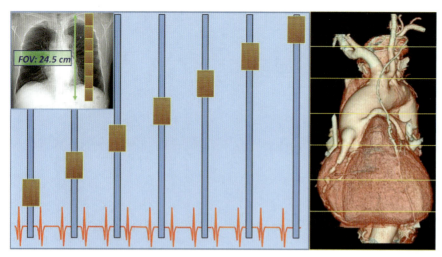

Fig. 14.8 Prospective ECG gating provides a sequential scan of the whole course of the grafts by acquiring a contiguous stack with a thickness of 35 mm (0.625 mm x 64 with an overlapping of 5 mm) every two heart beats, but with a consequent longer acquisition time

Exam Description: TAC TORACE — LightSpeed VCT

Report Dose

Series	Type	Scan Range (mm)	CTDIvol (mGy)	DLP (mGy-cm)	Phantom cm
3	Cine	39.500- 283.875	23.92	586.02	Body 32

Effective Dose: DLP x *K* = 586.02 x *0.017* = 9.96 mSv

Effective Dose: DLP x *K* = 586.02 x *0.014* = 8.20 mSv

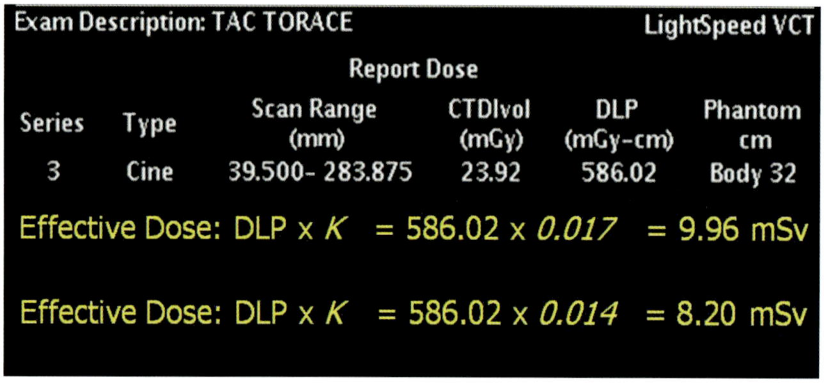

Fig. 14.9 Prospective ECG gating enables a significant reduction in radiation dose, with a total effective dose (ED) lower than 10 mSv for an in-situ LITA graft scan. The effective dose of CT examinations is estimated by a method proposed by the European working group for guidelines on quality criteria in CT [36, 37]

reconstructions and MIP, maximum intensity projections) are required for diagnostic purposes. The 3D reconstructions with volume rendering (VR) also play an important role, particularly in understanding the anatomy of grafts which can be complex and not immediately interpretable on native axial images. Lastly, curved multiplanar reconstructions (cMPR) may be used to give a 2D visualization of the entire graft and the distal native vessel, thus enabling an accurate identification and quantification of stenoses (Fig. 14.7). The technologic development of MDCT scanners in recent years has significantly strengthened the potential already demonstrated in scanners with 4 detector rows for the long-term follow-up of coronary bypass grafts. Table 14.1 presents the diagnostic accuracy of the technique in some of the major studies published in the literature. The advent of 16-MDCT and then of 64-MDCT has enabled not only an evaluation of bypass grafts, but also an evaluation of the native coronary circulation distal to the distal anastomoses of the grafts, as well as an improvement in the detail of the anastomoses themselves.

Moreover, recently developed prospective ECG-gating has a dedicated field of application in patients who have undergone surgical myocardial revascularization (Fig. 14.8), because of their usual medical therapy with beta-blockers. Prospective gating enables the application of the sequential scan protocol with the advantage of a lower radiation dose and wider anatomic coverage, but with the disadvantage of slightly lower longitudinal spatial resolution due to the contiguity of each image without overlapping, and increased sensitivity to arrhythmias (Fig. 14.9).

14.7 Conclusions

In general, the follow-up of patients who have undergone CABG surgery is one of the main areas of application of MDCT and should be associated as accurately as possible with the clinical findings of the patient and where available with the results of stress tests (ECG, echocardiography and scintigraphy). The main limitations of the

Table 14.1 Diagnostic accuracy of the technique reported in the literature

Study	Patients	Grafts	Arterial	Venous	Occlusion-CABG				Stenosis-CABG			
					Se	Sp	PPV	NPV	Se	Sp	PPV	NPV
4 slices												
Ropers [23]	65	182	20	162	97	98	97	98	75	92	71	93
Marano [24]	57	122	95	27	93	97.8	93	97.8	80	96	80	96
16 slices												
Martuscelli [25]	84	251	85	166	100	100	nr	nr	90	100	nr	nr
Schlosser [26]	48	131	40	91	-	-	-	-	96*	95*	81*	99*
Chiurlia [27]	52	166	49	117	100	100	nr	nr	96	100	nr	nr
Stauder [28]	20	50	16	34	nr	nr	nr	nr	98.5[a] 96.2[b]	93.9[a] 97.2[b]	91.8[a] 96.2[b]	98.9[a] 97.2[b]
Anders [29]	32	93	19	74	100	98	97	100	80-82	85-88	57-64	94-95
Kovacsik [30]	19	29	24	5	nr	nr	nr	nr	66.67	100	100	95.45
64 slices												
Pache [31]	31	93	22	71	nr	nr	nr	nr	97.8	89.3	90	97.7
Malagutti [32]	52	109	45	64	nr	nr	nr	nr	100	98.3	98	100
Ropers [33]	50	138	37	101	100	100	nr	nr	100	94	92	100
Dikkers [34]	35	69	52	17	100	100	100	100	100	98.7	75	100
Romagnoli [35]	77	212	97	115	100[a] 83.3[b]	100[a] 100[b]	100[a] 100[b]	100[a] 98.8[b]	94.4[a] 100[b]	98.4[a] 97.7[b]	96.9[a] 77.7[b]	96.7[a] 100[b]

Se, sensitivity; *Sp*, specificity; *NPV*, negative predictive value; *PPV*, positive predictive value; *, graft patency=grade 0 stenosis; *a*, venous graft; *b*, arterial graft; *nr*, not reported.

noninvasive study of coronary artery bypass grafts with MDCT are essentially related to the problems of heart rate and the number of surgical clips present along the course of arterial grafts. The problem of heart rate can be pharmacologically overcome with the use of ß-blocker and in part by using dual source scanners, which have already appeared on the market [38], or flat panel scanners, which are still under development [39]. In comparison to magnetic resonance imaging, MDCT is limited in being unable to provide functional/qualitative information about the flow in the studied grafts, although this limitation may be partially if not completely bypassed with a strong correlation between the morphologic and clinical findings of the patient.

References

1. Bourassa MG, Fisher LD, Campeau L et al (1985) Long-term fate of bypass grafts: the Coronary Artery Surgery Study (CASS) and Montreal Heart Institute experiences. Circulation 72:V71-V78
2. Campeau L, Enjalbert M, Lesperance J et al (1983) Atherosclerosis and late closure of aortocoronary saphenous vein grafts: sequential angiographic studies at 2 weeks, 1 year, 5 to 7 years, and 10 to 12 years after surgery. Circulation 68:II 1-7
3. Motwani JG, Topol EJ (1998) Aortocoronary saphenous vein graft disease: pathogenesis, predisposition, and prevention. Circulation 97:916-931
4. Cameron A, Davis KB, Green G, Schaff HV (1996) Coronary bypass surgery with internal thoracic artery grafts: effects on survival over a 15-year period. N Eng J Med 334:216-219
5. Eagle KA, Guyton RA, Davidoff R et al (2004) ACC/AHA 2004 guideline update for coronary artery bypass graft surgery: su mmary article.A report of the American College of Cardiology/American Heart Association Task Force on Practice Guidelines (Committee to Update the 1999 Guidelines for Coronary Artery Bypass Graft Surgery) Circulation 110:e340-437
6. Kennedy JW, Basley WA, Bunnel IL et al (1982) Mortality related to cardiac catheterization and angiography. Cath Cardiovasc Diagn 8:233-340
7. Davidson CJ (1997) Cardiac catheterization. In: Braunwald (ed) Heart disease: a textbook of cardiovascular medicine. WB Saunders, Philadelphia, pp 177-203
8. Topol EJ, Nissen SE (1995) Our preoccupation with coronary luminology. The dissociation between clinical and angiographic findings in ischemic heart disease. Circulation 92:2333-2342
9. Meurin P,Weber H, Renaud N et al (2004) Evolution of the postoperative pericardial effusion after day 15: the problem of the late tamponade. Chest 125:2182-2187
10. Katara AN, Samra SS, Bhandarkar DS (2003) Thoracoscopic window for a post-coronary artery bypass grafting pericardial effusion. Indian Heart J 55:180-181
11. Vargas F, Cukier A, Hueb W et al (1994) Relationship between pleural effusion and pericardial involvement after myocardial revascularization. Chest 105:1748-1752
12. Roy MC (1998) Surgical-site infections after coronary artery bypass graft surgery: discriminating site-specific risk factors to improve prevention efforts. Infect Control Hosp Epidemiol 19:229-233
13. Shammas NW (2000) Pulmonary embolus after coronary artery bypass surgery: a review of the literature. Clin Cardiol 23:637-644
14. Marano R, Storto ML, Merlino B et al (2005) A pictorial review of coronary artery bypass grafts at multidetector row CT. Chest 127:1371-1377
15. Calafiore AM, Di Giammarco G, Teodori G et al (1996) Left anterior descending coronary artery grafting via left anterior small thoracotomy without cardiopulmonary bypass. Ann Thorac Surg 61:1658-1663
16. Loop FD, Lytle BW, Cosgrove DM et al (1986) Influence of internal mammary artery graft on 10-year survival and other cardiac events. N Engl J Med 314:1-6
17. Carpentier A, Guermonprez JL, Deloche A et al (1973) The aorta-to-coronary radial artery bypass graft. A technique avoiding pathological changes in grafts. Ann Thorac Surg 16:111-121
18. Iaco AL, Teodori G, Di Giammarco G et al (2001) Radial artery for myocardial revascularization: long-term clinical and angiographic results. Ann Thorac Surg 72:464-468
19. Calafiore AM, Teodori G, Di Giammarco G et al (1995) Coronary revascularization with the radial artery: new interest for an old conduit. J Card Surg 10:140-146
20. Pym J, Brown PM, Charrette EJ et al (1987) Gastroepiploic-coronary anastomosis.A viable alternative bypass graft. J Thorac Cardiovasc Surg 94:256-259
21. Vincent JG, van Son JA, Skotnicki SH (1990) Inferior epigastric artery as a conduit in myocardial revascularization: the alternative free arterial graft. Ann Thorac Surg 49:323-325
22. Weininger M, Ritter C, Beer M et al (2006) Evaluation of the optimal image reconstruction interval for coronary artery imaging using 64-slice CT. Eur Radiology 16:6-L22 (abstract)
23. Ropers D, Ulzheimer S, Wenkel E et al (2001) Investigation of aortocoronary artery bypass grafts by multislice spiral computed tomography with electrocardiographic-gated image reconstruction. Am J Cardiol 88:792-795
24. Marano R, Storto ML, Maddestra N, Bonomo L (2004) Non-invasive assessment of coronary artery bypass graft with retrospectively ECG-gated four-row multi-detector spiral computed tomography. Eur Radiol 14:1353-1362
25. Martuscelli E, Romagnoli A, D'Eliseo A et al (2004) Evaluation of venous and arterial conduit patency by 16-slice spiral computed tomography. Circulation 110:3234-3238
26. Schlosser T, Konorza T, Hunold P et al (2004) Noninvasive visualization of coronary artery bypass grafts using 16-detector row computed tomography. J Am Coll Cardiol 44:1224-1229
27. Chiurlia E, Menozzi M, Ratti C et al (2005) Follow-up of coronary artery bypass graft patency by multislice computed tomography. Am J Cardiol 95:1094-1097
28. Stauder NI, Kuttner A, Schroder S et al (2006) Coronary artery bypass grafts: assessment of graft patency and native coronary artery lesions using 16-slice MDCT. Eur Radiol 16:2512-2520
29. Anders K, Baum U, Schmid M et al (2006) Coronary artery bypass graft (CABG) patency: assessment with high-resolution submillimeter 16-slice multidetector-row computed tomography (MDCT) versus coronary angiography. Eur J Radiol 57:336-344
30. Kovacsik HV, Battistella P, Demaria R et al (2006) Early postoperative assessment of coronary artery bypass graft patency and anatomy: value of contrast-enhanced 16-MDCT with retrospectively ECG-gated reconstructions. Am J Radiol 186:S395-S400
31. Pache G, Saueressig U, Frydrychowicz A et al (2006) Initial experience with 64-slice cardiac CT: noninvasive visualization of coronary artery bypass grafts. Eur Heart J 27:976-980
32. Malagutti P, Nieman K, Meijboom WB et al (2007) Use of 64-slice CT in symptomatic patients after coronary bypass surgery: evaluation of grafts and coronary arteries. Eur Heart J 28:1879-1885
33. Ropers D, Pohle FK, Kuettner A et al (2006) Diagnostic accuracy of noninvasive coronary angiography in patients after bypass surgery using 64-slice spiral computed tomography with 330-ms gantry rotation. Circulation 114:2334-2341; quiz 2334

34. Dikkers R, Willems TP, Tio RA et al (2006) The benefit of 64-MD-CT prior to invasive coronary angiography in symptomatic post-CABG patients. Int J Cardiovasc Imaging 26:369-377

35. Romagnoli A, Patrei A, Mancini A et al (2010) Diagnostic accuracy of 64-slice CT in evaluating coronary artery bypass grafts and of the native coronary arteries. Radiol Med 115:1167-1178

36. Bongartz G , Golding SJ, Jurik AG et al (2000) European Guidelines on Quality Criteria for Computed Tomography. EUR 16262. The European Commission's Study Group on Development of Quality Criteria for Computed Tomography. Luxembourg, Luxembourg: European Commission

37. Bongartz G, Golding SJ, Jurik AG et al (2004) CT quality criteria. Luxembourg, Luxembourg: European Commission, 2004

38. Goetti R, Leschka S, Baumüller S et al (2010) Low dose high-pitch spiral acquisition 128-slice dual-source computed tomography for the evaluation of coronary artery bypass graft patency. Invest Radiol 45:324-330

39. Gupta R, Cheung AC, Bartling SH et al (2008) Flat-panel volume CT: fundamental principles, technology, and applications. Radiographics 28:2009-2022

Myocardial Viability and Stress Perfusion

15

Tust Techasith, Brian Ghoshhajra, and Udo Hoffmann

15.1 Introduction

The role of noninvasive imaging for patients with suspected coronary artery disease (CAD) has expanded rapidly over the past few decades. The growth and refinement of noninvasive modalities have occurred in both anatomic imaging (cardiac computed tomography [CCT]) and functional imaging (stress echocardiography, nuclear stress myocardial perfusion imaging-MPI, and stress magnetic resonance imaging-MRI).

From the early days of CT, the pace of technologic advancement has been swift, with rapid improvement in temporal and spatial resolutions, expanding z-axis coverage, and radiation dose reduction technology. Despite these advances, the use of CT has been limited primarily to the anatomic domain, such as CCT or coronary calcium scoring.

Cardiac CT has been shown by several multicenter trials to have excellent diagnostic accuracy in the detection and exclusion of significant coronary stenosis as compared to invasive coronary angiography [1-3]. A high negative predictive value (>95%) makes CCT an excellent *rule-out* test. However, these data also demonstrated a limited positive predictive value of CCT (60-90% dependent on the prevalence of stenotic lesions) due to the inherent limitations related to its anatomic basis for detecting a significant stenosis. This diagnostic dilemma is most prominent in patients at high risk for CAD and patients with known CAD, who often demonstrate severe coronary calcification, which tends to limit the ability to exclude stenosis and often leads to overestimation of the extent of CAD [4, 5]. Furthermore, it has been established that the presence of anatomic lesions does not nec-

essarily correlate with functional abnormality, i.e. significantly impaired myocardial blood flow [6]. The shortcomings of an anatomically-based modality are further illustrated by numerous studies demonstrating that functional information - i.e. myocardial perfusion reserve and myocardial tissue viability - is incremental to anatomic assessment alone in both guiding immediate (diagnosis) and long-term (prognosis) clinical management [7-10].

Given the inherent limitations of anatomic imaging, many have attempted to combine CCT with functional studies such as positron emission tomography (PET) or single photon emission computed tomography (SPECT), drawing upon their complementary nature [11, 12]. While these studies demonstrated the incremental value of stress SPECT and PET, these modalities have their own limitations, including attenuation artifacts and limited spatial resolution. In addition, the patient is subjected to at least two diagnostic studies in order to arrive at the final result, which is not only inconvenient and expensive, but also carries an increased radiation burden.

Therefore, a need exists for an exam that combines anatomic and functional acquisition. Many recent studies have aimed to accomplish this with CT, specifically via pharmacologic stress myocardial CT perfusion (CTP) imaging. Thus far, these studies have demonstrated the feasibility of stress myocardial CTP and shown its incremental value to traditional CCT in the detection of significant coronary stenosis, potentially overcoming the limitations of CCT alone [13-16]. Others have attempted to evaluate myocardial viability via delayed contrast enhancement, with varying degrees of success. As CT technology continues to evolve, stress myocardial CTP is likely to play a prominent role in the evaluation of CAD due to the ease and comprehensiveness of its data acquisition. The remainder of this chapter will review the historical development and the current state of stress CT perfusion and myocardial viability CT examinations, various considerations in setting up the protocols, and future directions for the modality.

U. Hoffmann (✉)
Cardiac MR/PET/CT Program,
Massachusetts General Hospital and Harvard Medical School,
Boston, MA, USA

F. Cademartiri, G. Casolo, M. Midiri (eds.), *Clinical Applications of Cardiac CT*,
© Springer-Verlag Italia 2012

15.2 Historical Development of Perfusion Evaluation by CT

Within a few years of the invention of the CT scanner, numerous attempts were made to image the heart. In 1976, Adams et al. first reported the use of CT to the image canine myocardium ex vivo, the use of iodinated contrast to distinguish between myocardium and ventricular cavity, and, more importantly, the difference in attenuation between normal and infarcted myocardium [17, 18]. They suggested that a properly gated CT scanner can be employed as a noninvasive approach to the diagnosis of myocardial infarction. Further works by Higgins et al. confirmed the ability of CT to detect and even quantify areas of acute and chronic myocardial infarction based on attenuation differences [19-21]. Carlsson et al. subsequently described the presence of delayed enhancement in areas of infarcted myocardium in addition to the initial perfusion defect in a canine model [22]. Masuda et al. evaluated a series of 103 patients with known myocardial infarction and confirmed these two perfusion-related findings which is still used to characterize myocardial infarction today [23]. Around the same period of time, other investigators experimented with the use of CT in detecting myocardial ischemia as well. Cipriano et al. employed a canine model with balloon occluder to image acute myocardial ischemia in vivo and illustrated reduced attenuation in ischemic myocardium compared to normal myocardium, although the difference did not meet statistical significance [24].

Despite these initial results demonstrating the feasibility of CT as a modality to evaluate the myocardium, there were some technical limitations that held the modality back at that time, particularly the low temporal resolution and the inability to cover the heart quickly as only one slice could be acquired at a time. Over time, many technologic improvements, such as reliable ECG-gating mechanism, improved spatial and temporal resolutions, multidetector capability, and three-dimensional reconstructions have made CT a more suitable modality for the evaluation of myocardial perfusion and viability as Hoffmann et al. was able to illustrate in a porcine model using retrospectively gated CT in 2004 [25]. Subsequent efforts to use CT in cardiac imaging have focused on imaging of the coronary arteries, resulting in the establishment coronary CT as an exam with a uniformly high negative predictive value for significant coronary stenosis. However, the limitations of coronary CT as an anatomic modality have led to renewed interest in the use of CT to evaluate functional parameters such as myocardial tissue viability and to detect myocardial perfusion abnormality.

15.3 Current State of CT Perfusion and Viability

For evaluation of ischemic cardiomyopathy, recent efforts have focused on the simultaneous imaging of both the myocardium for stress perfusion reserve and the coronary arteries for anatomic stenosis, to provide complementary information that might overcome the shortcomings of CCT. In 2005, Kurata et al. evaluated this combined approach–the stress myocardial CTP–in a small cohort of patients under adenosine stress using 16-detector-row MDCT [26]. More than half of the coronary segments in this study were not evaluable, illustrating that the temporal resolution was insufficient. In 2007, George et al. illustrated the feasibility of stress myocardial CTP in canine models using 64-detector-row MDCT [27, 28]. Subsequent studies have evaluated stress myocardial CTP in multiple human cohorts, using various scanners, pharmacologic stress agents, imaging protocols, and reference standards. The findings of these studies generally support the preceding animal studies, demonstrating that CTP can be used to detect stress-related myocardial perfusion defects with favorable diagnostic characteristics.

George et al. evaluated CTP in 40 patients with abnormal SPECT. Using adenosine as the pharmacologic vasodilator stress agent, beta-blockers for heart rate control, and 64-detector-row MDCT or 256-detector-row MDCT for image acquisition [13], they demonstrated good per-vessel-territory sensitivity, specificity, positive predictive value (PPV), and negative predictive value (NPV) as compared to a combined quantitative coronary angiography (QCA) and SPECT criterion standard. Blankstein et al. evaluated stress myocardial CTP in the setting of adenosine stress with a first generation dual source CT (DSCT) which offers the advantage of significantly higher temporal resolution, allowing pharmacologic stress without beta-blockade, and simultaneous CCT acquisition [14]. The result showed that the modality is equivalent to SPECT in the detection of coronary artery stenosis as defined by QCA. Furthermore, the CCT obtained during the protocol was able to detect stenosis of 70% or more on QCA with excellent accuracy. Further analysis of the same patient cohort by Rocha-Filho et al. demonstrated incremental value of adding myocardial CTP to CCT, improving specificity and positive predictive value when compared to coronary CT alone [16]. Cury et al. employed a different stress agent, dipyridamole, with a 64-detector-row MDCT [15]. Their result confirmed that stress myocardial CTP is at least equivalent to SPECT in the detection of stenosis found on QCA. The specific findings of these studies evaluating patient cohorts are summarized in Table 15.1.

While numerous attempts to evaluate myocardial viability have been made since the advent of CT, this indication has not been well-established. The presence of delayed enhancement in myocardial infarction was first reported in the 1970s [22, 29, 30]. Masuda et al. subsequently showed that delayed enhancement alone is visualized in only half of patients with known myocardial infarction [23]. While the feasibility and prognostic value of cardiac MR evaluation for myocardial viability has been established [31, 32], studies evaluating the use of CT for viability have only shown moderate results[33-35]. Particularly, with regards to delayed enhancement, it is evident that CT has significantly lower signal-to-noise and contrast-to-noise ratios versus MRI [36]. Currently there is not enough literature to definitively support the use of delayed phase CT as a stand-alone evaluation for myocardial viability. Another approach, such as a combined evaluation of rest myocardial perfusion, delayed enhancement, and CT wall motion, have performed better for this purpose and may emerge as the best method for CT viability evaluation in the future [37]. Further research on the use of delayed enhancement CT for viability evaluation is needed.

15.4 Principles of Stress Perfusion and Viability CT Exam

There are a few principles that underlie the ability of CT to evaluate myocardial perfusion and viability. Stress myocardial CTP relies upon a flow differential between ischemic and nonischemic myocardium (i.e. *stress perfusion reserve*). A fundamental pretext is the direct relationship between the amount of iodinated contrast within the myocardium and myocardial attenuation as measured in Hounsfield Units (HU) [27]. Differences in myocardial perfusion will result in areas of differing CT attenuations. For example, an area of myocardium with decreased blood flow due to a functionally significant coronary artery stenosis will have lower attenuation than adjacent myocardium supplied by non-diseased vessel and appear as a distinct area of perfusion defect; this difference will be accentuated under physiologic or pharmacologic stress. When present, a perfusion defect can usually be detected visually; however, confirmation with region of interest (ROI) measurements can be helpful. Regarding the interpretation of a perfusion defect in the setting of stress and/or at rest, CTP is similar to nuclear MPI, with reversibility serving as the key distinguishing feature between stress-induced ischemia and myocardial infarction (Fig. 15.1).

Myocardial viability evaluation by CT includes morphologic evaluation and perfusion assessment. Morphologic findings of infarcted myocardium include myocardial thinning, left ventricular aneurysm, calcification, and fatty metaplasia. CT viability evaluation based on delayed contrast enhancement was first reported in a canine model and human cohorts early in the development of cardiac CT [22, 23]. These findings were further confirmed and established when the similar pharmacokinetics between iodinated contrast used in CT and gadolinium-based MR contrast in diseased myocardium were illustrated [38]. Time-dependent contrast patterns characterizing myocardial infarction have since been demonstrated with both contrast agents, with hypoenhancement seen at first-pass (due to decreased inflow to the infarcted myocardium) and increased enhancement at a delayed phase scan (secondary to increased distribution volume and altered contrast pharmacokinetics in myocardial scar tissue) [38, 39].

15.5 General Overview of CT Perfusion Exam

This section is meant as a general overview of stress myocardial CTP exam; specific considerations in setting up protocols can be found in the subsequent section. Full protocols from various feasibility studies have been previously published [13-15].

Stress myocardial CTP protocol is composed of stress and rest phase acquisitions, similar to a nuclear MPI exam (Fig. 15.2). These acquisitions can be used to evaluate both functional and anatomic information, although the coronary anatomy is preferentially evaluated using the rest phase acquisition for better image quality due to lower heart rate. Iodinated contrast is administered both in the stress and the rest acquisition, for a total of approximately 150 mL. Stress phase imaging is performed under pharmacologic stress agents; an additional intravenous catheter is placed in the opposite arm for the infusion of stress agents. For myocardial viability, a stress phase scan is less important; however, a delayed phase acquisition can be performed for delayed contrast enhancement evaluation for myocardial scar, using the contrast administered previously in the stress and the rest phase acquisition. Electrocardiogram (ECG) and blood pressure measurements are performed prior to scan acquisition to establish a baseline for patient monitoring during and after the completion of the protocol.

Scout images are acquired to localize the heart position. Contrast timing for image acquisition is determined. For the stress phase acquisition, infusion of pharmacologic stress agent is initiated. Once peak effect is reached, contrast is administered and images are

Table 15.1 Summary of selected human studies evaluating stress CT perfusion imaging

Study	Population	CTP Protocol	Reference Standard	Results	Conclusion
George et al. 2009 [13]	40 patients: - abnormal SPECT MPI - subset with invasive coronary angiography (n=27)	- beta blocker - adenosine stress - 64-detector MDCT (n=24) and 256-detector MDCT (n=16) - stress phase and rest phase	Combination: 50% or greater stenosis on QCA and matched territorial defect on SPECT	CCT/CTP: Per Vessel Territory → sensitivity 79% and specificity 91%	CCT/CTP combination can detect atherosclerosis causing perfusion defects when compared to QCA/SPECT
Blankstein et al. 2009 [14]	34 patients: - moderate to high risk SPECT MPI - all had invasive coronary angiography	- no beta blocker - adenosine stress - 64-detector DSCT - stress phase, rest phase, and delayed phase	50% or greater stenosis on QCA	CTP: Per Vessel Territory → sensitivity 79% and specificity 80% SPECT: Per-Vessel → sensitivity 67% and specificity 83%	CTP has comparable diagnostic characteristics to SPECT in the detection of stress-induced myocardial perfusion defects, with similar radiation dose.
Cury et al. 2010 [15]	36 patients: - abnormal SPECT MPI - subset with invasive coronary angiography (n=26)	- no beta blocker - dipyridamole stress - 64-detector MDCT - stress phase and rest phase	70% or greater stenosis on QCA	CTP: Per Vessel Territory → sensitivity 88% and specificity 79% SPECT: Per-Vessel → sensitivity 69% and specificity 76% Good agreement between CTP and SPECT (K=0.53)	Dipyridamole CTP is feasible with similar diagnostic characteristics to SPECT.

SPECT MPI, single photon emission computed tomography myocardial perfusion imaging; *QCA*, quantitative coronary angiography; *MPS*, myocardial perfusion scintigraphy.

15 Myocardial Viability and Stress Perfusion

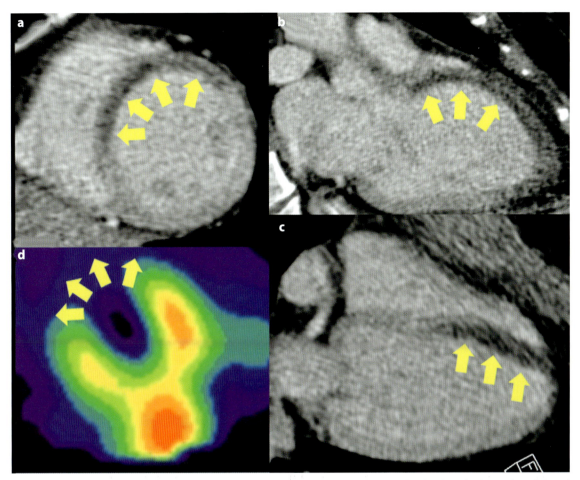

Fig. 15.1 Myocardial perfusion defect at first-pass CT performed due to failed interventional catheterization and suspicion of anomalous coronary artery. CT was performed to image coronary anatomy but revealed a large anterior and anteroseptal wall perfusion defect on short axis (**a**), 2-chamber (**b**), and 4-chamber (**c**) views. Thallium viability image subsequently revealed perfusion defect in the same territory (**d**)

acquired using the timing previously derived. Throughout the entire process, the patient's symptoms, heart rate, blood pressure, and ECG are closely monitored. The stress agent is stopped immediately (or reversed if using dipyridamole or regadenoson) after the images are acquired. There should be a period of delay after stress to allow the effects of the pharmacologic stress to resolve. For the rest acquisition, contrast is again administered and the images are acquired using similar timing. This acquisition can be used to assess the coronary arteries as well. Post-exam ECG and vital sign measurements are performed to ensure patient's safety. A delayed phase acquisition can be added to evaluate for delayed enhancement (i.e. scar at the site of myocardial infarct). This acquisition is performed approximately 7 to 10 minutes after the completion of the second acquisition. No additional contrast injection is necessary; the previously injected stress and rest phase contrast can be employed for the delayed scan. Of note, if myocardial viability is the sole purpose of the exam, stress phase examination may be omitted; instead, a combination of rest and delayed phases are sufficient to assess for infarct. This will allow optimization of late contrast enhancement timing through the use of a single contrast bolus instead of using the two separate smaller, temporally distinct contrast boluses from the stress and rest phase acquisitions.

15.6 Specific Considerations in CT Perfusion Exam

15.6.1 Pharmacologic Stress Agents

In feasibility trials of myocardial stress CTP, pharmacologic stress agents adenosine and dipyridamole were successfully used [13-15]. Both agents are vasodilators that induce differences in myocardial blood flow owing to the fact that normal coronary arteries dilate more than their diseased counterpart, leading to a flow differential in the downstream myocardium appearing as relative perfusion defects in the territory supplied by the diseased artery, both due to a relative increase and preferential flow (i.e. coronary steal phenomenon). Since both agents exert their effects through the adenosine receptors, they have been shown to have similar diagnostic characteristics in the detection of myocardial perfusion defect and also share similar side effect profile (reflex tachycardia) and contraindications (asthma, COPD, and advanced atri-oventricular block in the absence of pacemaker). Adenosine has a rapid onset and short duration of action, while the effects of dipyridamole last longer and often require reversal with an adenosine receptor antagonist such as aminophylline. Both agents are administered via infusion pump at previously established rates, 140 µg/kg/min infused over 3-4 minutes for adenosine and 0.56 mg/kg infused over 4-6 minutes for dipyridamole. Other pharmacologic stress agents such as dobutamine (β1 agonist) or regadenoson (adenosine receptor agonist subtype A2) have been used for stress echocardiography and nuclear stress MPI but have not been reported in studies evaluating stress myocardial CTP; future studies may support the conventional wisdom stating that these agents are suitable for this modality as well.

15.6.2 Sequence of Exams

A fundamental tradeoff is made when setting up a stress and rest CTP protocol with regard to the order of the stress vs. rest scan acquisitions. The main consideration is that the first scan will be a *cleaner* acquisition, and that the second acquisition can be contaminated by the recirculating contrast from the first scan, particularly when myocardial infarction is present. The contrast from the first scan will accumulate in areas of infarct (myocardial delayed enhancement) and interfere with the perfusion profile of the second scan in the sequence, leading to the underestimation or even a false negative result, depending on the degree of delayed enhancement contaminating the myocardium. For the patient population which CTP targets (high risk or known CAD), the predominant argument is that accurate stress phase images are preferred over rest phase images (stress phase followed by rest phase Fig. 15.2a), as the primary aim of CTP is to detect myocardial ischemia.

The opposite order of acquisition - rest phase followed by stress phase - (Fig. 15.2b) yields a *clean* rest phase at the expense of a slightly contaminated stress phase acquisition. This could potentially mask areas of ischemic myocardium, particularly in the setting of peri-infarct ischemia (which carries prognostic value and may benefit from revascularization). The benefits of perform-

ing rest phase acquisition first are realized when the patient has no evidence of CAD on a carefully-performed coronary CT (i.e. no coronary stenosis or calcification). In such a scenario, no further functional imaging is necessary (due to the established high negative predictive value of CT). This situation may arise frequently in a clinical setting, when patients with low probability of CAD are referred for coronary CT. Conversely, in cases of intermediate (40-70% luminal narrowing) or nondiagnostic segments (such as in the setting of calcification or stents) discovered at routine CCT, the stress phase may prove valuable in assigning significance to an otherwise uncertain lesion [16]. Such a protocol would allow a single diagnostic appointment.

It may be advantageous to stratify patients into low- and high-risk groups before deciding the order of a comprehensive protocol (Fig. 15.3). The low-risk group would undergo a rest phase scan first and only proceed to stress phase imaging in the positive or indeterminate cases, whereas the high risk group would start with the stress phase scan. Coronary calcium scoring may have a future role in risk stratification to the appropriate protocol.

15.6.3 Contrast and Timing for Image Acquisition

For proper timing of image acquisition either a test-bolus method or trigger-bolus method can be employed. For the test-bolus method, 10-15 mL of contrast is administered at 4-5 mL/s followed by 20 mL of saline flush. Time of peak contrast enhancement in the ascending aorta is measured and the image acquisition time is calculated by adding a few seconds, in order to achieve a sufficient level of contrast perfusion throughout the myocardium, from the subepicardial to the subendocardial layer and from base to the apex of the heart. In the trigger-bolus method, an attenuation-based threshold (HU) is set at a specific location and image acquisition commences once the threshold is met. For image acquisition, contrast is administered at a rate of 4-5 mL/s. For each acquisition (stress and rest), between 60-70 mL of contrast is administered. During stress acquisition, the contrast administration begins a few minutes after the infusion of pharmacologic stress agent started. The delayed phase acquisition does not require contrast, but employs contrast from previous phases.

15.6.4 Scan Settings

Images can be acquired with either retrospective ECG gating (usually with tube current modulation) or

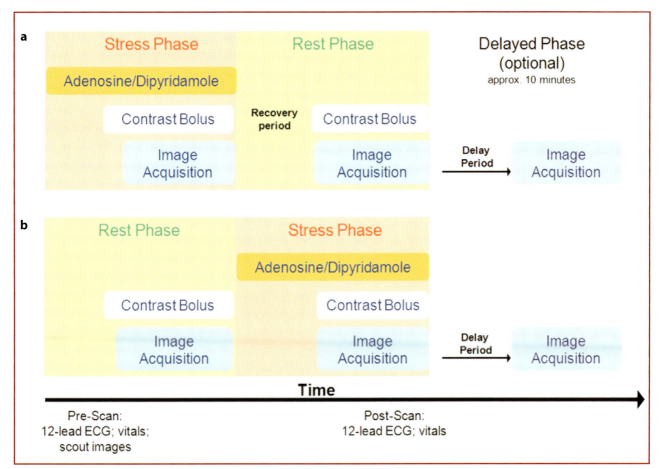

Fig. 15.2 CTP protocol design: order of scan acquisition. **a** Stress acquisition first and **b** Rest acquisition first

prospective ECG-triggered modes. Tube voltage and current can be adjusted according to body mass index (BMI) and body habitus, with 100 kV for BMI less than 30 kg/m^2 and 120 kV for BMI equal to or greater than 30 kg/m^2. Low kV is preferred due to the resulting higher CNR in the myocardium, when body habitus allows [40, 41]. With tube current modulation, the mA can vary depending on patient's body habitus, and modulated throughout the cardiac cycle, but at least one phase of peak mA should be prescribed. Peak mA is best centered in mid- to late-diastole for the least cardiac motion. Prospective triggering minimizes the radiation dose; however, this removes the redundancy in the data and may not be suitable for a patient with ectopy, particularly in scanners with a short z-axis coverage.

15.7 Image Processing

As with nuclear MPI, analysis of myocardial segments are best analyzed in true cardiac planes, according to the AHA 17-segment model [42]. This is accomplished by using a 3D-capable workstation, and reconstructing short- and long-axis (double-oblique) views of the left ventricle with multiplanar reconstruction software. Adjustment of certain reconstruction and viewing parameters during CTP interpretation can increase the diagnostic accuracy for the detection of true perfusion defects. Initial data indicate that the optimal reconstruction parameters are relatively thick MPR, diastolic phase short axis images [43]. Narrow viewing window (100-200HU) should be used centered at attenuation of around 100 HU. The use of multiphase data, when available, leads to increased specificity; true perfusion defects should persist throughout the cardiac cycle whereas minor artifacts are transient.

15.8 Conclusion and Future Directions

The initial investigations evaluating stress perfusion CT with 64-detector-row MDCT and newer scanners have been promising, illustrating comparable diagnostic characteristics to SPECT MPI/QCA and adding incremental value to coronary CTA alone in the detection of hemodynamically significant stenosis. The radiation exposure in such protocols has been reported to be similar to that of

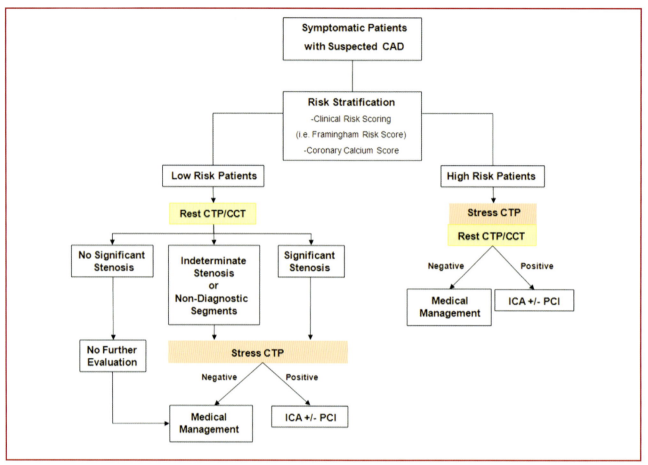

Fig. 15.3 Proposed algorithm for the use of myocardial CT perfusion exam

a traditional SPECT MPI exam but is likely to decrease as CT technology advances [14]. However, these preliminary results reflect single-center experiences in high-risk referral populations. Furthermore, these initial feasibility studies utilized varying CT protocols and the current literature is lacking of robust and standardized trials for CTP. Therefore, further studies in a wider patient population and in multicenter settings are warranted before CTP can be established as a viable clinical tool. Such investigation may focus on 64-detector-row MDCT as this is a widely available technology, albeit at a disadvantage to DSCT or wide-area detector scanners (such as 256- or 320-detector row CT).

Given the promising findings in initial stress perfusion CT trials, recently introduced technology such as dual energy and dynamic scan modes have also been investigated [44-47]. Dual energy CT (DECT) takes advantage of different spectral characteristics of various materials when penetrated by different X-ray energies; this allows for the mapping of iodine concentration within the myocardium - perhaps reflecting more precisely the degree of perfusion [48]. Initial investigation demonstrated that DECT had good sensitivity and specificity in detecting perfusion defects seen on SPECT [44]. These findings have subsequently been reinforced in the setting of adenosine stress using stress perfusion MRI and fractional flow reserve measurement as the criterion standard [49, 50]. Preliminary experiences with dynamic myocardial CT perfusion imaging also showed good promise in both animal models and human patients, allowing the derivation of myocardial blood flow based on time-attenuation curve (by acquiring multiple scans at successive time points and calculating the enhancement rates and input functions to inform perfusion reserve) [45-47]. This method has been shown to have good diagnostic characteristics compared to nuclear MPI [47]. Furthermore, the calculated myocardial blood flow was shown to have good correlation with fractional flow reserve measurement in an initial human subject and to add incremental value to CT alone in the detection of hemodynamically significant stenosis [46, 51]. However, radiation dose concern is a major issue for this particular scan mode. These specific scan modes are both in their infancy and further evaluation will be necessary; they are also limited to the latest scanners and are not widely available as of yet.

References

1. Meijboom WB, Meijs MF, Schuijf JD et al (2008) Diagnostic accuracy of 64-slice computed tomography coronary angiography: a prospective, multicenter, multivendor study. J Am Coll Cardiol 52:2135-2144
2. Miller JM, Rochitte CE, Dewey M et al (2008) Diagnostic performance of coronary angiography by 64-row CT. N Engl J Med 359:2324-2336
3. Budoff MJ, Dowe D, Jollis JG et al (2008) Diagnostic performance of 64-multidetector row coronary computed tomographic angiography for evaluation of coronary artery stenosis in individuals without known coronary artery disease: results from the prospective multicenter ACCURACY (Assessment by Coronary Computed Tomographic Angiography of Individuals Undergoing Invasive Coronary Angiography) trial. J Am Coll Cardiol 52:1724-1732
4. Pflederer T, Marwan M, Renz A et al (2009) Noninvasive assessment of coronary in-stent restenosis by dual-source computed tomography. Am J Cardiol 103:812-817
5. Pugliese F, Weustink AC, Van Mieghem C et al (2008) Dual source coronary computed tomography angiography for detecting in-stent restenosis Heart 94:848-854
6. Meijboom WB, Van Mieghem CA, van Pelt N et al (2008) Comprehensive assessment of coronary artery stenoses: computed tomography coronary angiography versus conventional coronary angiography and correlation with fractional flow reserve in patients with stable angina. J Am Coll Cardiol 52:636-643
7. Shaw LJ, Berman DS, Maron DJ et al (2008) Optimal medical therapy with or without percutaneous coronary intervention to reduce ischemic burden: results from the Clinical Outcomes Utilizing Revascularization and Aggressive Drug Evaluation (COURAGE) trial nuclear substudy. Circulation 117:1283-1291
8. Boden WE, O'Rourke RA, Teo KK et al (2007) Optimal medical therapy with or without PCI for stable coronary disease. N Engl J Med 356:1503-1516
9. Hachamovitch R, Hayes SW, Friedman JD, Cohen I et al (2003) Comparison of the short-term survival benefit associated with revascularization compared with medical therapy in patients with no prior coronary artery disease undergoing stress myocardial perfusion single photon emission computed tomography. Circulation 107:2900-2907
10. Kwong RY, Sattar H, Wu H et al (2008) Incidence and prognostic implication of unrecognized myocardial scar characterized by cardiac magnetic resonance in diabetic patients without clinical evidence of myocardial infarction. Circulation 118:1011-1020
11. Gaemperli O, Husmann L, Schepis T et al (2009) Coronary CT angiography and myocardial perfusion imaging to detect flow-limiting stenoses: a potential gatekeeper for coronary revascularization? Eur Heart J 30:2921-2929
12. Di Carli MF, Dorbala S, Curillova Z et al (2007) Relationship between CT coronary angiography and stress perfusion imaging in patients with suspected ischemic heart disease assessed by integrated PET-CT imaging. J Nucl Cardiol 14:799-809
13. George RT, Arbab-Zadeh A, Miller JM et al (2009) Adenosine stress 64- and 256-row detector computed tomography angiography and perfusion imaging: a pilot study evaluating the transmural extent of perfusion abnormalities to predict atherosclerosis causing myocardial ischemia. Circ Cardiovasc Imaging 2:174-182
14. Blankstein R, Shturman LD, Rogers IS et al (2009) Adenosine-induced stress myocardial perfusion imaging using dual-source cardiac computed tomography. J Am Coll Cardiol 54:1072-1084
15. Cury RC, Magalhaes TA, Borges AC et al (2010) Dipyridamole stress and rest myocardial perfusion by 64-detector row computed tomography in patients with suspected coronary artery disease. Am J Cardiol 106:310-315
16. Rocha-Filho JA, Blankstein R, Shturman LD et al (2010) Incremental value of adenosine-induced stress myocardial perfusion imaging with dual-source CT at cardiac CT angiography. Radiology 254:410-419
17. Adams DF, Hessel SJ, Judy PF et al (1976) Computed tomography of the normal and infarcted myocardium. AJR Am J Roentgenol 126:786-791
18. Adams DF, Hessel SJ, Judy PF et al (1976) Differing attenuation coefficients of normal and infarcted myocardium. Science 192:467-469
19. Siemers PT, Higgins CB, Schmidt W et al (1978) Detection, quantitation and contrast enhancement of myocardial infarction utilizing computerized axial tomography: comparison with histochemical staining and 99mTc-pyrophosphate imaging. Invest Radiol 13:103-109
20. Higgins CB, Siemers PT, Schmidt W, Newell JD (1979). Evaluation of myocardial ischemic damage of various ages by computerized transmission tomography. Time-dependent effects of contrast material. Circulation 60:284-291
21. Higgins CB, Sovak M, Schmidt W, Siemers PT (1979) Differential accumulation of radiopaque contrast material in acute myocardial infarction. Am J Cardiol 43:47-51
22. Carlsson E, Lipton MJ, Berninger WH et al (1977) Selective left coronary myocardiography by computed tomography in living dogs. Invest Radiol 12:559-562
23. Masuda Y, Yoshida H, Morooka N et al (1984) The usefulness of x-ray computed tomography for the diagnosis of myocardial infarction. Circulation 70:217-225
24. Cipriano PR, Nassi M, Ricci MT et al (1981) Acute myocardial ischemia detected in vivo by computed tomography. Radiology 140:727-731
25. Hoffmann U, Millea R, Enzweiler C et al (2004) Acute myocardial infarction: contrast-enhanced multi-detector row CT in a porcine model. Radiology 231:697-701
26. Kurata A, Mochizuki T, Koyama Y et al (2005) Myocardial perfusion imaging using adenosine triphosphate stress multi-slice spiral computed tomography: alternative to stress myocardial perfusion scintigraphy. Circ J 69:550-557
27. George RT, Silva C, Cordeiro MA et al (2006) Multidetector computed tomography myocardial perfusion imaging during adenosine stress. J Am Coll Cardiol 48:153-160
28. George RT, Jerosch-Herold M, Silva C et al (2007) Quantification of myocardial perfusion using dynamic 64-detector computed tomography. Invest Radiol 42:815-822
29. Higgins CB, Sovak M, Schmidt W, Siemers PT (1978) Uptake of contrast materials by experimental acute myocardial infarctions: a preliminary report. Invest Radiol 13:337-339
30. Higgins CB, Siemers PT, Newell JD, Schmidt W (1980) Role of iodinated contrast material in the evaluation of myocardial infarction by computerized transmission tomography. Invest Radiol 15:176-182
31. Choi KM, Kim RJ, Gubernikoff G et al (2001) Transmural extent of acute myocardial infarction predicts long-term improvement in contractile function. Circulation 104:1101-1107
32. Kim RJ, Wu E, Rafael A et al (2000) The use of contrast-enhanced magnetic resonance imaging to identify reversible myocardial dysfunction. N Engl J Med 343:1445-1453
33. Jacquier A, Boussel L, Amabile N et al (2008) Multidetector computed tomography in reperfused acute myocardial infarction. Assessment of infarct size and no-reflow in comparison with cardiac magnetic resonance imaging. Invest Radiol 43:773-781
34. Lessick J, Dragu R, Mutlak D et al (2007) Is functional improvement after myocardial infarction predicted with myocardial enhancement patterns at multidetector CT? Radiolog. 244:736-744
35. Rodriguez-Granillo GA, Rosales MA, Baum S et al (2009) Early assessment of myocardial viability by the use of delayed enhance-

36. Nieman K, Shapiro MD, Ferencik M et al (2008) Reperfused myocardial infarction: contrast-enhanced 64-Section CT in comparison to MR imaging. Radiology 247:49-56
37. Cury RC, Nieman K, Shapiro MD et al (2008) Comprehensive assessment of myocardial perfusion defects, regional wall motion, and left ventricular function by using 64-section multidetector CT. Radiology 248:466-475
38. Gerber BL, Belge B, Legros GJ et al (2006) Characterization of acute and chronic myocardial infarcts by multidetector computed tomography: comparison with contrast-enhanced magnetic resonance. Circulation 113:823-833
39. Flacke SJ, Fischer SE, Lorenz CH (2001) Measurement of the gadopentetate dimeglumine partition coefficient in human myocardium in vivo: normal distribution and elevation in acute and chronic infarction. Radiology 218:703-710
40. Keller MR, Kessler RM, Brooks RA, Kirkland LR (1980) Optimum energy for performing CT iodinated constrast studies. Br J Radiol 53:576-579
41. Mahnken AH, Bruners P, Muhlenbruch G et al (2007) Low tube voltage improves computed tomography imaging of delayed myocardial contrast enhancement in an experimental acute myocardial infarction model. Invest Radiol 42:123-129
42. Cerqueira MD, Weissman NJ, Dilsizian V et al (2002) Standardized myocardial segmentation and nomenclature for tomographic imaging of the heart: a statement for healthcare professionals from the Cardiac Imaging Committee of the Council on Clinical Cardiology of the American Heart Association. Circulation 105:539-542
43. Blankstein R, Rogers I, Cury R (2009) Practical tips and tricks in cardiovascular computed tomography: Diagnosis of myocardial infarction. J Cardiovasc Comput Tomogr 3:104-111
44. Ruzsics B, Schwarz F, Schoepf UJ et al (2009) Comparison of dual-energy computed tomography of the heart with single photon emission computed tomography for assessment of coronary artery stenosis and of the myocardial blood supply. Am J Cardiol 104:318-326
45. Mahnken AH, Klotz E, Pietsch H et al (2010) Quantitative Whole Heart Stress Perfusion CT Imaging as Noninvasive Assessment of Hemodynamics in Coronary Artery Stenosis: Preliminary Animal Experience. Invest Radiol 45:298-305
46. Bamberg F, Klotz E, Flohr T et al (2010) Dynamic myocardial stress perfusion imaging using fast dual-source CT with alternating table positions: initial experience. Eur Radiol 20:1168-1173
47. Ho KT, Chua KC, Klotz E, Panknin C (2010) Stress and rest dynamic myocardial perfusion imaging by evaluation of complete time-attenuation curves with dual-source CT. JACC Cardiovasc Imaging 3:811-820
48. Johnson TR, Krauss B, Sedlmair M et al (2007) Material differentiation by dual energy CT: initial experience. Eur Radiol 17:1510-1517
49. Ko SM, Choi JW, Song MG et al (2011) Myocardial perfusion imaging using adenosine-induced stress dual-energy computed tomography of the heart: comparison with cardiac magnetic resonance imaging and conventional coronary angiography. Eur Radiol 21:26-35
50. Ko BS, Cameron JD, Meredith IT et al (2011) Computed tomography stress myocardial perfusion imaging in patients considered for revascularization: a comparison with fractional flow reserve. Eur Heart J [Epub Ahead of print]
51. Bamberg F, Becker A, Schwarz F et al (2011) Detection of Hemodynamically Significant Coronary Artery Stenosis: Incremental Diagnostic Value of Dynamic CT-based Myocardial Perfusion Imaging Radiology 260:689-698

Evaluation of Cardiac Volumetric and Functional Parameters

16

Giancarlo Messalli, Giuseppe Runza, Ludovico La Grutta, Erica Maffei, Chiara Martini, Massimo Midiri, Jan Bogaert, and Filippo Cademartiri

16.1 Definition of Cardiac Volume and Function

The milestone definition of "Cardiac Function" has to be attributed to William Harvey, the discoverer of the circulation, who in 1628 stated: "The movement of the blood is constantly in a circle, and is brought about by the beat of the heart" [1, 2]. From a modern point of view, the main function of the heart is the delivery of oxygen to metabolizing tissues. Since oxygen delivery is dependent on (1) the oxygen-carrying capacity of blood, (2) the flow output from the heart, and (3) regional distribution of flow, then the heart is nowadays regarded as a pump with the function of supplying flow in blood vessels [2].

It is intuitive why a correct and reproducible assessment of functional parameters of the left and right ventricle is a fundamental step in establishing diagnosis, therapy and prognosis in patients with cardiac and pulmonary disease [3-8].

Different parameters reflect cardiac function but the overall parameter able to roughly indicate global systolic function is undoubtedly the ejection fraction (EF), which is the percentage of diastolic volume ejected by the ventricle during systole.

$$LVEF\ (\%) = [(EDV\text{-}ESV)/EDV] \times 100$$
$$RVEF\ (\%) = [(EDV\text{-}ESV)/EDV] \times 100$$

The importance of cardiac ejection fraction has been shown in numerous studies; in particular, left ventricular EF (LVEF) is commonly used to stratify risk in patients with suspected or known coronary artery disease and to assess functional recovery during medical therapy or after myocardial revascularization [9]. Therefore evaluation of EF is a fundamental step in routine cardiologic practice, and many methods are currently available hav-

ing a variable degree of accuracy and reproducibility [10-20].

Two-dimensional transthoracic echocardiography has been used for decades for EF measurement as a result of its noninvasiveness, low cost, ease of use, bedside availability and lack of ionizing radiation, but the method suffers from some drawbacks and poor intra- and interobserver reproducibility [21].

In the absence of a true noninvasive gold standard, in the last decade cardiac magnetic resonance imaging (MRI) has become the criterion standard in evaluating biventricular cardiac function; MRI has the ability to overcome some echo-related disadvantages, such as inadequate echocardiographic window, foreshortening due to improper alignment to the cardiac long axis and geometrical assumptions that often make EF unreliable, especially in patients with segmental wall motion abnormalities like in coronary artery disease [22].

Thanks to recent technologic advances, multidetector CT (MDCT) has proven its ability to produce optimal images for visualizing the coronary tree while providing global and regional left and right systolic function without geometrical assumptions and without the need to expose patients to a further dose of ionizing radiation and/or iodinated contrast material; furthermore CT images, characterized by high definition of endocardial contours, have allowed for reduction in analysis time and intra- and interobserver variability [19, 23].

Currently Doppler echocardiography remains the criterion standard noninvasive imaging technique to assess diastolic function [24].

16.2 Image Acquisition and Reconstruction

Dataset for cardiac function assessment can be obtained from the same acquisition used for coronary angiography except in the case of prospective gating; in this last case data are acquired just at a single point of cardiac cycle and multiphase temporal windows will not be available for the analysis. A retrospective gating is usu-

G. Messalli (✉)
Department of Radiology, SDN-IRCCS,
Naples, Italy

F. Cademartiri, G. Casolo, M. Midiri (eds.), *Clinical Applications of Cardiac CT*,
© Springer-Verlag Italia 2012

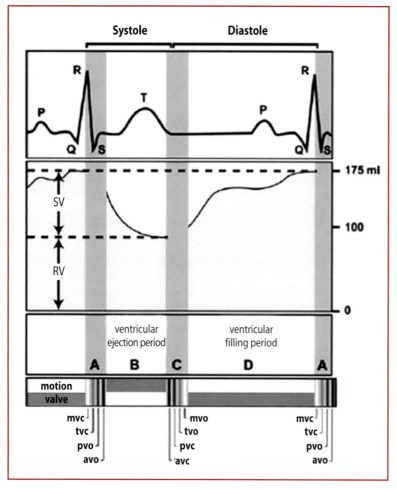

Fig. 16.1 Diagram illustrating the mechanical and electrical phenomena present during the cardiac cycle. The graph depicts left ventricular volume curve, electrocardiogram and valve motion. *A*, isovolumetric contraction phase; *B*, ventricular ejection period; *C*, isovolumetric relaxation phase; *D*, ventricular filling period; *mvc/mvo*, mitral valve closing/opening; *tvc/tvo*, tricuspid valve closing/opening; *pvo/pvc*, pulmonary valve opening/closing; *avo/avc*, aortic valve opening/closing; *SV*, stroke volume; *RV*, residual volume. (Modified from [5], with permission)

ally adopted with some tricks to reduce radiation exposure; nowadays it is possible to deliver maximum tube current just in mid diastole, with an important drop of effective dose and preserving superb definition of myocardial borders during the remaining cardiac phases [25-30]. In our experience an intravenous injection of 100 mL of iodinated contrast medium at a flow-rate of 2 gI/s, followed by 30 mL of saline chaser (same injection rate), starting at 150 HU increment (bolus tracking, ROI in ascending aorta), is able to furnish an adequate enhancement for coronary artery assessment and contemporary evaluation of right and left ventricular function [19]; different protocols are available for this aim, using up to a half dose of contrast medium [31].

After raw data acquisition, specific reconstructions are needed; we usually perform reconstructions each 5% of cardiac cycle, covering the whole left and right ventricles from base to apex using 8 mm MRP thick cardiac short axis reconstructions; this method reduces the time required for CT analysis with semi-automated software, and thus improves time efficiency which will be acceptable for practical use [32]. In our experience the choice of reconstruction kernel can influence time efficiency too; in particular an edge enhancement filter may help the semi-automated software in recognizing myocardial contours reducing the need of manual corrections (unpublished data). There is no evidence that *half scan* or *multisegmental* reconstruction algorithms may have an advantage on each other.

In the past years it was necessary to reconstruct the dataset in a short-axis plane before analysis; nowadays most of vendors have got over this issue by producing dedicated software able to skip this preliminary reconstruction and thus further accelerating volume assessment.

During the cardiac cycle there is a variability of cardiac volumes in the different phases (Fig. 16.1).

In clinical routine it is sufficient to calculate right and left ventricular volumes at maximal filling (end-diastole) and at maximal emptying (end-systole). From end-diastolic volume and end-systolic volume the main global systolic functional parameters can be deduced and then can be indexed for body surface area (BSA).

In theory we would need reconstructions only at 0% and 35% of the R-R interval, although more temporal windows can help in choosing the correct phase by reviewing images in cine-loop. The freezing of correct phases is dependent on the scanner temporal resolution, which can be different among different vendors; nowadays we have scanners able to reach a temporal resolution of 75 ms, still far from the temporal resolution of magnetic resonance, but very good to obtain a contained bias (<5%) for EF and other functional parameters calculation [19].

Optimal temporal resolution should be <50 ms, corresponding to isovolumetric relaxation at any heart rate; in the near future, reaching the above mentioned temporal resolution will provide a precise capture of correct end-systolic phase, and a contemporary freezing of the heart in a relative quiescent period for coronary artery assessment leading to a consequent further drastic drop in dose.

16.3   Image Analysis

Dedicated workstations are usually adopted for cardiac analysis and in particular for volume assessment. The first step is the correct choice of ED and ES phases. Semi-automated software can reliably identify the end-diastolic phase (acquired just at the R peak), corresponding to the ventricular maximum filling, but they often fail in identifying the end-systolic phase which should be visually assessed as the images displaying the smallest left and right ventricular cavity [33]. After correct identification of the end-diastolic and end-systolic phase, endocardial and epicardial borders are traced on the end-diastolic images with endocardial borders subsequently propagated to end-systole thanks to the aid of semi-automated software. Manual corrections are made where and when necessary. Though there are no absolute recommendations, it may be advisable to include the papillary muscles and trabeculations in the myocardium in patients with hypertensive diseases, hypertrophic cardiomyopathy, or myocardial storage diseases and to include the papillary muscles and trabeculations in the left ventricular cavity in the remaining cases. Regardless of the choice adopted, the same approach should be used for follow-up [34, 35]. The most apical LV and RV sections with a visible cavity are considered to be the apex, whereas the most basal section of LV surrounded by at least 50% of myocardium is considered to be the base [14]. The most basal section of right ventricle and of left ventricle are usually difficult to assess in a short axis plane, with most vendors implementing software able to allow contemporary views of long axes (Fig. 16.2).

Thanks to long axis views it is easier to trace the contour near tricuspid and mitral valve, and of the apex; further help can be provided by reviewing images in cine-loop.

After contour tracing, the software will finally compute the EDV, the ESV and all the other systolic functional parameters according to Simpson's rule [36]. The measurement of volume with Simpson's rule is based on the division of the object in sections of known thickness. The volume of the object is therefore equal to the sum of the volumes of the various sections and only the surface area (SA) and the thickness (T) of each section are required to determine the volume according to the formula:

$$LV\ Vol = \Sigma SA \times T$$
$$RV\ Vol = \Sigma SA \times T$$

Since it does not rely on any geometric assumptions, Simpson's method proves to be more accurate than other methods in determining global ventricular function [36]. In Figure 16.3 the LV is represented by a rotation ellipsoid and is divided into sections or circular discs. The sum of the volumes of the discs provides the measurement of LV volume.

Even though the shape of the LV is distorted, as in the case of an aneurysmal dilatation (Fig. 16.4), with Simpson's rule LV volume can still be calculated by summing the volume of the individual sections to obtain the measurement of the entire chamber.

The need to use volumetric methods such as Simpson's is even more important in the right ventricle because of its complex geometry; for this reason, the value of echocardiography and other imaging techniques which use geometric assumptions to estimate RV function and ejection fraction is limited [37]. To obtain a valid measurement of right ventricle volume, Simpson's method has to be associated with multiplanar evaluation because no single imaging plane is well suited for correct contour tracing.

A normal EF is considered >55% for both left and right ventricle, with an EF<50% being correlated with a worse prognosis [38].

As stated previously, from ED and ES Volumes, other parameters can be deduced.

SV is calculated as the difference between EDV and ESV:

$$SV\ (mL) = EDV - ESV$$

EF is calculated by dividing the SV for EDV x 100:

$$EF\ (\%) = SV/EDV\ x\ 100$$

Cardiac output (CO) represents the volume of blood pumped out of the heart in one minute and is calculated by multiplying the SV by the heart rate (HR):

$$CO\ (mL/min) = SV\ x\ HR$$

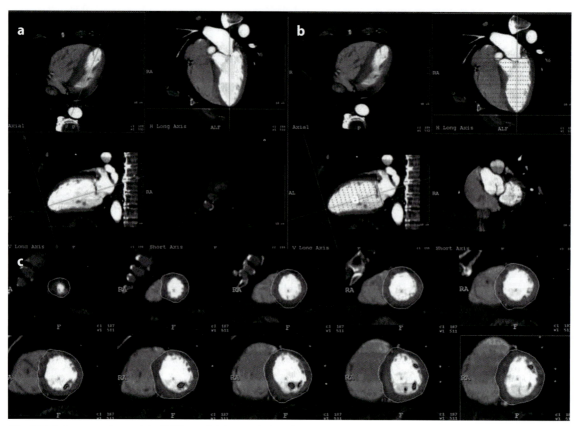

Fig. 16.2 Software package of the Brilliance 3.0.2 extended workstation dedicated to the analysis of left ventricular volume and function. After multiplanar reconstructions are done of the multiphase datasets (every 5-10% of the entire cardiac cycle) in the sagittal, coronal and axial planes, the elevated attenuation difference between the left ventricular myocardium and the contrast agent in the ventricle facilitates both the segmentation based on the differences in peak enhancement of the different structures and the consequent calculation of left ventricular volumes and global function. **a** Heart visualized in axial, sagittal and coronal planes. In the images in the axial and sagittal planes, the two orthogonal axes (*green lines*) can be rotated to obtain an axis parallel to the septum in the coronal plane, with apex-valvular plane direction. **b** Previous images after processing of the 14 contiguous slices (*dotted red lines*) perpendicular to the long axis of the left ventricle (*green line*).The *purple line* represents the valvular plane and the *green line* the apex of the heart. **c** The 14 contiguous slices in the short-axis from the valvular plane to the apex of the heart. The *yellow line* and the *purple line* represent the subepicardial borders and the subendocardial borders, respectively, which are automatically recognized by the software and can be remodeled manually and semiautomatically by the operator

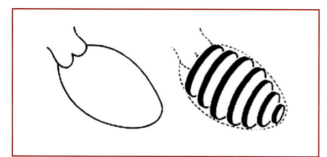

Fig. 16.3 Diagram illustrating Simpson' rule, according to which the left ventricle is represented by a series of circular sections

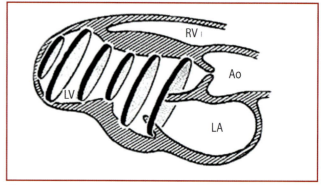

Fig. 16.4 Diagram illustrating Simpson's rule (*circular sections*) in the case of left ventricular aneurysm. *LV*, left ventricle; *Ao*, aorta; *LA*, left atrium; *RV*, right ventricle

Attention should be paid in furnishing SV and CO values, because in the presence of valve insufficiency these parameters are not reliable.

For calculation of ventricular mass, using the volumetric approach, on the same end diastolic stack of images the epicardial and endocardial contours are delineated as suggested previously (35). Taking into account

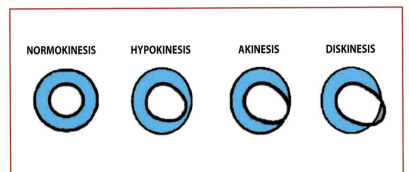

Fig. 16.5 Degrees of ventricular dysfunction for the qualitative evaluation of left ventricular regional wall function: regular regional wall motion is classified as normokinesis. Left ventricular wall motion disturbances are classified as hypokinesis (reduced regional systolic wall thickening); akinesis (absent regional systolic wall thickening); dyskinesis (outward movement of the LV wall segment during systolic contraction). (Modified from [5], with permission)

slice thickness and inter-slice distance, the volume included between epi- and endo-contour is multiplied for the specific density of myocardium (1.05 g/cm^3), obtaining the ED LV mass.

For regional function assessment, a visual analysis of multiphase dataset is usually performed. Dedicated workstations are able to visualize images in cine-loop, in the same manner as MRI, and allow for the assessment of left and right wall thickening and wall motion.

16.4 Clinical Value of Cardiac Function Measured with CT

Several studies using this approach have confirmed that 64 slice CT agrees well with MRI for LV and RV function assessment, and is more accurate than echocardiography and SPECT in EF estimation [31].

Nowadays 64-slice CT is considered a clinically acceptable and as robust in the evaluation of LV and RV function as MRI. It is very unlikely that CT can be used as a first-line investigation owing to exposure to ionizing radiation and intravenous iodinated contrast material. However, if the same raw data provided by CT coronary angiography is used to reconstruct a multiphase dataset, LV and RV function can be assessed without exposing the patient to any further dose of radiation or contrast material, and the anatomic study can be integrated with a functional study that has the same accuracy as MRI [19]. Cardiac CT can be used to assess LV function following myocardial infarction in patients with suboptimal echocardiography, in those with a pacemaker (an important factor in patients with heart disease) and/or other ferromagnetic materials, as well as in claustrophobic patients because cardiac CT is not limited by the same contraindications as MRI; thanks to these potentialities, CT reached a "7" and is finally considered appropriate for LV function assessment in patients with a poor echocardiographic window and for RV function in patients suspected for dysplasia [39].

Recent papers showed CT has a good accuracy also on regional systolic function assessment [31]. Even though a quantitative approach is preferable, for daily clinical use a visual analysis is often used to regionally score systolic wall thickening; Figure 16.5 shows different degrees of ventricular dysfunction.

A region of the LV or RV with reduced motility is defined hypokinetic. If motility is absent, the region is defined akinetic (Fig. 16.6), and outward movement during systolic contraction is defined dyskinetic (Fig. 16.7).

The MDCT evaluation of regional LV wall motion is performed with the standardized American Heart Association 17-segment model which is based on the division of the LV in three portions in the short axis: basal with 6 segments; mid-cavity with 6 segments; apical with 4 segments; the apex is considered segment 17 [40] (Fig. 16.8).

Preserved wall thickness is a good indicator of the presence of viable myocardium in the setting of a chronic infarction with a wall thickness <5mm suggestive of non viable tissue [41].

Before the cardiac performance in a patient can be defined as abnormal, the normal values for ventricular volumes, function, and mass, as well as their physiologic ranges, need to be known. Nowadays there are few papers dealing with this issue and in most cases normal values in cardiac MRI are used as reference just because CT was shown to provide a high correlation with measurements from MRI. It is nonetheless important to highlight that small differences between CT and MRI regarding measurements of EDV and ESV have been repetitively reported, which reinforces the need for modality-specific reference values [42]. Knowledge of normal distribution of left and right heart measurements and differences that exist between genders should assist the correct interpretation of disease states with cardiac CT [42].

In patients with coronary artery disease, myocardial function at rest is often within normal limits. However, during periods of increased oxygen consumption, the oxygen supply through a stenotic coronary artery might

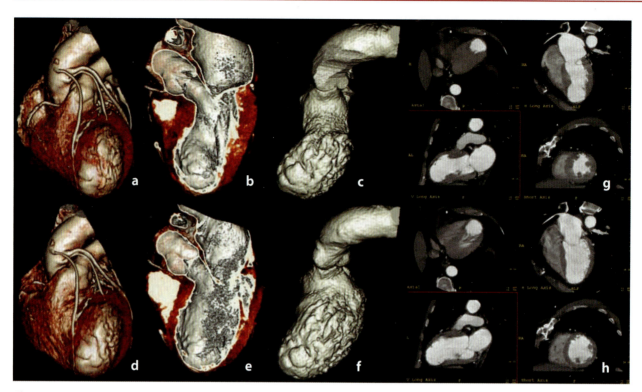

Fig. 16.6 Patient with three-vessel disease having undergone coronary artery bypass grafting surgery, with grafts to the left anterior descending coronary artery, the diagonal branch, the obtuse marginal branch and the right coronary artery. Different volume rendering techniques of the left ventricle in the end-systolic phase (**a-c**) and end-diastolic phase (**d-f**). The images depict thinning and systolic akinesis with significant post-infarction scarring in the anterolateral, inferoseptal and apical segments of the left ventricle, which can be identified as strips of subendocardial hypodensity due to perfusion deficit. The multiplanar reconstructions in the short-axis, long-axis and 4-chamber view in the end-systolic phase (**g**) and end-diastolic phase (**h**) depict a dilatation of the anterior half of the left ventricle in end-diastole

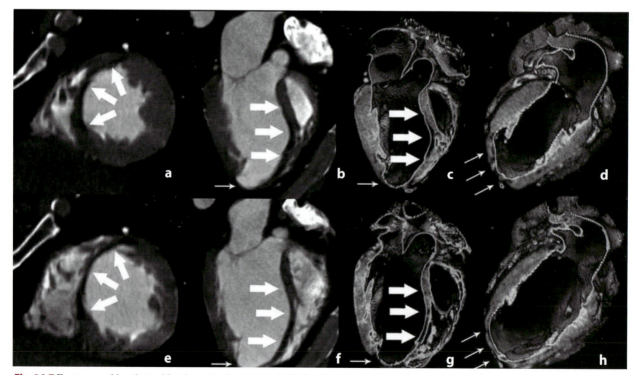

Fig. 16.7 Forty-year old patient with prior extensive myocardial infarction: short-axis and long-axis multiplanar reconstructions and volume rendering images in MDCT of the mid portion of the left ventricle in end-systolic phase (**a-d**) and end-diastolic phase (**e-h**), respectively, which demonstrate a postinfarction aneurysmal dilatation of the apex of the hear (*thin arrows*), subendocardial hypodensity and thinning of the walls and absent wall thickening of the left ventricular myocardium (*thick arrows*)

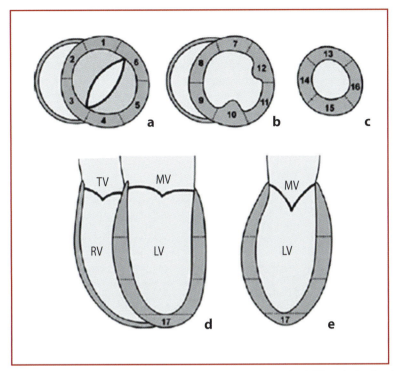

Fig. 16.8 A 17-segment model used for segment-based MR and MDCT analysis of regional left ventricular function: **a-c** short-axis planes (basal, mid-cavity and apical, respectively); **d** horizontal long-axis plane (4-chamber view); **e** long-axis vertical plane (2-chamber view). Left ventricular segments (*S*): anterior: S1, S7 and S13; anteroseptal: S2 and S8; inferoseptal: S3 and S9; inferior: S4, S10 and S15; inferolateral: S5 and S11; anterolateral: S6 and S12; septal: S14; lateral: S16; apical: S17. *RV*, right ventricle; *TV*, tricuspid valve; *LV*, left ventricle; *MV*, mitral valve. (Modified from [5], with permission)

be insufficient to cover the increased needs, leading to regional or more global myocardial ischemia. Nowadays CT can provide some clues in conditions of stress too, as demonstrated by recent publications showing cardiac CT is able to investigate perfusion defects in the same way as SPECT, with limited radiation dose [43-45].

16.5 Conclusions

Cardiac CT is able to obtain information regarding the state of the coronary tree and to correlate this information with the presence of pathologic wall thinning, loss of ventricular wall motion at rest and during stress and a possible reduction in EF, thus providing fundamental information on function and completing the diagnostic and prognostic cardiovascular evaluation of our patient. Cardiac CT is a powerful tool which can have an impact on health spending by avoiding exam duplication.

As the modality provides valuable information which is not limited to the coronary tree, and because of these capabilities and potentialities we think that it is better to speak of cardiac CT and not coronary CT and that functional cardiac information should always be furnished in our report.

References

1. Franklin KJ, editor (1933) A Short History of Physiology. London: Bale
2. Cohen-Solal A, Beauvais F, and Tan LB (2009) European Heart Journal 30:2962-2964
3. Moise A, Bourassa MG, Theroux P et al (1985) Prognostic significance of progression of coronary artery disease. Am J Cardiol 55:941-946
4. Emond M, Mock MB, Davis KB et al (1994) Long-term survival of medically treated patients in the Coronary Artery Surgery Study (CASS) registry. Circulation 90:2645-2657
5. Juergens KU, Fischbach R (2006) Left ventricular function studied with MDCT. Eur Radiol 16:342-357
6. de Feyter PJ, van Eenige MJ, Dighton DH et al (1982) Prognostic value of exercise testing, coronary angiography and left ventriculography 6-8 weeks after myocardial infarction. Circulation 66:527-536
7. Taylor GJ, Humphries JO, Mellits ED et al (1980) Predictors of clinical course, coronary anatomy and left ventricular function after recovery from acute myocardial infarction. Circulation 62:960-970
8. White HD, Norris RM, Brown MA et al (1987) Left ventricular end-systolic volume as the major determinant of survival after recovery from myocardial infarction. Circulation 76:44-51
9. Shaw LJ, Peterson ED, Kesler K et al (1996) A meta-analysis of predischarge risk stratification after acute myocardial infarction with stress electrocardiographic, myocardial perfusion, and ventricular function imaging. Am J Cardio 178:1327-1337
10. Bansal D, Singh RM, Sarkar M et al (2008) Assessment of left ventricular function: comparison of cardiac multidetector-row comput-

10. ed tomography with two-dimension standard echocardiography for assessment of left ventricular function. Int J Cardiovasc Imaging 24:317-325
11. Pouleur AC, le Polain de Waroux PB, Pasquet A et al (2008) Assessment of left ventricular mass and volumes by three- dimensional echocardiography in patients with or without wall motion abnormalities: comparison against cine magnetic resonance imaging. Heart 94:1050-1057
12. Heuschmid M, Rothfuss JK, Schroeder S et al (2006) Assessment of left ventricular myocardial function using 16-slice multidetector-row computed tomography: comparison with magnetic resonance imaging and echocardiography. Eur Radiol 16:551-559
13. Nicol ED, Stirrup J, Reyes E et al (2008) Comparison of 64-slice cardiac computed tomography with myocardial perfusion scintigraphy for assessment of global and regional myocardial function and infarction in patients with low to intermediate likelihood of coronary artery disease. J Nucl Cardiol 15:497-502
14. Wua YW, Tadamuraa E, Yamamuroa M et al (2008) Estimation of global and regional cardiac function using 64-slice computed tomography: a comparison study with echocardiography, gated-SPECT and cardiovascular magnetic resonance. Int J Cardiol 128:69-76
15. Stegger L, Heijman E, Schäfers KP et al (2009) Quantification of left ventricular volumes and ejection fraction in mice using PET, compared with MRI. J Nucl Med 50:132-138
16. Sugeng L, Mor-Avi V, Weinert L et al (2006) Quantitative assessment of left ventricular size and function side-byside comparison of real-time threedimensional echocardiography and computed tomography with magnetic resonance reference. Circulation 114:654-661
17. Puesken M, Fischbach R, Wenker M et al (2008) Global left-ventricular function assessment using dual-source multidetector CT: effect of improved temporal resolution on ventricular volume measurement. Eur Radiol 18:2087-2094
18. Salm LP, Schuijf JD, de Roos A et al(2006) Global and regional left ventricular function assessment with 16-detector row CT: comparison with echocardiography and cardiovascular magnetic resonance. Eur J Echocardiogr 7:308-314
19. Palumbo A, Maffei E, Martini C et al (2009) Functional parameters of left ventricle: comparison between cardiac MR and cardiac CT in a large population. Radiol Med 115:702-13
20. Jenkins C, Moir S, Chan J et al (2009) Left ventricular volume measurement with echocardiography: a comparison of left ventricular opacification, threedimensional echocardiography, or both with magnetic resonance imaging. Eur Heart J 30:98-106
21. Chuang ML, Hibberd MG, Salton CJ et al (2000) Importance of imaging method over imaging modality in noninvasive determination of left ventricular volumes and ejection fraction: assessment by two- and threedimensional echocardiography and magnetic resonance imaging. J Am Coll Cardiol 35:477-484
22. Maffei E, Messalli G, Palumbo A, Martini C, Seitun S, Aldrovandi A, Cuttone A, Emiliano E, Malagò R, Weustink A, Mollet N, Cademartiri F (2010) Left ventricular ejection fraction: real-world comparison between cardiac computed tomography and echocardiography in a large population. Radiol Med 115:1015-1027
23. Palazzuoli A, Cademartiri F, Geleijnse ML et al (2008) Left ventricular remodelling and systolic function measurement with 64 multi-slice computed tomography versus second harmonic echocardiography in patients with coronary artery disease: A double blind study. Eur J Radiol 73:82-88
24. Mandinov L, Eberli FR, Seiler C, Hess OM (2000) Diastolic heart failure. Cardiovasc Res 45:813-825
25. Hausleiter J, Meyer T, Hadamitzky M et al (2006) Radiation dose estimates from cardiac multislice computed tomography in daily practice: impact of different scanning protocols on effective dose estimates. Circulation 113:1305-1310

26. Alkadhi H, Stolzmann P, Scheffel H et al (2008) Radiation dose of cardiac dual-source CT: the effect of tailoring the protocol to patient-specific parameters. Eur J Radiol 68:385-391
27. Achenbach S, Anders K, Kalender WA (2008) Dual-source cardiac computed tomography: image quality and dose considerations. Eur Radiol 18:1188-1198
28. Jakobs TF, Becker CR, Ohnesorge B et al (2002) Multislice helical CT of the heart with retrospective ECG gating: reduction of radiation exposure by ECG-controlled tube current modulation. Eur Radiol 12:1081-1086
29. Stolzmann P, Scheffel H, Schertler T et al (2008) Radiation dose estimates in dual-source computed tomography coronary angiography. Eur Radiol 18:592-599
30. Pflederer T, Jakstat J, Marwan M et al (2010) Radiation exposure and image quality in staged low-dose protocols for coronary dual source CT angiography: a randomized comparison. Eur Radiol 20:1197-1206
31. Wu YW, Tadamura E, Yamamuro M, et al (2008) Estimation of global and regional cardiac function using 64-slice computed tomography: A comparison study with echocardiography, gated-SPECT and cardiovascular magnetic resonance. International Journal of Cardiology 128: 69-76
32. Suzuki S, Furui S, Kaminaga T, et al (2006) Accuracy and Efficiency of Left Ventricular Ejection Fraction Analysis, Using Multidetector Row Computed Tomography Effect of Image Reconstruction Window Within Cardiac Phase, Slice Thickness, and Interval of Short-Axis Sections. Circ J 70: 289 -296
33. Belge B, Coche E, Pasquet A et al (2006) Accurate estimation of global and regional cardiac function by retrospectively gated multidetector row computed tomography. Comparison with cine magnetic resonance imaging. Eur Radiol 16:1424-1433
34. Miller S, Simonetti OP, Carr J et al (2002) MR imaging of the heart with cine true fast imaging with steady-state precession: influence of spatial and temporal resolutions on left ventricular functional parameters. Radiology 223:263-269
35. Sievers B, Kirchberg S, Bakan A et al (2004) Impact of papillary muscles in ventricular volume and ejection fraction assessment by cardiovascular magnetic resonance. J Cardiovasc Magn Reson 6:9-16
36. Dulce MC, Mostbeck GH, Friese KK, Caputo GR, Higgins CB (1993) Quantification of the left ventricular volumes and function with cine MR imaging: comparison of geometric models with three-dimensional data. Radiology 188:371-376
37. Markiewicz W, Sechtem U, Higgins CB (1987) Evaluation of the right ventricle by magnetic resonance imaging. Am Heart J 113:8-15
38. Hamad MA, van Straten AHM, Schönberger JPAM et al (2010) Preoperative ejection fraction as a predictor of survival after coronary artery bypass grafting: comparison with a matched general population. Journal of Cardiothoracic Surgery 23:5-29
39. Taylor AJ, Cerqueira M, Hodgson JM (2010) ACCF/SCCT/ACR/ AHA/ASE/ASNC/NASCI/ SCAI/SCMR appropriate use criteria for cardiac computed tomography: a report of the American College of Cardiology Foundation Appropriate Use Criteria Task Force, the Society of Cardiovascular Computed Tomography, the American College of Radiology, the American Heart Association, the American Society of Echocardiography, the American Society of Nuclear Cardiology, the North American Society for Cardiovascular Imaging, the Society for Cardiovascular Angiography and Interventions, and the Society for Cardiovascular Magnetic Resonance. J Am Coll Cardiol 56:1864-1894
40. Cerqueira MD, Weissman NJ, Dilsizian V et al (2002) Standardized myocardial segmentation and nomenclature for tomographic imaging of the heart: a statement for healthcare professionals from the Cardiac Imaging Committee of the Council on Clinical Cardiology of the American Heart Association. Circulation 105:539-542

41. Baer FM, Theissen P, Schneider CA, et al (1994) Magnetic resonance imaging techniques for the assessment of residual myocardial viability. Herz 19:51-64
42. Stolzmann P, Scheffel H, Leschka S (2008) Reference values for quantitative left ventricular and left atrial measurements in cardiac computed tomography. Eur Radiol 18:1625-1634
43. Blankstein R, Shturman LD, Rogers IS, et al (2009) Adenosine-induced stress myocardial perfusion imaging using dual-source cardiac computed tomography J Am Coll Cardiol 54:1072-1084
44. Rocha-Filho JA, Blankstein R, Shturman LD, et al (2010) Incremental value of adenosine-induced stress myocardial perfusion imaging with dual-source CT at cardiac CT angiography Radiology 254:410-419
45. Ko SM, Choi JW, Song MG, et al 2011 Myocardial perfusion imaging using adenosine-induced stress dual-energy computed tomography of the heart: comparison with cardiac magnetic resonance imaging and conventional coronary angiography. Eur Radiol 21:26-35

Cardiac Veins and Pulmonary Veins

17

Maurizio Centonze, Giulia Casagranda, Maurizio Del Greco,
Andrea Laudon, Alessandro Cristoforetti, and Giandomenico Nollo

17.1 Introduction

In the field of noncoronary applications of cardiac CT the study of the cardiac and pulmonary veins is of great use for the cardiologist, the former particularly in patients with heart failure who require electrical resynchronization of the cardiac chambers (cardiac resynchronization therapy or biventricular pacing) and the latter in patients scheduled to undergo a catheter ablation procedure. Noninvasive cardiac imaging has the task of compiling an anatomic roadmap to render the interventional procedures more effective and efficient. Unlike the study of the coronary arteries, the aim is not to detect disease, but rather to accurately outline the regional anatomy, an objective which can be achieved thanks to the elevated spatial and temporal resolution of multidetector computed tomography (MDCT).

17.2 Cardiac Veins

17.2.1 Rationale Behind the Study of the Cardiac Veins with MDCT

The considerable interest in the cardiac venous system is justified by the increasing number of interventional procedures using these vessels (electrophysiologic studies with catheter implantation in the coronary sinus; ablation procedures of the accessory electrical circuits; coronary retroperfusion in high-risk or complicated angioplasty). Precise knowledge of the cardiac veins (CV) is crucial in biventricular pacing interventions for patients suffering from heart failure [1-4]. The failure rate of pacing-lead implantation is relatively high (from 5% to 12%) [4], with the main cause being the inability

to cannulate the coronary sinus and the lack of an appropriate vessel for implantation [4, 5]. Knowledge of the vascular anatomy, which is characterized by a high degree of individual variability, is therefore highly advantageous for the physician, who may orient the patient with unsuitable vascular anatomy towards mini-invasive surgery [5, 6]. Retrograde venography, which is performed as a rule in the setting of interventional procedures, is the criterion standard for the study of the CV and can provide good information on the number, location, diameter and angulation of the vessels [7]. However, the largest study on the topic to appear in the literature reports that conventional angiography is diagnostic only in 67% of patients due to inability to cannulate the coronary sinus or poor balloon occlusion causing backwash of the retrograde-injected contrast agent for the enhancement of the CV [8].

MDCT in contrast provides an optimal visualization of the entire cardiac venous system and thanks to volume rendering (VR) and multiplanar (MPR/MIP) images enables the indispensable measurements which render biventricular more effective and efficient [9-12]. In addition to being less invasive and subject to fewer complications than conventional angiography, MDCT can exclude patients with unsuitable anatomy from pacemaker implantation and reduce the duration of interventional procedures, thus increasing the possibility of selective cannulation of the target vessel – usually the left marginal vein – which is distributed in the area of greatest desynchronization of the left ventricle.

17.2.2 Anatomic Background

As mentioned above, the CV anatomy is highly variable [13-22]. Most of the CV flow into the coronary sinus, a wide venous channel varying in length but generally 2-3 cm, situated in the posterior portion of the right atrioventricular or coronary groove (Figs. 17.1, 17.2b). The coronary sinus empties into the right atrium, between the orifice of the inferior vena cava and the tricuspid valve. The opening of the coronary sinus may be guard-

M. Centonze (✉)
Radiology Unit,
"San Lorenzo" Hospital,
APSS Trento,
Trento, Italy

F. Cademartiri, G. Casolo, M. Midiri (eds.), *Clinical Applications of Cardiac CT*,
© Springer-Verlag Italia 2012

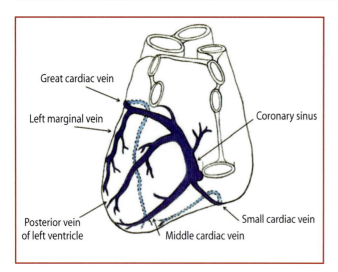

Fig. 17.1 Posterior view of the normal anatomy of the main cardiac veins

ed by a thin semilunar flap (Thebesian valve). The main tributaries of the coronary sinus are:

- *Great cardiac vein*: originates anteriorly at the apex of the heart and ascends in the interventricular groove parallel to the left anterior descending coronary artery. At the level of the origin of the latter the vein changes direction and follows the left atrioventricular groove alongside the left circumflex artery, and after having run across the diaphragmatic surface of the heart reaches the origin of the coronary sinus. During this long course it receives several branches draining the left atrium and both ventricles including the *left marginal vein* (Figs. 17.1, 17.2a, b).

- *Small cardiac vein*: runs in the coronary groove between the right cardiac chambers and empties into the terminal tract of the coronary sinus (Fig. 17.1).
- *Middle cardiac vein*: originates posterior to the apex of the heart and ascends in the interventricular groove parallel to the posterior descending artery, emptying into the terminal tract of the coronary sinus (Figs. 17.1, 17.2b).
- *Posterior vein of the left ventricle*: runs on the diaphragmatic surface of the left ventricle close to the middle cardiac vein. It normally empties into the coronary sinus, but an opening into the great cardiac vein is not uncommon (Figs. 17.1, 17.2b).
- *Minor veins*: these are a series of small-diameter vessels which include the oblique vein of the left atrium which empties into the coronary sinus and the anterior cardiac veins, generally 3-4, which drain the anterior wall of the right ventricle and empty directly into the right atrium.

17.2.3 Study Technique and Image Analysis

The international literature is rather limited regarding MDCT studies of the CV [9-12, 21, 23]. As a result, no study protocol has to date been universally accepted and validated, partly because most of the studies of the CV refer to patient populations in whom the main purpose of the MDCT study was the evaluation of the coronary arteries. In these studies attempts are made to avoid the enhancement of the CV with the optimal timing of contrast agent administration.

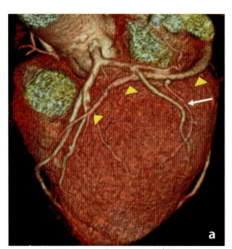
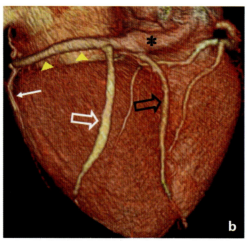

Fig. 17.2 Volume rendering image. The anterior view (**a**) clearly depicts the great cardiac vein (*yellow arrowheads*) which runs parallel to the left anterior descending coronary artery and then follows the left circumflex coronary artery; a thin left marginal vein at the level of the obtuse margin of the left ventricle (*white arrow*) can be appreciated. The posterior view (**b**) depicts the left posterior vein (*hollow white arrow*) ascending on the diaphragmatic surface of the left ventricle to empty into the great cardiac vein (*yellow arrowheads*) at the level where the latter drains into the coronary sinus (*black asterisk*). The middle cardiac vein (*hollow black arrow*) runs in the interventricular groove to join the preterminal tract of the coronary sinus

Table 17.1 Study protocol of cardiac veins with 64-MDCT

Parameter	Levels
Tube voltage	120-140 kV
Tube current	250-500 mAs
FOV	180-250 mm
Nominal slice thickness	64 x 0.5 or 1.5 mm
Effective slice thickness	1 or 2 mm
Reconstruction increment	0,5 or 1 mm
Rotation time	0.33-0.42 s
Pitch	Automatically adapted to patient's heart rate
Reconstruction filter	Smooth
Contrast agent	80-100 ml at 4-5 mL/s (preferred iodine concentration 370-400 mgI/mL)
Trigger	Automatic bolus tracking with ROI in descending aorta and additional delay of 10 s
Gating	Retrospective with reconstruction of 6 time windows of the ECG R-R interval (40, 50, 60, 70, 75 and 80%)

Regardless of the scanner available (4, 16, 64 detector rows), a collimation between 0.5 and 1.5 mm is sufficient for maintaining the radiation dose within acceptable levels thanks to the possibility of reducing the tube current (250 mA) without loss in image quality. In personal experience, the technical parameters reported in Table 17.1 for a 64-MDCT study are used.

Window level is set to include a volume extending from the tracheal bifurcation to the base of the heart. Depending on the patient's build and heart rate, the single breath-hold scan performed in the craniocaudal direction lasts between 6-10 s.

Contrast agent is administered with an 18-20 G needle through an antecubital access in the arm. Adequate enhancement is obtained with the injection of 80-100 mL of contrast agent, preferably with high iodine concentration (370-400 mgI/mL) at an injection rate of 4-5 mL/s. Once a region of interest (ROI) has been set in the lumen of the descending aorta, a series of dynamic scans are performed (one every 2 s) with low tube current (20-40 mAs) in the same position during which the bolus of contrast agent is injected. When the density within the ROI reaches a predefined threshold – preferably +100 HU – and after an additional 10 s delay the patient tray automatically shifts to the preset position for the beginning of the volumetric scan. This technique, known as bolus tracking, has the advantage of guaranteeing maximum enhancement of the target anatomy being studied, in this case the CV.

Retrospective gating involves the reduction of motion artifacts caused by the beating heart which otherwise would cause a loss in image quality enough to impede the recognition of the CV. Furthermore, since the diameter of the veins varies in the various phases of the cardiac cycle, being greatest in early diastole (Fig. 17.3), the earlier time windows of the R-R interval (from 40% to 60%) should be reconstructed, thus enabling the correct identification of the origin, course and size of the tributaries of the coronary sinus. However, the early diastolic windows are most affected by motion artifacts able to impede the recognition of the vessels, especially the smaller veins such as the left marginal. Therefore, the end-diastolic windows (from 70% to 80%) should also be reconstructed. One study suggests that optimal evaluation of the CV is achieved in the early diastolic phase in 61% of cases and in the end-diastolic phase in 39% of cases [9]. The image analysis phase is performed at the workstation with a software dedicated to cardiac applications. The native axial images are not particularly useful in the evaluation of the CV except for indicating the quality of the examination and identifying the presence of a Thebesian valve, which appears as a thin hypodense strip at the ostium of the coronary sinus, immediately posteroanteriorly and anchored to the dorsal wall of the vessel. In contrast, VR and MPR/MIP reconstructions are much more informative [9-12, 15-22]. The epicardial view provided by the former offers immediate information regarding the patient's venous anatomy (Figs. 17.3 and 17.4a, b), being able to establish the number, exact position, diameter, angulation and tortuosity of the CV and providing a reasonably intuitive evaluation of the pacing feasibility. The MPR/MIP reconstructions, especially the centerline views, enable a more accurate measurement of the distance between the coronary sinus ostium and the confluence of tributaries, as well as their angulation and diameter (Fig. 17.4c). This information is indispensable for the physician to improve the effectiveness and efficiency of the interventional procedure (Fig. 17.4d, e). Attention should especially be focused on the evaluation of the veins running on the posterolateral surface of the left ventricle – the portion of the cardiac chamber with the latest activation and therefore the most desynchronized – where the implantation of the pacing lead is capable of guaranteeing an improvement in ventricular function. A

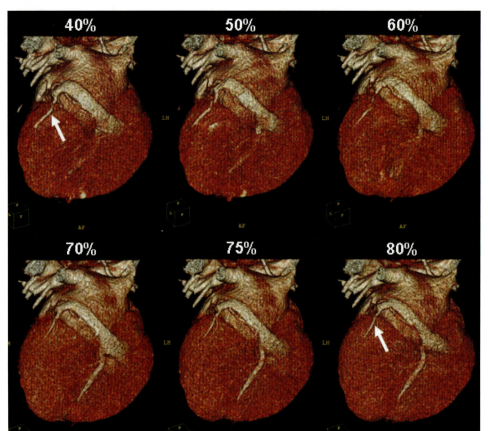

Fig. 17.3 Volume rendering images of 6 different time windows within the R-R interval which demonstrate the variations in diameter of the cardiac veins during the cardiac cycle. Worth noting is the left marginal vein (*white arrow*) which is of greater diameter in the early and mid-diastolic windows (40%, 50% and 60%) where however there are evident motion artifacts due to rapid ventricular filling. In the end-diastolic windows (70%, 75% and 80%) no motion artifacts are visible and therefore the vein is better recognizable but of smaller diameter

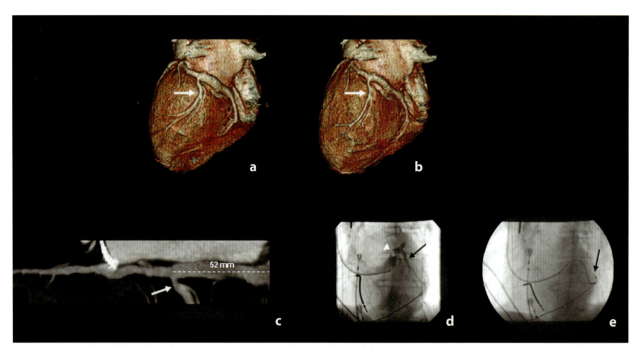

Fig. 17.4 The volume rendering images at 40% (**a**) and 75% (**b**) of the R-R interval depict a left marginal vein (*white arrow*) of moderate diameter. Since the early diastolic phase is better than the end-diastolic phase for the precise definition of the vascular anatomy, this time window is used for the centerline MPR/MIP reconstruction (**c**) which is used to calculate the distance of the vessel opening from the coronary sinus ostium (*dotted line*) and the confluence angle. In the angiographic study, after the identification of the target vessel (*black arrow* in **d**) the pacing lead is positioned (**e**). Despite the presence of balloon occlusion in the coronary sinus (**d**, *white arrowhead*) there is considerable backwash of the retrograde-injected contrast material

highly accurate evaluation of the target-vessel morphology should therefore be made, as this can influence both the choice of pacing lead to implant and the duration of the procedure. In a study by Jongbloed et al. [10], whereas the coronary sinus and the great and middle cardiac arteries were visualized in all 38 patients making up the study population, the posterior and marginal veins were visualized in 95% and 61% of cases, respectively. In another study conducted on 70 patients [9], the coronary sinus was recognized in 91% of patients, all of whom however had at least one vein corresponding to the posterior and marginal veins: 36% of patients had two veins and 45% of patients had more than two vessels. These findings are confirmed by another study [11] in which all the 54 patients examined had either a posterior or marginal vein, with the latter appearing more dominant in 55.6% of cases. A study comparing venography and MDCT found the noninvasive technique more accurate in identifying the CV, especially in the identification of the great cardiac vein – often poorly enhanced during the angiographic study – and the smaller vessels [12]. In a recent Italian study [20] on 84 patients, the lateral cardiac vein was visualized in 67% of cases and the overall vein visualization along the posterolateral wall of the left ventricle was one branch in 52%, two branches in 25% and three or more branches in 22% of cases. The left marginal vein is less frequently identified in patients with a history of myocardial infarction as compared with coronary artery disease patients and control patients (27% vs. 61% and 71%, respectively): this may hamper left ventricular lead positioning in cases of cardiac resynchronization therapy [15]. Furthermore, thanks to MPR/MIP reconstructions MDCT provided much more precise and repeatable measurements of the diameter of the veins than venography [9, 18, 22]. Moreover, thanks to its improved spatial resolution, 64-slice MDCT enables adequate detection of the left and right pericardiophrenic neurovascular bundles in relation to cardiac anatomy. In the setting of electrophysiologic interventions, MDCT before a procedure may elucidate anatomic relationships and help minimize inadvertent complications [19, 24].

Cardiac venous imaging with whole-heart magnetic resonance (MR) angiography has recently been described using developmental pulse sequences with or without intravascular contrast agents [25-29]. Both gradient echo (GRE) and steady-state free precession (SSFP) are viable sequences, although GRE provides more robust results with better contrast. Imaging during the early diastolic period is preferable as it coincides with the maximum size of the CV.

The combination of cardiac venous imaging, assessment of ventricular function and late gadolinium enhancement may be useful in the management of patients with left ventricular dysfunction being considered for cardiac resynchronization therapy.

The last frontier is represented by the use of segmentation tools, advanced image registration software, and high-fidelity images from MDCT and MR of the coronary sinus (CS), which are able to guide cardiac resynchronization therapy and improve implantation success.

17.3 Pulmonary Veins

17.3.1 Rationale Behind the Study of the Pulmonary Veins with MDCT

One of the most internationally validated *noncoronary* applications of cardiac CT is the evaluation of the pulmonary veins (PV) and the left atrium (LA) [30-37]. The electrical isolation of the PV from the LA with catheter ablation is in most cases an effective procedure for resolving atrial fibrillation (AF) failing to respond to pharmacologic treatment and a valid alternative to the more invasive and costly cardiosurgical procedure of atrial compartmentalization (Maze procedure) [30, 31]. With the use of various energy forms (radiofrequency, thermal waves, laser or ultrasound) at the level of the wall, linear transmural lesions are created which circumscribe the PV ostia, thus electrically isolating the LA from those regions capable of triggering AF. Percutaneous treatment is the new therapeutic frontier and is particularly effective in the form of paroxysmal AF (80% success rate at 1 year from procedure) [38, 39]. The precise placement of the ablation sites on the wall of the LA is crucial for both the success of the procedure and the reduction of complications, the most frequent of which is PV stenosis [40, 41]. These aims depend in great part on the understanding of the complex anatomy of this region, which is guaranteed by MDCT thanks to its high spatial and temporal resolution.

17.3.2 Anatomic Background

The PV convey oxygenated blood from the lungs to the LA. Usually there are four - two on each side - and they are destitute of valves. The PV arise from the capillary network of the alveoli which joining together form a single trunk for each pulmonary lobe. The vein draining oxygenated blood from the middle lobe usually joins with the superior lobe such that two veins, superior and inferior, leave each lung. However, the three right lobar veins frequently remain separate, thus creating the presence of an accessory vein, while in a certain number of

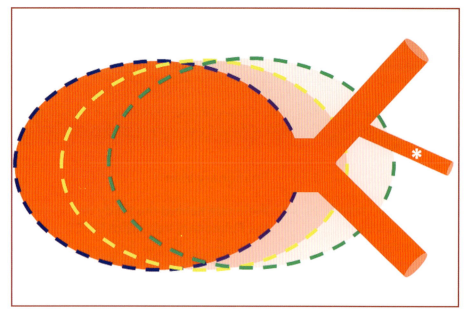

Fig. 17.5 Incorporation of the pulmonary veins by the left atrium during embryogenesis. Normal incorporation is characterized by typical anatomic morphology (*yellow dotted line*), whereas abnormal incorporation may be characterized by accessory veins (*green dotted line, over-incorporation*) or common trunks (*blue dotted line, under-incorporation*). In normal incorporation the accessory vein (*asterisk*) represents an early branching of pulmonary vein

cases the two lobar veins in the left lung join to form a single common trunk. A rarer occurrence is an accessory left vein (e.g. lingular vein), whereas no cases have been documented of a right common trunk. According to a respected theory of embryogenesis, this anatomic variability can be traced to the abnormal incorporation of the common PV in the LA which occurs around the seventh week of gestation [42]. Normal incorporation of the PV in the LA is characterized by the normal PV morphology, whereas abnormal incorporation can lead to accessory veins or common trunks (Fig. 17.5). The accessory PV are very common on the right [43, 44] and very rare on the left, while the opposite is true for common trunks, which are the most frequent anatomic variant (12-25%) and exclusive to the left side. In order to simplify reporting of the MDCT examination, one study proposed a classification of possible PV variants [45].

17.3.3 Study Technique and Image Analysis

The evaluation of the PV can be performed with a collimation greater than 1 mm, regardless of the scanner used, since the diameter of the vessels is considerable. With 64-MDCT the examination can be performed with the technical parameters presented in Table 17.2.

The volume to be studied extends from the tracheal bifurcation to the base of the heart in the craniocaudal direction. On the basis of the patient's build and heart rate, the scan time varies from 6 to 8 s and is performed in a single breath-hold. Contrast agent is administered with an 18-20 G needle cannula in an antecubital access in the arm with a dual-head injector: 70-80 mL of high iodine concentration (370-400 mgI/mL) contrast agent is injected at a rate of 4-5 mL/s, followed by 40 mL of physiologic solution at the same rate (bolus chaser). This set-up guarantees constant and optimal enhancement of the LA-PV complex and a reduction in the volume of contrast agent administered (from 20 to 40% less). The bolus chaser also considerably limits the attenuation caused by hyperconcentration of the contrast agent in the superior vena cava and in the right sections of the heart, thus eliminating the artifacts which can hamper the evaluation of the PV on this side. The bolus tracking ROI is positioned in the centre of the LA. Although retrospective gating is not mandatory, unlike in the study of the coronary arteries and CV, it is preferred when possible (sinus rhythm and heart rate lower than 90 bpm). Retrospective gating reduces artifacts due to cardiac motion and therefore improves image quality, which is particularly important in view of fusing the images with electroanatomic maps, which will be dealt with below. In order to keep the radiation dose of a gated examination within the levels of a non-gated examination, activating dose modulation is advisable, with the reconstruction of only the end-diastolic windows of the R-R (from 70% to 90%) which are capable of guaranteeing good quality images. The same examination technique is also used in follow-up, usually performed 1-3 months after the ablation procedure, with the aim of looking for possible complications such as PV stenosis. A workstation with software dedicated to cardiac examinations is used for image analysis. The analysis should follow a series of predetermined steps. First, the native 2 mm-thick axial images are examined for possible thrombi, which can be easily identified by the presence of filling defects. Thrombi,

Table 17.2 Study protocol of pulmonary veins with 64-MDCT

Parameter	Levels
Tube voltage	120-140 kV
Tube current	250 mAs
FOV	180-250 mm
Nominal slice thickness	64 x 1.5 mm
Effective slice thickness	2 mm
Reconstruction increment	1 mm
Rotation time	0.33-0.42 s
Pitch	If cardiac gating is used, automatically adapted to patient's heart rate
Reconstruction filter	Smooth
Contrast agent	70-80 ml at 4-5 mL/s (preferred iodine concentration 370-400 mgI/mL, followed by 40 mL of physiologic solution at the same rate)
Trigger	Automatic bolus tracking with ROI in left atrium
Gating	When possible, retrospective with reconstruction of 75% of the ECG R-R interval. Dose modulation

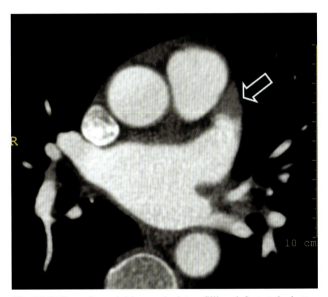

Fig. 17.6 The native axial image depicts a filling defect at the bottom of the left appendage (*arrow*) due to a thrombus, which contraindicates transcatheter ablation

which may also be detected by transesophageal echocardiography, are an absolute contraindication to catheter ablation procedures (Fig. 17.6). The axial images also depict the spatial orientation of the LA in relation to the other cardiac chambers, the knowledge of which is indispensable for the electrophysiologist when planning the percutaneous approach. More accurate and detailed information on the LA-PV complex is provided by the successive MPR/MIP reconstructions. With these images the anteroposterior, laterolateral and longitudinal axes of the LA can be calculated according to the method proposed by Ho [46], thus providing a precise picture of the size of the heart chamber on which the electrophysiologist will operate during catheter ablation. The MPR/MIP also depict the position and angulation of the interatrial septum, which needs to be perforated to allow the passage of the ablation catheter introduced intravenously into the LA. With regard to the PV, the MPR/MIP guarantee the reconstruction of the exact spatial orientation and direction of the vessel, thanks to the possibility of inclining a slab of variable thickness along its main axis (Figs. 17.7-17.11). This provides an accurate evaluation of the vessel diameter and morphology at the level of the ostium and above all to detect the presence of branching near the ostium (Figs. 17.7a,b; 17.8a,b). In the MPR/MIP images the presence of accessory veins, more common on the right, and common trunks on the left, can also be easily appreciated [35, 47]. This information is extremely relevant for the electrophysiologist whose system of electroanatomic mapping, despite being highly sophisticated, is unable to distinguish between early branching and accessory veins or common trunks. Precise knowledge of the ostial and preostial anatomy is crucial: catheter ablation should be limited to the electrical isolation of the ostia of all of the PV, including the accessory veins which are frequently the site of anomalous electrical circuits, and not penetrate within early branching or common trunks, since mistaken treatment can cause vessel stenosis with possible ischemia of the proximal pulmonary parenchyma [30, 31]. Lastly, the MPR/MIP images in parasagittal planes of the individual PV enable the accurate calculation of the circumference and the axes of the venous ostia, which is useful for the choice of the size and type of catheter to be used in the ablation procedure. In addition, these reconstruction planes also enable the evaluation of the ostial morphology. On the left side the PV ostia tend to be oval (craniocaudal axis > anteroposterior axis) whereas on the right side they

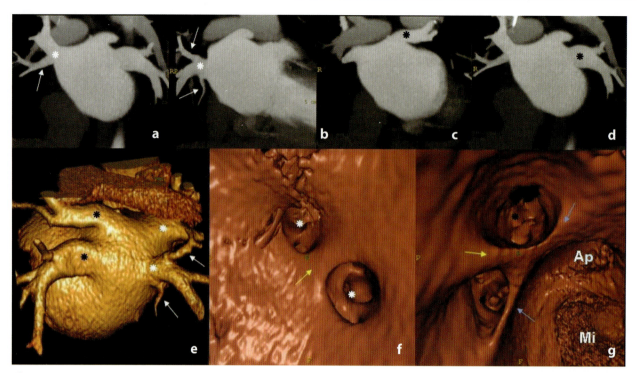

Fig. 17.7 Typical anatomy of the pulmonary veins. The MPR/MIP images reconstructed in the paracoronal planes along the main axis of the individual vessels (**a-d**) depict the two right pulmonary veins (**a**, **b** *white asterisks*) and the two left pulmonary veins (**c**, **d** *black asterisks*). Worth noting is the early branching at the venous ostium on the right side (*white arrows*), with classic branching inferiorly. The epicardial and endocardial views, provided by volume rendering (**e**) and virtual angioscopy (**f, g**) confirm the typical anatomic morphology. The *yellow arrows* indicate the saddle of myocardial tissue separating the pulmonary vein ostia on the right (**f**) and on the left (**g**). The *blue arrows* (**g**) indicate the thin myocardial ridge dividing the pulmonary veins from the appendage orifice (*Ap*). *Mi*, mitral plane

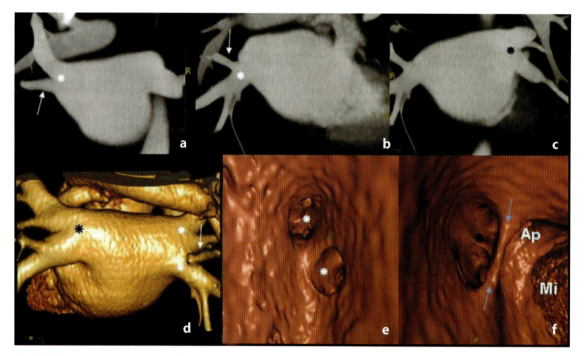

Fig. 17.8 Left common trunk. The MPR/MIP reconstructions depict two right veins (**a**, **b** *white asterisks*), both with early branching (*white arrows*) and a relatively short left common trunk (**c** *black asterisk*). The volume rendering (**d**) and virtual angioscopy (**e, f**) images confirm the anatomic variant. The ridge (**f** *blue arrows*) dividing the common trunk from the appendage orifice (*Ap*) can also be appreciated. *Mi*, mitral plane

17 Cardiac Veins and Pulmonary Veins

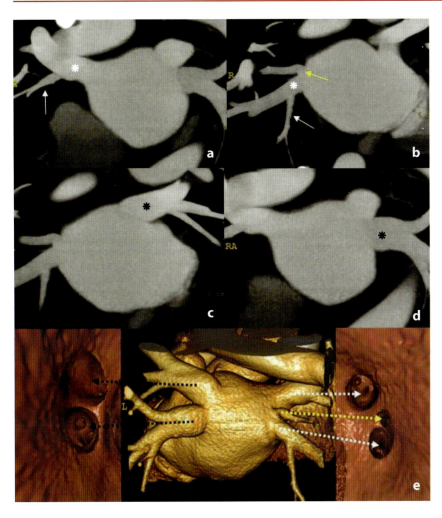

Fig. 17.9 Three right pulmonary veins and two left pulmonary veins. The MPR/MIP reconstructions depict three right pulmonary veins, the classic superior and inferior (**a**, **b** *white asterisks*) and a small accessory vein (**b** *yellow arrow*) which opens into the left atrium alongside the inferior vein. The white arrows indicate the early branching of the superior and inferior veins distinguishable from the accessory vein. Two distinct pulmonary veins can be appreciated on the left side (**c**, **d** *black asterisks*). In **e**, the volume rendering and virtual angioscopy images confirm the anatomic variant. The left panel indicates how the pulmonary veins on this side open into the atrium side by side but distinct from one another in comparison to Fig. 17.8f. In case of doubt the virtual angioscopy images are the best method for identifying the real anatomy of the left pulmonary veins

tend to be more rounded (craniocaudal axis = anteroposterior axis) [36, 45, 47, 48]. While the ostia of the superior PV are generally larger than the inferior ostia, there appears to be no statistically significant difference between the measurements of the PV ostia in patients with AF compared with the healthy population, even though due to LA remodeling there is a trend towards larger diameters in the former [32, 36, 47].

The last two steps of the analysis regard the VR reconstructions, which provide an intuitive epicardial view of the overall LA-PV complex [31], and the virtual angioscopy images (Voyager), which in contrast provide a view of the inside of the atrium (Figs. 17.7-17.11). With the latter view measurements can be made of the diameters of the PV ostia, as well as of the thickness of the myocardial tissue between the ostia (saddle) and between the PV ostia and the appendage orifice (ridge) (Figs. 17.7f, g; 17.8f). Lastly, the Voyager views enable the evaluation of the close relation between the left PV and the appendage orifice, a *critical* anatomic structure

given the limited thickness of its walls and therefore its elevated risk of perforation. The aim of PV postablation follow-up, which is usually performed 1-3 months after the procedure to avoid overestimation due to physiologic parietal edema which can appear in the first few days after the procedure, is to exclude the possible complications associated with the procedure, the most frequent being the abovementioned venous stenosis. The contraction and proliferation of the elastic lamina, caused by the application of energy directly in the vessel lumen, associated with chronic perivascular inflammation, can cause progressive venous stenosis. In rare cases, total occlusion can occur with the onset of symptoms of segmental pulmonary hypertension [30, 49]. The prevalence of stenosis in the various study populations varies from 1.5% to 42.4% [30, 34, 47, 50]. The PV most at risk of stenosis are the left PV, since the oval morphology in the ostial and preostial region facilitates contact between the anterior and posterior walls. In the native axial images the stenosis can be identified and quantified. The vessel

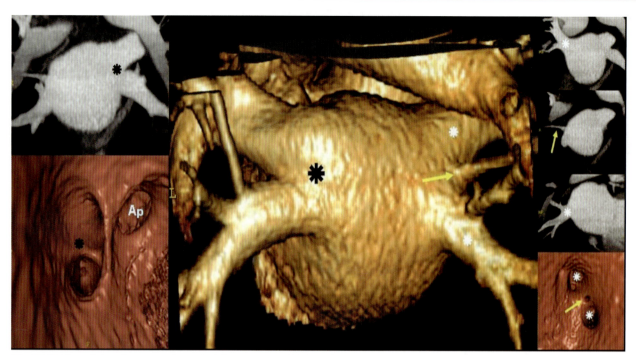

Fig. 17.10 Three right pulmonary veins and a left common trunk. The volume rendering image in the central panel clearly depicts the three right vessels, with an accessory vein (*yellow arrow*) between the two main veins (*white asterisks*), while the anatomy of the left pulmonary veins is more doubtful. In the lateral panels, the MPR/MIP reconstructions and the virtual angioscopy images confirm the right three-vessel anatomy and depict the left common trunk (*black asterisk*). *Ap*, appendage orifice

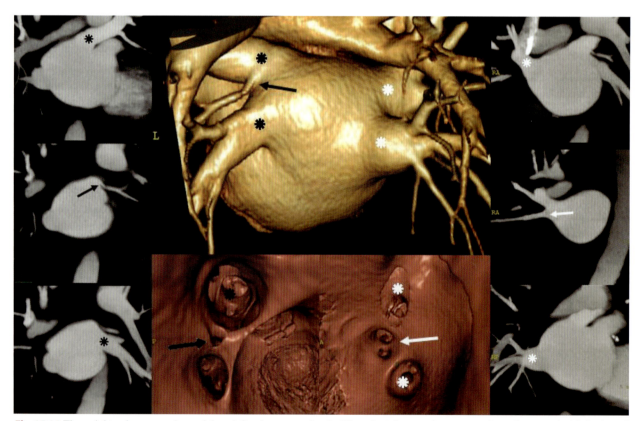

Fig. 17.11 Three right pulmonary veins and three left pulmonary veins. In this patient the complex anatomy is easily recognizable in the volume rendering image (*central panel above*) and the virtual angioscopy images (*central panel below*). On both sides an accessory vein (*white arrow right; black arrow left*) can be appreciated opening into the atrium between the two main veins (*white and black asterisks right* and *left*, respectively). In the lateral panels the MPR/MIP reconstructions in the paracoronal planes of the individual vessels clearly distinguish the accessory veins from branching. In this context, the extensive branching of the right inferior pulmonary artery in the lower right panel is of particular note

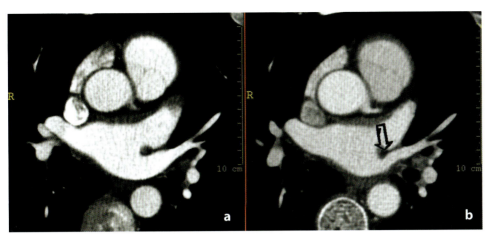

Fig. 17.12 Native axial images from MDCT studies for ablation: preprocedure (**a**) and postprocedure (**b**). The postprocedure image depicts a slight hourglass-like narrowing of the left superior pulmonary vein (*arrow*). The finding is compatible with nonsignificant stenosis

tends to have an *hourglass* shape, since the narrowing is situated only several millimeters from the ostium. The MDCT postablation images should be accurately compared with the corresponding preablation images to avoid errors of over- or underestimation (Fig. 17.12). If the follow-up examination is positive for stenosis, regular follow-up should be planned (3-6 months) and the option of performing a procedure of venous dilatation should be considered [51-53]. Lastly, other much rarer complications can be encountered in the PV (thrombosis, dissection), the pericardium (pericarditis, hemopericardium), the heart (perforations or parietal hematomas) and the esophagus (atrioesophageal fistula) [54].

A head-to-head comparison of contrast-enhanced MR and MDCT for the evaluation of LA-PV morphology provides similar and detailed anatomic and quantitative information before and after ablation of AF, without radiation exposure [53, 55-61]. Recently, some studies showed that LA-PV depiction with non-contrast-enhanced MR is feasible [62, 63]. The recent introduction of a delayed-enhancement cardiac MR sequence (DE-MR) allows for the noninvasive assessment of the location and extent of LA scarring following the ablation procedure [64]. Moreover, DE-MR provides a noninvasive means of assessing left atrial myocardial tissue in patients suffering from AF and insight into the progress of the disease. Preablation DE-MR holds promise for predicting responders to AF ablation and may provide a metric of overall disease progression. LA pre-ablation fibrosis and ablation related scarring are major predictors of success in rhythm control of AF: DE-MR examinations are extremely useful for stratifying AF patients in order to identify predictors of a successful procedure [65-69].

17.4 Integration of MDCT Images and Electroanatomic Maps

The integration of high spatial resolution images (MDCT or MR) with electroanatomic maps constructed in the operating room is a technique which has already demonstrated its potential in neurosurgery [70]. The development of the integration of anatomic images in the surgical field is in fact largely due to the efforts of neurosurgeons, who in the 1980s experimented with stereotactic systems for centering the operating field [71]. These early pioneering studies paved the way for modern surgery guided by both static and dynamic multimodal images which are widely used in many fields of classic surgical approaches and modern mini-invasive interventional procedures [72]. To achieve this aim a key component has been the ability to register images and maps acquired with different modalities, both prior to and during surgery, capable of describing not only the anatomy but also the specific functional properties of the organ subject to surgery. In cardiology, recent studies both in animal models [73] and in humans [74] have demonstrated the possibility of integrating electroanatomic maps and high-resolution three-dimensional images of cardiac anatomy. The main aim of this integration of multimodal images is to increase the effectiveness and efficiency of AF ablation treatment. As stated earlier, the treatment of arrhythmias with ablation of the PV ostia requires detailed information of the LA and the PV which cannot be obtained with traditional fluoroscopy. The availability of anatomic images as a roadmap for the movement of the radiofrequency catheter can shorten procedure times by optimizing the ablation lines and at the same time

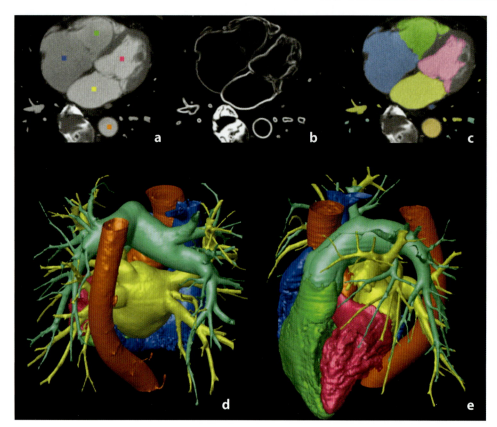

Fig. 17.13 Main phases of semi-automatic watershed segmentation. On the native axial MDCT image the operator marks the main structures to be segmented (**a**). The software processes the image and identifies the borders of the segments (**b**) and then classifies the structures according to the initial operator-defined settings (**c**). Posterior and left oblique anterior views of the three dimensional model of the segmented cardiovascular structures of the mediastinum (**d, e**). This segmentation technique enables the accurate identification and separation of the four cardiac chambers as well as the arterial and venous mediastinal vessels, with their reconstruction up to vessel diameters in the order of 1 mm

reduce the risk of radiation exposure and PV stenosis [35, 75, 76]. The integration of electroanatomic maps and anatomic images should also facilitate a more precise localization of the critical mechanisms which sustain AF [77, 78]. The creation of multimodal maps in which cardiac electric activity can be spatially represented with good anatomic detail is in fact considered particularly useful in the treatment of chronic forms of AF and AF in elderly patients, areas in which catheter ablation is still developing [79].

17.4.1 Segmentation

The fundamental prerequisite for performing effective registration is the segmentation of the image acquired with high spatial resolution imaging, i.e. the detailed separation and reconstruction of the anatomic structure of specific interest. These postprocessing operations can be done thanks to rather *simple* applications installed on the workstations supporting MDCT scanners. These programs are essentially based on the different degree of enhancement of the blood in the vessels and the cardiac chambers, although they often require significant manual input [80], which can be rather time consuming. In addition, the optimal segmentation of the target anatomy relies on a *dedicated* examination protocol (Table 17.2), which at the same time precludes or at least limits the possibility of the precise reconstruction and isolation of the adjacent cardiovascular structures.

With the development of more sophisticated techniques the segmentation of all of the cardiac chambers and the mediastinal vessels can be done relatively rapidly [74, 81] with minimal human intervention in the initial phase. The operator need only define several reference markers within the structures to be isolated (cardiac chambers, arterial and venous vessels) and an automatic procedure based on the watershed technique [82] applied to the degree of contrast performs complete segmentation (Fig. 17.13).

17.4.2 Registration and Fusion of Electroanatomic Maps

As mentioned earlier, the integration of electroanatomic maps and anatomic images (registration and fusion) is required by the electrophysiologist to fully appreciate the critical mechanisms of the arrhythmia and implement effective treatment. The process of registering elec-

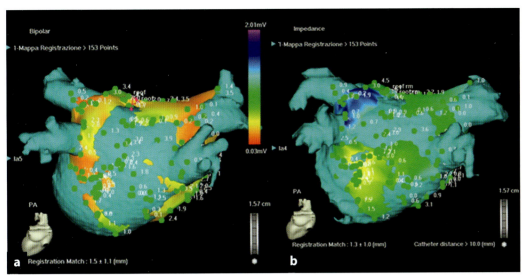

Fig. 17.14 Two examples of CARTO MERGE TM integration with MDCT (**a**) and MR (**b**) images of the same patient. The registration points are almost equivalent in the two maps

troanatomic maps on the MDCT images is based on a geometric transformation which aims at aligning around one hundred points distributed on the internal wall of the LA with the corresponding anatomic reconstruction obtained with MDCT. The registration phase proper takes place automatically with an iterative process in which the software performs continuous rotations and translations of the coordinate system of points to be aligned, thus minimizing the distance between them and the atrial surface [74]. After the registration phase interpolation algorithms are applied to continuously represent the electrical patterns of interest on that surface [83]. This process is known as fusion (Fig. 17.14). The construction of electroanatomic maps to be used in fusion requires knowledge of the exact spatial location of the catheter in the cardiac chamber. Since this is not possible with the simple use of fluoroscopy, navigation systems have been developed capable of acquiring electrical signals and associating them with fixed spatial coordinates, or during catheter ablation capable of storing the coordinates of the ablation points [78]. Several studies have demonstrated the feasibility of the registration and the potential clinical use of each of these systems [76, 78, 80]. In this setting, the most developed system is the CARTO-MERGE TM (Biosense-Webster Inc., Diamond Bar, CA), a software package capable of integrating electroanatomic data acquired with the NAVISTAR® catheter with MDCT images. To facilitate the alignment process a number of fiducial points are acquired in the most easily and precisely identifiable anatomic positions [84]. In the CARTO-MERGE TM procedure these fiducial points are paired with the corresponding positions of the MDCT images and the software is then launched to find the best alignment. Although different strategies may be adopted, to guarantee good registration and avoid alignment errors, acquiring the CARTO points well distributed on the atrial wall is advisable, including the appendage, the PV borders [76, 84] and several points on the aorta [85]. Although the technique is still not very diffuse, the different experiences are in accordance with an alignment error, measured as the distance between the mapping points and the MDCT surface, in the order of 2 mm. Several studies have also demonstrated the feasibility of integrating MDCT and MR images with real-time electroanatomic maps (CARTO MERGE TM or Navx-/Ensite-system) for guiding catheter ablation procedures for the treatment of AF [86-89] (Fig. 17.5).

A multicenter study established that image integration, in comparison with segmental PV isolation and circumferential PV isolation guided by three-dimensional electroanatomic mapping alone, significantly improves clinical outcome [90]; in a more recent study, image integration using CARTO-MERGE TM in patients undergoing catheter ablation for paroxysmal and persistent AF, failed to significantly improve the clinical outcome, although radiation exposure was reduced [91].

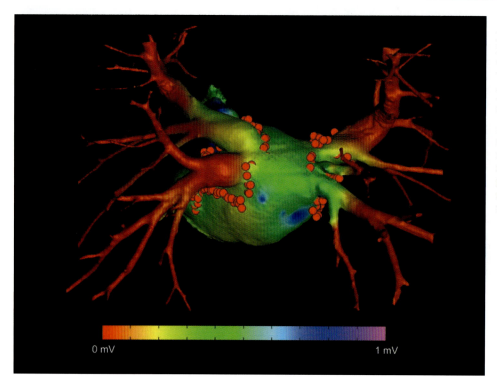

Fig. 17.15 Fusion of action potentials of the left atrium after pulmonary vein ablation. The color map indicates the distribution of action potentials on the atrial surface and in the preostial portions of the pulmonary veins. The image was obtained by integrating the previously segmented atrium with the electroanatomic map acquired with CARTO. The red dots indicate the ablation points registered with an automatic procedure on the 3D surface

References

1. Gras D, Mabo P, Tang T et al (1998) Multisite pacing as a supplemental treatment of congestive heart failure: preliminary results of the Medtronic Inc. InSync Study. Pacing Clin Electrophysiol 21:2249-2255
2. Daubert JC, Ritter P, Le Breton H et al (1998) Permanent left ventricular pacing with transvenous leads inserted into the coronary veins. Pacing Clin Electrophysiol 21:239-245
3. Abraham WT, Fisher WG, Smith AL et al (2002) Cardiac resynchronization in chronic heart failure. N Engl J Med 346:1845-1853
4. Abraham WT, Hayes DL (2003) Cardiac resynchronization therapy for heart failure. Circulation 108:2596-2603
5. Puglisi A, Lunati M, Marullo AG et al (2004) Limited thoracotomy as a second choice alternative to transvenous implant for cardiac resynchronization therapy delivery. Eur Hearth J 25:1063-1069
6. Ansalone G, Giannantoni P, Ricci R et al (2002) Doppler myocardial imaging to evacuate the effectiveness of pacing sites in patients receiving biventricular pacing. J Am Coll Cardiol 39:489-499
7. Melo WD, Prudencio LA, Kusnir CE et al (1998) Angiography of the coronary venous system. Use in clinical electrophysiology. Arq Bras Cardiol 70:409-413
8. Meisel E, Pfeiffer D, Engelmann L et al (2001) Investigation of coronary venous anatomy by retrograde venography in patients with malignant ventricular tachycardia. Circulation 104:442-447
9. Tada H, Kurosaki K, Naito S et al (2005) Three-dimensional visualization of the coronary venous system using multidetector row computed tomography. Circ J 69:165-170
10. Jongbloed MRM, Lamb HJ, Bax JJ et al (2005) Noninvasive visualization of the cardiac venous system using multislice computed tomography. J Am Coll Cardiol 45:749-753
11. Abbara S, Cury RC, Nieman K et al (2005) Noninvasive evaluation of cardiac veins with 16-MDCT angiography. AJA Am J Roentgenol 185:1001-1006
12. Muhlenbruch G, Koos R, Wildberger JE et al (2005) Imaging of the cardiac venous system: comparison of MDCT and conventional angiography. AJR Am J Roentgenol 185:1252-1257
13. Cademartiri F, Marano R, Luccichenti G et al (2004) Normal anatomy of the vessels of the heart with 16-row multislice computed tomography. Radiol Med 107:11-23
14. von Ludinghausen M (2003) The venous drainage of the human myocardium. Adv Anat Embryol Cell Biol 168:104
15. Van de Veire NR, Schuijf JD, De Kini J et al (2006) Noninvasive visualization of the cardiac venous system in coronary artery disease patients using 64-slice computed tomography. J Am Coll Cardiol 48:1832-1838
16. Kini S, Bis KG, Weaver L (2007) Normal and variant coronary arterial and venous anatomy on high-resolution CT angiography. AJR Am J Roentgenol 188:1665-1674
17. Butler J (2007) The emerging role of multi-detector computed tomography in heart failure. J Card Fail 13:215-226
18. Chen JJ, Lee WJ, Wang YC et al (2007) Morphologic and topologic characteristics of coronary venous system delineated by noninvasive multidetector computed tomography in chronic systolic heart failure patients. J Card Fail 13:482-488
19. Tops LF, Krishnàn SC, Schuijf JD et al (2008) Noncoronary applications of cardiac multidetector row computed tomography. JACC Cardiovasc Imaging 1:94-106
20. Lumia D, Laganà D, Canì A et al (2009) MDCT evaluation of the cardiac venous system. Radiol Med 114:837-851
21. Pontone G, Andreini D, Cortinovis S et al (2010) Imaging of cardiac venous system in patients with dilated cardiomyopathy by 64-slice computed tomography: comparison between non-ischemic and ischemic etiology. Int J Cardiol 144:340-343
22. Hua W, Ding LG, Zhang S et al (2010) Usefulness of previsualization of the cardiac venous system by 64-slice computed tomography in patients with heart failure underwent cardiac resynchronization therapy. Zhonghua Xin Xue Guan Bing Za Zhi 38:610-613

23. Hara T, Yamashiro K, Okajima K et al (2009) Improvement in the quality of the cardiac vein images by optimizing the scan protocol of multidetector-row computed tomography. Heart Vessels 24:434-439

24. Matsumoto Y, Krishnan S, Fowler SJ et al (2007) Detection of phrenic nerves and their relation to cardiac anatomy using 64-slice multidetector computed tomography. Am J Cardiol 100:133-137

25. Nezafat R, Han Y, Peters DC, Herzka DA et al (2007) Coronary magnetic resonance vein imaging: imaging contrast, sequence, and timing. Magn Reson Med 58:1196-1206

26. Rasche V, Binner L, Cavagna F et al (2007) Whole-heart coronary vein imaging: a comparison between non-contrast-agent- and contrast-agent-enhanced visualization of the coronary venous system. Magn Reson Med 57:1019-1026

27. Chiribiri A, Kelle S, Götze S et al (2008) Visualization of the cardiac venous system using cardiac magnetic resonance. Am J Cardiol 101:407-412

28. Younger JF, Plein S, Crean A et al (2009) Visualization of coronary venous anatomy by cardiovascular magnetic resonance. J Cardiovasc Magn Reson 11:26

29. Stoeck CT, Han Y, Peters DC et al (2009) Whole heart magnetization-prepared steady-state free precession coronary vein MRI. J Magn Reson Imaging 29:1293-1299

30. Ghaye B, Szapiro D, Dacher JN et al (2003) Percutaneous ablation for atrial fibrillation: the role of cross-sectional imaging. Radio Graphics 23:19-33

31. Lacomis JM, Wigginton W, Fuhrman C et al (2003) Multi-detector row CT of the left atrium and pulmonary veins before radiofrequency catheter ablation for atrial fibrillation. RadioGraphics 23:35-48

32. Schwartzman D, Lacomis J, Wigginton G (2003) Characterization of left atrium and distal pulmonary vein morphology using multidimensional computed tomography. J Am Coll Cardiol 41:1349-1357

33. Maksimovic R, Cademartiri F, Scholten M et al (2004) Sixteen-row multislice computed tomography in the assessment of pulmonary veins prior to ablative treatment: validation vs conventional venography and study of reproducibility. Eur Radiol 14:369-374

34. Cronin P, Sneider MB, Kazerooni EA et al (2004) MDCT of the left atrium and pulmonary veins in planning radiofrequency ablation for atrial fibrillation: a how-to guide. AJR Am J Roentgenol 183:767-778

35. Centonze M, Del Greco M, Nollo G et al (2005) The role of multidetector CT in the evaluation of the left atrium and pulmonary veins anatomy before and after radio-frequency catheter ablation for atrial fibrillation. Preliminary results and work in progress. Radiol Med 110:52-60

36. Jongbloed MR, Dirksen MS, Bax JJ et al (2005) Atrial fibrillation: multi-detector row CT of pulmonary vein anatomy prior to radiofrequency catheter ablation-initial experience. Radiology 234:702-709

37. Kim Y-H, Marom EM, Herndon JE et al (2005) Pulmonary vein diameter, cross sectional area and shape: CT analysis. Radiology 235:43-49

38. Pappone C, Rosanio S, Oreto G et al (2000) Circumferential radiofrequency ablation of pulmonary vein ostia: a new anatomic approach for curing atrial fibrillation. Circulation 102:2619-2628

39. Pappone C, Oreto G, Rosanio S et al (2001) Atrial electroanatomic remodeling after circumferential radiofrequency pulmonary vein ablation: efficacy of an anatomic approach in a large cohort of patients with atrial fibrillation. Circulation 104:2539-2544

40. Arentz T, Jander N, von Rosenthal J et al (2003) Incidence of pulmonary vein stenosis 2 years after radiofrequency catheter ablation of refractory atrial fibrillation. Eur Heart J 24:963-969

41. Dill T, Neumann T, Ekinci O et al (2003) Pulmonary vein diameter reduction after radiofrequency catheter ablation for paroxysmal atrial fibrillation evaluated by contrast-enhanced three-dimensional magnetic resonance imaging. Circulation 107:845-850

42. Chung B, Yucel EK, Rolnick J et al (2002) Morphology and variations of the pulmonary veins: classification and dimensions using 3D-CTA models (abstr). Radiology 225:155

43. Budorick NE, McDonald V, Flisak ME et al (1989) The pulmonary veins. Semin Roentgenol 24:127-140

44. Healey JE (1952) An anatomic survey of anomalous pulmonary veins: their clinical significance. Thorac Surg 23:433-444

45. Marom EM, Herndon JE, Kim Y-H et al (2004) Variations in pulmonary venous drainage to the left atrium: implications for radiofrequency ablation. Radiology 230:824-829

46. Ho SY, Sanchez-Quintana D, Cabrera JA et al (1999) Anatomy of the left atrium: implications for radiofrequency ablation for atrial fibrillation. J Cardiovascular Electrophysiol 10:1525-1533

47. Kato R, Lickfett L, Meininger G et al (2003) Pulmonary vein anatomy in patients undergoing catheter ablation of atrial fibrillation. Circulation 107:2004-2010

48. Wittkampf FH, Vonken EJ, Derksen R et al (2003) Pulmonary vein ostium geometry: analysis by magnetic resonance angiography. Circulation 107:21-23

49. Ravenel JG, McAdams HP (2002) Pulmonary venous infarction after radiofrequency ablation for atrial fibrillation. AJR Am J Roentgenol 178:664-666

50. Haissaguerre M, Jais P, Shah DC et al (2000) Electrophysiological end point for catheter ablation of atrial fibrillation initiated from multiple pulmonary venous foci. Circulation 101:1409-1417

51. Qureshi AM, Prieto LR, Latson LA et al (2003) Transcatheter angioplasty for acquired pulmonary vein stenosis after radiofrequency ablation. Circulation 108:1336-1342

52. Holmes DR Jr, Monahan KH, Packer D (2009) Pulmonary vein stenosis complicating ablation for atrial fibrillation: clinical spectrum and interventional considerations. JACC Cardiovasc Interv 2:267-276

53. Saremi F, Tafti M (2009) The role of computed tomography and magnetic resonance imaging in ablation procedures for treatment of atrial fibrillation. Semin Ultrasound CT MR 30:125-156

54. Preis O, Digumarthy SR, Wright CD et al (2007) Atrioesophageal fistula after catheter pulmonary venous ablation for atrial fibrillation: imaging features. J Thorac Imaging 22:283-285

55. Schmidt B, Ernst S, Ouyang F (2006) External and endoluminal analysis of left atrial anatomy and the pulmonary veins in three-dimensional reconstructions of magnetic resonance angiography: the full insight from inside. J Cardiovasc Electrophysiol 17:957-964

56. Mansour M, Refaat M, Heist EK et al (2006) Three-dimensional anatomy of the left atrium by magnetic resonance angiography: implications for catheter ablation for atrial fibrillation. J Cardiovasc Electrophysiol 17:719-723

57. Anselme F, Gahide G, Savouré A et al (2006) MR evaluation of pulmonary vein diameter reduction after radiofrequency catheter ablation of atrial fibrillation. Eur Radiol 16:2505-2511

58. Katoh M, Bücker A, Mühlenbruch G et al (2006) Impact of ECG gating in contrast-enhanced MR angiography for the assessment of the pulmonary veins and the left atrium anatomy. Rofo 178:180-184

59. Hauser TII, Peters DC, Wylic JV et al (2008) Evaluating the left atrium by magnetic resonance imaging. Europace 10 (Suppl 3):iii22-27

60. Allgayer C, Zellweger MJ, Sticherling C et al (2008) Optimization of imaging before pulmonary vein isolation by radiofrequency ablation: breath-held ungated versus ECG/breath-gated MRA. Eur Radiol 18:2879-2884

61. Hamdan A, Charalampos K, Roettgen R et al (2009) Magnetic resonance imaging versus computed tomography for characterization of pulmonary vein morphology before radiofrequency catheter ablation of atrial fibrillation. Am J Cardiol 104:1540-1546

62. Krishnam MS, Tomasian A, Malik S et al (2009) Three-dimen-

sional imaging of pulmonary veins by a novel steady-state free-precession magnetic resonance angiography technique without the use of intravenous contrast agent: initial experience. Invest Radiol 44:447-453

63. Hu P, Chuang ML, Kissinger KV et al (2010) Non-contrast-enhanced pulmonary vein MRI with a spatially selective slab inversion preparation sequence. Magn Reson Med 63:530-536

64. Peters DC, Wylie JV, Hauser TH et al (2007) Detection of pulmonary vein and left atrial scar after catheter ablation with three-dimensional navigator-gated delayed enhancement MR imaging: initial experience. Radiology 243:690-695

65. McGann CJ, Kholmovski EG, Oakes RS et al (2008) New magnetic resonance imaging-based method for defining the extent of left atrial wall injury after the ablation of atrial fibrillation. J Am Coll Cardiol 52:1263-1271

66. Badger TJ, Adjei-Poku YA, Marrouche NF (2009) MRI in cardiac electrophysiology: the emerging role of delayed-enhancement MRI in atrial fibrillation ablation. Future Cardiol 5:63-70

67. Peters DC, Wylie JV, Hauser TH et al (2009) Recurrence of atrial fibrillation correlates with the extent of post-procedural late gadolinium enhancement: a pilot study. JACC Cardiovasc Imaging 2:308-316

68. Oakes RS, Badger TJ, Kholmovski EG et al (2009) Detection and quantification of left atrial structural remodeling with delayed-enhancement magnetic resonance imaging in patients with atrial fibrillation. Circulation 119:1758-1767

69. Badger TJ, Daccarett M, Akoum NW et al (2010) Evaluation of left atrial lesions after initial and repeat atrial fibrillation ablation: lessons learned from delayed-enhancement MRI in repeat ablation procedures. Circ Arrhythm Electrophysiol 3:249-259

70. Grunert P, Darabi K, Espinosa J et al (2003) Computer-aided navigation in neurosurgery. Neurosurg Rev 26:73-99

71. Peters TM, Clark JA, Olivier A et al (1986) Integrated stereotaxic imaging with CT, MR imaging, and digital subtraction angiography. Radiology 161:821-826

72. Peters TM (2006) Image-guidance for surgical procedures. Phys Med Biol 51:505-540

73. Reddy VY, Malchano ZJ, Holmvang G et al (2004) Integration of cardiac magnetic resonance imaging with three-dimensional electroanatomic mapping to guide left ventricular catheter manipulation: feasibility in a porcine model of healed myocardial infarction. J Am Coll Cardiol 44:2202-2213

74. Nollo G, Cristoforetti A, Faes L et al (2004) Registration and fusion of segmented left atrium CT images with CARTO electrical maps for the ablative treatment of atrial fibrillation. Comput Cardiol 31:345-348

75. Del Greco M, Ravelli F, Cristoforetti A et al (2005) Fusion of electrical maps and MDCT images for validation of left atrium ablation points. Europace 7:14

76. Tops LF, Bax JJ, Zeppenfeld K et al (2005) Fusion of multislice computed tomography imaging with three-dimensional electroanatomic mapping to guide radiofrequency catheter ablation procedures. Heart Rhythm 2:1076-1081

77. Ravelli F, Faes L, Sandrini L et al (2005) Wave-similarity mapping shows the spatiotemporal distribution of fibrillatory wave complex-

ity in the human right atrium during paroxysmal and chronic atrial fibrillation. J Cardiovasc Electrophysiol 16:1071-1076

78. Packer DL (2005) Three-dimensional mapping in interventional electrophysiology: techniques and technology. Journal of Cardiovascular Electrophysiol 16:1110-1116

79. Wood MA, Ellenbogen KA (2006) Catheter ablation of chronic atrial fibrillation - the gap between promise and practice. New Engl J Med 354:967-969

80. Sra J, Krum D, Hare J et al (2005) Feasibility and validation of registration of three-dimensional left atrial models derived from computed tomography with a noncontact cardiac mapping system. Heart Rhythm 2:55-63

81. Disertori M, Marini M, Cristoforetti A et al (2005) Enormous biatrial enlargement in a persistent idiopathic atrial standstill. Eur Heart J 26:2276

82. Vincent L, Soille P (1991) Watershed in digital spaces: an efficient algorithm based on immersion simulations. IEEE Trans Pattern Anal Machine Intell 13:583-598

83. Nollo G, Cristoforetti A, Del Greco M et al (2004) Fusion of electroanatomic maps with 3D tomographic images of the left atrium and pulmonary veins in patients with atrial fibrillation. Eur Heart J 25:344

84. Sra J (2005) Registration of three dimensional left atrial images with interventional systems. Heart 91:1098-1104

85. Reddy VY, Malchano ZJ, Neuzil P et al (2005) Early clinical experience with Carto-merge for integration of 3D-CT imaging with real-time mapping to guide catheter ablation of atrial fibrillation. Heart Rhythm 2:160

86. Mikaelian BJ, Malchano ZJ, Neuzil P et al (2005) Images in cardiovascular medicine. Integration of 3-dimensional cardiac computed tomography images with real-time electroanatomic mapping to guide catheter ablation of atrial fibrillation. Circulation 112:35-36

87. Dong J, Dickfeld T, Dalal D et al (2006) Initial experience in the use of integrated electroanatomic mapping with three-dimensional MR/CT images to guide catheter ablation of atrial fibrillation. J Cardiovasc Electrophysiol 17:459-466

88. Bertaglia E, Brandolino G, Zoppo F et al (2008) Integration of three-dimensional left atrial magnetic resonance images into a real-time electroanatomic mapping system: validation of a registration method. Pacing Clin Electrophysiol 31:273-282

89. Kettering K, Greil GF, Fenchel M et al (2009) Catheter ablation of atrial fibrillation using the Navx-/Ensite-system and a CT-/MRI-guided approach. Clin Res Cardiol 2009 98:285-296

90. Bertaglia E, Bella PD, Tondo C et al (2009) Image integration increases efficacy of paroxysmal atrial fibrillation catheter ablation: results from the CartoMerge Italian Registry. Europace 11:1004-1010

91. Caponi D, Corleto A, Scaglione M et al (2010) Ablation of atrial fibrillation: does the addition of three-dimensional magnetic resonance imaging of the left atrium to electroanatomic mapping improve the clinical outcome? A randomized comparison of Carto-Merge vs. Carto-XP three-dimensional mapping ablation in patients with paroxysmal and persistent atrial fibrillation. Europace 12:1098-1104

Collateral Findings on Cardiac CT

18

Roberto Malagò, Camilla Barbiani, Andrea Pezzato, Ugolino Alfonsi, Erica Maffei, Roberto Pozzi Mucelli, and Filippo Cademartiri

18.1 Introduction

Noninvasive imaging of the coronary arteries is an important clinical application since cardiac computed tomography (CCT) has proven to be an accurate imaging alternative to conventional coronary angiography [1-4]. The technique has a significant clinical role to play in patients with low-to-intermediate pre-test probability of coronary artery disease (CAD) and negative or equivocal findings on exercise stress testing.

The growing number of indications for the technique is associated with increasing patient demands in terms of expectations and quality of life, with an associated increasing intolerance of highly invasive diagnostic procedures. The increasing demand of noninvasive study of the coronaries has lead to the emerging problem of non-cardiac collateral findings revealed during the CCT [5-7].

The presence of incidental findings during diagnostic examinations is a well known problem in all anatomic regions [1-3]. In most cases these findings are incidental without any significance, but in other cases they are indeterminate or clinically significant and require further investigation to reach a correct diagnosis. At the end of the cardiac-radiologic evaluation, therefore, the radiologist interpreting and reporting the examination should dedicate time to a second phase aimed at detecting any extracardiac findings.

18.2 Study Technique

A typical cardiac CT angiography study involves an initial pre contrast scan for calcium score and a second post contrast scan, the coronary angiography cardiac CT. Both of the scans are collimated to the mediastinum in the X and Y axes and extends from a plane passing below the aortic arch to the base of the heart, including a portion of the organs of the upper abdomen (Fig. 18.1).

This collimated FOV is required for optimal resolution when analyzing the coronaries. However the raw data contain information included in the whole gantry. When evaluating non coronary collateral findings reformatting the dataset with a FOV collimated not to the mediastinum but to the chest skin is recommended. This dataset does not require the thin collimation expected for the coronary analysis; instead a slice thickness of 1.0 mm is enough, with a reconstruction increment 0.5 mm and convolution filter medium-soft and sharp for evaluation in the mediastinal window (350W/50C), lung window (1400W/600C) and bone window (2000W/800C) (Fig. 18.1).

This procedure, including the additional reconstruction time and transfer of the dedicated dataset, adds about 3-4 min to the evaluation of the examination. This is compatible with normal routine clinical practice, representing only a minimal fraction of the reporting time of a cardiac CT examination.

According to all anatomic structures contained in the chest, extracoronary findings can be distinguished into the following districts:

Mediastinal organs
- Heart
- Aorta
- Esophagus

Lung
- Parenchyma
- Lymph node
- Tracheal-bronchial structures

Abdominal Organs
- Liver
- Adrenal glands
- Kidneys
- Spleen
- Stomach
- Colon

Other
- Spinal Column

R. Malagò (✉)
Department of Radiology,
"G.B. Rossi" University Hospital,
Verona, Italy

F. Cademartiri, G. Casolo, M. Midiri (eds.), *Clinical Applications of Cardiac CT*,
© Springer-Verlag Italia 2012

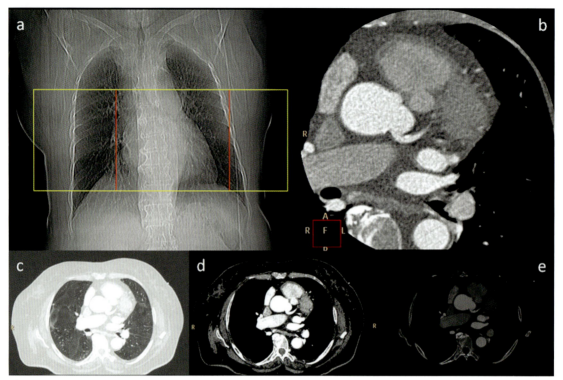

Fig. 18.1 Scout planar image in **a** of the chest showing the FOV collimated to the mediastinum (*red box*) for cardiac acquisitions (**b**). From the same raw data the FOV can be enlarged to the skin of the chest (*yellow box*) thus analyzing collateral findings in lung (**c**), mediastinal (**d**) and bone tissue window settings (**e**)

- Ribs
- Diaphragm
- Breast

All these districts can present multiple different alterations and abnormalities which should be identified and mentioned in the report (Table 18.1).

All incidental noncardiac collateral findings have to be recorded and scored as:
1. minor (no clinical significance; not necessary to report);
2. mild (uncertain clinical significance; preferably mentioned in the report);
3. major (further investigated is compulsory; mandatory to report).

Examples of minor and mild collateral findings are shown in Fig. 18.2, whereas major findings which should be reported for further investigations are depicted in Figs. 18.3-18.6.

18.3 Discussion

Given that CCT scans are usually performed to detect atherosclerotic disease, it is remarkable that incidental pathologic changes in organs and structures which were not the target organs of the examination can be found in almost every patient.

Many previous studies have already described this aspect presenting large single center series [6, 8].

Cademartiri et al. retrospectively reviewed 670 cases collecting 1,234 non cardiac findings, divided into nonsignificant 332 (26.9%), mild 821 (66.53%) and compulsory for further investigation 81 (6.56%). A total of 81 patients (12.08%) had significant noncardiac disease requiring clinical or radiologic follow-up. Among these, newly discovered diseases were revealed in two patients (2.46%).

The most recent papers on this issue by MacHaalany [8] and Onuma [9] show parallel results, reporting a high prevalence of 58.8% of noncardiac findings, 35.5% of them nonsignificant. Another relevant study was published by Hunold et al. in 2001 [5] but it was performed with EBCT. In the 1812 consecutive patients undergoing EBCT cardiac studies, the authors reviewed only the mediastinal windows, but also encountered the cardiac findings such as mitral valve or pericardiac disease. In his study Hunold reported 38% of noncoronary findings as located in the heart or pericardium. Moreover, abnormalities included in his study were a large number of minor, relatively insignificant abnormalities, such as scars, granulomata, atelectasis, degenerative arthritis, and rib fractures. Considering 1812 patients 67% were

18 Collateral Findings on Cardiac CT

Table 18.1 Collateral findings according to the main non coronary structures of the chest and upper abdomen

Structure	Incidental findings
Parenchyma	Emphysematous bubbles, Emphysema, Calcified pulmonary nodules, Pulmonary nodules <1 cm, Pulmonary nodules >1 cm, Edema, Atelectasis (basal+apical lobes), Coils embolising a lung lobe, Lung cancer, Lung metastasis, Lung infection
Pleura	Multiple pleural calcific thickening, Low/medium degree pleural effusion, Severe pleural effusion, Retraction, Calcifications, Thickening, Mesothelioma,
Vascular	Embolism
Bronchi	Tracheal/bronchial calcifications
Lymph node	Hilar calcified, Hilar nodal consolidation, Mediastinal Lymph Nodes >1 cm
Liver	Hepatomegaly, Liver calcifications, Liver cysts, Ascites, Hepatic metastasis, Hepatic angioma (single+multiple)
Gallbladder	Stones
Biliary Tree	Dilatation
Kidney	Tumor
Pancreas	Calcifications, Masses
Adrenal	Hyperplasia
Spleen	Accessory spleen, Splenic calcification, Splenomegaly, Lesions
Thyroid	Goitre
Esophagus	Esophageal wall thickening, Esophageal varicose veins
Thymus	Thymic remnants
Diaphragm	Diaphragmatic calcifications, Diaphragmatic elevation, Diaphragmatic thickening, Diaphragmatic relaxation, Hiatal hernia
Aorta	Aortic calcification, Aortic elongation, Aortic ectasia, Atheroma, Aortic stent, Thrombotic aneurysm, Aortic arch dissection, Chronic aortic dissection, Aortic thrombus
Spine	Vertebral arthrosis, Vertebral cyst, Vertebral bone thickening, Scoliosis, Vertebral angioma, Vertebral metastasis
Breast	Mastectomy (R+L), Mastectomy with bilateral prosthesis, Breast nodules/calcifications
Bone	Cyst, Rib lytic lesion, Rib bone thickening lesion, Metastasis, Lytic lesion,
Mediastinum	Pectum excavatum, Mediastinal shift, Lipoma of the thoracic wall, SVC thrombosis, SVC duplication, Azygos lobe

R, right; *L*, left; *SVC*, superior vena cava.

located in the lungs, mediastinum or upper abdomen, but only 2% were considered significant and underwent further analyses. In our study we also described minor lesions which made up 26.5 % of all lesion counted. In the 1326 patients studied with EBCT by Horton et al. [10], 103 (7.8%) had significant extracardiac disease requiring clin-

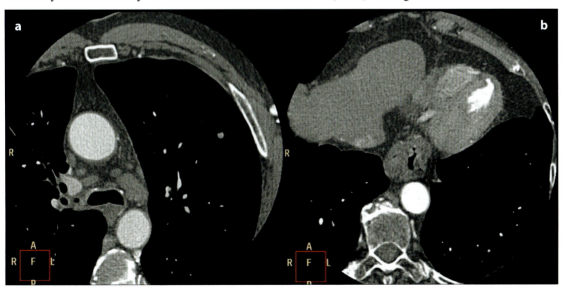

Fig. 18.2 Main examples of minor (mediastinal lymph nodes in **a**) and mild (hiatal hernia in **b**) incidental finding which should be preferably mentioned in the report for complete analysis of the dataset

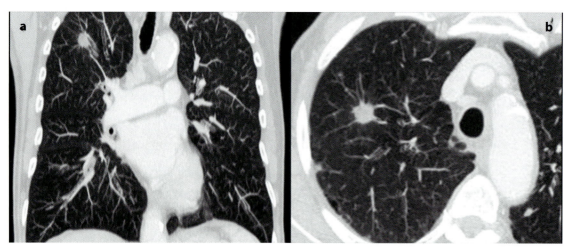

Fig. 18.3 Lung window setting with large FOV (**a**, **b**) in this by-pass patient shows a solitary proliferative nodule located at the apex of the right lung

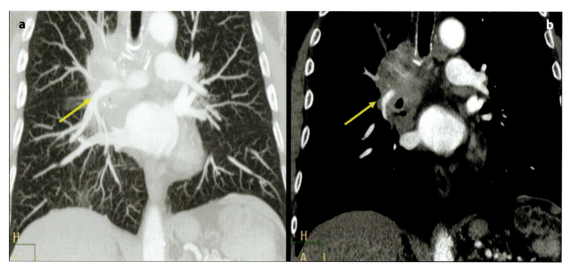

Fig. 18.4 Lung and mediastinal window settings chest show a large hilar carcinoma invading the main right pulmonary artery (*arrows* in **a**, **b**) and the ipsilateral bronchus

ical or imaging follow-up. These included 53 patients with noncalcified lung nodules < 1 cm, 12 patients with lung nodules > 1 cm, 24 patients with infiltrates, 7 patients with indeterminate liver lesions, 2 patients with sclerotic bone lesions, 2 patients with breast abnormalities, 1 patient with polycystic liver disease, 1 patient with esophageal thickening and 1 patient with ascites.

In conclusion many MDCT-CA studies are interpreted by radiologists or cardiologists who evaluate only the heart and the coronaries [11]. However, in addition to this information, examinations of the volume acquired with different window settings can demonstrate the presence of portions of the lungs, bony thorax, and the very first part of the upper abdomen. Using this field of view, most of the right and left lung over that section is visualized, thus making possible the identification and diagnosis of important noncardiac findings which can in some cases be significant.

18.4 Cardiac Incidental Findings in the Context of Chest CT

When performing chest CT without or with intravenous contrast material administration, abnormalities related to the coronary arteries and the heart can be detected. This is not a trivial observation since the chest CT is often performed for suspected thoracic disease and the heart may the source of symptoms even though this is not immediately evident from the clinical information collected.

For instance, cardiomegaly can be easily appreciated

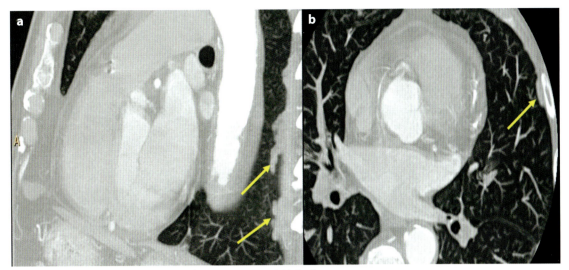

Fig. 18.5 Lung window setting in **a** and **b** depicting pleural thickenings

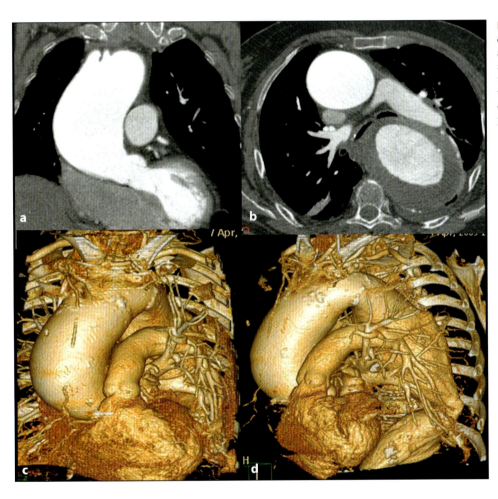

Fig. 18.6 MPR reformatting in coronal (**a**) and axial (**b**) plane and 3D VR images in **c** and **d** show a large aortic aneurysm which compresses the trachea and the main left bronchus thus explaining the chest pain and dyspnea of the patient

on chest CT, as well as different types of calcifications (Table 18.2). This approach has several implications both for patients undergoing chest CT for generic chest diseases and even more so for patients undergoing high resolution CT of the chest for screening purposes. In the latter case collateral cardiac findings may have the same importance as noncardiac findings. In addition they may need further investigation.

Table 18.2 Cardiac collateral findings on chest CT

Parameter	With CM	Description
Cardiomegaly	NO	Easily assessed by measuring normal proportions
Ventricular dilatation/hypertrophy	YES	Assessed by measuring normal proportions
Atrial dilatation	NO	Easily assessed by measuring normal proportions
Coronary Calcifications	NO	Can be visualized and also quantified using soft-medium convolution kernels
Heart Valve Calcifications	NO	Can be easily visualized
Pericardial calcifications	NO	Can be easily visualized
Pericardial thickening	NO	Can be visualized
Cardiac Thrombi	YES	Easy when thrombi are located in the left ventricle
Previous Myocardial Infarction	NO/YES	Hypodense layers within left ventricle wall

CM, contrast material.

References

1. Cademartiri F, Nieman K, Mollet N et al (2003) [Non-invasive 16-row spiral multislice computed tomography coronary angiography after one year of experience]. Ital Heart J Suppl 4:587-593
2. Cademartiri F, Runza G, Marano R et al (2005) Diagnostic accuracy of 16-row multislice CT angiography in the evaluation of coronary segments. Radiol Med 109:91-97
3. Pugliese F, Mollet NR, Runza G et al (2006) Diagnostic accuracy of non-invasive 64-slice CT coronary angiography in patients with stable angina pectoris. Eur Radiol 16:575-582
4. de Feyter P, Mollet N, Nieman K et al (2004) Noninvasive visualisation of coronary atherosclerosis with multislice computed tomography. Cardiovasc Radiat Med 5:49-56
5. Hunold P, Schmermund A, Seibel RM et al (2001) Prevalence and clinical significance of accidental findings in electron-beam tomographic scans for coronary artery calcification. Eur Heart J 22:1748-1758
6. Cademartiri F, Malago R, Belgrano M et al (2007) Spectrum of collateral findings in multislice CT coronary angiography. Radiol Med 112:937-948
7. Law YM, Huang J, Chen K et al (2008) Prevalence of significant extracoronary findings on multislice CT coronary angiography examinations and coronary artery calcium scoring examinations. J Med Imaging Radiat Oncol 52:49-56
8. Machaalany J, Yam Y, Ruddy TD et al (2009) Potential clinical and economic consequences of noncardiac incidental findings on cardiac computed tomography. J Am Coll Cardiol 54:1533-1541
9. Onuma Y, Tanabe K, Nakazawa G et al (2006) Noncardiac findings in cardiac imaging with multidetector computed tomography. J Am Coll Cardiol 48:402-406
10. Horton KM, Post WS, Blumenthal RS, Fishman EK (2002) Prevalence of significant noncardiac findings on electron-beam computed tomography coronary artery calcium screening examinations. Circulation 106:532-534
11. Rumberger JA (2006) Noncardiac abnormalities in diagnostic cardiac computed tomography: within normal limits or we never looked! J Am Coll Cardiol 48:407-408

Reporting in Cardiac CT

19

Erica Maffei, Chiara Martini, Udo Hoffmann, and Filippo Cademartiri

19.1 Introduction

The report is probably the most important part of cardiac computed tomography (CCT) and usually it is the last stage of the procedure. It should collect all the information concerning the patient's history and radiologic/clinical judgment together with images. A structured report is mandatory for a good CCT lab. The referring clinicians expect a report that they can understand and from which they can extrapolate the relevant information needed for patient care. Common criteria and language are therefore important, as it is for other imaging modalities (echocardiography, cardiac magnetic resonance imaging, nuclear cardiology, conventional coronary angiography - CAG), whenever possible. This will become more important from now on since CCT will be able to provide information on inducible ischemia and viability.

19.2 Requirements for Reporting (Table 19.1)

General principles are related to the exploitation of the full potential of the technique in terms of hardware and software. All tools for image processing should be used in order to avoid misinterpretation of artifacts and doubtful findings. Information delivery should be extended to stenosis and plaques.

19.3 Post-processing Techniques (Table 19.2)

All post processing techniques are important. Some of them are more suitable for diagnosis (axial images, multiplanar reformats, curved reformats) while others are more suitable for documentation (maximum intensity projections and volume rendering). However, there is a lot of flexibility between different techniques and they are all available at the same time when operating with CCT datasets. The user should be well trained in post-processing techniques and know all the advantages and disadvantages of each tool.

19.4 Parameters Included in the Report (Tables 19.3-19.5)

19.4.1 Patient Data

This part of the report includes demographics and database information.

19.4.2 CCT Scan

This part of the report should describe the hardware used for CCT (e.g. name, model, detector width, number of slice/rotation and tube configuration), the contrast material administered (i.e. volume, rate, type), ECG synchronization method (defining in which phase of the cardiac cycle images were acquired and/or reconstructed. This section should also mention which types of reformatting were performed for image analysis.

19.4.3 Medication

When preparing the patients, usually oral and/or intravenous drugs are administered. The type, route and dose of drugs should be noted.

E. Maffei (✉)
Cardiovascular Imaging Unit,
"Giovanni XXIII" Hospital,
Monastier di Treviso (TV), Italy

F. Cademartiri, G. Casolo, M. Midiri (eds.), *Clinical Applications of Cardiac CT*,
© Springer-Verlag Italia 2012

Table 19.1 Principles and requirements for CT reporting. (Modified from Raff GL et al., 2009)

Type	Principles and Requirements	Relevance
Hardware	Interpretation on 3-dimensional workstations equipped with dedicated software.	+++
	Images reviewed in the appropriate post-processing formats.	+++
	Interpreters should customize image reconstructions when appropriate.	+++
Quality	Data set should be previewed for artifacts.	+++
	Non-contrast studies should be reviewed prior to contrast studies.	+
	The coronary tree should be examined systematically.	+++
	Lesions should be reviewed in 3-dimensions.	++
Approach	Assess lesions for extent and quality of plaque, not just for stenosis severity.	+++
	Extra-coronary cardiac and thoracic anatomy should be always examined.	++

Table 19.2 Post-processing techniques for CCT reporting. (Modified from Raff GL et al., 2009)

Post-processing technique	Image analysis	Key images for report
Axial images	Required	Not required
Multi-planar reformation (MPR)	Required	Required
Maximum intensity projection (MIP)	Required	Required
Curved MPR (cMPR)	Not required but recommended	Not required but recommended
Volume-rendered (VR) reconstructions	Not required	Not required but recommended

Table 19.3 AHA coronary artery segment classification. (Modified from Raff GL et al., 2009)

Segment no.	Segment name	Abbreviation	Description
1	Proximal RCA	pRCA	Origin of the RCA (right coronary artery) to one-half the distance to the acute margin of heart
2	Mid RCA	mRCA	pRCA to the acute margin of heart
3	Distal RCA	dRCA	mRCA to origin of the PDA (posterior descending artery)
4	PDA from the RCA	r-PDA	PDA from RCA
16	PLB from the RCA	l-PLB	PLB (posterior-lateral branch) from RCA
5	Left Main	LM	Origin of Left Coronary to bifurcation into LAD (left anterior descending artery) and LCX (left circumflex artery)
6	Proximal LAD	pLAD	Origin of LAD to first large septal or D1 (first diagonal)
7	Mid LAD	mLAD	End of proximal LAD to one-half the distance to the apex
8	Distal LAD	dLAD	End of mid LAD to end of LAD
9	Diagonal 1	D1	First diagonal branch D1
10	Diagonal 2	D2	Second diagonal branch D2
11	Proximal LCX	pCX	End of LM to the origin of the OM1 (first obtuse marginal)
12	1st Obtuse Marginal	OM1	First OM1 traversing the lateral wall of the left ventricle
13	Mid and distal LCX	mCX	Traveling in the AV groove, distal to the first obtuse marginal branch to the end of the vessel or origin of the L-PDA (left posterior descending artery)
14	2nd Obtuse Marginal	OM2	Second marginal OM2
15	PDA from the LCX	l-PDA	PDA from LCX
17	Intermediate Branch	IMB	From LM between the LAD and LCX in case of a trifurcation
18	PLB from the LCX	l-PLB	PLB from Lcx

19.4.4 Heart Rate

Heart rate (mean and range) during the scan should be noted in the report as it represents direct evidence of image quality.

19.4.5 Coronary Calcium Score

When performed (alone or in combination with CCT), the coronary calcium score should always be mentioned since it is a well recognized prognosticator and indirect-

19 Reporting in Cardiac CT

Table 19.4 Reporting Requirements for CCT. (Modified from Raff GL et al., 2009)

Section	Description	Importance
Clinical Data		
General	Clinical Indication for the procedure and date	+++
Demographics	Name, date of birth, sex, referring clinician, height, weight	+++
History	Symptoms, risk factors, previous relevant diagnostic tests	+++
Scan		
Description	Scan type (eg, CT coronary angiography, calcium scoring, ventricular function, pulmonary vein, other)	++
Equipment	Scanner type, number of detectors, rotation time	++
Acquisition	Gating method	+++
	Tube voltage, dose modulation (if used)	+++
	Estimated radiation dose	++
Reconstruction	Slice thickness	
	Slice increment, reconstruction filter, phases of cardiac cycle	+++
Medications	Contrast type, volume and rate	+++
	b-blockers, nitroglycerin, or any other, if given	+++
Pt parameters	Complication(s), if present	+++
	Heart rate, arrhythmia, if present	++
Results		
Quality	Overall quality	+
	Presence and type of artifact and effect on interpretation	+++
	Coronary arteries	+++
	Calcium score (if calcium scan performed)	+++
	Coronary anomalies (origins and course), if present	+++
	Stenosis location and severity	+++
	Uninterpretable segments, arteries, or overall study	+++
	Stenosis plaque type: Calcified, noncalcified, mixed	+++
	Stenosis extent: Ulceration, length, ostial or branch involvement,	++
	Positive remodeling, tortuosity	+
	Use of SCCT stenosis severity classification	++
	Use of SCCT axial coronary segmentation model	++
	Calcium score percentile (if calcium scan performed)	++
	Use of AHA or CASS coronary segment model	+++
Non coronary vessels	Abnormalities of aorta, vena cavae, pulmonary veins/arteries	++
	Pulmonary vein morphology and ostia sizes	+++*
Cardiac chambers	Chamber dilation, masses, thrombus, shunts, etc etc	+++
	LV size and volume	+++
	LA volume	+++*
	RV size and volume	+++++
Function	LV wall motion (17 segment model)	++
Myocardium	LV ejection fraction (if functional data obtained)	+++
	End-diastolic LV wall thickness	++
Valves	Abnormal thickness, calcification, effusion	++
Pericardium	Abnormal aortic and mitral valve calcification, thickness	++
Chest	Abnormal Chest structure	+++
Conclusions	Coronary interpretation	+++
	Abnormal non-coronary cardiac findings	+++
	Abnormal non-cardiac findings	++
	Non-coronary cardiac interpretation (ventricular function, etc)	++
	Correlation to other or prior cardiac studies	++
	Clinical recommendations	+
Images	Representative coronary segments	++

*Mandatory for pre-ablation studies. *LV*, left ventricle; *RV*, right ventricle; *LA*, left atrium

Table 19.5 Stenosis Grading for CCT. (Modified from Raff GL et al., 2009)

	Qualitative	Method 1	Method 2
0	Normal Absence of plaque and luminal stenosis	Normal Absence of plaque and luminal stenosis	Normal Absence of plaque and no luminal stenosis
1	Minimal Plaque with negligible impact on lumen	Minimal Plaque with 25% stenosis	Mild Plaque with <39% stenosis
2	Mild Plaque with no flow-limiting stenosis	Mild 25%–49% stenosis	Moderate 40%–69% stenosis
3	Moderate Plaque with possible flow-limiting disease	Moderate 50%–69% stenosis	Severe 70%–99% stenosis
4	Severe Plaque with probable flow-limiting disease	Severe 70%–99% stenosis	Occluded
5	Occluded	Occluded	-

ly an indicator of confidence, since a progressively higher calcium score decreases specificity for significant obstructive CAD.

19.4.6 Coronary Arteries

First, the presence of normal anatomy vs. anatomical variants vs. coronary anomalies should noted (Fig.19.1). Then a segment-by-segment description of the coronary artery tree should be provided defining for each segment the presence of plaques (type and remodeling) and their impact of lumen (stenosis). Within these vessels, a brief description of any plaque causing non trivial luminal narrowing should be included (Table 19.5). It should be noted whether the plaque is predominantly calcified, non calcified, or mixed.

19.4.7 Cardiac Morphology

The presence of abnormalities at the level of cardiac chambers (e.g. size), myocardial wall thickness, cardiac valves (thickening, calcifications) should be described. The pericardium should also be described when pericardial effusion and/or thickening and/or pericardial calcifications are present. Cardiac masses and thrombi should also be described concerning site, anatomic relationship, morphology and patterns of contrast enhancement.

19.4.8 Cardiac Function

When retrospective ECG gating is applied, global and regional LV/RV function can be calculated. This is

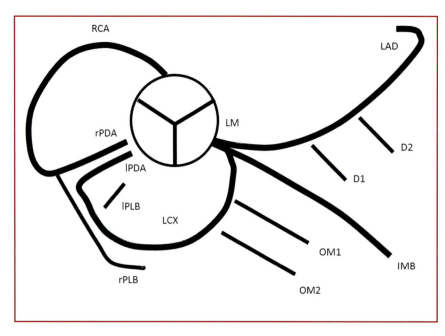

Fig. 19.1 AHA coronary artery segment classification. *RCA*, right coronary artery; *rPDA*, right posterior descending artery; *rPLB*, right posterior lateral branch; *LM*, left main; *LAD*, left anterior descending; *D1*, diagonal 1; *D2*, diagonal 2; *IMB*, intermediate branch; *LCX*, left circumflex; *OM1*, 1st obtuse marginal; *OM2*, 2nd obtuse marginal; *lPLB*, left posterior lateral branch; *lPDA*, left posterior descending artery. (Modified from Raff GL et al., 2009)

important especially if there are abnormalities related to a possible diagnosis.

19.4.9 Chest

All other structures comprised within the field of view should be assessed (i.e. aorta, mediastinum, lung parenchyma, pleura). Incidental findings may occur and sometimes may explain the symptoms leading the patient to CCT.

19.4.10 Overall Quality

When the quality of the CCT scan is suboptimal or less in a way that may compromise the confidence of coronary artery assessment, the user should mention it in the report. This is also valid when there are unassessable coronary segments.

19.4.11 Conclusions

At the end of the report a brief summary/conclusion of the results and the relationship with the indication for CCT should be written. This is important for addressing the specific questions and to indicate what may happen next.

19.5 Stenosis quantification

Stenosis quantification in CCT is semi-quantitative (Table 19.5). There is at the moment moderate consensus on how to grade stenosis. This is a tricky task since the clinicians may decide to send the patient directly to CAG or not depending on the degree of stenosis detected at CCT.

Suggested Readings

Achenbach S (2008) Quantification of coronary artery stenoses by computed tomography. JACC Cardiovasc Imaging 1(4):472-474

Budoff MJ, Achenbach S, Berman DS et al (2008) American Society of Nuclear Cardiology; Society of Atherosclerosis Imaging and Prevention; Society for Cardiovascular Angiography and Interventions; Society of Cardiovascular Computed Tomography. Task force 13: training in advanced cardiovascular imaging (computed tomography) endorsed by the American Society of Nuclear Cardiology, Society of Atherosclerosis Imaging and Prevention, Society for Cardiovascular Angiography and Interventions, and Society of Cardiovascular Computed Tomography. J Am Coll Cardiol 51:409-414

Cheng V, Gutstein A, Wolak A et al (2008) Moving beyond binary grading of coronary arterial stenoses on coronary computed tomographic angiography: insights for the imager and referring clinician. JACC Cardiovasc Imaging. 1:460-471

Hoe JW, Toh KH (2007). A practical guide to reading CT coronary angiograms-how to avoid mistakes when assessing for coronary stenoses. Int J Cardiovasc Imaging 23:617-33

LaBounty TM, Kim RJ, Lin FY et al (2010) Diagnostic accuracy of coronary computed tomography angiography as interpreted on a mobile handheld phone device. JACC Cardiovasc Imaging 3:482-490

LaBounty TM, Leipsic J, Srichai MB et al (2010) What is the optimal number of readers needed to achieve high diagnostic accuracy in coronary computed tomographic angiography? A comparison of alternate reader combinations. J Cardiovasc Comput Tomogr 4:384-390

Meijboom WB, Van Mieghem CA, van Pelt N et al (2008) Comprehensive assessment of coronary artery stenoses: computed tomography coronary angiography versus conventional coronary angiography and correlation with fractional flow reserve in patients with stable angina. J Am Coll Cardiol 52:636-643

Pugliese F, Hunink MG, Gruszczynska K et al (2009) Learning curve for coronary CT angiography: what constitutes sufficient training? Radiology 251:359-368

Raff GL, Abidov A, Achenbach S et al (2009) Society of Cardiovascular Computed Tomography. SCCT guidelines for the interpretation and reporting of coronary computed tomographic angiography. J Cardiovasc Comput Tomogr 3:122-136

Schroeder S, Achenbach S, Bengel F et al (2008) Working Group Nuclear Cardiology and Cardiac CT; European Society of Cardiology; European Council of Nuclear Cardiology. Cardiac computed tomography: indications, applications, limitations, and training requirements: report of a Writing Group deployed by the Working Group Nuclear Cardiology and Cardiac CT of the European Society of Cardiology and the European Council of Nuclear Cardiology. Eur Heart J 29:531-556

Training and Implementation in Cardiac CT

20

Erica Maffei, Chiara Martini, and Filippo Cademartiri

20.1 Introduction

Cardiac CT (CCT) is one of the major diagnostic innovations in cardiac imaging in the new millennium. It is the only tool able to noninvasively directly assess coronary artery disease (CAD).

Besides technologic issues cardiac CT (CCT) has several implications concerning implementation and training. Implementation may appear an easy task, especially from a radiologic perspective, since it could seem another type of vascular examination. In reality, the workflow and operational features with CT sections are significantly affected by CCT layout.

20.2 Training

Training in CCT is a major challenge. Several American and European scientific societies have defined adequate training for appropriate certification as 6 months' cumulative experience and 400 patient examinations, of which 100 should be reviewed while the procedure is ongoing and 300 in the presence of an expert examiner. However, these criteria were defined arbitrarily in 2005 and without having preliminarily assessed the real difficulty in guaranteeing that the diagnostic performance achieved is the one expected on the basis of results reported in the literature.

In a study by Pugliese et al. (2009) the authors verified whether intensive training for 1 year in a highly specialized center and with a high patient turnover enabled operators to achieve the expected diagnostic accuracy. The conclusion of the study was that one year is not sufficient. Based on this evidence there is currently the need to structure intensive and relatively long training courses in centers that fulfill the necessary requirements for whoever intends to carry out these diagnostic examinations (Fig. 20.1).

Another training area concerns pharmacology. For stress MRI the presence of a cardiologist is needed to administer the stressor drugs (i.e. dipyridamole, dobutamine, adenosine). In this case a heart which potentially has obstructed coronary arteries is subjected to stress and the aim is to detect acute iatrogenic myocardial ischemia. However, this must be performed under the expert guidance of a cardiologist or alternative medical professional able to manage complications associated with the procedure. With the upcoming application of stress CCT these requirements will become more important and will probably constitute training requirements.

During CCT the main drugs administered are beta-blockers. Available scientific evidence to date indicates an excellent safety profile for these drugs in expert centers. The presence of a cardiologist does not therefore appear to be a determining factor for the preparation and monitoring of patients undergoing CCT.

20.3 Implementation

The implementation of CCT requires a great deal of investment in technology and human resources and typically requires a long timeframe (Fig. 20.2). The technologic investments are extensive because the equipment needed to achieve adequate diagnostic standards is extremely costly. Moreover, constant improvements and changes in the reference standards leads to relatively rapid technologic obsolescence and thus the need for continuing investment.

The investment in human resources is particularly onerous in this case because professionals able and willing to dedicate themselves for at least one year (see Section 20.2 Training) to training and learning are needed. Although this can happen in a few specialization schools and centers, it is nevertheless frequently difficult to dedicate a resource for an entire year to CCT alone.

E. Maffei (✉)
Cardiovascular Imaging Unit,
"Giovanni XXIII" Hospital,
Monastier di Treviso (TV), Italy

F. Cademartiri, G. Casolo, M. Midiri (eds.), *Clinical Applications of Cardiac CT*,
© Springer-Verlag Italia 2012

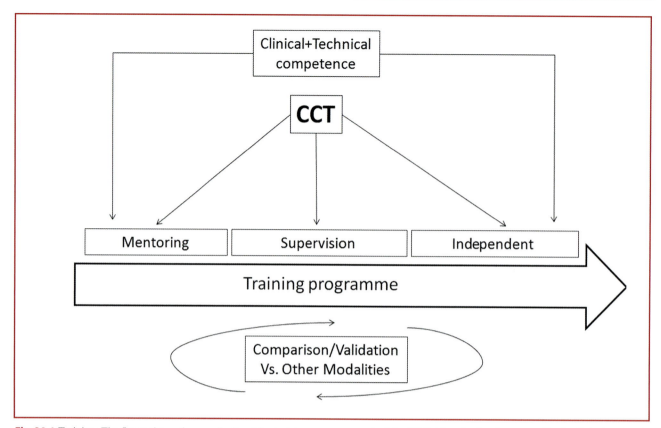

Fig. 20.1 Training. The figure shows the complexity of the training program required for CCT. After the development of basic clinical and technical competence the trainees should be exposed to a high number of CCT examinations with mentoring followed by supervision. In this phase it is important to expand the information collection to other imaging modalities to better understand the strength and limitations of CCT and perform internal validation of findings. At the end the trainees should perform the examination and reporting independently and constantly update clinical and technical competence. *CCT*, cardiac computed tomography

In addition to purely radiologic investment, the implementation of CCT requires at least equivalent investment of an organizational and management nature concerning the work-up of patients (i.e. collaboration and sharing of indications with nuclear medicine, cardiology and cardiac surgery departments, with other medical divisions focused on cardiologic aspects, with accident & emergency etc.), the ability to guarantee not only an elective service but also service in emergency situations (i.e. training is needed for >1 person among the radiologic staff), the sharing of information systems through which to convey pertinent cardiologic information (i.e. electronic departmental directories, cardiologic RIS/PACS systems), technician and nursing personnel. These factors are able to ensure the successful implementation of CTCA in a hospital situation and should be applied and managed in an appropriate way.

20.4 Integration

Besides training and implementation there is another chapter of a CCT program that requires planning. This is the integration between clinical aspects and other imaging modalities (Fig. 20.2). With the wide variety of imaging modalities available CCT should be managed to play the role in which it allows the optimization of resources and time. Low dose CCT is easily able to rule out obstructive CAD, thus avoiding multiple and repeated examination. It also provides relevant morphologic and prognostic information. In this context, the role CCT may play is probably a major one. More evidence is required in this field, although we can expect a very fast growth in CCT usage worldwide.

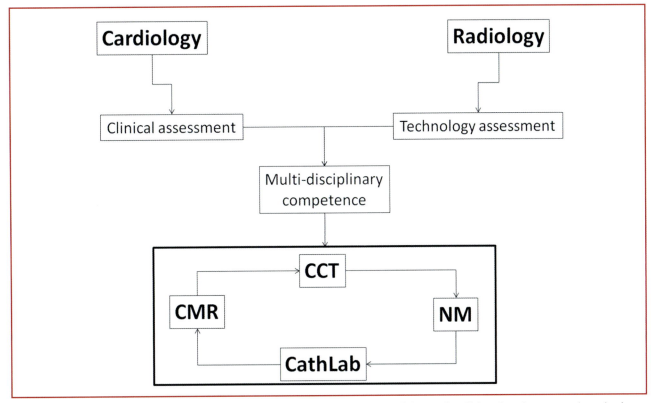

Fig. 20.2 Implementation. Full implementation of CCT requires the efforts from both radiology and cardiology in order to create the optimal conditions for the development of multidisciplinary competence. This competence can be managed by a cardiovascular imaging team in cooperation. *CCT*, cardiac computed tomography; *CMR*, cardiac magnetic resonance; *NM*, nuclear medicine

20.5 Conclusions

Adequate training is a key factor for the success of a CCT program. The logistics and implementation are also demanding.

Suggested Readings

Achenbach S (2008) Quantification of coronary artery stenoses by computed tomography. JACC Cardiovasc Imaging 1:472-474

Budoff MJ, Achenbach S, Berman DS et al (2008) American Society of Nuclear Cardiology; Society of Atherosclerosis Imaging and Prevention; Society for Cardiovascular Angiography and Interventions; Society of Cardiovascular Computed Tomography. Task force 13: training in advanced cardiovascular imaging (computed tomography) endorsed by the American Society of Nuclear Cardiology, Society of Atherosclerosis Imaging and Prevention, Society for Cardiovascular Angiography and Interventions, and Society of Cardiovascular Computed Tomography. J Am Coll Cardiol 51:409-414

Cheng V, Gutstein A, Wolak A et al (2008) Moving beyond binary grading of coronary arterial stenoses on coronary computed tomographic angiography: insights for the imager and referring clinician. JACC Cardiovasc Imaging 1:460-471

Hoe JW, Toh KH (2007) A practical guide to reading CT coronary angiograms—how to avoid mistakes when assessing for coronary stenoses. Int J Cardiovasc Imaging 23:617-633

LaBounty TM, Kim RJ, Lin FY et al (2010) Diagnostic accuracy of coronary computed tomography angiography as interpreted on a mobile handheld phone device. JACC Cardiovasc Imaging 3:482-490

LaBounty TM, Leipsic J, Srichai MB et al (2010) What is the optimal number of readers needed to achieve high diagnostic accuracy in coronary computed tomographic angiography? A comparison of alternate reader combinations. J Cardiovasc Comput Tomogr 4:384-390

Meijboom WB, Van Mieghem CA, van Pelt N et al (2008) Comprehensive assessment of coronary artery stenoses: computed tomography coronary angiography versus conventional coronary angiography and correlation with fractional flow reserve in patients with stable angina. J Am Coll Cardiol 52:636-643

Pugliese F, Hunink MG, Gruszczynska K et al (2009) Learning curve for coronary CT angiography: what constitutes sufficient training? Radiology 251:359-368

Raff GL, Abidov A, Achenbach S et al (2009) Society of Cardiovascular Computed Tomography. SCCT guidelines for the interpretation and reporting of coronary computed tomographic angiography. J Cardiovasc Comput Tomogr 3:122-136

Schroeder S, Achenbach S, Bengel F, et al (2008) Working Group Nuclear Cardiology and Cardiac CT; European Society of Cardiology; European Council of Nuclear Cardiology. Cardiac computed tomography: indications, applications, limitations, and training requirements: report of a Writing Group deployed by the Working Group Nuclear Cardiology and Cardiac CT of the European Society of Cardiology and the European Council of Nuclear Cardiology. Eur Heart J 29:531-556

Section IV
Technique

CT and CT Angiography - Basics

21

Erica Maffei, Chiara Martini, and Filippo Cademartiri

21.1 Introduction

The development of spiral computed tomography (CT) has seen the transformation from single slice to multislice scanners with 2, 4, 8, 16, 32, 40 and 64 detector rows with single or dual-source [1-9]. The most significant improvements include the increase in gantry rotation speed and consequent increase in temporal resolution, the increase in spatial resolution in the longitudinal axis, which is made possible by the use of thin collimations with broad volumetric acquisitions.

Noninvasive vascular imaging is an important application and cardiac CT angiography (CCT) has proven to be a valid alternative to digital subtraction angiography [3, 10-20]. Compared with the conventional examination, the dynamic CCT technique involves a number of additional variables which can influence the examination. The technique is made up of the following elements: the features related to image formation (scan and reconstruction parameters of the images) on the one hand and the geometry and timing of the bolus of contrast agent (infusion parameters, the volume and concentration of the bolus, the delay between delivery and the beginning of the scan) on the other. The latter are covered in another chapter.

With the optimization of these factors the selective visualization of the vessels studied can be obtained with the greatest possible spatial resolution.

Given the differences in the process of image formation between single-slice and multislice scanners, the techniques of administration and synchronization of the bolus of contrast agent need to be consequently adapted.

This chapter aims to define the fundamental parameters regarding image formation and the use of contrast agent, which are relevant for performing the CCT examination. CCT scans are formulated with single-slice and multislice spiral scanners.

E. Maffei (✉)
Cardiovascular Imaging Unit,
"Giovanni XXIII" Hospital,
Monastier di Treviso (TV), Italy

21.2 Spiral CT Angiography Technique

21.2.1 Factors Related to Image Formation

Image formation in CCT is determined by the scan and reconstruction parameters (Table 21.1). The optimization of these parameters aims to obtain the maximum possible spatial resolution in the longitudinal axis (z-axis), thus limiting image noise and stair-step artifacts. These are caused by the effects of aliasing, which produce the typical stair-step appearance associated with inclined surfaces in multiplanar reconstructions [21-24].

Collimation: this is the width of the X-ray beam in the longitudinal axis. In single-slice scanners the collimation is mainly defined by a collimator which determines the width of the X-ray beam which will strike the single row of detectors (Fig. 21.1a).

In multislice scanners the X-ray source is collimated with the width equivalent to the sum of the size of t he detectors (Fig. 21.1b, c). The geometry and thickness of the detector rows depends on the scanner and determines the minimum slice thickness and the number of slices per rotation (Fig. 21.1d). A thin collimation produces high spatial resolution in the longitudinal plane or z-axis (craniocaudal direction) and an increase in image noise [25].

Feed: this is the speed the table advances during the scan and is generally expressed per gantry rotation, although it can also be expressed per second.

Pitch: this corresponds to the table feed per rotation divided by the collimated detector width of all detector rows. It can be expressed as the ratio of the table feed per rotation either to the nominal section thickness or to the collimated beam thickness at isocenter. In the case of a single detector scanner the definitions equal each other. In multislice scanners, however, they are different, since the first provides a value which can be interpreted only by knowing the number of detector rows used, while the second provides a value relative to the data sampling along the z-axis (Fig. 21.2). In other words, the

F. Cademartiri, G. Casolo, M. Midiri (eds.), *Clinical Applications of Cardiac CT*,
© Springer-Verlag Italia 2012

Table 21.1 CCT protocols with different scanner generations in the study of the abdominal aorta and/or visceral vessels

Parameters	Single slice	4 slices	16 slices	64 slices
Scan				
Detectors	1	4	16	64 (32x2)
Collimation (mm)	3	1	0.75	0.6 (voxel 0.4 mm^3)
Tube voltage (kV)	120	120	120	120
Tube current (mAs)	140	140	140	140
Rotation time (ms)	750	500	500-420	330
Feed (mm/rotation)	4.5-6.0	4.0-6.0	12.0-18.0	19.2
Detector pitch	1-1.5	4-6	16-24	32
X-ray beam pitch	1-1.5	1-1.5	1-1.5	1
Scan time for 30 cm (s)	50-37.5	37.5-25	12.5-8.8	7
Reconstruction				
Effective slice thickness (mm)	3	1	0.75	0.6
Reconstruction increment (mm)	1	0.6	0.5	0.4
Field of view (mm)	250-300	250-300	250-300	250-300
Convolution kernel	medium	medium	medium	medium
Window (width/level)	600/200	600/200	600/200	600/200
Contrast agent				
Volume (mL)	140	120	100	80
Injection rate (mL/s)	4	4	4	4
Injection time (s)	35	30	25	20
Concentration (mgI/mL)	300-400	300-400	300-400	300-400
Bolus chaser (physiologic solution)	50 mL @ 4mL/s	50 mL @ 4mL/s	50 mL @ 4mL/s	50 mL @ 4mL/s
Venous access	antecubital	antecubital	antecubital	antecubital
Total administration time/ contrast agent+bolus chaser	35/47.5	30/42.5	25/37.5	20/32.5

pitch expresses the distance between the information used for image reconstruction. Generally speaking, a lower pitch produces greater image quality, greater scan times and greater spatial resolution [26].

Rotation time: this is the time required for the gantry supporting the radiation tube and the row of detectors to perform a rotation of 360°. A fast rotation time produces a faster scan time, with greater temporal resolution. High temporal resolution is vital in cardiac applications and coronary CCT, since it overcomes motion artifacts due to the beating heart.

Field of view (FOV) and matrix: this is the relationship between the real size and the pixel size of the image. An image can be divided into elementary units: the pixels (picture elements). The matrix defines the number of pixels which make up the image. With a constant matrix, an enlargement of the image sees a proportional increase in the size of its pixels. A smaller FOV will produce a depiction of the structures with smaller pixels and an increase in spatial resolution (Fig. 21.3). With the matrix remaining constant, a larger FOV will produce a decrease in the size of the same structures, which will be represented by larger pixels and a reduced spatial resolution.

Reconstruction increment: this parameter defines the distance between the two reconstructed slices. The slices are contiguous when this value equals the collimation (single-slice scanners) or the effective slice thickness (multislice scanners). The slices are superimposed when the reconstruction increment is lower than the slice thickness (Fig. 21.4). The overlapping of slices produces an increase in longitudinal spatial resolution by minimizing stair-step artifacts.

Effective slice thickness: multislice scanners can perform scans with thin collimations and slices which are later reconstructed with thicknesses different but always equal to or greater than the width of the detector (Fig. 21.5). This parameter is important for the data management and display of images. For example, in the case of a CT chest examination performed for suspected acute pulmonary embolism, a 16-MDCT acquisition with 0.75 mm collimation can be reconstructed with a 1 mm slice thickness for viewing on the screen and for multiplanar reconstructions. An additional reconstruction of the images with an effective slice thickness of 5 mm can be used for film image display.

21 CT and CT Angiography - Basics

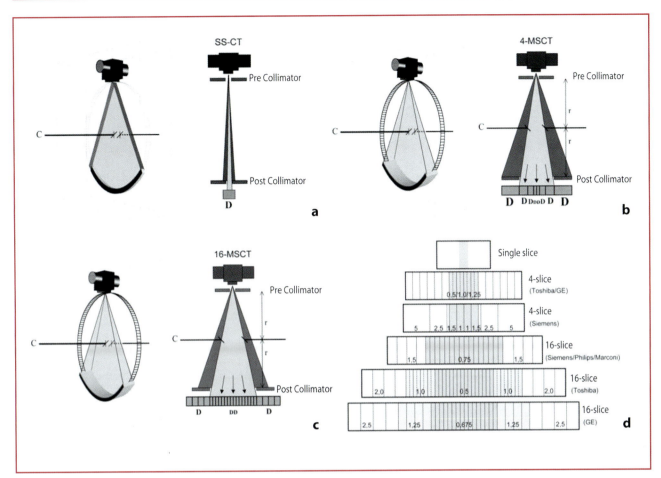

Fig. 21.1 The geometry of the X-ray beam in single-slice (**a**), 4-slice (**b**) and 16-slice (**c**) CT scanners are shown in relation to the detector width in the z-axis. Of significant interest is the maximum beam width between 4-slice and 16-slice scanners which is only modestly increased by the effective increase in the number of detectors (**d**). *SS-CT*, single-slice computed tomography; *4-MSCT*, 4-multislice computed tomography; *16-MSCT*, 16-multislice computed tomography; *C*, cone; *D*, detector; *r*, ray

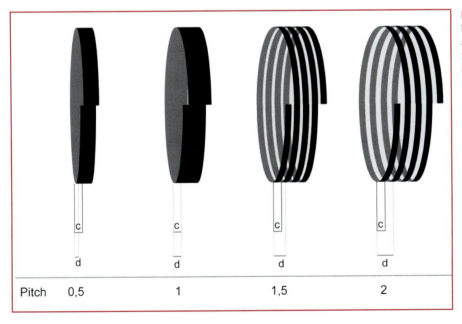

Fig. 21.2 Pitch is the relationship between table feed during a 360° rotation and collimation (c). By varying the table feed, the distance (d) between two points at 360° of rotation changes in the z-axis

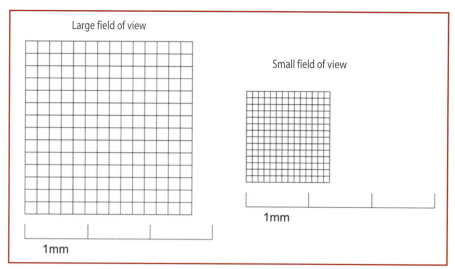

Fig. 21.3 With a constant matrix (in CT scanners where it is equal to 512x512 pixels) a reduction in the field of view produces a reduction in the size of the pixels and therefore an increase in spatial resolution in the scan plane

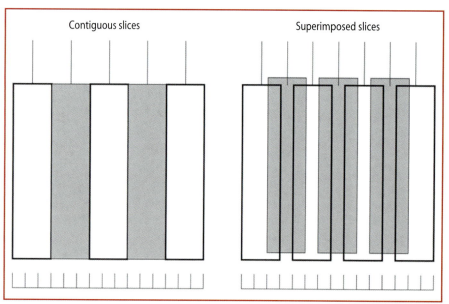

Fig. 21.4 The reconstruction increment describes the position of and therefore the mutual distance between the slices reconstructed in the z-plane. When the reconstruction increment is the same as the effective slice thickness slices are contiguous, whereas if it is lower the slices are superimposed. The ideal condition for CCT is an overlap between 50% and 70% of the effective thickness of the slice itself

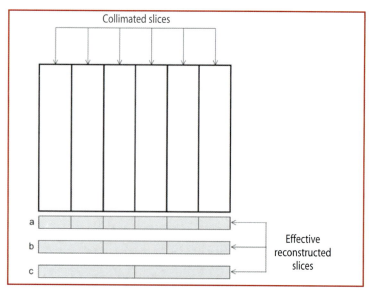

Fig. 21.5 With multislice scanners the reconstructed slice thickness can be the same or greater than the collimation used. Therefore, with the acquisition of a dataset with 0.75 mm collimation additional datasets can be obtained with greater effective slice thicknesses, such as 1 mm, 2 mm, 3 mm and so on

21 CT and CT Angiography - Basics

Table 21.2 Algorithm for the application of CCT protocols with single-slice scanners

1. Establish the scan volume
2. Establish the maximum duration of the scan time for the required kVp and mAs or for the maximum breath-hold capacity of the patient
3. Calculate the table speed (table movement in mm/s) and the table feed (speed/rotation time) for the faster rotation speed
4. Choose the thinnest slice allowed with a pitch (feed/collimation) less than or equal to 2
5. The scan duration and the use of bolus synchronization techniques (test bolus and bolus tracking) determine the injection rate of the contrast agent

Table 21.3 Algorithm for the application of CCT protocols with 4-slice scanners

1. Establish the scan volume
2. Choose the necessary spatial resolution in the z-axis (collimation 0.5, 1.0/1.25 or 2.0/2.5 mm)
3. Establish the maximum duration of the scan in the case of chest or abdominal CTA requiring breath-hold
4. Based on the scan volume, the collimation and the scan time, the pitch can be calculated (pitch = scan volume/(scan time x rotation time x number of detectors x collimation))
5. The scan duration and the use of bolus synchronization techniques (test bolus and bolus tracking) determine the injection rate of the contrast agent

Table 21.4 Algorithm for the application of CCT protocols with 16-slice scanners

1. Establish the scan volume
2. Choose the necessary spatial resolution in the z-axis (collimation 0.75/1.5 mm)
3. The scan duration and the use of bolus synchronization techniques (test bolus and bolus tracking) determine the injection rate of the contrast agent

Table 21.5 Algorithm for the application of CCT protocols with 64-slice scanners

1. Establish the scan volume
2. Choose the necessary spatial resolution in the z-axis (collimation 0.5/0.6 mm)
3. The scan duration and the use of bolus synchronization techniques (test bolus and bolus tracking) determine the injection rate of the contrast agent

Convolution filter (kernel): this is a reconstruction algorithm which attenuates or highlights the presence of certain image characteristics. For example, although they tend to increase image noise, high-frequency detail enhancing (sharp) kernels with their improvement in edge definition are generally used to more clearly visualize high-contrast structures (e.g. pulmonary parenchyma and bone).

21.3 Protocols (Tables 21.2-21.5; Fig. 21.6)

21.3.1 CCT with Single-slice Spiral Scanners

Single-slice CCT is limited by the need to obtain high spatial resolution in the z-axis with a broad scan volume in times compatible with patient breath-hold. These three factors essentially depend on collimation and pitch. In general, a thin collimation and high pitch is preferable to wide collimation and low pitch. Long scan times imply motion or respiratory artifacts, venous return and a longer injection of contrast agent.

21.3.2 CCT with 16-slice Spiral Scanners

Sixteen-slice CT scanners have reduced the limitations linked to the time required to perform the scan. The influence of pitch is limited. The significant features of 16-slice scanners include the geometry of the X-ray fan beam, the increased power of the radiation tube, and the speed of data transfer from the rotating system to the computer buffers receiving the raw data [1, 2, 27, 28].

21.3.3 CCT with 64-slice Spiral Scanners

Sixty-four-slice CT scanners eliminate the limitations related to the time required for performing the examina-

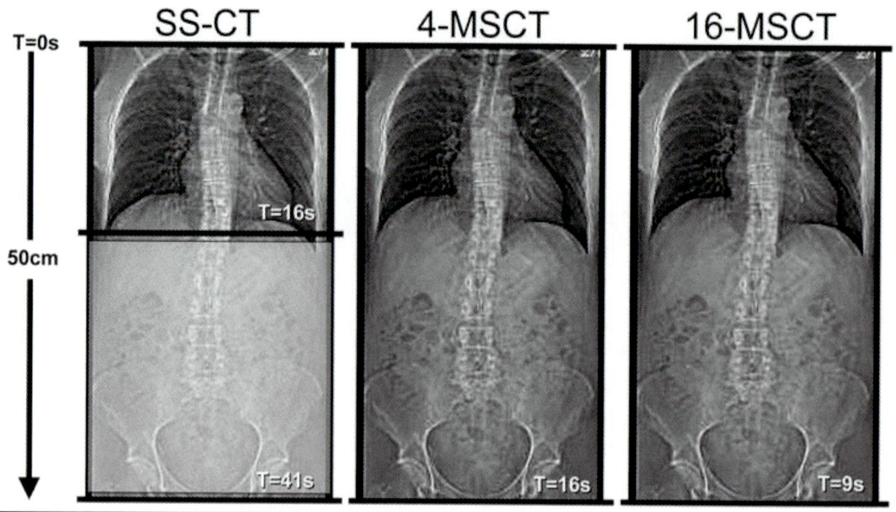

Fig. 21.6 Examples of the performance of different CT scanners. The figure depicts several examples of thoracoabdominal scans performed with single-slice, 4-slice and 16-slice scanners with the relative scan times and possible parameters. *T*, time; *ESW*, effective slice width; *HR-CCT*, high resolution CT angiography

	SS-CT	4-MSCT	16-MSCT
Collimation	8mm	4x2.5 mm	16x1.5 mm
Pitch	1.5	1.5	1.5
Rotation Time	1000ms	500ms	500ms
ESW	8mm	3,4,5,6,7,8, or 10mm	2,3,4,5,6,7,8, or 10mm
HR-CTA	111s (with collimation 3mm)	36s (with collimation 1mm)	18s (with collimation 0.75mm)

tion. Pitch has no influence except for the purposes of obtaining an improved signal-to-noise ratio or in the management of obese patients.

21.3.4 CCT with >64-slice Spiral Scanners

Recently, all vendors introduced a new generation of CT scanners with >64 slice. The scanners range from 256 to 640 slices depending on design and hardware upgrade. The limitations concerning coverage are basically absent using these types of scanners. The issues are mainly related to scan speed. In fact, the scanners are so fast in finishing the scan range that it has become possible to miss the proper first pass arterial phase for CT angiography. On the other hand, thanks to their high speed these scanners have made perfusion imaging possible.

21.3.5 Image Reconstruction

The use of 16-slice scanners shifts the vital stage of the examination to the image reconstruction phase. For example, the reconstruction of a scan with a collimation of 0.75 mm can be done with an effective slice thickness of 1.0 mm (this reduces image noise and improves the quality of multiplanar reconstructions, MIP and volume rendering) and a reconstruction increment of 0.5-0.6 mm. A second dataset can be reconstructed for film image display, usually with 3 mm thickness and contiguous slices. Additional reconstructions can be dedicated to regions of interest, such as stenoses with lower effective thicknesses (0.75 mm), more marked overlapping (0.4 mm), and high-frequency filters (sharp and/or dedicated kernels) to study the characteristics of atherosclerotic plaque (composition and calcifications) and the presence of stents (position and patency).

21.4 Discussion

Spiral CT scanners are able to acquire data volumes and reconstruct images in arbitrary points in the z-axis, thus modifying the imaging approach from exclusively in the axial plane to volumetric imaging (Fig. 21.7). With single-slice scanners the acquisition (scan) phase and the reconstruction phase are relatively concomitant in clinical practice, with the exception of some cases such as the algorithms for bone and lung parenchyma applied to scans performed for the visualization of soft tissue.

This approach is dictated by hardware/software limitations (elevated reconstruction time of the individual image) and by the low spatial resolution of the scanners.

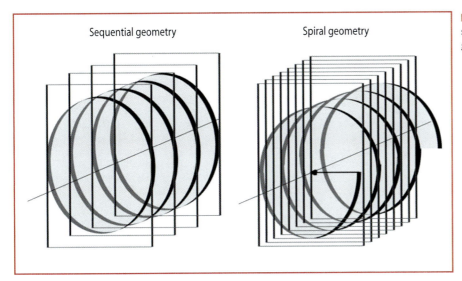

Fig. 21.7 Example of typical sequential scan geometry compared with spiral geometry

With the advent of multislice scanners the scan and reconstruction phases have become progressively separate. The introduction of 16-slice scanners further tipped the emphasis towards the management of data produced by the spiral CT scanners. Indeed the number of collimation protocols has been reduced to two or three, reconstruction times are shorter and the availability of postprocessing instruments has increased.

In the setting of CCT and CT in general, image postprocessing is the final and perhaps the most important phase. There are fundamentally two features influencing the effectiveness of this phase: the first is the processing speed of the workstation data, and the second is the skill of the operator in processing the data volume. Current computer speeds are capable of easily managing dataset >500 images (i.e. >250 Mb).

The limitation remains the analysis of the information by the operator. The use of a workstation is therefore crucial for visualizing all of the images and for performing three-dimensional reconstructions, since it is unthinkable that a radiologist analyze 500 images on conventional film. The time required for an expert operator to evaluate a thoracoabdominal angiographic scan acquired with a 16-slice scanner of a patient with multiregional vascular disease and abdominal aortic aneurysm can easily reach an hour or more. This is due to the amount of data to analyze and the quantity of information contained in a high-resolution dataset. This increase in information for each scan tends to increase the reporting time. The superabundance of information especially of processing techniques creates an evident medical-legal problem, since the same dataset can be examined in a variety of ways. The possibility of memorizing the parameters with which the dataset was visualized and processed has been met with reservation. However, there are limits to the standardization of the examination.

References

1. Flohr T, Stierstorfer K, Bruder H et al (2002) New technical developments in multislice CT - Part 1: Approaching isotropic resolution with sub-millimeter 16-slice scanning. Rofo 174:839-845
2. Flohr T, Bruder H, Stierstorfer K et al (2002) New technical developments in multislice CT, Part 2: sub-millimeter 16-slice scanning and increased gantry rotation speed for cardiac imaging. Rofo 174:1022-1027
3. Nieman K, Cademartiri F, Lemos PA et al (2002) Reliable noninvasive coronary angiography with fast submillimeter multislice spiral computed tomography. Circulation 106:2051-2054
4. Flohr T, Stierstorfer K, Raupach R et al (2004) Performance evaluation of a 64-slice CT system with z-flying focal spot. Rofo 176:1803-1810
5. Nikolaou K, Flohr T, Knez A et al (2004) Advances in cardiac CT imaging: 64-slice scanner. Int J Cardiovasc Imaging 20:535-540
6. Scheffel H, Alkadhi H, Plass A et al (2006) Accuracy of dual-source CT coronary angiography: first experience in a high pre-test probability population without heart rate control. Eur Radiol 16:2739-2747
7. Achenbach S, Ropers D, Kuettner A et al (2006) Contrast-enhanced coronary artery visualization by dual-source computed tomography–initial experience. Eur J Radiol 57:331-335
8. Flohr TG, McCollough CH, Bruder H et al (2006) First performance evaluation of a dual-source CT (DSCT) system. Eur Radiol 16:256-268
9. Johnson TR, Nikolaou K, Wintersperger BJ et al (2006) Dual-source CT cardiac imaging: initial experience. Eur Radiol 16:1409-1415
10. Achenbach S, Ulzheimer S, Baum U et al (2000) Noninvasive coronary angiography by retrospectively ECG-gated multislice spiral CT. Circulation 102:2823-2828
11. Chung JW, Park JH, Im JG et al (1996) Spiral CT angiography of the thoracic aorta. Radiographics 16:811-824
12. Cinat M, Lane CT, Pham H et al (1998) Helical CT angiography in the preoperative evaluation of carotid artery stenosis. J Vasc Surg 28:290-300

13. de Monye W, van Strijen MJ, Huisman MV et al (2000) Suspected pulmonary embolism: prevalence and anatomic distribution in 487 consecutive patients. Advances in New Technologies Evaluating the Localisation of Pulmonary Embolism (ANTELOPE) Group. Radiology 215:184-188

14. Horton KM, Fishman EK (2000) 3D CT angiography of the celiac and superior mesenteric arteries with multidetector CT data sets: preliminary observations. Abdom Imaging 25:523-525

15. Marro B, Valery CA, Bitard A et al (2000) Intracranial aneurysm on CTA: demonstration using a transparency volume-rendering technique. J Comput Assist Tomogr 24:96-98

16. Luboldt W, Straub J, Seemann M et al (1999) Effective contrast use in CT angiography and dual-phase hepatic CT performed with a subsecond scanner. Invest Radiol 34:751-760

17. Rubin GD, Napel S (1997) Helical CT angiography of renal artery stenosis. AJR Am J Roentgenol 168:1109-1111

18. Rubin GD, Shiau MC, Leung AN et al (2000) Aorta and iliac arteries: single versus multiple detector-row helical CT angiography. Radiology 215:670-676

19. Rubin GD, Zarins CK (1995) MR and spiral/helical CT imaging of lower extremity occlusive disease. Surg Clin North Am 75:607-619

20. Rieker O, Duber C, Schmiedt W et al (1996) Prospective comparison of CT angiography of the legs with intraarterial digital subtraction angiography. AJR Am J Roentgenol 166:269-276

21. Yen SY, Rubin GD, Napel S (1999) Spatially varying longitudinal aliasing and resolution in spiral computed tomography. Med Phys 26:2617-2625

22. Fleischmann D, Rubin GD, Paik DS et al (2000) Stair-step artifacts with single versus multiple detector-row helical CT. Radiology 216:185-196

23. Brink JA, Heiken JP, Wang G et al (1994) Helical CT: principles and technical considerations. RadioGraphics 14:887-893

24. Wang G, Vannier MW (1994) Stair-step artifacts in three-dimensional helical CT: an experimental study. Radiology 191:79-83

25. Wang G, Vannier MW (1994) Spatial variation of section sensitivity profile in spiral computed tomography. Med Phys 21:1491-1497

26. Wa ng G, Vannier MW (1997) Optimal pitch in spiral computed tomography. Med Phys 24:1635-1639

27. Fuchs T, Krause J, Schaller S et al (2000) Spiral interpolation algorithms for multislice spiral CT—part II: measurement and evaluation of slice sensitivity profiles and noise at a clinical multislice system. IEEE Trans Med Imaging 19:835-847

28. Schaller S, Flohr T, Klingenbeck K et al (2000) Spiral interpolation algorithm for multislice spiral CT—part I: theory. IEEE Trans Med Imaging 19:822-834

CT of the Heart: Scan Technique

22

Erica Maffei, Chiara Martini, and Filippo Cademartiri

22.1 Introduction

For several years now computed tomography (CT) scanners have been available which enable the simultaneous acquisition of 64 slices per rotation. The technology has been updated such CT scanners are now available which are equipped with up to 320 slices and dual source.

The additional improvement in spatial and temporal resolution of this new equipments has already provided excellent results in the field of cardiac imaging. In the future the optimization of protocols will enable cardiac computed tomography angiography (CCT) to reach levels of diagnostic accuracy similar to those of invasive techniques.

22.2 64-slice Computed Tomography

The most important components of a CT system are the X-ray tube and the system of detectors. The combination of a fast rotation time and multislice acquisitions is particularly important for cardiac applications [1, 2]. The latest generation of 64-slice CT meets these requirements. They are able to acquire 64 submillimeter slices per rotation and routinely achieve excellent image quality and the visualization of small-diameter vessels of the coronary circulation, combining isotropic spatial resolution (0.4 mm³) with gantry rotation speeds of 0.33 s. They also redefine the CT methodology of analyzing coronary plaque and evaluating stent lumens.

Until a few years ago CT systems had only a single row of detectors, which meant that for each rotation they were able to acquire only one slice. These systems were followed by others known as multislice or multidetector-row, featuring many detector rows positioned in a two-dimensional array. During a rotation numerous contigu-

ous slices are acquired. As a result, a broader region of the body can be acquired in the same timeframe, with an improvement in image quality. This also has the advantage of drastically reducing examination times, which is an important factor given that thoracic and abdominal examinations require the patient to maintain breath-hold to guarantee image quality is not compromised by chest motion. The clinical impact of the new technology lies in the improvement in image quality in terms of both spatial and temporal resolution. The improvement in spatial resolution regards numerous features of noninvasive coronary imaging:

- it increases the ability to visualize small-diameter vessels (e.g. the distal coronary branches) [3];
- it increases the ability to quantify calcium in that it reduces blooming artifacts;
- it enables the reduction of blooming artifacts in stents and therefore enables the visualization of the stent lumen;
- it improves the definition of the presence of coronary plaques and better quantifies their characteristics (volume, attenuation, etc.).

The improvement in temporal resolution influences many other aspects of noninvasive coronary imaging:

- it increase the ability to freeze images in the cardiac cycle;
- it enables additional reconstruction windows to be found within the cardiac cycle;
- it increases the performance of the system when left ventricular function needs to be evaluated
- it reduces scan time.

The technical characteristics of each scanner vary according to the model and their technological development is ongoing and rapid. The precise temporal resolution of the images obtained by CT scanners depends on many factors: gantry rotation speed, size and position of the field of view in the scan volume, and the image reconstruction and post-processing algorithms. In reality, the data acquired at half a rotation of the gantry are enough to reconstruct a single tomographic image. The temporal resolution of the latest CT scanners therefore approximate 165 ms [4-6].

E. Maffei (✉)
Cardiovascular Imaging Unit,
"Giovanni XXIII" Hospital,
Monastier di Treviso (TV), Italy

F. Cademartiri, G. Casolo, M. Midiri (eds.), *Clinical Applications of Cardiac CT*,
© Springer-Verlag Italia 2012

This can be enough to obtain images of the heart during the diastolic phase (when cardiac motion is at a minimum) free of obvious motion artifacts if the heart rate (HR) is <70 beats per minute.

22.3 Patient Selection

22.3.1 Inclusion Criteria

Normally inclusion criteria for the scan are HR<70 bpm (spontaneous or induced by beta-blockers) and ability to maintain breath-hold for a period compatible with the scan time [2, 3, 7]. Both these criteria are aimed at avoiding motion artifacts. In the first case the problem derives from residual motion of the coronary artery present in each phase of the cardiac cycle. In conditions of bradycardia the diastolic interval is longer, which translates into an increased duration of end-diastole, when the heart and the coronary arteries are almost motionless. Even though CCT can be diagnostic with a higher HR, motion artifacts progressively reduce the number of segments which can be correctly visualized [8]. The second criterion aims to avoid artifacts associated with respiratory motion. Evidently the respiratory motion of the patient during the scan can drastically affect the quality and quantity of information acquired.

22.3.2 Exclusion Criteria

Patients with a HR = 70 bpm, known allergies to iodinated contrast agent, renal insufficiency (serum creatinine >120 mmol/L), pregnancy, respiratory failure, unstable clinical conditions and severe heart failure are excluded from the CCT study.

The problems associated with an elevated HR have been described above. When a patient reports having had a slight or intermediate allergic reaction to iodinated contrast agent in the past the scan can be performed after desensitization with antihistamines and corticosteroids. In the advent of renal insufficiency, the administration of contrast agent may be better tolerated if an iso-osmolar agent is used and/or if the patient is adequately hydrated prior to contrast agent injection [9]. In pregnancy and in infants the scan should only be performed when the diagnostic information cannot be obtained in any other way. Respiratory failure and unstable clinical conditions can impede appropriate breath-hold during the scan. Patients with severe heart failure are generally unable to maintain the supine position and have an elevated HR, which as stated above is a contraindication to CCT. Due to their conditions, there is an absolute contraindication to the extemporaneous administration of beta-blockers in these patients.

22.4 Scan Parameters for CCT

The ideal protocol enables high spatial resolution (thin collimation), high temporal resolution (fast gantry rotation) and low radiation dose (prospective modulation of the tube current synchronized to the ECG [10]) compatible with a good signal-to-noise ratio. The main protocols are covered in another chapter, so the following sections are limited to outlining some general principles.

Regardless of the number of slices used, spatial and temporal resolution need to be as high as possible, all the while remaining compatible with the other scan parameters. The final objective is to obtain a scan during an easily performed breath-hold.

The duration of the scan is essentially linked to the number of slices and the pitch: generally <0.5 and more often <0.3. This allows for the oversampling of data which characterizes CT of the heart. Multisegment reconstructions should be avoided, partly because there is no evidence to suggest they are able to compensate for a poor relationship between effective temporal resolution (i.e. the width of the reconstruction time window) and HR. This relationship is favorable when the duration of the diastolic phase enables the time window to be placed in a moment of the cardiac cycle when the coronary arteries are motionless long enough for the X-ray tube to complete a 180° rotation. The tube current is modulated and managed to reduce the radiation dose, even though an elevated tube current generally produces better contrast resolution.

22.5 Retrospective Gating

The acquisition of image data in CCT is continuous during the cardiac cycle, such that the data corresponding to the phase when cardiac motion is at a minimum need to be retrospectively extracted to minimize blurring and motion artifacts (Fig. 22.1) [5, 6]. This process is called cardiac gating (Fig. 22.2). Once the data have been acquired they can be reconstructed with retrospective gating in any phase of the cardiac cycle by shifting the initial point of the image reconstruction window relative to the R-wave. Therefore, the combination of z-interpolation and cardiac gating enable a stack of parallel tomographic images to be generated which represent the heart in the same phase of the cardiac cycle [5, 6]. A real optimization of retrospective gating is yet to be achieved.

To obtain images in the diastolic phase, some opera-

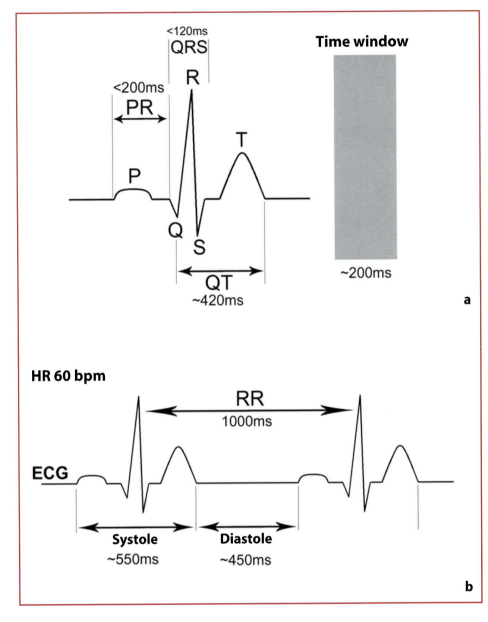

Fig. 22.1 Baseline ECG in MDCT coronary angiography. The cardiac cycle is composed of a systole and a diastole. Systole involves contraction of the atria, followed by contraction of the ventricles. The synchronized contraction is guided by a conducting system which arises from the sinoatrial node in the right atrium. The impulse then propagates to the atrioventricular node via the walls of the atria. From the atrioventricular node the impulse is transmitted via the conducting system across the septum and the ventricular walls. This phenomenon is depicted by the ECG trace, which shows the typical sequence of waves (**a**) P-wave (atrial contraction), QRS complex (ventricular contraction), T-wave (ventricular repolarization). Normally the P-R interval is <120 ms, the QRS complex is <80 ms and the Q-T interval is ~320 ms. Therefore, the duration of a complete systolic contraction with repolarization wave is ~550 ms. The diastolic period is ~450 ms. This means that for a HR of 60 bpm systole and diastole account for 55% and 45% of the cardiac cycle, respectively (**b**). The ~200 ms windows for the ECG retrospectively gated reconstruction obtainable with MDCT coronary angiography is generally placed in the diastolic phase (**a**). The most generally favorable position extends from mid- to end-diastole just prior to the P-wave. *QRS*, QRS complex; *PR*, PR interval; *T*, T wave; *P*, P wave; *Q*, Q wave; *S*, S wave; *QT*, QT interval; *RR*, RR interval; *ECG*, electrocardiogram

tors reconstruct the images in relation to the phase (i.e. a percentage) of the cardiac cycle (typically between 50% and 60% of the R-R interval), whereas others use the time window of the absolute interval prior to the peak of the next R-wave (typically 350-400 ms) [11, 12]. Multiple reconstructions are usually performed in different time windows, and the physician/technician successively selects the dataset where motion artifacts are minimal, paying particular attention to the visualization of the right coronary artery [13]. In CCT different time windows can be optimized and used in the same patient for the visualization of the left and right coronary arteries [4, 12, 13].

Improving the temporal resolution of the CCT scan by increasing gantry rotation speed is subject to obvious limitations. To overcome these difficulties new data post-processing strategies have been proposed to further increase temporal resolution. With the simultaneous acquisition of multiple slices and the relative overlapping of the volume acquired, multisegment reconstructions can be created.

In a multisegment reconstruction data acquired in the same cardiac phase but from different cardiac cycles are combined in a single image. In this case the temporal resolution will depend on the number and size of the segments used for the creation of a single image, but it will be higher that derived from a single segment [5]. This technique is sensitive to variations in beat-per-beat HR

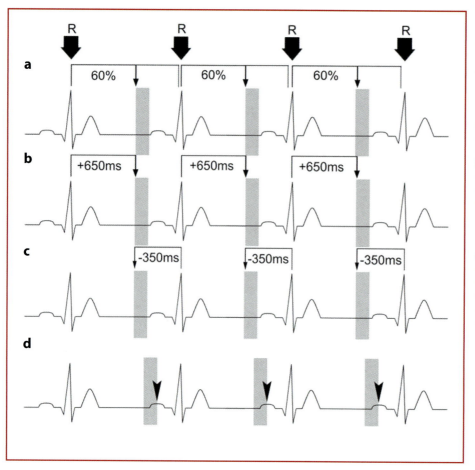

Fig. 22.2 Retrospective cardiac gating techniques. The figure depicts different strategies for cardiac gating in MDCT coronary angiography.
a Probably the most widely used strategy: percentage relative delay. The software calculates the distance from one R-wave to the next and positions the time window at a defined point based on the percentage of the entire R-R interval.
b Absolute delay. With this strategy the time window is placed according to a fixed delay time after the previous R-wave. **c** Absolute reverse delay. With this strategy the time window is placed with a fixed time delay prior to the next R-wave.
d With this strategy the final portion of the time window is positioned at the peak of the P-wave. The aim of this approach is to "strike" the final moment of cardiac akinesia prior to systolic contraction

and the current implementation of these algorithms does not always improve image quality [14].

22.6 Prospective ECG Triggering

Prospective ECG triggering, a technique which has already been available for several years, has recently been re-introduced into clinical practice (Fig. 22.3). With this technique images are acquired in a sequential manner only during the phase of interest in the cardiac cycle (i.e. during diastole) resulting in a dramatic reduction of the radiation dose. This technique has been utilized for many years in electron beam computed tomography (EBCT), widely used in North America and Asia, for risk stratification through quantification of coronary calcium (Calcium Score). The value of EBCT lies in its very high temporal resolution (50-100 ms) which means that it does not require all the phases of the cardiac cycle to freeze the movement of the coronaries during a heartbeat. The 4- and 16-detector row CT scanners have temporal resolutions of 250 ms and 200 ms, respectively, and thus cannot utilize prospective ECG triggering. With the 64-detector row CT scanner generation the temporal resolution has come down to 165-175 ms, thus enabling better management of heart rate. With this scanner generation it has been possible to re-introduce prospective ECG triggering in patients with very slow and regular heart rates. Prospective ECG triggering technique in use today is an improved version of the former in that it permits the width of the diastolic acquisition window to be adapted as appropriate. In this way the CT operator can modify the temporal acquisition window at his discretion in order to perform additional image reconstructions in the diastolic phase as necessary. The radiation dose reduction permitted by prospective ECG triggering is significant, in fact, it is usually possible to reduce the effective dose to less than 5 mSv (see Chapter 26).

22.7 Image Reconstruction

When the scan is performed in a correctly indicated patient and the inclusion/exclusion criteria have been satisfied, image reconstruction can be easily performed and the dataset obtained proves free from motion artifacts.

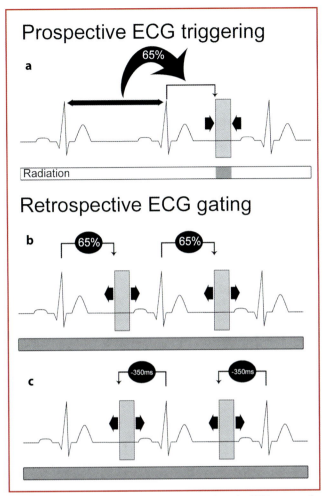

Fig. 22.3 Scan technique for CCT. Scan technique in CCT are mostly related to synchronization techniques. **a** Prospective (sequence) ECG triggering ("step-and-shoot"). **b**, **c** Retrospective (spiral) ECG gating. *CCT*, cardiac computed tomography angiography

According to the literature, the techniques able to provide diagnostic images are based on few reconstructions concentrated from the mid- to end-diastole (the time windows are positioned at about 400 ms prior to the next R-wave or at 60% of the R-R interval). A variety of approaches can be used for the reconstructions. At least four different strategies can be listed (Fig. 22.4):

1. relative delay strategy, whereby the delay time is a percentage of the R-R interval [15];
2. absolute delay strategy, whereby the delay time is constant after the previous R wave [15];
3. absolute reverse delay strategy, whereby the delay time is constant prior to the next R-wave [15];
4. end of the time window positioned at the peak of the P-wave [16].

There is no evidence to suggest that one method is better than the others. All four strategies can be used, but this will largely depend on the degree of experience of the operator and to a lesser extent on the capabilities of the software/hardware, the type of change in the HR and the time available for the reconstructions. The phase of the cardiac cycle which provides the most information is between mid- and end-diastole, since at the end of the contraction of the heart coronary artery motion is at a minimum.

Other reconstruction parameters are relevant for obtaining an image of diagnostic quality. The effective slice thickness is usually slightly wider than the minimum possible collimation so as to improve the signal-to-noise ratio of the image. The reconstruction increment should be about 50% of the effective slice thickness so as to improve spatial resolution and the overlap in the z-axis. The field of view should be as small as possible to include the entire heart, so as to fully exploit the image matrix which is constant (512x512 pixels). The convolution kernel should be half way between noise and image quality. In general, medium convolution kernels are used for coronary artery imaging. When the coronary arteries are highly calcified or stents are present, sharper convolution kernels may be used: although they tend to increase image noise, they usually improve the visualization of the vessel wall or the structure of the stent and its lumen.

22.8 Image Evaluation

There is still no standardized technique for the evaluation of CCT images. In terms of repeatability, the performance of CCT is currently operator-dependent [17].

The evaluation is generally performed with the American Heart Association classification in 15 or 16 coronary segments [18]. With this classification in mind, the operator carefully observes the clinically more important segments (Fig. 22.5).

The studies conducted to date have demonstrated the ability of CCT to identify significant stenoses, which are defined as a reduction in lumen diameter = 50% [2, 3, 7]. The evaluation is always done in a semi-quantitative fashion. The first step is to observe the axial images by scrolling the dataset to evaluate whether there are any pertinent findings which do not regard the coronary arteries. At the same time, the location of the cardiac structures can be checked (e.g. the great thoracic vessels, the cardiac valves, the atria, the ventricles, etc.), including the coronary arteries to identify the presence of significant morphologic anomalies.

The next step involves the evaluation of the multiplanar reconstructions (MPR).

For each vessel there is a dedicated plane which facilitates its correct and complete visualization. The main

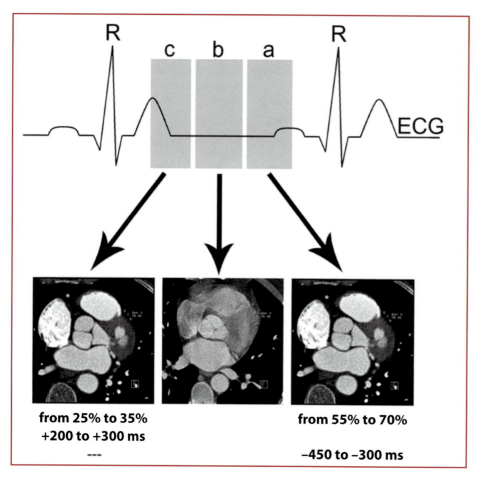

Fig. 22.4 Positioning the reconstruction time window. Several principles need to be borne in mind regarding the positioning of the time window when performing image reconstruction in MDCT coronary angiography. The operator should concentrate on three main areas of the ECG trace. The first (a) is the end-diastolic phase. In this phase the ventricle has completed filling, just prior to atrial systole and motion is at a minimum. The second phase (b) is the early-mid diastolic phase. In this phase the heart is filling and there is generally residual motion which does not allow adequate coronary artery imaging. The third phase (c) is end-systole. In this phase the heart is in isovolumetric contraction and motion is at a minimum. The images obtained in this phase can be just as valid as those obtained at end-diastole and in a number of cases even better. *R*, R wave; *ECG*, electrocardiogram; *ms*, milliseconds

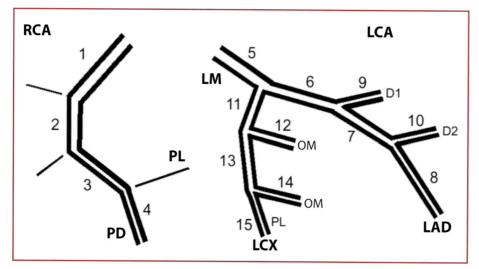

Fig. 22.5 Classification of coronary artery segments. The figure shows a diagram of the coronary tree divided into 15 segments according to the modified American Heart Association classification [18]. The classification includes most of the segments with diameter greater than 1.5 mm. *LCA*, left coronary artery; *LCX*, left circumflex coronary artery; *LAD*, left anterior descending coronary artery; *LM*, left main coronary artery; *OM*, obtuse marginal branch; *RCA*, right coronary artery; *D1*, first diagonal branch; *D2*, second diagonal branch; *PL*, posterolateral branch; *PD*, posterior descending branch

planes for the evaluation of the coronary arteries are: (1) the plane parallel to the atrioventricular groove, which enables the longitudinal visualization of the right coronary artery and the left circumflex artery; and (2) the plane parallel to the interventricular groove, which enables the visualization of the left anterior descending coronary artery. Once the best evaluation plane has been obtained, in the event the vessel has a tortuous course, the reconstruction algorithm for maximum intensity projections (MIP) can be used. If vascular calcifications are absent or present in only minimal quantities, an MIP with a thickness between 5 mm and 8 mm is usually excellent, whereas if the calcifications are present in great quantity, the slice thickness needs to be reduced to 3 mm. Manually or automatically tracing the centerline of the vascular lumen to produce curved MPR reconstruction may be useful when the vessel is only partially visualized, but also when it can be completely visualized in a plane. When dedicated software is used, the resulting image may be rotated 360° on its own axis. At the same time a cross-sectional plane of the vessel is visualized. This modality of visualization is particularly useful for the evaluation of stenoses with a semi-quantitative system. Volume rendering images are usually reconstructed to obtain a global view and for teaching purposes.

22.9 Limitations of CCT

Patients with a HR higher than 70 bpm should not undergo CCT. Only patients with slightly irregular cardiac rhythms can be included (e.g. early beat, atrial fibrillation, left bundle-branch block, prolonged QRS complex, HR lower than 40 bpm, etc.). In this case the scan should not be performed with ECG-controlled tube current modulation [10]. In the presence of an abnormal HR the location of the period with lowest dose will be variable and can be included within diastole.

In addition, the presence of rhythm irregularities, with the exclusion of low HR (<40 bpm), does not allow the application of multisegment reconstruction algorithms [19, 20]. This is due to the variability in diastolic filling which hampers the combination of data originating from contiguous cardiac cycles.

22.10 Newer Generations of CT Scanners and CCT

Current state-of-the-art CT technology is based on different hardware philosophies. In some cases more detector rows (up to 320) have been introduced, while other companies have developed CT scanners with two X-ray sources. At the same time all vendors developed solutions to improve spatial/contrast resolution using multiple sampling in the longitudinal axis and dual-energy capabilities. Currently, the implementation of dual energy capabilities is at the beginning and cardiac applications are not yet standardized in this field.

Another great innovation in the field of image reconstruction is the implementation of iterative reconstructions. These reconstructions are more similar to direct calculations of attenuation as compared to filtered back-projection. Using iterative reconstructions is able to sig-

nificantly improve image quality and border detection and/or reduce image noise. The latter may allow a significant (10-20%) reduction in radiation dose with preserved image quality.

22.11 Conclusions

The recent development and technologic research in cardiologic imaging with CT is integrating and profoundly changing the diagnostic protocol of the patient with suspected coronary artery disease, for whom percutaneous coronary angiography has for long been the imaging modality of absolute diagnostic value. It should nonetheless be borne in mind that although CCT is a promising technique, it is the sole domain of highly skilled operators. The clinical outcome of the technique is in fact closely associated with the optimization of each step of the procedure.

References

1. Flohr TG, Schoepf UJ, Kuettner A et al (2003) Advances in cardiac imaging with 16-section CT systems. Acad Radiol 10:386-401
2. Nieman K, Cademartiri F, Lemos PA et al (2002) Reliable noninvasive coronary angiography with fast submillimeter multislice spiral computed tomography. Circulation 106:2051-2054
3. Ropers D, Baum U, Pohle K et al (2003) Detection of coronary artery stenoses with thin-slice multidetector row spiral computed tomography and multiplanar reconstruction. Circulation 107:664-666
4. Achenbach S, Ulzheimer S, Baum U et al (2000) Noninvasive coronary angiography by retrospectively ECG-gated multislice spiral CT. Circulation 102:2823-2828
5. Ohnesorge B, Flohr T, Becker C et al (2000) Cardiac imaging by means of electrocardiographically gated multisection spiral CT: initial experience. Radiology 217:564-571
6. Kachelriess M, Kalender WA (1998) Electrocardiogram-correlated image reconstruction from subsecond spiral computed tomography scans of the heart. Med Phys 25:2417-2431
7. Mollet NR, Cademartiri F, Nieman K et al (2004) Multislice spiral computed tomography coronary angiography in patients with stable angina pectoris. J Am Coll Cardiol 43:2265-2270
8. Nieman K, Rensing BJ, van Geuns RJ et al (2002) Non-invasive coronary angiography with multislice spiral computed tomography: impact of heart rate. Heart 88:470-474
9. Aspelin P, Aubry P, Fransson SG et al (2003) Nephrotoxic effects in high-risk patients undergoing angiography. N Engl J Med 348:491-499
10. Jakobs TF, Becker CR, Ohnesorge B et al (2002) Multislice helical CT of the heart with retrospective ECG gating: reduction of radiation exposure by ECG-controlled tube current modulation. Eur Radiol 12:1081-1086
11. Nieman K, Oudkerk M, Rensing BJ et al (2001) Coronary angiography with multi-slice computed tomography. Lancet 357:599-603
12. Georg C, Kopp A, Schroder S et al (2001) [Optimizing image reconstruction timing for the RR interval in imaging coronary arteries with multi-slice computerized tomography]. Rofo 173:536-541
13. Hong C, Becker CR, Huber A et al (2001) ECG-gated reconstruct-

ed multi-detector row CT coronary angiography: effect of varying trigger delay on image quality. Radiology 220:712-717

14. Flohr T, Ohnesorge B (2001) Heart rate adaptive optimization of spatial and temporal resolution for electrocardiogram-gated multislice spiral CT of the heart. J Comput Assist Tomogr 25:907-923

15. Cademartiri F, Luccichenti G, Marano R et al (2003) Non-invasive angiography of the coronary arteries with multislice computed tomography: state of the art and future prospects. Radiol Med (Torino) 106:284-296

16. Sato Y, Matsumoto N, Kato M et al (2003) Noninvasive assessment of coronary artery disease by multislice spiral computed tomography using a new retrospectively ECG-gated image reconstruction technique. Circ J 67:401-405

17. Cademartiri F, Mollet NR, Lemos PA et al (2004) Standard vs. user-interactive assessment of significant coronary stenoses with multislice computed tomography coronary angiography. Am J Cardiol 94:1590-1593

18. Austen WG, Edwards JE, Frye RL et al (1975) A reporting system on patients evaluated for coronary artery disease. Report of the Ad Hoc Committee for Grading of Coronary Artery Disease, Council on Cardiovascular Surgery, American Heart Association. Circulation 51:5-40

19. Dewey M, Laule M, Krug L et al (2004) Multisegment and halfscan reconstruction of 16-slice computed tomography for detection of coronary artery stenoses. Invest Radiol 39:223-229

20. Halliburton SS, Stillman AE, Flohr T et al (2003) Do segmented reconstruction algorithms for cardiac multi-slice computed tomography improve image quality? Herz 28:20-31

Patient Preparation for Cardiac CT

23

Erica Maffei, Chiara Martini, and Filippo Cademartiri

23.1 Introduction

In the setting of the technical requirements for performing an effective cardiac CT angiography (CCT) study, patient preparation plays a crucial role. Inadequate patient preparation can influence all the following phases of the procedure, and in the end affect the diagnostic result of the study. The concept of preparation for the examination should be seen in its broadest sense. It should include patient selection, pharmacologic management and the delivery of explicit patient instructions.

23.2 Rationale for Proper Patient Preparation in CCT

An optimal patient preparation is the key factor for a good CCT. In fact, proper preparation is the pre-condition for optimized image quality and "as low as reasonably achievable" (ALARA) radiation dose (Fig. 23.1, 23.2). In order to use the latest CCT protocols that allow a dramatic radiation dose reduction, even below 1 mSv (as compared to 10-20 mSv of previous years), it is mandatory to reduce heart rate as low as possible. Of course this must be done in safe conditions. Safe conditions means continuous ECG control, blood pressure control and absence of absolute contraindications to specific drugs. This is particularly important when heart rate management is performed intravenous (IV).

23.3 Patient Selection

Patient selection is influenced by two main features: compliance with the concept of diagnostic appropriateness and compliance with the inclusion/exclusion criteria

E. Maffei (✉)
Cardiovascular Imaging Unit,
"Giovanni XXIII" Hospital,
Monastier di Treviso (TV), Italy

of the examination defined on the basis of shared experience.

23.3.1 Appropriateness

The current indications for CCT are in constant development (see Chapter 31) [1]. Nonetheless it should be absolutely clear that an examination performed without the correct indication, regardless of whether it is technically suitable, can in the best of cases lead to unnecessary exposure to radiation and nephrotoxic contrast agent, and in the worst to an unnecessary invasive procedure (e.g. false positive examination due to severe coronary calcifications). The operator should therefore be obliged to verify the foundation of the indication and the clinical information available at the time of the examination. Fragmentary or deficient information will make it very difficult to complete a report of diagnostic quality which is truly useful for the patient.

23.3.2 Inclusion Criteria

Normally inclusion criteria for the scan are HR<65-70 bpm (spontaneous or pharmacologically induced) and ability to maintain breath-hold for a period compatible with the scan time [2-4]. Both these criteria are aimed at avoiding motion artifacts. In the first case the problem derives from residual motion of the coronary artery present in each phase of the cardiac cycle. In conditions of bradycardia the diastolic interval is longer, which translates into an increased duration of end-diastole when the heart and the coronary arteries are almost motionless. Even though CCT can be diagnostic with a higher HR, motion artifacts progressively reduce the number of segments which can be correctly visualized [5]. The second criterion aims to avoid artifacts associated with respiratory motion. Evidently the respiratory motion of the patient during the scan can drastically affect the quality and quantity of information acquired.

F. Cademartiri, G. Casolo, M. Midiri (eds.), *Clinical Applications of Cardiac CT*,
© Springer-Verlag Italia 2012

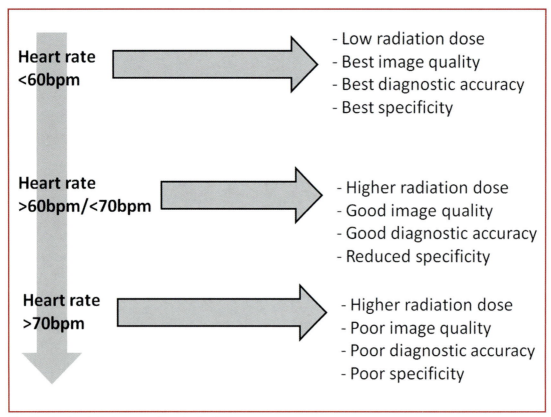

Fig. 23.1 Rationale for heart rate lowering in CCT

23.3.3 Exclusion Criteria

Patients with a HR = 65-70 bpm, known allergies to iodinated contrast agent, renal insufficiency (serum creatinine >120 mmol/L), pregnancy, respiratory failure, unstable clinical conditions and severe heart failure are excluded from the CCT scan. Actually not all these are absolute contraindications. As in other fields, the cost-benefit ratio associated with the need for diagnostic information with respect to the potential induced harm varies from situation to situation. For example, in a very young patient (18-30 years) with atypical pain and very low cardiovascular risk for whom a cardiovascular examination is requested as a screening test for competitive sports, a CCT scan would be inappropriate in the absence of clear evidence of ischemia obtained with other techniques which do not use ionizing radiation. However, CCT using low radiation protocols (<1 mSv) may be an option in this cohort.

In the low-risk critical patient, with low cardiac output and signs of perioperative acute myocardial infarction, avoiding a probably negative conventional coronary angiography in favor of CCT is definitely of benefit to the patient.

When a patient reports having had a slight or intermediate allergic reaction to iodinated contrast agent in the past, the scan can be performed after desensitization with antihistamines and corticosteroids. In the advent of renal insufficiency, the administration of contrast agent may be better tolerated if an iso-osmolar agent is used and/or if the patient is adequately hydrated prior to contrast agent injection [6]. In pregnancy and in infants the scan should only be performed when the diagnostic information cannot be obtained in any other way. Respiratory failure and unstable clinical conditions can impede appropriate breath-hold during the scan. Patients with severe heart failure are generally unable to maintain the supine position and have an elevated HR, which as stated above is a contraindication to CCT. Due to their conditions, there is an absolute contraindication to the extemporaneous administration of beta-blockers in these patients.

23.3.4 Borderline Situations

Patients with a HR higher than 70 bpm should not undergo CCT. Only patients with slightly irregular cardiac rhythms can be included (e.g. early beat, atrial fibrillation, left bundle-branch block, prolonged QRS complex,

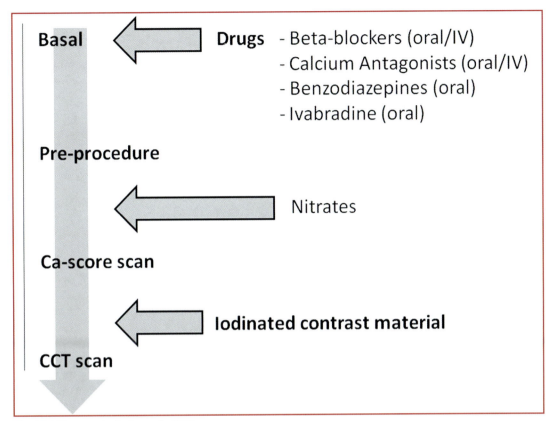

Fig. 23.2 Pharmacological steps in CCT

HR less than 40 bpm, etc.). In this case the scan should not be performed with ECG-controlled tube current modulation [7]. In the presence of an abnormal HR the location of the period with lowest dose will be variable and can be included within diastole. In addition, the presence of rhythm irregularities, with the exclusion of low HR (<40 bpm), does not allow the application of multisegment reconstruction algorithms [8, 9]. This is due to the variability in diastolic filling which hampers the fusion of data from contiguous cardiac cycles.

One favorable situation for the CCT scan even in the presence of an elevated HR (>70 bpm) occurs when the ejection fraction is low and/or the ventricles hypokinetic. In these conditions even with a HR of 80-90 bpm images of high diagnostic quality can be obtained, especially if the end-diastolic and end-systolic windows can be used. Nonetheless a significant amount of experience is required to achieve images of high diagnostic quality in these conditions.

23.4 Pharmacologic Management

For the entire period ranging from the first trials with 4-slice CCT to the most recent 320-slice scanners, the use of pharmacologic agents to reduce HR has been a constant feature [2-4, 10-24]. The agents can be administered to the patient prior to the scan to reduce HR and include (Table 23.1):

- beta-blockers;
- calcium antagonists;
- benzodiazepine;
- nitrates;
- ivabradine.

23.4.1 Beta-blockers

Orally: 45-60 min prior to the scan, metoprolol-tartrate with a dose between 50 and 200 mg.

Intravenously: esmolol is characterized by a very short duration of action and is definitely the agent of choice. The intravenous administration with pressure and ECG monitoring enable the reference HR to be reached rapidly, thus facilitating patient throughput. Other beta-blockers with a longer plasma half-life can be used intravenously, such as metoprolol, atenolol and propranolol. The latter in particular has a longer lasting effect. Prudent administration should also take into account a short period of monitoring after the examination.

Table 23.1 Pharmacology and CCT. The table shows the spectrum of drugs that can be employed for CCT with their indication, target, effect and pharmacology

Class	Compound	Indication	Target	Effects	Peak	½ life	Dose
Beta-Blockers	Atenolol IV	Hypertension; Angina Pectoris; Arrhythmias; Early treatment of AMI; LV failure	Blockers of beta adrenergic receptors	Bradycardia; Anti-arrhythmic; LV contraction depression; arteriolar and bronchial constriction	5 min	6 h	5 mg
	Metoprolol Oral	Hypertension; Angina Pectoris; Arrhythmias; Early treatment of AMI; LV failure	Blockers of beta adrenergic receptors	Bradycardia; Anti-arrhythmic; LV contraction depression; arteriolar and bronchial constriction	1.5-4 h	3-7 h	100 mg
	Propranolol IV	Hypertension; Angina Pectoris; Arrhythmias; Early treatment of AMI; LV failure	Blockers of beta adrenergic receptors	Bradycardia; Anti-arrhythmic; LV contraction depression; arteriolar and bronchial constriction	5 min	2 h	5 mg
	Esmolol IV	Hypertension; Arrhythmias; Intensive care	Blockers of beta adrenergic receptors	Bradycardia; Anti-arrhythmic; LV contraction depression; arteriolar and bronchial constriction	30 sec	9 min	0.5 mg/kg
Coronary Dilators	Isosorbide Di-nitrates sub-lingual tablets	Angina Pectoris; LV failure	Relaxant of smooth muscle including coronary arteries	Arterial and venous dilatation	1-3 min	5-10 min	0.3 mg
Calcium Antagonists	Verapamil IV	Hypertension; Angina Pectoris; Arrhythmias	Blockers of Calcium channels (slow)	Bradycardia; LV contraction depression	5 min	3-4.5 h	5 mg
	Diltiazem IV	Hypertension; Angina Pectoris; Arrhythmias	Blockers of Calcium channels (slow)	Bradycardia; LV contraction depression	5 min	3-4 h	5 mg
Benzo-diazepines	Lorazepam Oral	Anxiety Sedation	Enhancer of GABA action	Anxiolytic; Slight respiratory depression	1 h	40-100 h	0.5-1 mg (20-40 drops)
	Diazepam Oral	Anxiety Sedation Muscle relaxant Anti-convulsivant	Enhancer of GABA action	Anxiolytic; Slight respiratory depression	30-120 min	Biphasic; 3 h with a long elimination phase (20-50 h)	2 mg (10 drops)

IV, intra-venous; *LV,* left ventricle; *h,* hours; *min,* minutes; *GABA,* gamma-aminobutyric acid.

23.4.2 Calcium Antagonists

These are generally used in the event of contraindications to beta-blockers. They are more difficult to handle.

23.4.3 Benzodiazepine

Sometimes the emotive aspect of "anticipation" of the examination is overriding, especially in younger patients. In these cases short half-life benzodiazepine (Lorazepam) can be administered to reduce pre-examination anxiety.

23.4.4 Nitrates

To further facilitate the optimal visualization of the coronary arteries nitrates may also be administered (isosorbide dinitrate; orally, sublingually, spray) which in patients without excessive atherosclerosis produces a dilatation of the coronary arteries which proves particularly useful in the distal branches, where CCT has the greatest difficulty visualizing normal conditions.

Whenever negative chronotropic agents are administered, and especially if administered intravenously, ECG and pressure monitoring must be available. The early recognition of changes in the patient's condition enables administration to be halted and therapy with pharmacologic antagonists to be undertaken where necessary, thus avoiding complications.

23.4.5 Ivabradine

A new drug that has a selective effect on heart rate without any impact on contractility is Ivabradine. At the moment it can be administered orally but soon it will be available for IV administration. It is quite safe, it can be administered in association or on top of beta-blockers and it is very powerful in reducing heart rate. Ivabradine is highly recommended and will soon become the main alternative to beta-blockers and the main drug for heart rate lowering in CCT.

23.5 Instructions for the Examination

An expert operator (whether a nurse, radiology technician or radiologist) must provide the patient with thorough instructions. This may take only a few seconds or several minutes. Spending one minute more instructing the patient, particularly regarding breathing maneuvers,

can make the difference between a perfect examination and a very difficult if not impossible examination to interpret and report. Moreover, the explanation and understanding of the instructions also serve to reassure the patient and gain their utmost cooperation. Sometimes a lower HR may be achieved simply due to the reassurance the patient receives.

The instructions should begin with the operator describing to the patient how the procedure is performed. Once the procedure has been described, in the presence of ECG monitoring (and pressure monitoring if negative chronotropic agents have been administered), the operator should perform a trial breath-hold to verify that the patient does not perform an excessive Valsalva maneuver and that the diaphragm remains still. To do so the operator should place one hand at the epigastric level to feel the thoracoabdominal motion.

23.6 Patient Preparation Algorithm

It has been shown that an elevated HR negatively influences the performance and success of the scan in terms of diagnostic quality [25]. The best method for reducing HR is undoubtedly pharmacologic. This is nonetheless more difficult in patients with a HR >90 bpm. An optimal study of the coronary arteries requires that the HR is lower than 70 bpm. For an evaluation of the myocardium, the pericardium, the anatomy of the great vessels or myocardial function, the study can be performed in patients with higher HR or with atrial fibrillation, provided the ventricular response is low.

Once the HR has been optimized the variability should be evaluated. In addition, a test should be performed to evaluate whether the patient's breath-hold is compatible with the scan time. With 64-slice scanners or above the breath-hold is generally 10 s or less and in most cases compatible with a stable breath-hold, except in critical and/or uncooperative patients. If at the end of the breath-hold the HR remains stable, the patient may undergo the examination. In some cases early beats may be observed. These are not an absolute contraindication to the examination if the software used allows editing of the ECG after the scan. When this correction cannot be made, the information registered at the premature beat will be lost. In this case the patient should not undergo the diagnostic procedure.

23.7 Conclusions

Optimal patient preparation is based on good knowledge of the clinical conditions associated with coronary artery disease and those independent of it, as well as appropriate knowledge of the mechanisms of action and the absolute and relative contraindications of the drugs used. Obtaining the best from this phase of the examination, and therefore from all the following phases which are influenced by it, can only be achieved when working in a highly specialized setting and in a team with a solid background in clinical cardiology. In addition, optimal patient preparation allows the radiation dose to be reduced.

References

1. Hendel RC, Patel MR, Kramer CM et al (2006) ACCF/ACR/SCCT/SCMR/ASNC/NASCI/SCAI/SIR 2006 appropriateness criteria for cardiac computed tomography and cardiac magnetic resonance imaging: a report of the American College of Cardiology Foundation Quality Strategic Directions Committee Appropriateness Criteria Working Group, American College of Radiology, Society of Cardiovascular Computed Tomography, Society for Cardiovascular Magnetic Resonance,American Society of Nuclear Cardiology, North American Society for Cardiac Imaging, Society for Cardiovascular Angiography and Interventions, and Society of Interventional Radiology. J Am Coll Cardiol 48:1475-1497
2. Nieman K, Cademartiri F, Lemos PA et al (2002) Reliable noninvasive coronary angiography with fast submillimeter multislice spiral computed tomography. Circulation 106:2051-2054
3. Ropers D, Baum U, Pohle K et al (2003) Detection of coronary artery stenoses with thin-slice multi-detector row spiral computed tomography and multiplanar reconstruction. Circulation 107:664-666
4. Mollet NR, Cademartiri F, Nieman K et al (2004) Multislice spiral computed tomography coronary angiography in patients with stable angina pectoris. J Am Coll Cardiol 43:2265-2270
5. Nieman K, Rensing BJ, van Geuns RJ et al (2002) Non-invasive coronary angiography with multislice spiral computed tomography: impact of heart rate. Heart 88:470-474
6. Aspelin P, Aubry P, Fransson SG et al (2003) Nephrotoxic effects in high-risk patients undergoing angiography. N Engl J Med 348:491-499
7. Jakobs TF, Becker CR, Ohnesorge B et al (2002) Multislice helical CT of the heart with retrospective ECG gating: reduction of radiation exposure by ECG-controlled tube current modulation. Eur Radiol 12:1081-1086
8. Dewey M, Laule M, Krug L et al (2004) Multisegment and halfscan reconstruction of 16-slice computed tomography for detection of coronary artery stenoses. Invest Radiol 39:223-229
9. Halliburton SS, Stillman AE, Flohr T et al (2003) Do segmented reconstruction algorithms for cardiac multi-slice computed tomography improve image quality? Herz 28:20-31
10. Achenbach S, Giesler T, Ropers D et al (2001) Detection of coronary artery stenoses by contrast-enhanced, retrospectively electrocardiographically-gated, multislice spiral computed tomography. Circulation 103:2535-2538
11. Nieman K, Oudkerk M, Rensig BJ et al (2001) Coronary angiography with multislice computed tomography. Lancet 357:599-603
12. Kuettner A, Trabold T, Schroeder S et al (2004) Noninvasive detection of coronary lesions using 16-detector multislice spiral computed tomography technology: initial clinical results. J Am Coll Cardiol 44:1230-1237
13. Martuscelli E, Romagnoli A, D'Eliseo A et al (2004) Accuracy of thin-slice computed tomography in the detection of coronary stenoses. Eur Heart J 25:1043-1048
14. Hoffmann MH, Shi H, Schmitz BL et al (2005) Noninvasive coronary angiography with multislice computed tomography. JAMA 293:2471-2478
15. Achenbach S, Ropers D, Pohle FK et al (2005) Detection of coronary artery stenoses using multidetector CT with 16 x 0.75 collimation and 375 ms rotation. Eur Heart J 26:1978-1986
16. Garcia MJ, Lessick J, Hoffmann MH (2006) Accuracy of 16-row multidetector computed tomography for the assessment of coronary artery stenosis. JAMA 296:403-411
17. Raff GL, Gallagher MJ, O'Neill WW, Goldstein JA (2005) Diagnostic accuracy of noninvasive coronary angiography using 64-slice spiral computed tomography. J Am Coll Cardiol 46:552-557
18. Leschka S, Alkadhi H, Plass A et al (2005) Accuracy of MSCT coronary angiography with 64-slice technology: first experience. Eur Heart J 26:1482-1487
19. Mollet NR, Cademartiri F, van Mieghem CA et al (2005) High-resolution spiral computed tomography coronary angiography in patients referred for diagnostic conventional coronary angiography. Circulation 112:2318-2323
20. Fine JJ, Hopkins CB, Ruff N, Newton FC (2006) Comparison of accuracy of 64-slice cardiovascular computed tomography with coronary angiography in patients with suspected coronary artery disease. Am J Cardiol 97:173-174
21. Ropers D, Rixe J,Anders K et al (2006) Usefulness of multidetector row spiral computed tomography with 64- x 0.6-mm collimation and 330-ms rotation for the noninvasive detection of significant coronary artery stenoses. Am J Cardiol 97:343-348
22. Nikolaou K, Knez A, Rist C et al (2006) Accuracy of 64-MDCT in the diagnosis of ischemic heart disease. AJR Am J Roentgenol 187:111-117
23. Schuijf JD, Pundziute G, Jukema JW et al (2006) Diagnostic accuracy of 64-slice multislice computed tomography in the noninvasive evaluation of significant coronary artery disease. Am J Cardiol 98:145-148
24. Mollet NR, Cademartiri F, Krestin GP et al (2005) Improved diagnostic accuracy with 16-row multi-slice computed tomography coronary angiography. J Am Coll Cardiol 45:128-132
25. Cademartiri F, Runza G, Mollet NR et al (2005) Impact of intravascular enhancement, heart rate, and calcium score on diagnostic accuracy in multislice computed tomography coronary angiography. Radiol Med (Torino) 110:42-51

Contrast Material Administration in Cardiac CT

24

Erica Maffei, Chiara Martini, and Filippo Cademartiri

24.1 Introduction

Despite the advent of highly advanced scanner generations that offer a procedural robustness that has never been reached before, contrast agent administration remains one of the most crucial aspects of cardiac computed tomography (CCT). CCT has substantially improved over the past years with faster gantry rotation, more powerful X-ray tubes, dedicated interpolation algorithms, and – last but not least – the introduction of dual-source CT in 2006.

As one of the consequences of this technical evolution, CCT angiography has become an established technique for minimally-invasive imaging and has together with MR angiography replaced a high percentage of diagnostic catheter angiographies. Fundamental advantages of the newest CT scanners are related to three cornerstones, i.e. shorter scan time, larger scan range and improved spatial resolution.

Faster image acquisitions can obviously be of advantage. With 64-slice CT scanners imaging of the entire aorta can easily be performed in a single breath-hold and scan ranges the size of the whole body using true submillimeter resolution are also feasible today. However, modern CCT procedures are less forgiving in terms of contrast applications as one can overrun the bolus or miss it completely if injection regimens are not adapted to scanner capabilities.

24.2 General Principles of Attenuation in Computed Tomography

The CT image consists of a matrix of voxels (usually 512 x 512). The mean attenuation value of a single voxel is usually expressed in a scale of Hounsfield unit (HU).

The fixed point of this scale is the attenuation of water, which is defined as 0 HU. The attenuation of air (-1000 HU) and dense bone (+1000 HU) limit the scale in the human body. The physical attenuation behavior of certain tissues or structures in CT depends on their density and the atomic number of dominating atoms in the region of interest. In the context of intravascular contrast agents, the only feasible element for providing high contrast and an acceptable low rate of adverse events is iodine, thanks to its high atomic number and low toxicity. However, the K-edge of iodine – the energy level at which the optimal attenuation of a certain element shows – lies far beneath the conventional energies used in CT, thus leading to a theoretical suboptimal dose-attenuation relationship. Lowering kV energies makes it possible to come closer to the K-edge.

24.3 Bolus Geometry

Bolus geometry is the pattern of enhancement, measured in a region of interest (ROI), plotted on a time(s)/attenuation (Hounsfield Units - HU) diagram, after intravascular injection of contrast material. Enhancement is calculated by subtracting the attenuation value in an unenhanced baseline scan from the attenuation values in the enhanced scans.

The optimal bolus geometry for CCT is an immediate rise in the enhancement of the studied artery to a high maximum value of enhancement (high HU) just before the start of the acquisition of CT data and a steady-state in which the enhancement does not alter during data acquisition. However, the actual bolus geometry is different from the optimal one. After intravascular injection of contrast material with a fixed injection rate there is a steady increase in enhancement, the top of the curve will be reached after the end of contrast material injection, followed by a steady decline in enhancement. Normally CCT will be performed during the upslope and downslope of the enhancement curve (Fig. 24.1).

E. Maffei (✉)
Cardiovascular Imaging Unit,
"Giovanni XXIII" Hospital,
Monastier di Treviso (TV), Italy

F. Cademartiri, G. Casolo, M. Midiri (eds.), *Clinical Applications of Cardiac CT,*
© Springer-Verlag Italia 2012

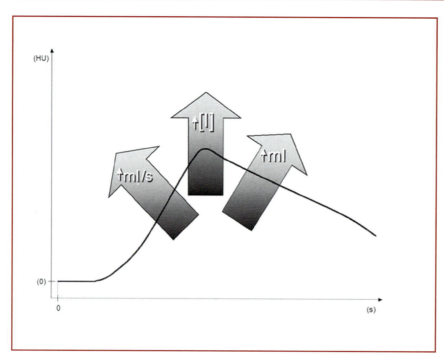

Fig. 24.1 The parameters used for the administration of contrast agent significantly influence the shape of the enhancement curve. An increase in injection rate (mL/s) produces an increase in PME and a decrease in tPME. An increase in iodine concentration (I) only produces an increase in PME. An increase in the volume of contrast agent (mL) produces an increase in both PME and tPME. *PME*, peak of maximum enhancement; *tPME*, time to reach PME

The actual bolus geometry can be characterized by several parameters: peak of maximum enhancement in HU (PME) and time to peak of maximum enhancement in seconds (tPME). The time(s)/attenuation (HU) curve generates other parameters, but these are less important.

24.4 Parameters Influencing Bolus Geometry

24.4.1 Demographics

The tPME is not significantly affected by age, weight, height, body surface, blood pressure, heart rate, and gender while PME is not affected by age and gender.

24.4.2 Clinical Conditions

A reduction in cardiac output determines a higher PME and longer tPME in the arterial bolus geometry. Circulation time is increased and contrast material pools in the venous system.

24.4.3 CM Volume, Rate and Iodine Concentration (Fig. 24.1)

A higher volume of contrast material determines higher PME and a longer tPME while a higher rate produces a proportionally higher PME and earlier tPME with a shift of the time/attenuation curve upwards and leftwards. A higher iodine concentration determines an increase in PME alone.

The relations between described parameters are independent of each other.

24.4.4 Bolus Chaser

A bolus chaser is a saline solution pushed through the injection line immediately after the injection of the main bolus. Bolus chaser is usually administered by a parallel power injector technique. Using a bolus chaser determines a reduction in the need for contrast volume (approximately -20/40%) and a washout of right cardiac chambers with a reduction in streak artifacts. Dual-injection and/or mixed injection of saline and contrast material are allowed by contemporary injector hardware. The advantage is that it is possible to decide at different time points how much contrast/saline is administered.

24.4.5 Injection Site

Two typical peripheral sites of injection of contrast material for CCT have been used: (1) an antecubital vein (directly draining into the deep venous circulation of the arm); (2) a forearm vein, which is part of the superficial venous plexus. It is better to inject contrast material in

24 Contrast Material Administration in Cardiac CT

the antecubital vein since the compound can run directly to the heart without any spread into the superficial plexus of the forearm.

24.5 Prediction of Bolus Geometry

24.5.1 Bolus Tracking

In bolus tracking technique a region of interest (ROI) is plotted inside the lumen of an artery close to the region which has to be studied and a trigger attenuation value (threshold) is arbitrarily chosen before starting the CCT data acquisition. A single level low-dose dynamic scan is performed at determined intervals of time during the injection of contrast material. When the contrast material arrives at the level of the ROI, the change in attenuation is detected and a CT scan is started after reaching the triggering threshold. The CT scanner needs 4-5 seconds to give the patient breathing instructions. The threshold should be 80-100 HU above the baseline level of the ROI.

24.5.2 Test Bolus

In test bolus technique a ROI is plotted inside the lumen of an artery close to the region which has to be studied. A small amount of contrast material (10-15 mL) at the same rate of the main bolus is injected while a single level low-dose dynamic scan is performed at determined intervals of time. When the contrast material arrives inside the lumen of the artery at the level of the ROI the test bolus geometry is assessed and the time between the start of the test bolus injection and a determined point of the time/attenuation curve of the test bolus is used as delay time for the injection of the main bolus. Test bolus has a different geometry than the main bolus which is related to the lack of injection power after the injection of the test bolus which determines a pooling of the test bolus in the venous system. Usually it needs 4-6 seconds to be added to the delay calculated from test bolus.

24.6 Impact of Bolus Management on Diagnostic Accuracy

A higher intravascular attenuation determines a higher diagnostic accuracy for the detection of significant coronary artery stenosis. This is more important for patients with higher Body Mass Index, in smaller patients (i.e. their coronary arteries are also small), in patients with higher calcium burden or stents (i.e. calcium/stent can obscure coronary lumen). All the strategies to increase intra-vascular attenuation should carried out when CCT is performed. For plaque detection we know that a higher intra-vascular attenuation determines an increased non calcified plaque attenuation. The clinical impact of this is still unknown.

24.7 Perfusion and Delayed Enhancement

A recent application of CCT includes myocardial perfusion and delayed enhancement for viability. For these applications the same rationale of gadolinium in cardiac MRI is applied. Good contrast enhancement is important both for perfusion and delayed enhancement, although it is more important for the latter. In fact, contrast resolution of CCT is lower as compared to cardiac MR and for this reason delayed scans are more noisy. A highly concentrated CM is mandatory to reach the higher intramyocardial concentration of iodine and the best pooling. To help with both perfusion and delayed enhancement there are some preliminary experiences with dual energy CT scanning. By selecting the proper energy differential it is possible to increase contrast resolution of CT imaging to achieve a better detection of iodine pools.

24.8 Contrast Material and Radiation Dose Reduction

Currently, radiation dose reduction in CCT is one of the main goals. Together with main hardware and software solutions, also contrast material can be used to reduce radiation dose. In fact, low-kV CT scanning it is one of the methods to reduce radiation dose (see Chapter 26). The K-edge of iodine is much closer to 100 kV and 80 kV as compared to 120 kV. This means that at lower kV energies the attenuation/detection of iodine improves, and this happens in a non linear way. Using higher iodine concentration allows the vascular concentration of iodine to be increased and therefore the CT attenuation. This determines a steep increase of the vascular signal which ultimately results in an increased contrast/noise (Fig. 24.2).

24.9 Recommendations

Ideally an iodine delivery rate (IDR) ≥2.0 grI/sec should be reached for optimal CCT. This can be achieved by means of a high/very high injection rate and/or a high/very high iodine concentration. It is possible to reach the goal even using a concentration of 300 mgI/mL, however, the injection rate needed will be high-

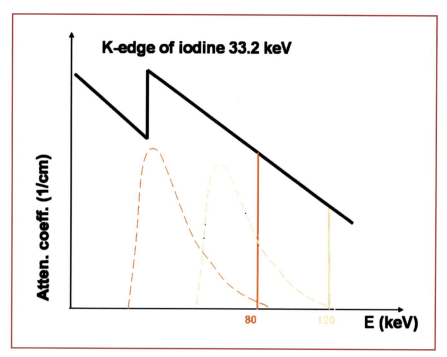

Fig. 24.2 Relationship between Iodine K-edge and kV delivered. The figure shows the modification of the attenuation profile of iodine by using lower kV settings. The attenuation peak is closer to the K-edge of iodine with a better contrast/noise

Table 24.1 Relationship between iodine concentration and injection rate

IDR	320 mg I /mL	350 mg I /mL	370 mg I /mL	400 mg I /mL
1.0 g I / s	3.1 mL / s	2.9 mL / s	2.7 mL / s	2.5 mL / s
1.25 g I / s	3.9 mL / s	3.6 mL / s	3.4 mL / s	3.1 mL / s
1.5 g I / s	4.7 mL / s	4.3 mL / s	4.1 mL / s	3.8 mL / s
1.75 g I / s	5.5 mL / s	5.0 mL / s	4.7 mL / s	4.4 mL / s
2.0 g I / s	6.2 mL / s	5.7 mL / s	5.4 mL / s	5.0 mL / s
2.25 g I / s	7.0 mL / s	6.4 mL / s	6.1 mL / s	5.6 mL / s
2.5 g I / s	7.8 mL / s	7.1 mL / s	6.8 mL / s	6.25 mL / s

An IDR ≥2.0gI/s is considered the goal for improved diagnostic accuracy. The part in yellow shows the injection rate required for different iodine concentration. *IDR*, iodine delivery rate.

er and this will require a good venous access for safety to avoid extravasation. It is, instead much easier to use a high iodine concentration (370-400 mgI/mL) and a medium-high injection rate (Table 24.1). Always remember that compounds with high viscosity need to be administered after preliminary heating at 38° to avoid venous extravasation.

Acknowledgements
Concerning the introductory paragraphs of this chapter, we gratefully acknowledge the authors of the previous edition.

Suggested Readings

Cademartiri F, de Monye C, Pugliese F et al (2006) High iodine concentration contrast material for noninvasive multislice computed tomography coronary angiography: iopromide 370 versus iomeprol 400. Invest Radiol 41:349-353

Cademartiri F, La Grutta L, Runza G et al (2007) Influence of convolution filtering on coronary plaque attenuation values: observations in an ex vivo model of multislice computed tomography coronary angiography. Eur Radiol 17:1842-1849

Cademartiri F, Maffei E, Palumbo AA et al (2008) Influence of intracoronary enhancement on diagnostic accuracy with 64-slice CT coronary angiography. Eur Radiol 18:576-583

Cademartiri F, Mollet N, van der Lugt A et al (2004) Non-invasive 16-row multislice CT coronary angiography: usefulness of saline chaser. Eur Radiol 14:178-183

Cademartiri F, Mollet NR, Lemos PA et al (2006) Higher intracoronary attenuation improves diagnostic accuracy in MDCT coronary angiography. AJR Am J Roentgenol 187:430-433

Cademartiri F, Mollet NR, Runza G et al (2005) Influence of intracoronary attenuation on coronary plaque measurements using multislice computed tomography: observations in an ex vivo model of coronary computed tomography angiography. Eur Radiol 15:1426-31

Cademartiri F, Mollet NR, van der Lugt A et al (2005) Intravenous contrast material administration at helical 16-detector row CT coronary angiography: effect of iodine concentration on vascular attenuation. Radiology 236:661-665

Cademartiri F, Nieman K, van der Lugt A et al (2004) Intravenous contrast material administration at 16-detector row helical CT coronary angiography: test bolus versus bolus-tracking technique. Radiology 233:817-823

Cademartiri F, van der Lugt A, Luccichenti G et al (2002) Parameters affecting bolus geometry in CTA: a review. J Comput Assist Tomogr 26:598-607

Principles of Cardiac CT Scan Protocol Optimization

25

Erica Maffei, Chiara Martini, and Filippo Cademartiri

25.1 Introduction

The scan protocols in cardiac computed tomography (CCT) are rather varied and in constant evolution due to the rapid development of multislice technology [1, 2]. Providing absolute indications which are valid for all scanners is no simple matter. The protocols are also influenced by the logic behind the positioning of the time windows and image reconstruction. The skill and experience of the operator also play a crucial role in the selective optimization of the study protocols, especially when the techniques become complex and the administration of intravenous contrast agent is applied.

Even in the absence of absolute indications, a number of general guidelines can be followed and applied to the scanner available, or examples of protocols used by expert operators can be used as a reference and adapted to the specific situation. In this chapter we will follow the first of these approaches, since general guidelines are easier to summarize and extend to all operators.

25.2 General Principles for the Optimization of CCT Protocols

The optimization of CCT protocols is based on several parameters which are decisive for image quality and therefore diagnostic accuracy. It should however be emphasized that an *attractive* image is not necessarily diagnostic, and vice-versa an *unattractive* image is not necessarily nondiagnostic. This observation takes into consideration the significant difference in approach existing between radiologists and clinicians (in this case cardiologists). The attractive three dimensional volume rendering images produced by CCT appeared at the end of the 1990s, kindling a great deal

of interest. Since then numerous validation studies have been carried out to quantify their diagnostic accuracy in detecting coronary stenosis >50%. However, 10 years later the clinical implementation of the technique still needs to undergo a validation of its effectiveness in terms of how and how much this new technique improves diagnostic imaging and in end effect the prognosis of the patient who undergoes the examination.

This information can only be extrapolated from multicenter longitudinal studies which also evaluate clinical outcome and above all compare this with other techniques used in routine clinical practice.

The optimization of the study protocol should therefore focus on the *attractive* image while bearing in mind that the most important aspect is immediate diagnostic outcome and long-term prognosis.

The fundamental criteria for a CCT image are (Table 25.1) [1-3]:

1. rapid acquisition of the data volume in the arterial phase;
2. high arterial intravascular attenuation;
3. high image contrast.
4. minimum radiation dose

These four criteria are expressed as follows.

Rapid Acquisition of the Data Volume in the Arterial Phase
This depends to a large extent on the generation of scanner used. The greater the number of slices then the faster the scan will be completed.

Elevated Arterial Intravascular Attenuation
This depends on the modality of intravenous contrast agent administration and the modality of synchronizing the delivery of the bolus during data acquisition.

Elevated Image Contrast
Many factors influence the level of image contrast, although the main ones are the tube current and the characteristics of the tissue being studied. In general, a CCT scan requires medium-high parameters from the scanner and the administration of contrast agent.

E. Maffei (✉)
Cardiovascular Imaging Unit,
"Giovanni XXIII" Hospital,
Monastier di Treviso (TV), Italy

F. Cademartiri, G. Casolo, M. Midiri (eds.), *Clinical Applications of Cardiac CT*,
© Springer-Verlag Italia 2012

Table 25.1 General hardware requirements for CCT

Parameter	Description	Reason
Scanner type/generation	≥64-slice/rotation	To provide the basic condition for proper CCT
Spatial resolution	High	To visualize the small and tortuous coronary arteries using small voxels
Temporal resolution	High	The heart beats and therefore diagnostic quality images need to be obtained in a relatively motionless phase of the cardiac cycle
Contrast resolution	High	Coronary plaques are of mixed density – high (calcium) and intermediate (fibrofatty tissue)
Scan duration	Low	To avoid respiratory motion
Synchronization	Retrospective	To avoid cardiac motion; more suitable in patients with high and/or irregular heart rate
	Prospective	To avoid cardiac motion; more suitable in patients with low and stable heart rate
Image reconstruction	Thin	To use the high spatial resolution
Convolution filtering	Adaptive	To be adapted to patients' related noise and to the need for visualization of particular structure (e.g. calcifications, stents,...)
Radiation dose reduction/modulation software	Required	To use and tailor the radiation dose to each patient

Minimum Radiation Dose

Contemporary CCT requires that diagnostic performance is obtained with a level of radiation exposure that is lower as compared to the past (see Chapter 26). Recent CT technologies allows a faster acquisition that paired with aggressive heart rate control can create the conditions for the need of less radiation. Of major importance is the preserved diagnostic performance. For no reason radiation dose should be lowered when a deterioration of image quality and diagnostic accuracy may be expected.

25.3 Parameter Optimization

The optimization of the CCT scan is probably the most delicate procedure (Fig. 25.1). Numerous parameters compete to obtain an image of diagnostic quality [1-3]:
- the scanner used;
- peak tube current in the reconstructed time window;
- patient breathing;
- patient heart rate;

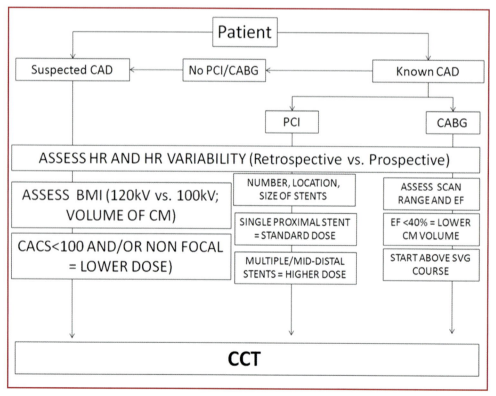

Fig. 25.1 Decision algorithm. *CAD*, coronary artery disease; *CCT*, cardiac CT; *CACS*, coronary artery calcium score; *BMI*, body mass index; *PCI*, percutaneous coronary intervention; *CABG*, coronary artery bypass graft; *CM*, contrast material; *EF*, ejection fraction; *SVG*, saphenous vein graft

- patient circulation time;
- synchronization between contrast agent administration and data acquisition;
- modality of contrast agent administration.

If we focus our attention on the technical requirements for performing CCT we can see that all of the available parameters have been brought to the maximum available values (Table 25.1).

A good CCT study requires optimal technical parameters on all fronts. The greater performance of the latest generation of scanners in fact is derived from the development guided by the optimization of the CCT scans.

A good CCT study, therefore, requires that the collimation/individual slice thickness be as thin as possible, the tube current be as high as possible in the reconstruction time window used, the reconstruction time window be as short as possible and the intravascular attenuation be as high as possible.

25.4 Special Cases

Although it has been emphasized that CCT requires maximum parameters to provide the best images possible, there are some cases where the protocol can be optimized according to clinical indication. For example, when the indication is given to evaluate coronary anomalies at the origin, having all the parameters at maximum will certainly not be necessary since the main information will be located at the origin of the coronary arteries and the images obtained will merely need to visualize origin and course.

An evaluation of the left atrium and the pulmonary arteries will not require elevated parameters to visualize the coronary arteries so that protocols with lower doses of radiation and contrast agent can be selected.

In contrast, the opposite will be true in certain cases, i.e. parameters will need to be at their absolute maximum. This is the case of the obese or very large patient, when stents are present at the level of the coronaries or intracardiac devices have been implanted (mechanical valves, pacemakers, defibrillators, etc.).

25.5 Conclusions

In conclusion, optimization of the CCT study can be achieved following a number of general guidelines. However, the operator will need to optimize and weigh up the clinical indication case by case with respect to the technical requirements to obtain the most from the scanner available.

Acknowledgements
We would like to thank the following colleagues for their assistance and for having provided opinions and indications regarding the protocols used: Maurizio Centonze, Gianluca Pontone, Andrea Romagnoli, Carlo Tedeschi, Giuseppe Runza, Roberto Malagò, Ludovico La Grutta, Rolf Raaijmaakers, Sara Seitun, Matteo Romano, Manuel Belgrano, Francesca Pugliese, Nico R. Mollet, Stephan Achenbach, Joanne Schuijf, Jeroen Bax, Alessandro Palumbo, Erica Maffei.

References

1. Cademartiri F, Malagutti P, Belgrano M et al (2005) Non-invasive coronary angiography with 64-slice computed tomography. Minerva Cardioangiol 53:465-472
2. Cademartiri F, Runza G, Belgrano M et al (2005) Introduction to coronary imaging with 64-slice computed tomography. Radiol Med (Torino) 110:16-41
3. Cademartiri F, van der Lugt A, Luccichenti G et al (2002) Parameters affecting bolus geometry in CTA: a review. J Comput Assist Tomogr 26:598-607

Management of Radiation Dose in Cardiac CT

26

Erica Maffei, Chiara Martini, and Filippo Cademartiri

26.1 Introduction

Cardiac computed tomography (CCT) has been one of the major innovations in diagnostic medicine over the past 10 years [1]. Technological developments have seen rapid evolution of scanner design and potential since the early days of 4-slice scanners. Radiation dose has been for several years a limitation of CCT (Tables 26.1, 26.2) [2]. Currently we are seeing the complete implementation of low radiation dose CCT [3-5]. One of the main issues of CCT which has thus far limited the widespread application of this modality is fading out. At the same time clinical applications are expanding together with reliability [6-9].

26.2 Technology

State of the art CT today utilizes equipment designed to use a variety of hardware approaches. After a relatively long period (i.e. up to the 64-detector row scanner generation) in which CT development for cardiologic applications was defined in terms of the number of detector rows and the gantry rotation time, scanner manufacturers began diversifying in terms of their approaches to innovation (Table 26.3). Some vendors increased the number of slices, while others introduced dual source [10-20]. Detector technology is also developing with different solution for improvement of spatial resolution and/or allowing dual-energy selective scans.

26.3 Strategies for Radiation Dose Reduction

The standard scan mode for CCT was the spiral technique at low pitch (0.2-0.35) (Table 26.4). The radiation dose was approximately 3/5-fold as compared to analogous anatomic coverage of the thorax using a standard protocol. With 64-detector row technology the mean effective dose is approximately 12 mSv (range 8-18) in a phase in which the prospective technique is already in use [21, 22]. Images in CCT have to be of the highest image quality in mid-to-end diastolic phase and for this reason heart rate has to be as low as possible (<60-65bpm) (Fig. 26.1).

26.3.1 Automatic Exposure Control

At the moment in which the CT equipment performs the scan it is possible to acquire the longitudinal attenuation profile of the patient. It is also possible to obtain the axial attenuation profile, i.e. the difference in attenuation between the anteroposterior and laterolateral positions of the gantry detector system [23]. In this way the number of photons needed to obtain images of diagnostic quality can be calculated based on the conformation and individual anatomy of the patient at every point along the longitudinal axis [23]. This technique is referred to as automatic exposure control (AEC). The radiation dose reduction achievable using this technique is often as much as 33% [23].

26.3.2 Prospective ECG-triggered Current Modulation

The first strategy for dose reduction involves prospective ECG-triggered modulation of the tube current (milliAmperes). This technique involves reducing the dose during the phase of the cardiac cycle in which it is

E. Maffei (✉)
Cardiovascular Imaging Unit,
"Giovanni XXIII" Hospital,
Monastier di Treviso (TV), Italy

F. Cademartiri, G. Casolo, M. Midiri (eds.), *Clinical Applications of Cardiac CT*,
© Springer-Verlag Italia 2012

Table 26.1 Comparison between radiation dose

Source	Dose
Background radiation (range)	3/year (1-10)
Stress ECG - Stress Echo-Cardiography - Stress CMR	0
Chest X-ray – 2 projections (range)	0.1 (0.05-0.24)
Screening Chest CT (low dose)	0.3-1.0
Standard Chest CT	3-8
Standard Abdominal CT	8-20
SPECT Tc^{99} (stress-rest)	10-15
SPECT Thal^{201} (stress-rest)	41
SPECT Rb^{82}	5
PET F^{18} - FDG	14
CAG diagnostic (range)	7 (2-16)
CAG interventional - coronary arteries (range)	15 (9-29)
CAG interventional - radiofrequency ablation (range)	20 (7-57)

Numbers correspond to mSv unless otherwise specified. The radiation dose numbers are collected from various published studies and should be considered as representative values [2]. *CAG*, conventional coronary angiography; *SPECT*, single-photon emission computed tomography; *CMR*, cardiac magnetic resonance; *ECG*, electrocardiogram; *Tc*, technetium; *Thal*, thallium; *Rb*, rubidium; *F^{18} FDG*, fluorodeoxyglucose; *mSv*, milliSievert.

Table 26.2 Ranges of radiation dose for CCT depending on scan protocols

Technique	120 kV	100 kV
Retrospective ECG gating, Spiral, No pulsing	25 mSv	18 mSv
Retrospective ECG gating, Spiral, Pulsing	13 mSv	9 mSv
Retrospective ECG gating, Spiral, Extreme Pulsing	5 mSv	3 mSv
Prospective ECG triggering (step-and-shoot)	3 mSv	2 mSv
High Pitch Spiral (Flash)	1.4 mSv	0.9 mSv

mSv, milliSievert.

Table 26.3 Scan and Reconstruction parameters with different equipment generations

Scan	Sensation 64	Definition as+	Definition ds	Definition flash
Tubes/Sources	1	1	2	2
Slices/rot (Detectors)	64 (32)	128 (64)	64 (32)	128 (64)
Total slice/rot (spiral mode)	64	128	128	256
Slice Collimation	0.6 mm	0.6 mm	0.6 mm	0.6 mm
Tube voltage	120 kV	120 kV	120 kV	120 kV
Total tube load (maximum)	180 mAs/rot	212 mAs/rot	413 mAs/rot	528 mAs/rot
Rotation time	330 ms	300 ms	330 ms	285 ms
Effective temporal resolution	165 ms	150 ms	83 ms	75 ms
Effective spatial resolution	0.3x0.3x0.4 mm	0.3x0.3x0.4 mm	0.3x0.3x0.4 mm	0.3x0.3x0.4 mm
Reconstruction				
Effective slice width	0.6-0.75 mm	0.6-0.75 mm	0.6-0.75 mm	0.6-0.75 mm
Reconstruction increment	0.3-0.4 mm	0.3-0.4 mm	0.3-0.4 mm	0.3-0.4 mm
FOV	140-180 mm	140-180 mm	140-180 mm	140-180 mm
Convolution Kernel	Medium	Medium	Medium	Medium
Contrast Material				
Synchronization	TB/BT	TB/BT	TB/BT	TB/BT
Region of Interest (ROI)	AAo	AAo	AAo	AAo
Threshold in the ROI	+100HU	+100HU	+100HU	+100HU
Pre-delay	10 s	10 s	10 s	10 s

(*cont.*) →

Table 26.3 (*continued*)

CM Volume	80-120 mL	80 mL	80 mL	60 mL
CM Rate	4-6 mL/s	4-6 mL/s	5-6 mL/s	5-6 mL/s
Iodine concentration	320-400 mgI/mL	320-400 mgI/mL	320-400 mgI/mL	320-400 mgI/mL
IDR	2 grI/s	2 grI/s	2 grI/s	2 grI/s
Bolus chaser	40 mL @ 4-6 mL/s	40 mL @ 5-6 mL/s	40 mL @ 4-6 mL/s	40 mL @ 5-6 mL/s
Venous Access	Antecubital	Antecubital	Antecubital	Antecubital

^The end-systolic spot is available in spiral mode. *TB*, test bolus; *BT*, bolus tracking; *AAo*, ascending aorta; *FOV*, field of view; *Hu*, Hounsfield unit; *ECG*, electrocardiogram; *ROI*, region of interest; *CM*, contrast material; *IDR*, iodine delivery rate.

Table 26.4 Relative impact of dose reduction techniques on CCT global dose

Dose reduction technique	% reduction*	Notes
Prospective ECG-triggered modulation	<50%	HR<65 bpm and stable condition
Automatic exposure control	~33%	Always
Low kilo-voltage (BMI<30 = 100kV; BMI<25 = 80kV)	50%	In patients with medium-small build
Prospective ECG triggering	>50%	With HR<65 bpm and stable condition
Dual/Single-beat with prospective ECG triggering and high-pitch spiral prospective ECG triggering	>80%	With HR <60 bpm and stable condition
Iterative reconstructions	15-25%	Always

*With respect to the standard spiral Retrospective ECG gating protocol. *BMI*, body mass index; *HR*, heart rate; *ECG*, electrocardiogram.

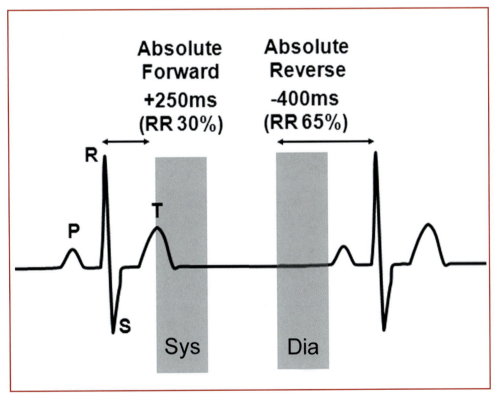

Fig. 26.1 Temporal windows with best image quality on CCT. The cardiac cycle offers two main temporal windows ("spots") for image reconstruction with reduced residual motion. The most used in end-diastolic phase (Dia) while the least used in end-systolic (Sys). *ECG*, electrocardiogram; *CCT*, cardiac computed tomography

not possible or at best unlikely that diagnostic images will be obtained (i.e. during systole; Fig. 26.2). A dose reduction of up to 50% depending on heart rate can often be achieved with this technique (i.e. the lower the heart rate the greater the achievable dose reduction) [24]. The dose reduction obtained can be further improved by as much as 43% with more recent software [25]. The advantage of this approach is that it makes possible a spiral

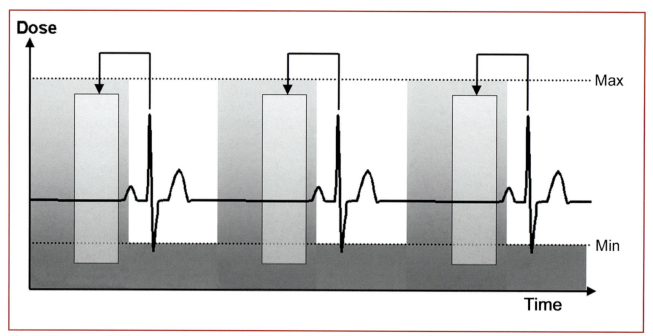

Fig. 26.2 Prospective ECG-triggered tube current modulation. During spiral retrospective ECG gated CCT scan mode mAs can be modulated during the cardiac cycle in order to use the peak mAs only in the mid-to-end-diastolic phase (i.e. where images are more likely to be of diagnostic quality). *CCT*, cardiac computed tomography; *Min*, minimum dose (4-20% of the peak dose); *Max*, maximum/peak dose

scan in which the correspondence between the temporal window expected and that effectively reconstructed is maintained. This technique is influenced by variations in heart rate and even more by arrhythmia (e.g. premature heart beats). Therefore modern software is equipped with modulation suppression systems when significant variations of cardiac rhythm occur.

26.3.3 Low Kilovoltage

Diagnostic quality in CCT scan can be achieved at 100 kV rather than at the traditional 120-140 kV. However, this can be achieved only if the global attenuation of the patient, expressed as body mass index (BMI), is <28 [26, 27]. To note is that the BMI is a surrogate of the attenuation of the patient at the level of the lower thorax and that notable discrepancies may exist between the patient's BMI and the effective attenuation in that anatomical region (e.g. in women whose BMI is within the normal range but who have abundant mammary tissue). The principal advantages of using 100 kV are the reduced radiation dose and the increased intravascular attenuation for a given administered concentration of iodine. The attenuation of iodine is greater at 100 kV than at the more conventional 120-140 kV. However, at 100 kV an increase in image noise also occurs which must be countered by an increase in milliAmperes (mAs). A dose reduction of 47-53% can be achieved with this technique [26, 27].

26.3.4 Retrospective ECG Gating and Prospective ECG Triggering

CCT is typically performed using a spiral scanning technique with retrospective ECG gating [1]. There are numerous advantages to this approach, in particular the possibility to reconstruct any phase of the cardiac cycle as and when appropriate in a consistent manner (Fig. 26.3). Nevertheless, as we have seen, a very low pitch (0.2-0.35) needs to be used in order to over-sample the information and this results in a concomitant increase in the radiation dose [1]. For this reason prospective ECG triggering, a technique which has already been available for several years, has recently been re-introduced into clinical practice. With this technique images are acquired in a sequential manner only during the phase of interest in the cardiac cycle (i.e. during diastole) resulting in a dramatic reduction of the radiation dose [4, 22, 28-31]. This technique has been utilized for many years in electron beam computed tomography (EBCT), widely used in North America and Asia, for risk stratification through quantification of coronary calcium (calcium score). The value of EBCT lies in its very high temporal resolution (50-100ms) which means that it does not require all the

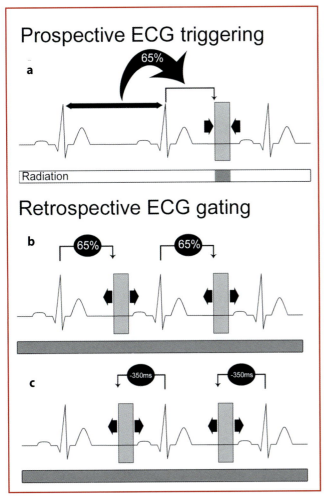

Fig. 26.3 Synchronization/scan techniques in CCT. Main techniques for synchronization between imaging and cardiac cycle in CCT are: **a** Prospective ECG triggering also known as "step-and-shoot" which is based on axial scanning; **b, c** Retrospective ECG gating also known as "spiral" or "low-pitch" technique. *CCT*, cardiac computed tomography; *ECG*, electrocardiogram; *ms*, milliseconds

phases of the cardiac cycle to freeze the movement of the coronaries during a heartbeat. The 4- and 16-detector row CT scanners have temporal resolutions of 250 ms and 200 ms, respectively, and thus cannot utilize prospective ECG triggering. With the 64-detector row CT scanner generation the temporal resolution has come down to 165-175 ms enabling better management of the cardiac frequency by CT operators (Fig. 26.4). With this scanner generation it has been possible to re-introduce prospective ECG triggering in patients with very slow and regular cardiac frequencies [4, 28-31]. The prospective ECG triggering technique in use today is an improved version of the former in that it enables the width of the diastolic acquisition window to be adapted as appropriate. In this way the CT operator can modify the temporal acquisition window at his discretion in order to perform additional image reconstructions in the diastolic phase as necessary. The radiation dose reduction permitted by prospective ECG triggering is significant, in fact, it is usually possible to reduce the effective dose to less than 5 mSv [4, 28-31]. With certain equipment and dose reduction strategies it is possible to reduce the dose to less than 2 mSv [28, 29].

26.3.5 High Pitch Spiral Prospective ECG Triggering

A very recently introduced technique is spiral prospective ECG triggering at high pitch (Fig. 26.5) [15, 16, 18, 32]. This technique utilizes totally innovative scan geometry in which the scan is performed with the table moving at high speed (pitch >3) and with the ECG-triggered acquisition carried out prospectively [15, 16, 18, 32]. With this approach acquisitions can be performed during multiple adjacent and partially overlapping temporal windows during the same cardiac cycle. The overall scan time is approximately 270-340 ms while the individual temporal windows are approximately 70-75 ms [15, 16, 18, 32].

The effective radiation dose is approximately 0.8 mSv for a single cardiac scan [15, 16, 18, 32]. However, this technique is appropriate only in patients with very low and regular heart rates (≤60bpm). A further disadvantage of the technique is that it allows the acquisition of only a single series of images without any possibility of varying the temporal acquisition window. Nevertheless, the very high temporal resolution achievable allows images of high diagnostic quality to be obtained which are analogous to those of previous techniques under equivalent operating conditions (low and regular heart rates).

26.3.6 Iterative Reconstructions

The ideal approach to image reconstruction in CT is the so-called exact approach in which the attenuation values of the pixels/voxels are reconstructed using all the information available [33]. However, as yet this type of reconstruction has not been utilized on commercially available equipment or in clinical practice. The reconstructions normally performed in CT are characteristically approximation algorithms (retroprojection filtered). This approach is necessary to improve reconstruction times in order to make the reconstructions clinically utilizable. The largest manufacturers of CT equipment are on the point of making iterative reconstruction algorithms avail-

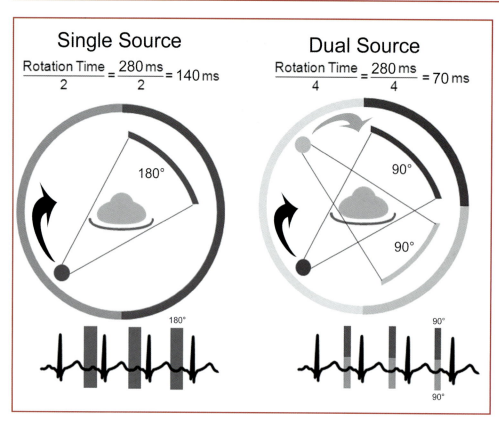

Fig. 26.4 Rationale of dual source CT scanners for CCT. In CCT temporal resolution is the most important parameter. This is because an image requires 180° of rotation to collect all the information. Therefore, with conventional CT systems (single source) the only way to increase temporal resolution is to increase gantry rotation time. Temporal resolution improves image quality and makes possible a reduction in radiation dose. To improve temporal resolution it is also possible to use two sources (and two detectors) perpendicular to each other. With this geometry the 180° of information can be obtained with a rotation of 90°. The result is twice the temporal resolution for the same gantry rotation time. *CCT*, cardiac computed tomography

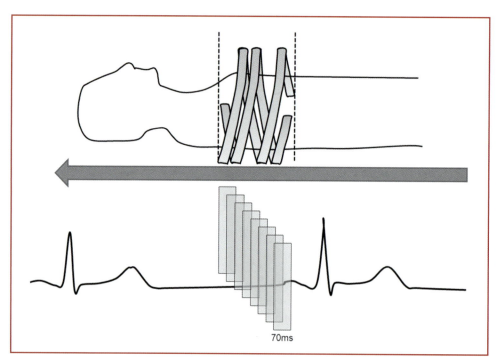

Fig. 26.5 Principle of high-pitch prospective ECG triggering technique (Flash) in CCT. With dual source CT scanners temporal resolution is significantly improved. Given current standards (i.e. 70 ms) it is possible to perform a CCT by concentrating and overlapping the temporal windows within the same mid-to-end diastolic phase. This technique requires a very high pitch (~3.0). The result is a very low-dose (~1mSv) single heart beat CCT. The technique is feasible only in patients with stable and low (<60bpm) heart rate. *CCT*, cardiac computed tomography

able on state-of-the-art commercial equipment. The practical benefits that these algorithms will bring about are notable. For example, these algorithms will allow markedly increased spatial resolution and contrast over that which we are currently used to [33]. This translates into the possibility to use lower radiation doses than those currently needed to obtain equivalent image quality [33].

26.3.7 Additional Considerations Concerning Dose and Management of the Cost-Benefit Relationship

Given the techniques described above, it is clear that the radiation dose problem in CCT is decidedly multifactorial. To a large extent it depends on the technology available. However, without a means to manage the heart rate even the most advanced scanners cannot be utilized to their full capacity, thus leading to results which may not be what was expected. It is therefore essential that professionals who dedicate themselves to CCT are equipped and able to manage patient heart rates using pharmacologic means [34].

There are many drugs used in CCT and these are not restricted to beta-blockers. Among the various types of drug are calcium-antagonists which are used if patients are contraindicated for beta-blockers (e.g. patients with documented asthma), nitroderivates which are given immediately before the scan to dilate the coronary tree, lidocaine which is used to suppress frequent extra-systoles, and benzodiazepines which are used to limit emotional disturbance during the examination of particularly anxious patients.

In addition there are also those drugs of cardiologic relevance which are used in emergency situations (i.e. atropine, adrenaline, etc). In the future such drugs may become more extensively used for CCT in patients with acute thoracic pain. For all these reasons it is clear that constant collaboration with a cardiologist is required and that the pharmacologic competency described goes beyond that needed in conventional radiology. However, it is necessary to note that the ever-increasing use of CCT makes it difficult to always have a cardiologist available during an examination. Resources are typically limited and, importantly, most radiologists necessarily already have the pharmacologic skills needed to carry out a complete CCT procedure, apart from perhaps in exceptional cases where urgent reanimation is needed.

Radiation dose management must also take into account other factors such as the dimensions and age of the patient. It is worth underlining that if patients with BMI >28-30 undergo CCT then the radiation dose should be increased. Otherwise the examination should not be performed to avoid patients needlessly being exposed to pointless radiation. The age of the patient is another important factor to bear in mind when assessing the radiologic risk associated with the procedure. Among the population typically at risk of CAD (men >50 years, women >60 years) the cumulative damaging (stochastic) effects of radiation exposure is clearly much lower than in young patients. Particular attention must be placed on young patients and in particular on young women [35].

Nevertheless, as we will see in the next section, there is practically no evidence for cancerous effects of radiation at the doses typically used in CCT.

A common criticism of CCT from the cardiologic world has been that the radiation dose needed for CCT is greater than that necessary for conventional diagnostic coronary angiography (CAG). Current and future CT technology demonstrates that this is no longer the case [36, 37].

26.4 Practical and Clinical Applications of CCT at Low Radiation Dose

At the current state of technological evolution it is possible to perform CCT using an effective radiation dose of 0.8 mSv [15-18, 32]. Images of the thorax with contrast medium can be acquired with an effective dose of 1-3 mSv. There are two main consequences due to this technology development:

1. Any CT of the thorax can become a CCT examination. The radiation dose necessary in any case should not be greater than that utilized routinely for thoracic CT carried out for suspected pulmonary embolism.
2. Given the low radiation dose and the high diagnostic reliability of CCT, it can be envisaged as a first line diagnostic tool.

26.5 Conclusions

In conclusion, new CCT technology paves the way for further paradigm shifts in diagnostic imaging. After the first paradigm shift that led to the possibility of studying the coronary arteries noninvasively, a further shift involves a possible extension of cardiologic studies using CT to all patients referred for thoracic CT without recourse to additional radiation dose.

References

1. Cademartiri F, Runza G, Belgrano M et al (2005) Introduction to coronary imaging with 64-slice computed tomography. Radiol Med 110:16-41
2. Gerber TC, Carr JJ, Arai AE et al (2009) Ionizing radiation in cardiac imaging: a science advisory from the American Heart Association Committee on Cardiac Imaging of the Council on Clinical Cardiology and Committee on Cardiovascular Imaging and Intervention of the Council on Cardiovascular Radiology and Intervention. Circulation 119:1056-1065
3. Nieman K, Oudkerk M, Rensig BJ et al (2001) Coronary angiography with multislice computed tomography. Lancet 357:599-603
4. Shuman WP, Branch KR, May JM et al (2008) Prospective versus retrospective ECG gating for 64-detector CT of the coronary arteries: comparison of image quality and patient radiation dose. Radiology 248:431-437

5. Pugliese F, Mollet NR, Hunink MG et al (2008) Diagnostic performance of coronary CT angiography by using different generations of multisection scanners: single-center experience. Radiology 246:384-393

6. Hendel RC, Patel MR, Kramer CM et al (2006) ACCF/ACR/SCCT/SCMR/ASNC/NASCI/SCAI/SIR 2006 appropriateness criteria for cardiac computed tomography and cardiac magnetic resonance imaging: a report of the American College of Cardiology Foundation Quality Strategic Directions Committee Appropriateness Criteria Working Group, American College of Radiology, Society of Cardiovascular Computed Tomography, Society for Cardiovascular Magnetic Resonance, American Society of Nuclear Cardiology, North American Society for Cardiac Imaging, Society for Cardiovascular Angiography and Interventions, and Society of Interventional Radiology. J Am Coll Cardiol 48:1475-1497

7. Bluemke DA, Achenbach S, Budoff M et al (2008) Noninvasive coronary artery imaging: magnetic resonance angiography and multidetector computed tomography angiography: a scientific statement from the american heart association committee on cardiovascular imaging and intervention of the council on cardiovascular radiology and intervention, and the councils on clinical cardiology and cardiovascular disease in the young. Circulation 118:586-606

8. Schroeder S, Achenbach S, Bengel F et al (2008) Cardiac computed tomography: indications, applications, limitations, and training requirements: report of a Writing Group deployed by the Working Group Nuclear Cardiology and Cardiac CT of the European Society of Cardiology and the European Council of Nuclear Cardiology. Eur Heart J 29:531-556

9. Fox K, Garcia MA, Ardissino D et al (2006) Guidelines on the management of stable angina pectoris: executive summary: the Task Force on the Management of Stable Angina Pectoris of the European Society of Cardiology. Eur Heart J 27:1341-1381

10. Min JK, Swaminathan RV, Vass M et al (2009) High-definition multidetector computed tomography for evaluation of coronary artery stents: comparison to standard-definition 64-detector row computed tomography. J Cardiovasc Comput Tomogr 3:246-251

11. Hein PA, Romano VC, Lembcke A et al (2009) Initial experience with a chest pain protocol using 320-slice volume MDCT. Eur Radiol 19:1148-1155

12. Lembcke A, Hein PA, Borges AC, Rogalla P (2009) One-stop-shop cardiac diagnosis in a single heart beat using 320-slice computed tomography: ascending aortic aneurysm, hypertrophic cardiomyopathy and mixed valvular heart disease. Eur J Cardiothorac Surg 35:726

13. Steigner ML, Otero HJ, Cai T et al (2009) Narrowing the phase window width in prospectively ECG-gated single heart beat 320-detector row coronary CT angiography. Int J Cardiovasc Imaging 25:85-90

14. Rybicki FJ, Otero HJ, Steigner ML et al (2008) Initial evaluation of coronary images from 320-detector row computed tomography. Int J Cardiovasc Imaging 24:535-546

15. Hausleiter J, Bischoff B, Hein F et al (2009) Feasibility of dual-source cardiac CT angiography with high-pitch scan protocols. J Cardiovasc Comput Tomogr 3:236-242

16. Achenbach S, Marwan M, Schepis T et al (2009) High-pitch spiral acquisition: a new scan mode for coronary CT angiography. J Cardiovasc Comput Tomogr 3:117-121

17. Cademartiri F (2009) Cardiac CT: the missing piece of the puzzle. Eur Radiol 19:2584-2585

18. Lell M, Marwan M, Schepis T et al (2009) Prospectively ECG-triggered high-pitch spiral acquisition for coronary CT angiography using dual source CT: technique and initial experience. Eur Radiol 19:2576-2583

19. Efstathopoulos EP, Kelekis NL, Pantos I et al (2009) Reduction of the estimated radiation dose and associated patient risk with prospective ECG-gated 256-slice CT coronary angiography. Phys Med Biol 54:5209-5222

20. Bardo DM, Asamato J, Mackay CS, Minette M (2009) Low-dose coronary artery computed tomography angiogram of an infant with tetralogy of fallot using a 256-slice multidetector computed tomography scanner. Pediatr Cardiol 30:824-826

21. Hausleiter J, Meyer T, Hermann F et al (2009) Estimated radiation dose associated with cardiac CT angiography. Jama 301:500-507

22. Malago R, D'Onofrio M, Baglio I et al (2009) Choice strategy of different dose-saving protocols in 64-slice MDCT coronary angiography. Radiol Med 114:1196-1213

23. Francone M, Napoli A, Carbone I et al (2007) Noninvasive imaging of the coronary arteries using a 64-row multidetector CT scanner: initial clinical experience and radiation dose concerns. Radiol Med 112:31-46

24. Jakobs TF, Becker CR, Ohnesorge B et al (2002) Multislice helical CT of the heart with retrospective ECG gating: reduction of radiation exposure by ECG-controlled tube current modulation. Eur Radiol 12:1081-1086

25. Weustink AC, Mollet NR, Neefjes LA et al (2009) Preserved diagnostic performance of dual-source CT coronary angiography with reduced radiation exposure and cancer risk. Radiology 252:53-60

26. Feuchtner GM, Jodocy D, Klauser A et al (2009) Radiation dose reduction by using 100-kV tube voltage in cardiac 64-slice computed tomography: A comparative study. Eur J Radiol 75:51-56

27. Bischoff B, Hein F, Meyer T et al (2009) Impact of a reduced tube voltage on CT angiography and radiation dose: results of the PROTECTION I study. JACC Cardiovasc Imaging 2:940-946

28. Stolzmann P, Leschka S, Scheffel H et al (2008) Dual-source CT in step-and-shoot mode: noninvasive coronary angiography with low radiation dose. Radiology 249:71-80

29. Scheffel H, Alkadhi H, Leschka S et al (2008) Low-dose CT coronary angiography in the step-and-shoot mode: diagnostic performance. Heart 94:1132-1137

30. Hirai N, Horiguchi J, Fujioka C et al (2008) Prospective versus retrospective ECG-gated 64-detector coronary CT angiography: assessment of image quality, stenosis, and radiation dose. Radiology 248:424-430

31. Pontone G, Andreini D, Bartorelli AL et al (2009) Diagnostic accuracy of coronary computed tomography angiography: a comparison between prospective and retrospective electrocardiogram triggering. J Am Coll Cardiol 54:346-355

32. Ertel D, Lell MM, Harig F et al (2009) Cardiac spiral dual-source CT with high pitch: a feasibility study. Eur Radiol 19:2357-2362

33. Penfold SN, Rosenfeld AB, Schulte RW, Schubert KE (2009) A more accurate reconstruction system matrix for quantitative proton computed tomography. Med Phys 36:4511-4518

34. Maffei E, Palumbo AA, Martini C et al (2009) "In-house" pharmacological management for computed tomography coronary angiography: heart rate reduction, timing and safety of different drugs used during patient preparation. Eur Radiol 19:2931-2940

35. Einstein AJ, Sanz J, Dellegrottaglie S et al (2008) Radiation dose and cancer risk estimates in 16-slice computed tomography coronary angiography. J Nucl Cardiol 15:232-240

36. Herzog BA, Wyss CA, Husmann L et al (2009) First Head-to-Head Comparison of Effective Radiation Dose from Low-Dose CT with Prospective ECG-Triggering versus Invasive Coronary Angiography. Heart 95:1656-1661

37. Raff GL, Chinnaiyan KM, Share DA et al (2009) Radiation dose from cardiac computed tomography before and after implementation of radiation dose-reduction techniques. Jama 301:2340-2348

Artifacts in Cardiac CT

27

Roberto Malagò, Andrea Pezzato, Camilla Barbiani, Ugolino Alfonsi, Erica Maffei, Filippo Cademartiri, and Roberto Pozzi Mucelli

27.1 Introduction

The reliability, simplicity and repeatability of the scan make CT a very interesting modality for noninvasive diagnostic imaging of the coronary arteries. The success of the technique is also due to the considerable technologic development of spiral multidetector CT (MDCT) scanners, which has produced elevated spatial and temporal resolution, indispensable parameters for the study of the heart and the coronary tree. These structures are in fact characterized by significant and rapid motion, as well as vessels with millimetric diameters and tortuous course, and until a few years ago were considered beyond the capabilities of CT.

The diagnostic power of the technique is nonetheless linked to an understanding by the radiologist of the potential artifacts which may be generated and the methods for reducing or where possible avoiding them. An artifact is generally described as a distortion or an error in an image which is not associated with the structure to be represented. In CT the term artifact indicates any systematic discrepancy between the CT numbers in the reconstructed image and the real attenuation coefficients of the object to be represented [1, 2].

Therefore, three broad categories of artifacts can be distinguished:

1. Artifacts intrinsic to the method, the geometry of the scanner or the physical properties of the technique. The use of black-and-white film, for example, generates images in black and white. This determines a distortion of the native color image with a loss of important information which due to intrinsic limitations of the technique is produced in gray-scale, thus producing an altered perception of the object being examined.
2. Artifacts generated during the implementation of the technique. For example, in a camera, an overly long exposure time will produce a blurred image if the object being photographed is moving at a speed greater than the shutter speed of the camera (Fig. 27.1).
3. The coronary evaluation is performed by multiplanar reconstructions. Errors during reconstruction can occur because of inadequate or insufficient phase selection. At the workstation, automatic tools for segmentation may produce errors.

27.2 Image Parameters

CT images are prone to generating artifacts since they are the product of millions of independent detector measurements obtained from objects (patients) with characteristics which may be suboptimal and influenced by numerous extrinsic factors. Reconstruction techniques are based on the assumption that all of the measurements are mutually coherent, such that any measurement error is transferred as an error in the image.

CT imaging of the coronary arteries requires elevated spatial and temporal resolution, since the arteries are small, have a tortuous course and are subject to continuous motion due to the contraction of the heart and respiratory motion [3]. This implies that the technique has precise prerequisites in terms of spatial, temporal and contrast resolution which cannot always be met. Despite optimal spatial resolution, motion artifacts can often be observed, especially in the right coronary artery.

This is one of the major causes of impoverishment of scan quality, which in some cases can render the images uninterpretable. The recent introduction of dual-source CT systems, characterized by temporal resolution below 100 ms (e.g. 83 ms with a rotation time of 330 ms) is aimed at bringing the speed of data acquisition in line with the speed of the moving coronary arteries. As Achenbach et al. [3] have shown the speed of coronary artery motion varies considerably in different planes during the cardiac cycle with broad variations between the three coronary arteries and among the population.

R. Malagò (✉)
Department of Radiology,
"G.B. Rossi" University Hospital,
Verona, Italy

F. Cademartiri, G. Casolo, M. Midiri (eds.), *Clinical Applications of Cardiac CT*,
© Springer-Verlag Italia 2012

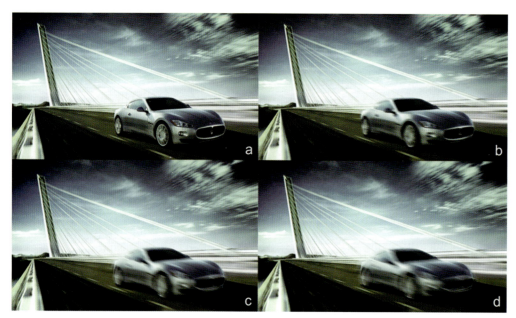

Fig. 27.1a-d Temporal resolution: for the image not to appear out of focus the shutter speed needs to be greater than the speed of the object. The ratio between the image acquisition speed and the speed of the object to be depicted determines the degree of blurring of the acquired image. Ideally the acquisition speed should be greater than the object depicted. In cardiac CT the degree of blurring depends in a similar way on heart rate and the reconstruction algorithm

This underlies the need to *freeze* the motion of the heart and reconstruct the images from the data originating from those phases of the cardiac cycle where vessel motion is at a minimum. To obtain artifact-free images of the coronary arteries the following features are required: a fast acquisition (short temporal resolution), small voxels (elevated spatial resolution in the X-,y- and z-axes) and elevated photon attenuation (optimal contrast resolution). An adequate understanding of artifacts is required to prevent them during the data acquisition phase, or in the event they have already been created, to recognize them, eliminate them or interpret them.

27.2.1 Temporal Resolution

In cardiac CT, the temporal resolution is the time required for the acquisition of the data needed for the generation of an image [4]. With regard to organs in motion, if an object is moving at a certain speed, a sharp image can only be obtained if the acquisition time/speed required to obtain the image is less than or equal to the speed of the object.

The temporal resolution in CT systems depends largely on the gantry rotation speed and the geometry of the image reconstruction algorithm. The image reconstruction algorithms are dependent on the segments available for the reconstruction of an image. The 180° required to generate an image can be obtained from a single cardiac cycle (single segment reconstruction) or from several consecutive cardiac cycles (multisegment reconstruction). The lower the speed of the object, the better the image quality will be. Therefore, in theory, a single segment algorithm is preferable, especially in the event of a low heart rate (HR) (<70 bpm). For a higher HR (>70 bpm), a multisegment algorithm can improve image quality [5-10]. Nonetheless, the clinical utility of multisegment algorithms has not been demonstrated, nor have comparative studies with single segment algorithms been done to verify their diagnostic impact. Using a fixed time window (single segment algorithm), the parameter which can be modified is the speed of the object. This is why the use of negative chronotropic agents (beta-blockers, calcium antagonists) is recommended to reduce HR prior to the acquisition.

27.2.2 Spatial Resolution

Spatial resolution is the ability to distinguish two adjacent objects as distinct from one another (Fig. 27.2). Spatial resolution in turn depends on many factors related to the type of scanner in use. Most of the parameters influencing spatial resolution (size of the focal spot, size of the detector, distance between the focal spot and the detector, number of projections) cannot be modified by the operator. Nonetheless, other parameters can be modified so it is therefore possible to intervene in the reconstruction phase (reconstruction thickness, reconstruction increment, field of view, convolution kernels) to obtain the maximum possible spatial resolution allowed by the scanner.

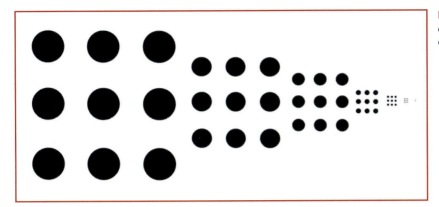

Fig. 27.2 Spatial resolution: this is the ability to distinguish two adjacent objects as distinct from one another

27.2.3 Contrast Resolution

Contrast resolution is the ability to discriminate between two adjacent objects on the basis of their respective attenuation values (Fig. 27.3). Contrast resolution is influenced by factors such as detector sensitivity and the attenuation characteristics of the patient. The parameters which can be modified include radiation beam properties (milliamperage for intensity and voltage for the beam energy), slice thickness and convolution kernels. In the end analysis, these parameters contribute to modulating the noise of the native reconstruction image (axial image). Noise has a broad influence on general image quality, and when excessive significantly compromises contrast resolution [11, 12]. Noise is discussed in the following sections.

Lastly, the manner in which images are visualized should be considered. Contrast between objects can in fact be improved simply by adjusting parameters relative to image processing, such as window settings (Fig. 27.4). Even the size of the display and the distance between screen and observer can influence the perception of contrast.

27.3 MDCT Coronary Angiography

27.3.1 Patient Preparation and Technical Optimization Protocol to Reduce and/or Avoid Artifacts

With 16- or 64-slice scanners, an optimal study of the coronary arteries requires a HR below 65 bpm obtained with the administration of negative chronotropic agents prior to performing the scan. If a dual-source scanner is used this preparation is not always necessary.

In patients undergoing the examination for the study of the myocardium, the pericardium, the anatomy of the

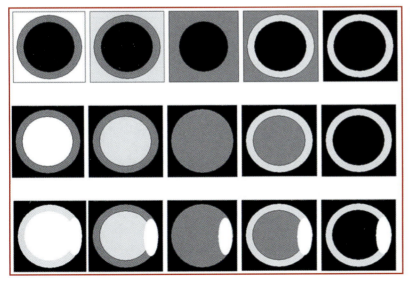

Fig. 27.3 Contrast resolution: this is defined as the ability of a technique to distinguish objects when their imaging characteristics are similar. The diagram to the right shows various situations of positive and negative contrast. The appearance of the structure studied varies with the changes in the relative enhancement

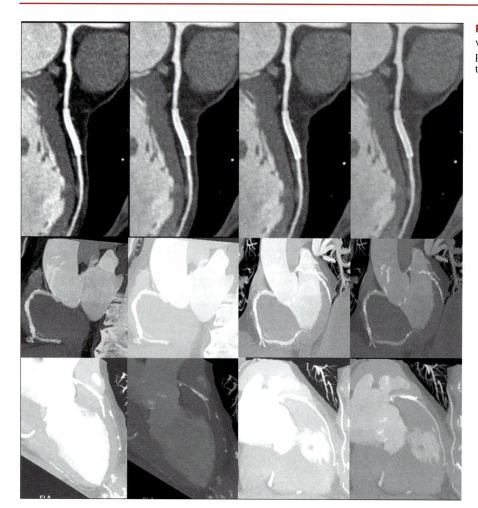

Fig. 27.4 Examples of how the window settings influence the perception of objects with respect to their surroundings

great vessels or myocardial function, the examination may be performed with a higher HR or with atrial fibrillation, provided that it is of low ventricular response. Once the patient has been placed on the CT table the ECG electrodes are positioned. The placement of the electrodes away from muscular surfaces avoids irregularities in the baseline ECG due to muscle contraction when the arms are positioned above the head for the scan. In this phase the sinus rhythm of the ECG trace should be observed, as well as the variation in HR with varying respiration. A breath-hold test should also be performed to assess whether the duration is compatible with the scan time. It should also be established that the patient holds their breath without performing the Valsalva maneuver. The high pressure which is generated during this maneuver can reduce the flow of contrast material through the subclavian vein and the pressure may compromise the patient's ability to remain motionless. In addition, patients may also have difficulty remaining immobile when the breath-hold is too deep.

It has been reported that supplementary oxygenation seems to help dyspneic patients to hold their breath for longer. Preoxygenation could also be useful for extending breath-hold particularly in cases of large scan volumes, thus increasing image quality [13]. In some cases patients may move voluntarily due to the sudden feeling of warmth passing through their body (due to the contrast agent) which may cause coughing or sneezing. The operator should explain to the patient the type of sensations they are likely to experience during the scan to prevent this inconvenience. If at the end and during the breath-hold the HR remains stable, the patient may proceed with the examination. In some cases, however, premature beats may be observed. These are not an absolute contraindication to the examination if the software used allows editing of the ECG after the scan. When this correction cannot be made, the information registered at the premature beat will be lost. In this case the patient should not proceed with the examination.

27.4 Catalogue of Artifacts, Methods for Avoiding Them and Possible Remedies

27.4.1 Motion Artifacts

Motion artifacts are generated by voluntary and/or involuntary and/or intrinsic motion of either the patient or an organ comprising a part of the body region being examined.

- Type I: Voluntary. A typical example is the interruption of breath-hold by the patient during the scan phase.
- Type II: A typical example is the slow diaphragmatic drift during patient breath-hold.
- Type III: A typical example is the natural motion of the coronary arteries which generates an artifact due to the inappropriate ratio between vessel speed and acquisition speed of the raw data (temporal resolution).

Type I artifacts are generally due to errors or failed compliance by the patient and they generate clear and severe changes in image quality. Voluntary motion artifacts can be distinguished from the artifacts related to cardiac motion in that in the former the artifact is present in the anterior thoracic wall, along the border of the heart (Fig. 27.5a) [14].

Type II motion artifacts can be generated by involuntary diaphragmatic drift. This phenomenon occurs shortly after the beginning of a standard breath-hold and varies from patient to patient. It occurs due to the progressive relaxation of the diaphragm which moves in a caudocranial direction. Since the movement is slow, progressive and in only one direction, it tends not to have a significant influence on the diagnostic quality of the image. The only possible consequence is an increase in the anomalous acquisition of data, between the stack of consecutive images in the case of a multisegment reconstruction, with the consequent formation of the stair-step artifact. Since the movement is involuntary, little can be

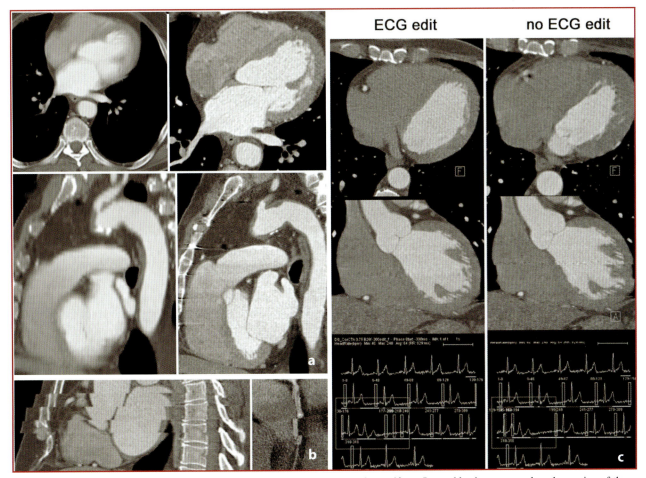

Fig. 27.5a-c Blurring and stair-step artifact: the typical appearance of two motion artifacts. Image blurring occurs when the motion of the cardiac structures is greater than the temporal resolution of the scanner. The stair-step artifact instead is due to an interruption in breath-hold

done to avoid it. Even a short scan time (<10 sec) can only reduce the effect of diaphragmatic drift.

Artifacts of this type can have various appearances and correcting them with reconstruction techniques or post processing can be very difficult or impossible. They may cause blurring or overlapping of the various sections, or their appearance may be similar to artifacts produced by variations in HR after a long phase of breath-hold [14].

In reconstructed images type III motion artifacts tend to have a typical appearance: blurring and stair-step. Blurring occurs when the speed of the moving cardiac structure exceeds the temporal resolution of the scanner, due to an elevated HR or an inadequate reconstruction time window for that particular coronary artery. As stated above, the right coronary artery has the highest speed and greatest degree of mobility in the three planes in space, followed by the left circumflex, the left main and the left anterior descending coronary arteries [3]. A significant negative correlation has been reported between HR and image quality [15] (Fig. 27.5b).

Irregular cardiac rhythms are not an absolute contraindication for CT coronary angiography, whereas irregular cardiac rhythms characterized by an elevated ventricular response (>70 bpm) heightens the problems described for an elevated HR. A slightly irregular cardiac rhythm with an average HR <70bpm can be optimized in most cases (if the system has a software application which enables ECG editing) during the image reconstruction phase. Extrasystoles can be considered slight rhythm alterations and are not absolute contraindications to CT coronary angiography, provided they are not very frequent (more than every two beats) (Fig. 27.5c).

In patients with accelerated HR (>70-75 bpm) or marked arrhythmias the administration of negative chronotropic agents (beta-blockers - see administration protocol) is advisable. The reduction in HR and normalization of the cardiac cycle contribute to controlling or eliminating these artifacts.

Often multiple datasets need to be reconstructed, each one being specific for the evaluation of a single coronary artery. The stair-step artifact derives from the inconsistent spatial geometry among the stack of images reconstructed for each cardiac cycle. The artifact generally appears in sagittal and coronal planes as a drift in the axial plane of the information contained in the stacks of contiguous images. A physiologic phenomenon which can generate this artifact is a variation in HR during breath-hold [15, 16]. To reduce its appearance the duration of the apnea needs to be reduced. To do so setting a FOV limited to the anatomic region of interest is advisable, thus reducing the scan time (this is not always possible in the evaluation of bypass grafts, which generally require a greater anatomic coverage than the evaluation of native coronary arteries).

Several manufacturers have proposed a number of measures to compensate for motion artifacts: overscan acquisition modality, correction software and cardiac gating.

Overscan: the reconstruction of the images at the scan periphery is aided by acquiring projection measurements over a greater extent than that required for image production. This is due to the fact that the maximum discrepancy between the data acquisitions occurs between the first and last view of the 360° dataset. Some models use this modality, which involves the acquisition of an extra 10% of a rotation which is added to the standard 360°. The extra measurements are then *weighted* and used to reduce the severity of the motion artifacts [11, 17].

Correction software: used in most scanners, correction software automatically performs a weighting of the initial and distal scans and reduces their contribution to the final image. However, this processing tends to increase image noise [2, 17].

Cardiac gating: the synchronization of data acquisition with the ECG trace enables images of the heart in (relative) immobility to be obtained. The reconstructions only use the data from the phase of the cardiac cycle with the least motion. This avoids the appearance of severe motion artifacts caused by the rapid and extensive motion of the heart [11, 17, 18].

27.4.2 Noise

Noise in a CT image is the variability of attenuation values around the mean of the pixels in a homogeneous region of interest (ROI). Noise can in fact be measured with the standard deviation of the attenuation values measured in an ROI positioned in the area being evaluated (Fig. 27.6).

Noise can be compared to the fog seen outside a window. The clarity of the view becomes progressively hazy and the outline of objects increasingly fuzzy in relation to the number and density of the water molecules in the air (Fig. 27.7).An ideal scanner should produce an image with low or absent noise such that, for example, the attenuation of a vessel lumen remains constant in all of the adjacent voxels along the vessel itself. The scanners currently on the market are able to produce relatively noise-free images, but at the price of an elevated radiation dose to the patient.

One of the main factors influencing noise is the tube current-time product (mAs). Increasing mAs will increase the number of photons striking the patient and therefore the detector, thus increasing the SNR. Another factor

27 Artifacts in Cardiac CT

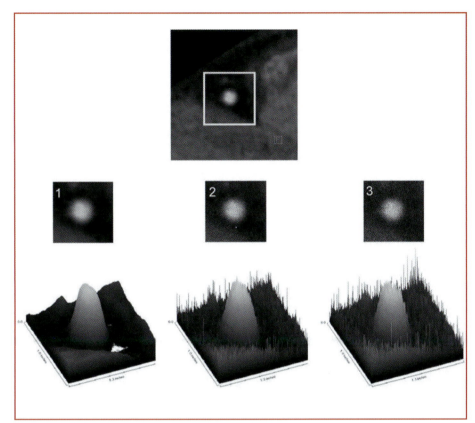

Fig. 27.6 Noise: graphic representation of image noise. The box represents a region of interest (ROI) obtained from a reference image at the level of the mid segment of the right coronary artery. The attenuation values of the area within the individual ROIs (*1-3*) are depicted in the attenuation graphs. The increase in noise causes a progressively broader oscillation of the attenuation values. This example explains why noisy images can be difficult to evaluate

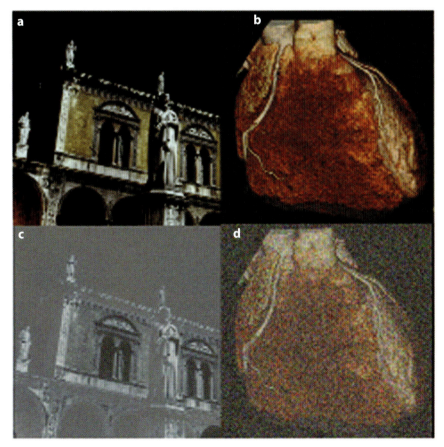

Fig. 27.7 Noise can be compared to the fog seen outside a window. The clarity of the view becomes progressively hazy and the outline of objects increasingly fuzzy in relation to the number and density of water molecules in the air. A cardiac CT scan can become too noisy when the ratio between X-ray attenuation due to the patient and the dose delivered is too high. The images reconstructed from an excessively noisy dataset cannot be improved (**a-d**)

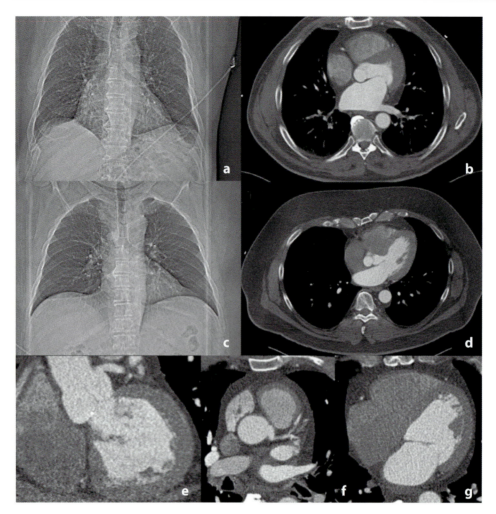

Fig. 27.8 CT coronary angiography of an obese patient. In patients with high body weight and/or high body mass index, the power of the scanner should be exploited to the maximum to produce diagnostic quality images. In this example of a patient with a bodyweight >100 kg the parameters used were 970 mAs with a rotation time of 330 ms. The images produced at various levels and in various planes are of diagnostic quality (**a-g**)

influencing noise is the photon absorption by the patient. In patients with normal bodyweight the radiation dose should be regulated on the basis of the characteristics of each scanner. In general, this depends on the operator's experience and the predefined protocols. Ideally scanners should be used with the minimum dose possible, a fact however which tends to reduce image quality. Indeed, when the ratio between radiation dose and absorption by the patient is too low the image will be noisy to the extent of no longer being diagnostic [12, 19].

There are conditions where it is necessary to increase the dose to avoid the noise artifact, such as in obese patients, with a significant proportion of soft tissue in the chest, or in the case of women with massive breasts. (Figs. 27.8, 27.9). A thick layer of fat determines a high absorption and therefore a smaller number of photons reach detectors. In both cases the inspection of the patient before the examination, or the preliminary view of the scanogram preceding the contrast phase should be sufficient to identify cases where is necessary to increase the radiation dose. It is not possible to provide default values of mAS as these depend on the patient and the technical specifications of the scanner (rotation time, power of the X-ray tube, etc.). As a general rule, the milliAmpere should be increased by 15-20% in case of obese patients or women with massive breasts [20].

27.4.3 Partial Volume Effects

27.4.3.1 Partial Volume

Partial volume (also known as volume averaging) is an artifact which occurs in all the voxels of all images whenever two or more objects with different attenuation values are present in a single voxel. This will occur when the voxels are larger than the structure to be depicted. For example, in a 0.33 mm^2 voxel a structure with a sub millimeter thickness, such as vessel endothelium or the fibrous cap of an atherosclerotic plaque cannot be depicted. These structures are therefore represented as part of

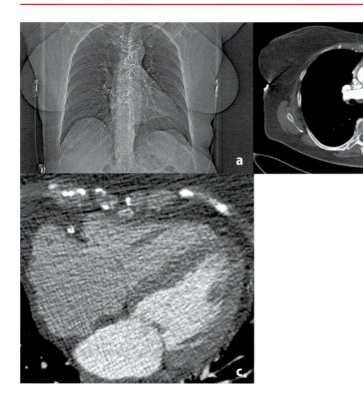

Fig. 27.9 CT coronary angiography of a patient with large breasts. The relationship between absorption by the patient and dose delivered should be optimized case by case. In this example, an adequate regulation of the scan parameters enabled diagnostic quality images to be obtained despite the considerable thickness of the subcutaneous tissue surrounding the heart (a-c)

the surrounding structures, making up part of the vessel wall or the plaque. The final appearance of the voxel situated in the plane where the endothelium lies will therefore be the result of the average attenuation of the surrounding structures present (Fig. 27.10) [12, 21].

Another type of partial volume effect, which is conceptually different from volume averaging, occurs when a dense object is only partially included within the X-ray beam and only when the x-ray tube-detector system is in determined position. The inconsistency between various views causes artifacts which appear as shading in the images. Acquiring thinner sections helps to avoid this artifact [12, 17].

27.4.3.2 Interpolation and Filters

Interpolation is an algorithm which calculates the attenuation between contiguous pixel/voxel according to precise mathematic formulae. It is the algorithm forming the basis of image reconstruction in spiral systems and it is used for creating data and filling in information gaps between two known points. There are however certain conditions where this can create artifacts. This is particularly evident in those areas of images where there are significant attenuation differences. Good examples are the sharp-edge transition between air and soft tissue in pulmonary parenchyma and between calcium and soft tissue in the coronary artery walls [11].

Partial volume and interpolation cause the blooming effect which can appear in the presence of calcium, contrast agent, surgical clips and stents in the coronary arteries. These structures with elevated attenuation appear much larger than they really are because in the image reconstruction they are depicted as being part of the structures of the adjacent voxels and are inserted in them. The use of convolution kernels can modulate this effect (Fig. 27.11).

Convolution kernels are reconstruction algorithms which determine the relationship between spatial resolution and image noise. They are applied to the raw data in the reconstruction phase and are designed to sharpen the contours of structures with different attenuation values. This process seeks to reestablish the balance between the need for interpolation to fill in the information gaps (which renders the image homogeneous) and the need for an adequate visualization of contours (which renders the image sharper). Unfortunately increasing convolution kernels increase image noise. It is therefore the task of the operator to identify the best balance between kernel and noise to obtain images of diagnostic quality [11, 12, 22] (Fig. 27.12).

27.4.4 Beam Hardening Artifacts

Beam hardening artifacts occur when part of the radiation spectrum is completely absorbed by an object with

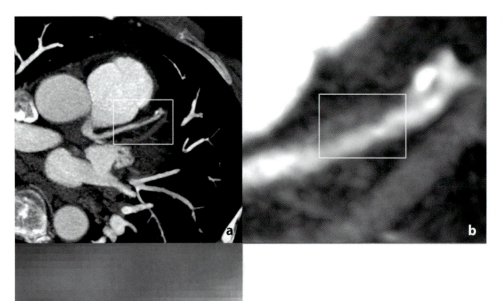

Fig. 27.10 Partial volume is an artifact which occurs in all the voxels of an image when two adjacent structures have different attenuation values. The progressive enlargement of the wall demonstrates how a microscopic structure such as the endothelium cannot be distinguished (**a-c**)

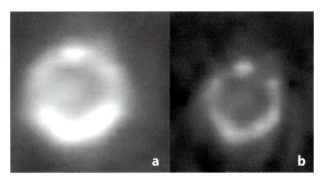

Fig. 27.11 Blooming caused by partial volume (averaging) in a stent. Due to the blooming effect high attenuation structures such as metal stents appear much thicker than they actually are (**a**, **b**). The use of a kernel reduces the blooming effect, thus enabling a more precise evaluation

extremely high attenuation values. The effect can be compared to an X-ray shied. When an X-ray beam passes through a material or tissue, it becomes *harder*, i.e. its energy increases because the low-energy photons are more easily absorbed than the high-energy photons. This causes beam hardening artifacts. The weight of the artifact increases progressively with the degree of attenuation, until a shadow of attenuation appears on the opposite side of the object (Fig. 27.13) [21, 23, 24].

Beam hardening artifacts can give rise to two effects: the cupping artifact and the appearance of dark bands or stripes between dense objects of the image (streak artifact). If we consider an X-ray beam which passes through a homogeneous cylindrical phantom, the attenuation of the beam will be greater (the beam will be harder) at the center than at the edges. The detector will therefore be struck by a more intense (harder) beam than it would be by a direct beam (not hardened by intervening material/tissue). The outcome is an attenuation profile which is different from the profile of an ideal beam and which displays the characteristic cupping artifact. If instead we consider a heterogeneous phantom, the images derived from it will be characterized by the presence of dark bands between the denser areas. This occurs because the beam passing though one of the objects in one position of the tube-detector system is softer than in another position where it passes through two or more dense objects (streak artifact) [17] (Fig. 27.13, Panel 1).

In cardiac imaging these types of artifacts can occur in different situations:

I. pacemaker leads, metal valvular prostheses, metal surgical clips, indicators of the site of bypass grafts (metal clips), metal sternal sutures and coronary stents. In such cases, where metal foreign bodies with a high attenuation factor are present, the metal artifact will be produced (Fig. 27.13, Panel 2);

II. the bolus of contrast agent in the superior vena

27 Artifacts in Cardiac CT

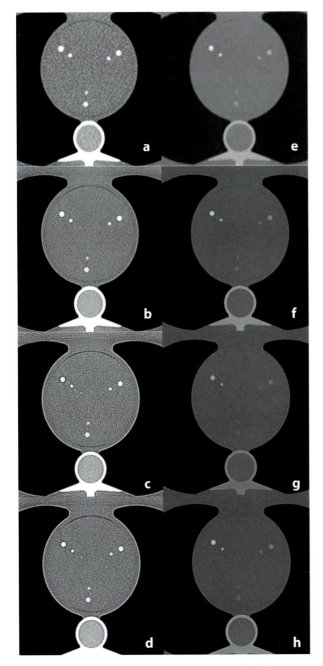

Fig. 27.12 Example of a phantom reconstructed with different convolution kernels (respectively -from **a-d** and **e-h** with kernels increasing from smooth to sharp) and different window settings (**a-d** with soft-tissue window, **e-h** with bone window)

cava and the right atrium can cause a beam hardening artifact, rendering the interpretation of the more cranial scans of the heart in the anatomic region of the right coronary artery more difficult (Fig. 27.13, Panel 3); Similar artifacts can be generated by anatomic structures filled with contrast agent which overlie the region being studied. Examples are bypass grafts crossing the anterior mediastinum, the atrial appendage and cardiac veins;

III. the presence of calcified atherosclerotic plaque can impair correct evaluation of the vessel lumen [25]. These high-attenuation spots appear larger than they really are, obscuring the vessel lumen and altering the visual perception of the residual diameter of the vessel (Fig. 27.13, Panel 4).

IV. artifacts produced by low-attenuation objects (such as bubbles of air accidentally introduced into the pulmonary artery during the administration of contrast agent or in the mediastinum during surgery) (Fig. 27.13, PaneI 5);

V. the position of the patient plays an important role in the generation of beam hardening artifacts. An examination performed with the patient's arms place by their sides will produce this artifact. Even if the arms remain outside the FOV; their presence affects some protection measurements, albeit partially, giving rise to shading or streaking and corrupting image quality (out-of-field artifact). Similar effects can occur with other dense objects such as probes filled with contrast material, wires or electrodes situated outside the FOV [17] (Fig. 27.13, PaneI 6).

The use of nonmetal surgical materials and an optimal reconstruction window contribute to reducing these kinds of artifacts. The patient should be invited to remove all metal objects. When this is not possible (e.g. prosthetic devices, metal sutures), attempts should be made to exclude them from the volume of acquired data. Osseous structures should also be excluded, and the most appropriate FOV should always be selected. In addition, increasing the scan parameters (especially the voltage) and selecting thinner slices to reduce the portion of artifact produced by partial volume can also be useful.

27.4.5 Contrast Agent Artifacts

The visualization of small-diameter vessels like the coronary arteries can be improved with intense endovascular contrast enhancement. The alteration of the parameters regulating the contrast agent (volume, injection rate, use of saline solution, circulation time) causes contrast agent artifacts.

Volume: the causes of poor enhancement are generally related to an inadequate administration and/or quality of the contrast agent. A technical error in the administration procedure is generally the cause of the non visualization of the contrast agent in the great vessels of the chest.

Speed: various studies have reported the advantages of the use of contrast agents with high concentrations of iodine (>350 mg/mL) and a high injection rate (>4.5 mg/mL) for increasing the visibility and therefore the

Panel 1

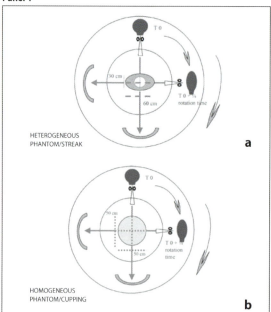

Panel 2

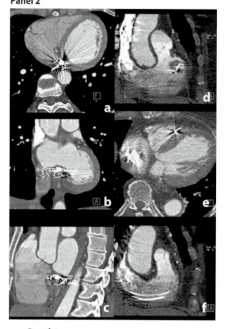

Panel 3

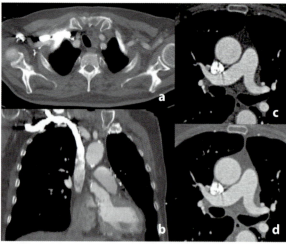

Panel 4

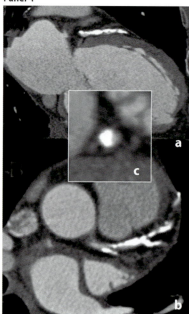

Panel 5

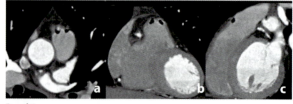

Panel 6

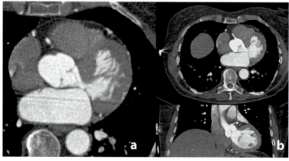

Fig. 27.13 Panel 1 Geometry/homogeneity of the object and type of artifact. **Panel 2** Beam hardening due to pacemaker. The presence of the metal lead is the cause of the artifact. The use of higher voltage and thinner slices can reduce the partial volume effect. **Panel 3** Beam hardening in the superior vena cave. The presence of hyperconcentrated contrast agent causes the beam hardening and produces the artifact. **Panel 4** Example of severely calcified plaque in the left anterior descending coronary artery depicted in a longitudinal view curved multiplanar image (**a**, **b**) and cross-sectional view (**c**). **Panel 5** Air bubbles within the leaflets of the pulmonary valve. **Panel 6** Streak artifact due to a metal object outside the field of view

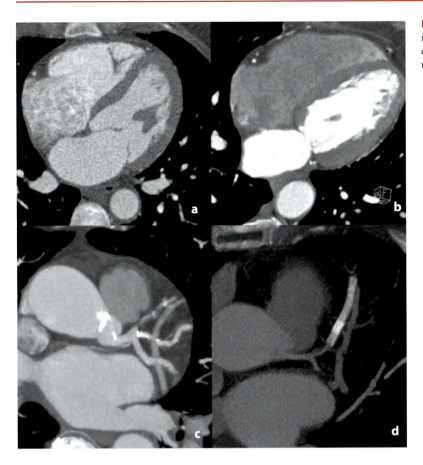

Fig. 27.14 Examples of how the administration of intravenous contrast agent can influence image quality, causing filling (**a**) or no filling (**b**) of the right ventricle and the cardiac veins (**c, d**)

diagnostic accuracy of the vessels, particularly in those containing low blood volume [26-31].

Saline solution: the use of a bolus of saline solution following the injection of contrast agent (bolus chaser) has the effect of pushing the contrast agent through the veins and maintaining it compact throughout its endovascular course. This produces optimal levels of attenuation in the coronary arteries and a minimum attenuation in the superior or vena cava and the right cardiac chambers. The bolus chaser reduces beam hardening artifacts and is advantageous especially for the visualization of the right coronary artery, which is subject to considerable beam hardening artifacts when hyper concentrated contrast agent is found in the superior vena cava and the right cardiac chambers (Fig. 27.14a,b).

Circulation time: another important aspect to bear in mind is the synchronization between the delivery of contrast agent to the target vessels and the beginning of data acquisition. If the synchronization is suboptimal, images will be obtained with possible artifacts due to the presence of contrast agent in unwanted anatomic structures (cardiac veins, pulmonary veins, pulmonary arteries, etc.) which can superimpose one another and impair or even obstruct the visualization of the coronary arteries (Fig. 27.14c) [27, 29, 32].

27.5 Artifacts from Poor Positioning of the Time Window

27.5.1 Artifacts from Irregularities in the Cardiac Cycle (Arrhythmias)

Obtaining a good-quality dataset of images without motion artifacts is highly dependent on the correct positioning of the time window within the cardiac cycle. The fundamental approach can be summarized as follows. At the completion of the acquisition the operator should perform a reconstruction in the mid- to end-diastolic phase, usually 400 ms before the next R-wave, or at 70% of the R-R interval.

There are two possible reasons why images may be suboptimal in these datasets: (1) the dataset is of good quality but one or more segments are characterized by residual motion; (2) the dataset is not of diagnostic quality and there is residual motion along the entire coronary tree. In the first case the operator should perform additional reconstructions in similar phases (-350/-450 ms or 55/65%). In the second case the operator should perform a multiphase reconstruction (i.e. 10-20 reconstructions every 5-10% of the R-R interval) of the entire cardiac

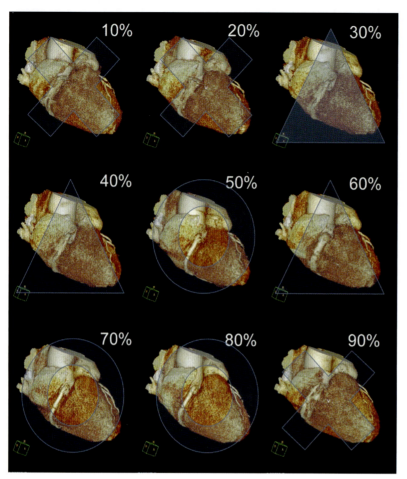

Fig. 27.15 Time windows: examples of volume rendering images reconstructed in different phases of the cardiac cycle. Artifact-free images can only be obtained in certain moments of the cardiac cycle when the coronary arteries are almost motionless

cycle to determine which is the best interval for positioning the reconstruction window (Fig. 27.15).

This second solution is usually adopted in the spiral retrospective acquisition, and in most cases diagnostic images can be obtained in at least one phase, even with relatively high HR or irregular heartbeat and even arrhythmias with low ventricular response.

When a portion of the reconstructed volume seems to be completely lost and no significant motion artifacts are observable in the other images, the ECG trace should be re-examined (ECG editing) to verify whether premature and/or ectopic beats are present [9, 33, 34].

ECG editing can be obtained only in spiral retrospective acquisitions covering the entire duration of the cardiac cycle. Modern dose reduction acquisition systems involving axial prospective acquisitions (step & shoot and snapshot) do not allow editing because the volume is acquired in only one phase of the cardiac cycle, usually the diastolic phase. Therefore, arrhythmias can cause severe motion or stair step artifacts rendering the examination non diagnostic and this cannot be corrected. In order to use prospective acquisitions a regular rhythm is a prerequisite; the HR, limited to less than 60 bpm in 16- 64 slice scanners, may be greater in the latest generation of CT systems, dual-source or 256 slices, which include software for the detection of rhythm irregularities during the scan. In any case the best way to avoid these artifacts is to reduce the heart rate and monitor the ECG before the test in order to choose the most efficient method of acquisition

27.5.2 Artifacts from Technical Errors: Data Loss

When the ECG signal is weak and noisy, the automatic synchronization software may have difficulty correctly recognizing the R-wave. The operator therefore should always check the quality of the ECG signal and the ECG synchronization prior to beginning the reconstructions.

An elevated HR (>70 bpm) is more likely to produce residual motion artifacts. In these cases a bi- or multisegment algorithm can be applied to increase temporal resolution [6, 9].These algorithms vary slightly from one manufacturer to the next, but they are all based on the reconstruction of a single image from two or more cardiac cycles. The use of this algorithm in theory could overcome the relative lack of temporal resolution in the

27 Artifacts in Cardiac CT

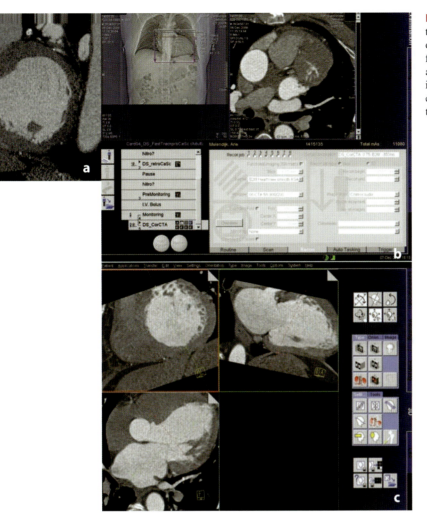

Fig. 27.16 Examples of interpolation artifacts (**a**) showing the lack of sufficient data for the successful reconstruction of the image and artifacts due to the incorrect initiation of the scan (**b,c**) with a consequent loss of a portion of the left main coronary artery

presence of an elevated HR. However, multisegment reconstructions have not yet proven effective in compensating for that relative shortfall. This is because they are based on a temporal and geometric assumption which in reality rarely occurs, i.e. that each cardiac cycle is exactly the same as the previous cardiac cycle and that during the different phases of myocardial contraction and relaxation the coronary arteries follow exactly the same trajectory and end up in exactly the same points in space. According to the fundamental notions of cardiac physiology, in baseline conditions the heart tends to rhythmically fill and contract but with slight pre- and post load variations which translate into slight differences in the position of the various points of the object in space. Patient breath-hold during the cardiac cycle also induces a variation in intrathoracic pressure which in turn produces a variation in the resistance to the flow of venous blood towards the heart from the brain, the upper limbs and the abdominal and pelvic regions. It is therefore understandable that minor differences may be present between each individual cardiac cycle, thus impairing the fusion of information from different cycles (Fig. 27.16).

Data can be lost when the length of the scan is inappropriately regulated. The main reasons for data loss are correlated with the scan range being too short or with a discrepancy between the depth of breath-hold during the scanogram and during the contrast enhancement phase. In the worst instance the cranial portion of the volume is lost, making the evaluation of the left main and the proximal branches impossible. Data loss can also occur when the scan finishes too early, with the loss of a part of the posterior descending artery.

The settings for scan length should be slightly increased to avoid these problems. If a real-time patient tray position display is available, the operator should set the scan length longer than necessary and interrupt the scan as soon as the entire cardiac volume has been acquired.

Another factor which can influence data loss is pitch, especially in patients with considerable variations in HR.

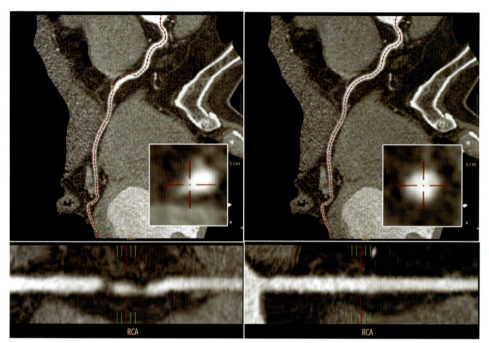

Fig. 27.17 Reconstruction artifact: the focus of the centerline on curved multiplanar reconstructions used for coronary evaluation has to be carefully checked as automated systems can produce disruption of vessel lumen (*on the left*) which can be confused with stenosis.
The simple manual reposition of the centerline (*on the right*) can correct this artifact

The new MDCT systems automatically calculate pitch on the basis of the HR recorded prior to the scan. In the event of significant variations in HR, manually setting pitch for a HR lower than the average recorded HR is advisable to avoid the formation of gaps between contiguous image sections. Such gaps can occur when the real HR is lower than the HR measured prior to the scan and on which the automatic pitch setting is based [14, 35].

Modern dual-source CT scanners allow high-pitch scans (3.2) with high temporal resolution (up to 75 ms) while maintaining high image quality, equivalent to the quality obtained by single-source scanners with a pitch of 1.0. The resulting reduction in acquisition time may offer a clinical advantage with trauma and pediatric patients.

In addition, the ECG-triggered prospective applications already used for patients with low heart rate in 64 slice devices can be extended in case of HR above 60 bpm because of the possibility to scan the entire heart volume in a single heartbeat, with a significant reduction in dose [36].

27.5.3 Reconstruction and Post-processing Artifacts

Software applications dedicated to the evaluation of cardiac CT examinations provided by the manufacturers include systems for the automatic reconstruction of the coronary tree in order to immediately provide curved multiplanar reconstructions (cMPR) needed for the diagnosis of coronary artery stenosis.

Such systems are, however, far from perfect and are certainly not free from assessment errors. Artifacts generated by these systems can simulate stenoses and lead the less experienced radiologist into error.

Curved multiplanar reconstructions used for coronary artery evaluation are obtained by obtaining a centerline in the vessel lumen; all the points of this centerline should fall within the center of the circle formed by the axial section of the vessel itself. The focus of this line must be carefully corrected by the operator, because automated systems are often deceived by normal anatomic conditions such as bifurcations, variations, kinking etc., producing disruptions of the vessel lumen which can be confused with stenosis. The simple manual repositioning of the centerline can quickly correct this artifact (Fig. 27.17).

Automatic reconstruction systems work better with high quality examinations. In this case they would be a time saver for the expert user, who can easily recognize and correct these artifacts [37].

27.5.4 MDCT Artifacts

There is another group of artifacts which arise from the incorrect functioning of the scanner at the time of data acquisition or during the reconstruction process.

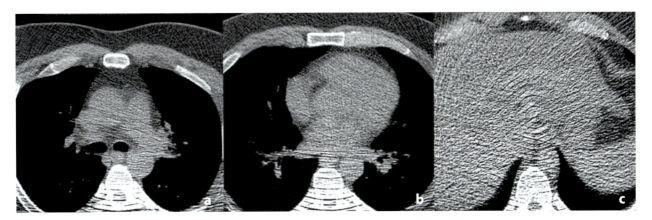

Fig. 27.18 Examples of artifacts produced by detector malfunction (**a-c**)

27.5.4.1 Ring Artifact

This occurs when a detector fails to function correctly or is not correctly calibrated with the rest of the system. Since the detector is inserted into a rotating system, a *non-reading* or a false reading at each angular view of the tube-detector system will appear as a uniform circular artifact. This artifact is not always visible in that its visualization depends on the width of the window (less evident with broad windows). When it is visible it can rarely be mistaken for a pathologic finding (Fig. 27.18). The deterioration in image quality is greater when central detectors rather than peripheral detectors are involved, with the presence of dark shading at the center of the image. Given their physical characteristics as independent units, solid-state detectors tend to be more prone to generating this type of artifact than gaseous detectors, which in contrast are made up of a single ionizing chamber [12, 17, 21]. Nonetheless, technical development has preferred the use of solid-state detectors as they are more stable. Modern scanners are therefore equipped with correction software which recognize, reduce and/or correct reading errors of individual detectors.

27.5.4.2 Cone Artifact

When the object being studied rapidly changes shape and/or position along the z-axis, the process of spiral interpolation and reconstruction produces artifacts in the form of image distortion. Studies performed on cone phantoms (whose diameter decreases in the z-axis), or on phantoms inclined at 45° on the patient table (which changes position in the z-axis), have shown that the shape of the sections in the axial images is distorted (and does not appear circular as it should) precisely due to the interpolation algorithm. With each rotation the detectors intersect the reconstruction plane at a different point, such that the contribution to the image formation changes since it is provided by parts of the cone with a greater diameter at one point in the rotation and a lesser diameter at another point.

This artifact can be reduced by using a low pitch, a 180° interpolation rather than 360° interpolation and thin-slice acquisitions. The introduction of modern MDCT systems which apply these parameters has reduced this effect which at any rate is of little importance in cardiac imaging. These artifacts are in fact more common in the liver, the kidneys and the skull - where an axial image may be preferable (organs with an approximately conic shape - cone artifact) - and in the ribs (which change position in the z-axis - rod artifact) [21, 35].

27.5.4.3 Helical (Windmill) Artifact

The spiral interpolation process in multidetector scanners has however produced a more complex distortion of the axial images, in that more detector rows intersect the reconstruction plane with each rotation. This produces the typical *windmill* appearance - radial bands which rotate around a high-attenuation structure along the volume. The intensity of the artifact, and therefore the number of windmill blades, depends on the pitch, since an increase in pitch corresponds to a greater number of detectors intersecting the reconstruction plane with each rotation (Fig. 27.19). Since the cause of the problem is to be found in inadequate and/or under sampling (aliasing), the traditional approaches aimed at reducing this effect based on the reduction of pitch and the increase of reconstructed slice thickness are ineffective, particularly in the peripheral regions outside of the isocenter.

27.5.4.4 Cone Beam Effect (Artifact)

The increase in the number of detectors has created the need for a broader collimation and therefore a change in the profile of the X-ray beam. Unlike the fan-shape of pre-

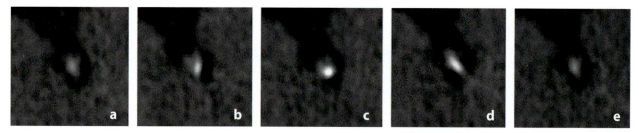

Fig. 27.19 Examples of windmill artifacts associated with the different position of the tube-detector system during different phases of the cardiac cycle. The same tract of the right coronary artery displays small lines spreading out from its lumen in different directions (**a-e**)

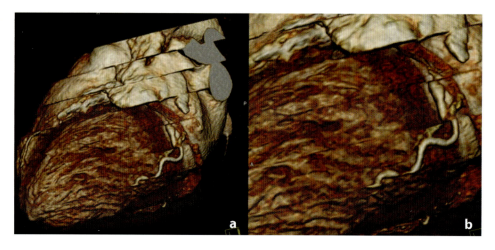

Fig. 27.20 Examples of stair-step artifacts in volume rendering images (**a**, **b**)

vious generations, the beam has taken on the appearance of a cone. The data registered by each detector per rotation are no longer lying in the same ideal plane as occurs with single-slice systems, rather they correspond to a volume between cones, such that points seen in one view may not be seen at 180°. This generates an artifact similar to a partial volume effect which is more pronounced for the external detectors than the internal detectors registering data lying almost in a single plane. The intensity of the effect is proportional to the number of detectors, which is why new dedicated reconstruction algorithms needed to be incorporated in multislice devices, effectively replacing those used in scanners with 4 detector rows [1, 2, 21].

27.5.4.5 Stair-Step and Zebra Artifact

This artifact occurs along the contours of structures in multiplanar and 3D reconstructions when an acquisition is performed with a wide collimation and no slice overlap. The artifact is typical in non spiral systems, less marked in spiral systems which enable reconstructions of overlapping sections, and almost nonexistent in modern multidetector scanners with isotropic voxels and which perform acquisitions with sub millimeter slices. In cardiac CT this artifact can also be found in the latest generation of scanner using axial ECG gated acquisitions as dose-saving protocols. Shaded stripes can also appear in multiplanar and 3D reconstructions due to spiral interpolation, which generates heterogeneous noise in the z-axis [17, 39] (Fig. 27.20).

27.6 Conclusions

The operator needs to be aware that artifacts are always present in CT imaging which are linked to the fundamental physical principles of CT itself. Added to these are the artifacts associated with the organ (the heart) being studied. With the improved spatial and temporal resolution of the most recent scanners and the increasingly sophisticated reconstruction algorithms, possibly together with new hardware resolutions, there will likely be a reduction in artifactual effects in CT imaging of the coronary arteries in the future.

References

1. Hsieh J (2003) Image artifacts: appearences, causes and corrections., in Computer tomography: principles, design, artifacts and recent advances SPIE Press. Bellingham, Wash pp 167-240

2. Seeram E (2001) Image quality. In: Computed tomography: physical principles, clinical applications and quality control Saunders: Philadelphia PA, pp 174-179

3. Achenbach S, Ropers D, Holle J et al (2000) In-plane coronary arterial motion velocity: measurement with electron-beam CT. Radiology 216:457-463

4. Cademartiri F, Luccichenti G, Marano R et al (2003) Spiral CT-angiography with one, four, and sixteen slice scanners. Technical note. Radiol Med 106:269-283

5. Cademartiri F, Runza G, Belgrano M et al (2005) Introduction to coronary imaging with 64-slice computed tomography. Radiol Med (Torino) 110:16-41

6. Dewey M, Laule M, Krug L et al (2004) Multisegment and halfscan reconstruction of 16-slice computed tomography for detection of coronary artery stenoses. Invest Radiol 39:223-229

7. Cademartiri F, Mollet NR, Runza G et al (2006) Improving diagnostic accuracy of MDCT coronary angiography in patients with mild heart rhythm irregularities using ECG editing. AJR Am J Roentgenol 186:634-638

8. Desjardins B, Kazerooni EA (2004) ECG-gated cardiac CT. AJR Am J Roentgenol 182:993-1010

9. Hoffmann MH, Shi H, Manzke R et al (2005) Noninvasive coronary angiography with 16-detector row CT: effect of heart rate. Radiology 234:86-97

10. Kopp AF, Schroeder S, Kuettner A et al (2001) Coronary arteries: retrospectively ECG-gated multi-detector row CT angiography with selective optimization of the image reconstruction window. Radiology 221:683-688

11. Prokop M, Galanski M et al (2003) Principles of CT, Spiral CT and Multislice CT., in Spiral and Multislice Computed Tomography of the Body Thieme Verlag: Stuttgart-New York

12. Barnes G, Lakshminarayanan A (1998) Conventional and Spiral Computed Tomography: Physical Principles and Image Quality Considerations, in Computed Body Tomography with MRI Correlation, S.S. Lee JKT, Stanley RJ, Heiken JP, Editor Lippincott Williams & Wilkins

13. Enzweiler CN, Kivelitz DE, Wiese TH et al (2000) Coronary artery bypass grafts: improved electron-beam tomography by prolonging breath holds with preoxygenation. Radiology 217:278-283

14. Choi HS, Choi BW, Choe KO et al (2004) Pitfalls, artifacts, and remedies in multi-detector row CT coronary angiography. Radiographics 24:787-800

15. Hong C, Becker CR, Huber A et al (2001) ECG-gated reconstructed multi-detector row CT coronary angiography: effect of varying trigger delay on image quality. Radiology 220:712-717

16. Mao SS, Oudiz RJ, Bakhsheshi H et al (1996) Variation of heart rate and electrocardiograph trigger interval during ultrafast computed tomography. Am J Card Imaging 10:239-243

17. Barrett JF, N Keat (2004) Artifacts in CT: recognition and avoidance. Radiographics 24:1679-1691

18. Flohr T, Prokop M, Becker C et al (2002) A retrospectively ECG-gated multislice spiral CT scan and reconstruction technique with suppression of heart pulsation artifacts for cardio-thoracic imaging with extended volume coverage. Eur Radiol 12:1497-1503

19. Prokop M, Galanski M et al (2003) Radiation Dose and Image Quality., in Spiral and Multislice Computed Tomography of the Body Thieme Verlag: Stuttgart - New York

20. Cademartiri F (2005) Artifacts, in Computed Tomography of the Coronary Arteries, K.G.P. de Fayter PJ, Editor Taylor & Francis

21. Prokop M, Galanski M et al (2003) Image Analysis., in Spiral and Multislice Computed Tomography of the Body Thieme Verlag: Stuttgart - New York

22. Cademartiri F, Runza G, Mollet NR et al (2005) Influence of increasing convolution kernel filtering on plaque imaging with multislice CT using an ex-vivo model of coronary angiography. Radiol Med (Torino) 110:234-240

23. Rollano-Hijarrubia E, Stokking R, van der Meer F, Niessen WJ (2006) Imaging of small high-density structures in CT A phantom study. Acad Radiol 13:893-908

24. Watzke O, Kalender WA (2004) A pragmatic approach to metal artifact reduction in CT: merging of metal artifact reduced images. Eur Radiol 14:849-856

25. Nieman K, Oudkerk M, Rensing BJ et al (2001) Coronary angiography with multi-slice computed tomography. Lancet 357:599-603

26. Cademartiri F, de Monye C, Pugliese F et al (2006) High iodine concentration contrast material for noninvasive multislice computed tomography coronary angiography: iopromide 370 versus iomeprol 400. Invest Radiol 41:349-353

27. Cademartiri F, Nieman K, van der Lugt A et al (2004) Intravenous contrast material administration at 16-detector row helical CT coronary angiography: test bolus versus bolus-tracking technique. Radiology 233:817-823

28. Mollet NR, Cademartiri F, de Feyter PJ (2005) Non-invasive multislice CT coronary imaging. Heart 91:401-417

29. Cademartiri F, Mollet N, van der Lugt A et al (2004) Non-invasive 16-row multislice CT coronary angiography: usefulness of saline chaser. Eur Radiol 14:178-183

30. Fleischmann D (2003) Use of high-concentration contrast media in multiple-detector-row CT: principles and rationale. Eur Radiol 13:14-20

31. Becker CR, Hong C, Knez A et al (2003) Optimal contrast application for cardiac 4-detector-row computed tomography. Invest Radiol 38:690-694

32. Cademartiri F, van der Lugt A, Luccichenti G et al (2002) Parameters affecting bolus geometry in CTA: a review. J Comput Assist Tomogr 26:98-607

33. Leschka S, Wildermuth S, Boehm T et al (2006) Noninvasive Coronary Angiography with 64-Section CT: Effect of Average Heart Rate and Heart Rate Variability on Image Quality. Radiology 24:378-385

34. Leschka S, Husmann L, Desbiolles LM et al (2006) Optimal image reconstruction intervals for non-invasive coronary angiography with 64-slice CT. Eur Radiol 16:1964-1972

35. Wilting JE, Timmer J (1999) Artefacts in spiral-CT images and their relation to pitch and subject morphology. Eur Radiol 9(2): p. 316-322

36. Flohr TG, Leng S, Yu L, Aiimendinger T (2009)Dual-source spiral CT with pitch up to 3.2 and 75 ms temporal resolution: image reconstruction and assessment of image quality. Med Phys 36:5641-5653

37. Kroft LJ, de Roos A, Geleijns J (2007) Artifacts in ECG-synchronized MDCT coronary angiography. AJR Am J Roentgenol 189:581-591

38. Kyriakou Y, Kachelriess M, Knaup M et al (2006) Impact of the z-flying focal spot on resolution and artifact behavior for a 64-slice spiral CT scanner. Eur Radiol 16:1206-1215

39. Taguchi K, Aradate H (1998) Algorithm for image reconstruction in multi-slice helical CT. Med Phys 25:550-561

40. Taguchi K, Aradate H, Saito Y et al (2004)The cause of the artifact in 4-slice helical computed tomography. Med Phys 31:2033-2037

41. Silver M (2003) Wind-mill artifact in multislice CT. Proc SPIE 5032:1918-1927

Section V

Clinical Applications

Diagnostic and Prognostic Value

28

Joanne D. Schuijf, Jacob M. van Werkhoven, Jeroen J. Bax, and Ernst E. van der Wall

28.1 Clinical Background

In a patient presenting with suspected coronary artery disease (CAD), imaging tests serve several important purposes. The first clinical goal is to establish whether the patient has CAD, and if so, to determine its severity and extent. Accordingly, in combination with clinical characteristics, the imaging test should result in a change of probability of disease. Secondly, the test should provide information on the likelihood of future major cardiovascular events. Lastly, the observations should have impact on therapeutic management and ultimately help clinicians to improve patient outcome.

Accordingly, the clinical value of an imaging test can be divided into:

- Diagnostic value and impact on disease probability
- Prognostic performance
- Impact on patient management and outcome

Since its introduction, the diagnostic value of cardiac CT angiography (CCT) to detect significant CAD (defined as a stenosis ≥50% luminal narrowing) has been evaluated extensively against conventional coronary artery angiography (CAG). In addition, the technique has been shown to allow visualization of the vessel wall, and thus detection of plaque in the absence of significant stenosis. Interestingly, data are emerging suggesting that the presence and extent of both plaque and significant stenoses on CCT are predictive of cardiovascular events. In contrast however, the precise implications of such observations and how they should change clinical management remain largely unknown. Accordingly, due to the current lack of data concerning the impact of coronary CCT on patient outcome, the current chapter will focus only on the diagnostic and prognostic value of CCT.

28.2 Diagnostic Value

28.2.1 Diagnostic Accuracy in Detecting Significant CAD

The diagnostic performance of 64-row CCT to detect significant CAD (defined as a stenosis ≥50% luminal narrowing) has been evaluated against CAG in numerous single-center studies. In addition, several meta-analyses as well as multicenter trials have been published [1-5]. As shown in Figure 28.1, a recent meta-analysis combining data from 13 studies with 875 patients enrolled, showed a sensitivity, specificity, positive and negative predictive value of 98%, 91%, 93%, and 97%, respectively [1]. Similar findings were observed in the multicenter ACCURACY trial, enrolling 230 patients across 16 centers in the US [2]. In this population with a low prevalence of CAD (≈25%) a sensitivity and specificity of respectively 95% and 83% were achieved. Corresponding positive and negative predictive values were 64% and 99%, respectively. Overall, these investigations strengthen the notion that CCT is an accurate technique to detect the presence of significant coronary stenosis. Moreover, the consistent high negative predictive values indicate that CCT may be an attractive technique to rule out CAD noninvasively. However, it should be noted that the positive predictive value tends to be limited. In particular, diagnostic accuracy is reduced in the presence of extensive calcifications [6, 7]. As a consequence, patients with a higher likelihood of CAD may be considered less suitable candidates for CCT [8]. Moreover, due to the high prevalence of significant CAD in this population, the value of CCT to rule out significant CAD will be highly limited as well [9]. A similar notion holds true for patients with known CAD. The presence of atherosclerosis has been previously established in these patients and further management, including the decision for revascularization, is most frequently based on the presence of recurrent ischemia [10].

J.D. Schuijf (✉)
Department of Cardiology,
Leiden University Medical Center,
Leiden, The Netherlands

F. Cademartiri, G. Casolo, M. Midiri (eds.), *Clinical Applications of Cardiac CT*,
© Springer-Verlag Italia 2012

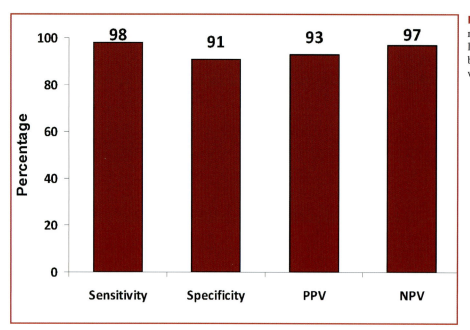

Fig. 28.1 Diagnostic accuracy of 64-row CCT to detect a stenosis ≥50% luminal narrowing on a patient basis, based on meta-analysis of 13 studies with 875 enrolled patients [1]

28.2.2 Impact on Disease Probability

For a diagnostic test to be clinically useful, it should not only have high diagnostic accuracy but should also be able to change the probability of disease. While positive and negative predictive values are commonly used for this purpose, it should be noted that these remain dependent of the pretest probability of the studied population. This issue was recently addressed by Meijboom et al. [8]. In total, 254 symptomatic patients were stratified according to pre-test probability of CAD and were studied with both 64-slice CCT and CAG. As a result of the different pre-test probabilities as well as the different diagnostic performances of CCT across these groups, a substantial difference was observed in the estimated post-test probability of significant CAD after CCT. Indeed, while a negative CCT study was able to reduce the post-test probability to 0% in patients with a low and intermediate pre-test probability, post-test probability remained high (17%) in patients with a high pre-test probability. Similarly, a positive CCT study was able to increase the post-test probability to 96% and 88% in patients with a high and intermediate pre-test probability, respectively. However, in patients with a low pre-test probability, post-test probability remained intermediate (68%) after a positive CCT study.

In a subsequent step, the same group explored the clinical utility of CCT as compared to stress testing (exercise ECG and myocardial perfusion imaging [MPI]) in relation to pre-test probability in 517 patients [11]. Across all groups, the authors observed that stress testing was less accurate than CCT. In patients with a low pre-test probability of disease, stress testing and CCT were performed similarly. In over 70% of patients a negative study was obtained, which was able to reduce post-test probability to below 5% (4% for stress testing, 0% for CCT). In patients with a high pre-test probability on the other hand, both stress testing and CCT were shown to be of limited value. Although a negative CCT study was superior as compared to a negative stress test in reducing post-test probability (12% for CCT versus 81% for stress testing), this reduction was insufficient to no longer require further testing. Moreover, a negative study was obtained in only 13% of patients, suggesting that use of noninvasive testing would only result in unnecessary layered testing in this population. Indeed, the highest benefit was obtained in patients with an intermediate pre-test probability. Whereas stress testing was unable to either reduce or increase post-test probability sufficiently, CCT was able to either confirm (post-test probability 94% after a positive test) or exclude CAD (post-test probability 1% after a negative test) with high certainty. Data are summarized in Figure 28.2.

28.2.3 Moving Beyond Significant Stenosis: Detection of Plaque

In the majority of studies addressing the diagnostic accuracy and clinical impact of CCT, the presence of significant CAD - as identified on CAG - has been used. However, it should be noted that fundamental differ-

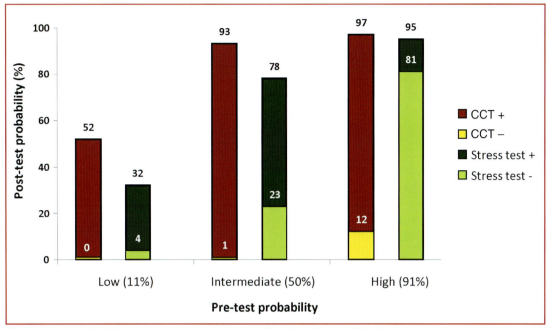

Fig. 28.2 Impact of CCT and stress testing on the probability of significant CAD. Bar graph showing the post-test probability of CAD in relation to the pre-test probability for both CCT (positive study indicated in red, negative study in yellow) and stress testing (positive study indicated in dark green, negative study in light green) [11]

ences exist between CCT and CAG. Due to restrictions in spatial resolution, lesions cannot be graded as precisely as they can with CAG. Particularly in the presence of extensive calcifications or borderline lesions, accurate assessment of lesion significance is difficult, as illustrated in Figure 28.3. Moreover, while CAG is based on luminography, CCT is a tomographic technique that provides information on both lumen and plaque. Accordingly, the performance of CCT may be better for the detection of any atherosclerotic lesions than for strict significant stenosis assessment. This issue was recently addressed by van Velzen et al. who performed a direct comparison of the diagnostic accuracy of CCT for the detection of *significant stenosis* (with CAG as the criterion standard) as well as for the detection of *atherosclerosis* (using intravascular ultrasound (IVUS) as the criterion standard) in 100 patients [12]. In line with previous literature, the authors found a high negative predictive value of 100% for the presence of significant stenosis (Table 28.1). However, a limited positive predictive value of 81% was observed, since 9 patients were incorrectly classified as having a significant stenosis. Importantly, when the endpoint was changed from significant stenosis on CAG to the presence of atherosclerosis on IVUS, the performance of CCT improved and an excellent diagnostic accuracy was observed. Moreover, further evaluation of false positive lesions revealed that plaque burden on IVUS was similar to lesions with significant narrowing on CAG (true positive lesions). These findings indicate that while false positive lesions on CCT may be indeed nonsignificant in terms of luminal narrowing, they nevertheless harbor substantial plaque burden. In terms of prognosis therefore, these lesions may still be relevant. At the same time, these observations highlight that CCT allows superior rule-out of any clinically relevant atherosclerosis. It is conceivable that this finding may also have important implications for risk stratification.

28.3 Prognostic Value

28.3.1 Prognostic Value of Stenosis Severity and Plaque Extent

Importantly, data concerning the prognostic value of CCT are rapidly emerging. While initial reports consisted of only small cohorts with relatively limited follow-up, data from larger registries are now rapidly emerging. Min et al. reported on the association between all-cause mortality and the extent of significant CAD on CCT in 1,127 patients [13]. During a follow-up period of 15.3 ± 3.9 months, a relation between increasing severity of significant CAD on CCT and worsened survival was demonstrated. Importantly, patients without significant stenosis on CCT were shown to have excellent survival (mortality rate at 1.5 years of 0.3%).

Several studies also explored the prognostic implications of nonsignificant plaque. In a small study evaluat-

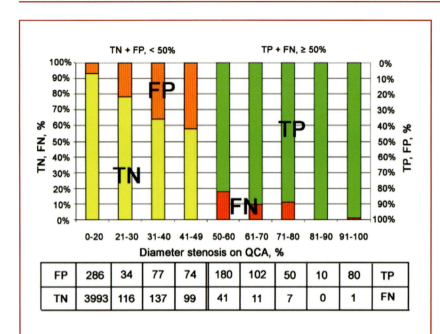

Fig. 28.3 Diagnostic performance of CCT on a segmental basis in relation to the degree of diameter stenosis on QCA. Most often, overestimated (false positive lesions, FP) and underestimated (false negative, FN) lesions were lesions classified between 40% to 60% luminal narrowing on QCA. (Reproduced from [4], with permission from Elsevier)

Table 28.1 Diagnostic accuracy of CCT for detection of significant stenosis and atherosclerosis. (Adapted from [12])

	Segmental analysis	Vessel analysis	Patient analysis
Detection of significant stenosis (≥50% luminal narrowing on invasive coronary angiography)			
Sensitivity	57/58 (98%, 95%-100%)	47/47 (100%)	38/38 (100%)
Specificity	435/452 (96%, 94%-97%)	158/172 (92%, 88%-96%)	53/62 (85%, 78%-93%)
PPV	57/74 (77%, 69%-85%)	47/61 (77%, 67%-88%)	38/47 (81%, 71%-90%)
NPV	435/436 (99.7%, 99%-100%)	158/158 (100%)	53/53 (100%)
Diagnostic accuracy	492/510 (96%, 95%-98%)	205/219 (94%, 90%-97%) 9	1/100 (92%, 86%-96%)
Detection of atherosclerosis (≥40% plaque burden on cross-sectional area on intravascular ultrasound			
Sensitivity	343/346 (99%, 98%-100%)	172/173 (99%, 98%-100%)	93/93 (100%)
Specificity	179/182 (98%, 97%-100%)	45/46 (98%, 94%-100%)	7/7 (100%)
PPV	343/346 (99%, 98%-100%)	172/173 (99%, 98%-100%)	93/93 (100%)
NPV	179/182 (98% (97%-100%)	45/46 (98 %, 94%-100%)	7/7 (100%)
Diagnostic accuracy	522/528 (99%, (98%-99.7%)	218/219 (99%, 99%-100%)	100/100 (100%)

ing first year event rates after CCT in 100 patients, Pundziute et al. noted slightly but significantly increased event rates in patients with nonsignificant plaque as compared to patients with completely normal coronary arteries [14]. Similar findings were reported by Shaw et al., showing that particularly in women the extent of nonsignificant CAD on CCT was an important independent predictor of all-cause mortality [15].

These observations were recently confirmed by a meta-analysis summarizing data from 18 studies with a total of 9,592 included patients [16]. Pooled annualized event rates increased from 0.17% for patients with a normal CCT study to 8.8% in patients with significant stenosis on CCT. Interestingly, as shown in Figure 28.4, the analysis also revealed that although overall risk was low, patients with nonsignificant stenosis nevertheless fared worse than patients with completely normal coronary arteries.

Thus far the majority of studies assessing the prognostic role of CCT focused on luminal stenosis severity and therefore used a relatively simple classification of CAD (normal, nonsignificant CAD or significant CAD). However, information regarding plaque extent, morphology and composition can be extracted from CCT and may provide additional information [13, 17]. In a report

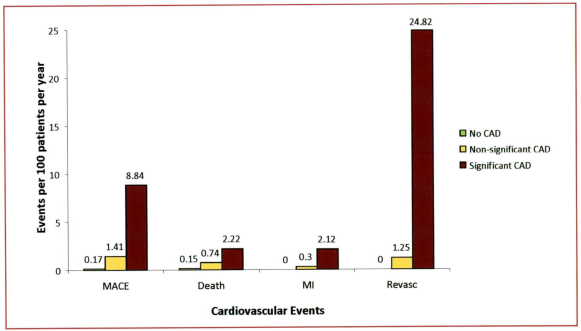

Fig. 28.4 Percentage of annualized event rates for combined major adverse cardiac events (MACE), death (all-cause), myocardial infarction (MI), and revascularization (Revasc), stratified by CCT. Data are based on meta-analysis of 18 studies with a total of 9,592 patients included. (Adapted from [16])

by van Werkhoven et al., noncalcified plaque was shown to provide incremental predictive value over the presence of significant stenosis [18]. Moreover, Motoyama et al. showed that the combination of low attenuation plaque and positive remodeling was a strong predictor of events [19]. In patients with lesions displaying both features, event rate was 22%, whereas only 3.7% of patients with lesions with one feature and 0.5% of patients without lesions positive for either features experienced an event ($p<0.001$). While these observations are promising, data integrating plaque composition with stenosis severity for risk stratification are currently scarce and further investigations are required.

28.3.2 Incremental Value of Other Risk Assessment Tools

Several studies have addressed the incremental prognostic value of CCT over baseline risk assessment and other imaging tests. Hadamitzky et al. followed 1,256 patients with suspected CAD for a median period of 18 months after CCT for the occurrence of events, in order to compare the predictive value of significant CAD on CCT to baseline Framingham risk assessment [20]. In line with previous studies, the presence of significant CAD was a strong predictor of events. Moreover, the event rate in patients without obstructive CAD was significantly lower than predicted by the Framingham risk score. The value of CCT to predict outcome incremental to other noninvasive modalities has been evaluated as well. In a large study (2,538 patients) with relatively long-term follow-up (up to 12 years), CCT-derived plaque burden was shown to have independent and incremental value for the prediction of all-cause mortality over baseline risk stratification and coronary calcium scoring [21]. Similar findings were reported by Rubinshtein et al. [22] as well as van Werkhoven et al. [23]. In contrast, a recent study by Schmermund et al. was unable to show incremental benefit from CCT over coronary calcium scoring in patients without significant CAD [24]. At present, data comparing the prognostic performance of CCT against MPI, which is the most commonly applied imaging technique for risk stratification, are scarce. A matched cohort comparison study by Shaw et al. showed that the extent of CAD on CCT had similar predictive value for mortality as the percentage of ischemic myocardium on MPI [17]. Moreover, in a direct comparison by van Werkhoven et al., CCT and MPI were found to be synergistic, suggesting that the combination of these techniques may allow better risk prediction than either technique alone [18].

28.4 Summary and Future Perspective

CCT has emerged as a highly accurate modality for the diagnosis of significant CAD. Particularly in patients with an intermediate pre-test probability, the technique allows clinicians to rule out CAD noninvasively with high diagnostic certainty. In these patients the probability of having significant CAD is reduced to virtually zero in case of a negative CT angiogram. However, the positive predictive value is relatively limited, resulting in frequent overestimation of the degree of stenosis. While the technique is commonly used to establish the presence or absence of significant stenosis, further differentiation can be performed into presence or absence of atherosclerosis as well as plaque type. Interestingly, the severity of CAD as detected by CCT has been demonstrated to have prognostic value, incremental to baseline risk stratification as well as other imaging techniques. In this setting, the characterization of plaque beyond significant stenosis may provide enhanced prognostic value. In particular, the absence of any plaque on CCT has been shown to portend excellent prognosis.

Thus far, the majority of prognostic data have been obtained in patients clinically referred for CCT because of chest pain complaints. Indeed, it remains important to realize that the use of CCT in asymptomatic patients at lower risk solely for the purpose of screening is considered inappropriate and may only trigger unnecessary invasive evaluations [25, 26]. Additional studies in large cohorts are needed to evaluate the predictive value of certain CCT characteristics in dedicated patient populations. Moreover, such studies should aim to further establish whether the use of CCT is cost-effective and may even result in improved patient outcome.

References

1. Abdulla J, Abildstrom SZ, Gotzsche O et al (2007) 64-multislice detector computed tomography coronary angiography as potential alternative to conventional coronary angiography: a systematic review and meta-analysis. Eur Heart J 28:3042-3050
2. Budoff MJ, Dowe D, Jollis JG et al (2008) Diagnostic performance of 64-multidetector row coronary computed tomographic angiography for evaluation of coronary artery stenosis in individuals without known coronary artery disease: results from the prospective multicenter ACCURACY (Assessment by Coronary Computed Tomographic Angiography of Individuals Undergoing Invasive Coronary Angiography) trial. J Am Coll Cardiol 52:1724-1732
3. Hamon M, Biondi-Zoccai GG, Malagutti P et al (2006) Diagnostic performance of multislice spiral computed tomography of coronary arteries as compared with conventional invasive coronary angiography: a meta-analysis. J Am Coll Cardiol 48:1896-1910
4. Meijboom WB, Meijs MF, Schuijf JD et al (2008) Diagnostic accuracy of 64-slice computed tomography coronary angiography: a prospective, multicenter, multivendor study. J Am Coll Cardiol 52:2135-2144
5. Miller JM, Rochitte CE, Dewey M et al (2008) Diagnostic performance of coronary angiography by 64-row CT. N Engl J Med 359:2324-2336
6. Brodoefel H, Reimann A, Burgstahler C et al (2008) Noninvasive coronary angiography using 64-slice spiral computed tomogra-

phy in an unselected patient collective: effect of heart rate, heart rate variability and coronary calcifications on image quality and diagnostic accuracy. Eur J Radiol 66:134-141
7. Meijs MF, Meijboom WB, Prokop M et al (2009) Is there a role for CT coronary angiography in patients with symptomatic angina? Effect of coronary calcium score on identification of stenosis. Int J Cardiovasc Imaging 25:847-854
8. Meijboom WB, van Mieghem CA, Mollet NR et al (2007) 64-slice computed tomography coronary angiography in patients with high, intermediate, or low pretest probability of significant coronary artery disease. J Am Coll Cardiol 50:1469-1475
9. Henneman MM, Schuijf JD, van Werkhoven JM et al (2008) Multi-slice computed tomography coronary angiography for ruling out suspected coronary artery disease: what is the prevalence of a normal study in a general clinical population? Eur Heart J 29:2006-2013
10. Hachamovitch R, Rozanski A, Hayes SW et al (2006) Predicting therapeutic benefit from myocardial revascularization procedures: aremeasurements of both resting left ventricular ejection fraction and stress-induced myocardial ischemia necessary? J Nucl Cardiol 13:768-778
11. Weustink AC, Mollet NR, Neefjes LA et al (2010) Diagnostic accuracy and clinical utility of noninvasive testing for coronary artery disease. Ann Intern Med 152:630-639
12. van Velzen JE, Schuijf JD, de Graaf FR et al (2010) Diagnostic performance of non-invasive multidetector computed tomography coronary angiography to detect coronary artery disease using different endpoints: detection of significant stenosis vs. detection of atherosclerosis. Eur Heart J 32:637-645
13. Min JK, Shaw LJ, Devereux RB et al (2007) Prognostic value of multidetector coronary computed tomographic angiography for prediction of all-cause mortality. J Am Coll Cardiol 50:1161-1170
14. Pundziute G, Schuijf JD, Jukema JW et al (2007) Prognostic value of multislice computed tomography coronary angiography in patients with known or suspected coronary artery disease. J Am Coll Cardiol 49:62-70
15. Shaw LJ, Min JK, Narula J et al (2010) Sex differences in mortality associated with computed tomographic angiographic measurements of obstructive and nonobstructive coronary artery disease: an exploratory analysis. Circ Cardiovasc Imaging 3:473-481
16. Hulten EA, Carbonaro S, Petrillo SP et al (2010) Prognostic Value of Cardiac Computed Tomography Angiography A Systematic Review and Meta-Analysis. J Am Coll Cardiol 57:1237-1247
17. Shaw LJ, Berman DS, Hendel RC et al (2008) Prognosis by coronary computed tomographic angiography: matched comparison with myocardial perfusion single-photon emission computed tomography. J Cardiovasc Comput Tomogr 2:93-101
18. van Werkhoven JM, Schuijf JD, Gaemperli O et al (2009) Prognostic value of multislice computed tomography and gated single-photon emission computed tomography in patients with suspected coronary artery disease. J Am Coll Cardiol 53:623-632
19. Motoyama S, Sarai M, Harigaya H et al (2009) Computed tomographic angiography characteristics of atherosclerotic plaques subsequently resulting in acute coronary syndrome. J Am Coll Cardiol 54:49-57
20. Hadamitzky M, Freissmuth B, Meyer T et al (2009) Prognostic value of coronary computed tomographic angiography for prediction of cardiac events in patients with suspected coronary artery disease. JACC Cardiovasc Imaging 2:404-411
21. Ostrom MP, Gopal A, Ahmadi N et al (2008) Mortality incidence and the severity of coronary atherosclerosis assessed by computed tomography angiography. J Am Coll Cardiol 52:1335-1343
22. Rubinshtein R, Halon DA, Gaspar T et al (2008) Cardiac computed tomographic angiography for risk stratification and prediction of late cardiovascular outcome events in patients with a chest pain syndrome. Int J Cardiol 137:108-115

23. van Werkhoven JM, Schuijf JD, Gaemperli O et al (2009) Incremental prognostic value of multi-slice computed tomography coronary angiography over coronary artery calcium scoring in patients with suspected coronary artery disease. Eur Heart J 30:2622-2629

24. Schmermund A, Elsasser A, Behl M et al (2010) Comparison of prognostic usefulness (three years) of computed tomographic angiography versus 64-slice computed tomographic calcium scanner in subjects without significant coronary artery disease. Am J Cardiol 106:1574-1579

25. Taylor AJ, Cerqueira M, Hodgson JM et al (2010) ACCF/SCCT/ACR/AHA/ASE/ASNC/NASCI/SCAI/SCMR 2010 appropriate use criteria for cardiac computed tomography: a report of the American College of Cardiology Foundation Appropriate Use Criteria Task Force, the Society of Cardiovascular Computed Tomography, the American College of Radiology, the American Heart Association, the American Society of Echocardiography, the American Society of Nuclear Cardiology, the North American Society for Cardiovascular Imaging, the Society for Cardiovascular Angiography and Interventions, and the Society for Cardiovascular Magnetic Resonance. J Am Coll Cardiol 56:1864-1894

26. Choi EK, Choi SI, Rivera JJ et al (2008) Coronary computed tomography angiography as a screening tool for the detection of occult coronary artery disease in asymptomatic individuals. J Am Coll Cardiol 52:357-365

Screening and High CV Risk Patients

29

Giancarlo Casolo

29.1 Introduction

Sudden death, myocardial infarction and heart failure contribute significantly to cardiovascular mortality in the general population and are a common manifestation of coronary artery disease [1]. Acute coronary syndrome (ACS) and sudden death may represent the first manifestation of CAD in about 50% of patients. Furthermore, while the hospital mortality of patients with ACS has greatly improved in the past 20 years, out of hospital deaths are not declining. The main problem is therefore our poor ability to recognize those patients before the appearance of the manifestation of CAD. In fact, while it is relatively easy to identify and treat a patient with symptomatic CAD this is not true for the other individuals. It is therefore of paramount importance to identify those patients at risk of developing an acute manifestation of CAD prior to any clinical event. Although a significant coronary stenosis can often develop prior to ACS, it is clear now that about 50% of the acute events are caused by the complication of nonstenotic coronary segments [2, 3].

Stroke and its complications contribute significantly to cardiovascular (CV) events and risk. The link between acute manifestations of CAD and stroke is atherosclerosis.

Strategies aiming to decrease the risk of cardiovascular events in the general population focus on the ability to identify those factors or those plaque characteristics that can favor or anticipate the acute manifestations of CAD or stroke. Predicting CV events is a difficult task for modern cardiology and prevention and a fascinating field of intensive clinical and epidemiological investigation.

29.2 Aim of Screening and Methodology

In order to decrease the number of subjects that will develop a CV event the first objective would be to identify those factors favoring and boosting atherosclerosis and those triggering the events. The main CV risk factors were definitely identified several years ago and have prompted action for those that are modifiable [4]. Several efforts have been made to improve the risk prediction that has therefore assumed a central role in the field of CVD prevention. However, evaluating the risk of asymptomatic individuals is a difficult task.

Five- and 10-year risk estimates have been widely adopted and are most often based on multivariable regression equations derived from the Framingham cohorts in which the levels of traditional risk factors are assigned to predict CAD events. There are several others systems to predict the CV risk beyond the Framingham-based equations; the most widely used for clinical practice guidelines are the European Systematic COronary Risk Evaluation (SCORE) algorithm and the Prospective Cardiovascular Munster (PROCAM) [5-7].

The lifetime risk of CHD and its various manifestations has been calculated for the Framingham Heart Study population at different ages. In nearly 8000 persons initially free from clinical evidence of CHD, the lifetime risk of developing clinically manifest CAD at age 40 was 48.6% for men and 31.7% for women; At age 70, the lifetime risk of developing CHD is 34.9% for men and 24.2% for women [8].

The available predictive tools, however, provide a method for forecasting a long term rather a near-term CAD risk. In this view they may serve as a basis for decision making about institution of lipid-lowering drug therapy and a useful mean for risk communication with patients rather than a short-term risk assessment tool for CV events. The ability to forecast near-term risk of ACS or sudden cardiac death would help identify those asymptomatic, apparently healthy individuals who are in imminent danger of a CV event. At present there are

G. Casolo (✉)
Cardiology Unit,
Versilia Hospital,
Lido di Camaiore (LU), Italy

F. Cademartiri, G. Casolo, M. Midiri (eds.), *Clinical Applications of Cardiac CT*,
© Springer-Verlag Italia 2012

several approaches involving biomarkers, genetic testing, imaging, proteomics, etc. [9].

In spite of their large implementation and use the score risk charts do not accurately predict cardiovascular risk. A risk factor is a probabilistic concept that applies to a population, not to a specific individual. This is due to the fact that atherosclerosis is a multifactorial disease where the weight of a single risk factor may not be so relevant to grant a strong association with its development. This explains the so-called Rose's paradox, which underlines the fact that for many diseases as well as for CV risk prediction the large majority of cases arise from the mass of the population with risk factor values around the average rather than from those with the highest expression of the risk factor [10]. The concordance statistic, an index of predictive discrimination of statistical models based on the rank correlation between predicted and observed outcomes is a widely used statistical method to evaluate the discriminatory accuracy of a test at the individual level. At best, the discriminatory capability of the traditional risk score is around 60%, being 50% the chance.

29.3 How to Screen Adult Asymptomatic Individuals for CV Risk

By using the traditional approach a significant amount of subjects at the population level fall within the intermediate risk of events. The analysis of such a population indicates that over 60% of men belonging to the Framingham heart study and a large number of subjects from the Norwegian population have an intermediate risk of events when stratified according to the risk scores used [11, 12]. Furthermore, about 31% of asymptomatic U.S. men and 7% of asymptomatic U.S. women age 40 to 79 years without diabetes will fall into the intermediate-risk category [13].

Keeping in mind the above mentioned limitation of the CV risk assessment based only on the use of the traditional risk score charts it should be of paramount importance to have access to new markers of risk or new strategies that may improve our ability to identify patients at risk of events.

29.4 Adding New Markers to Risk Prediction Models

The most likely opportunity to improve the traditional model is the use of additional risk factors to reclassify those in the intermediate-risk group to either high- or low-risk. A large number of biomarkers have been suggested to screen patients: leukocyte count, impaired fasting glucose, peridotontal disease, homocysteine level, lipoprotein a level, hs-CRP level. However, the evidence is insufficient to determine the magnitude of any reduction in CV events by using nontraditional risk factors. This lack of knowledge represents a critical gap in the evidence for benefit from screening with these markers. Although using hs-CRP and ABI to screen men and women with intermediate Framingham CAD risk would reclassify some into the low-risk group and others into the high-risk group, the evidence is insufficient to determine the ultimate effect on the occurrence of CAD events and CAD-related deaths [13-16].

29.5 Imaging to Improve the Risk Reclassification

An alternative way to evaluate the CV risk of asymptomatic adults is to look for subclinical atherosclerosis. The evidence of the presence and extent of atherosclerosis may identify the risk of a patient better than any available score based only on established risk factors. In fact atherosclerosis begins to develop early in life and progresses with time, but the speed of progression is, to a large extent, unpredictable and differs markedly among seemingly comparable individuals. Also, at every level of risk factor, the amount of atherosclerosis and the vulnerability to acute events varies greatly. Finally, the observed event rate may differ several fold among populations predicted to have similar risk by risk factor scoring [17-19]. It can be concluded that there is a relationship between risk factors and atherosclerosis, but this link is not very pronounced. This view, strongly recommended by some authors [20], has been translated into guidelines; the first SHAPE guidelines suggest performing an imaging test. The aim of this testing is to detect signs or equivalents of atherosclerosis possibly in the asymptomatic and subclinical stage, in order to provide the evidence-based prevention measures to an otherwise untreated or undertreated population.

The AHA/ACC guidelines for the assessment of CV risk in asymptomatic adults [21] have implemented part of this concept for the first time. Carotid intima-media thickness on ultrasound, as well as ankle-brachial index, appear to be reasonable tests with a IIA level of evidence in asymptomatic adults at intermediate risk. For the first time calcium score becomes a recommended test .with the same indications and level of evidence. The importance of calcium scoring in this context goes beyond the scope of this chapter. Briefly, the information obtained from calcium scoring is considered relevant, as it reflects the presence, extent and aggressiveness of coronary atherosclerosis. It is a simple and repeatable test, with low inter- and intra-observer variability. Unfortunately calcium score increases with age and show a partial loss of its predictive value in the oldest subjects. Nevertheless it is considered useful information, and very important for reclassifying asymptomatic adults at moderate risk of CV events.

These same guidelines do not recommend coronary computed tomography angiography for cardiovascular risk assessment in asymptomatic adults.

29.6 Atherosclerosis and Clinical Events

Because atherosclerosis is also common among otherwise normal individuals, there is an elusive link between acute events and atherosclerosis. Furthermore, the demonstration of atherosclerosis in peripheral vascular beds does not correctly identify those with significant coronary lesions. Although at high risk for CV events patients with peripheral atherosclerosis do not necessarily develop CAD related events.

As already stated although a significant coronary stenosis can often develop prior to ACS, it is clear now that about 50% of the acute events are caused by the complication of nonstenotic coronary segments [2]. This and other observations have supported the hypothesis of the existence of plaques prone to rupture or erosion compared to others that do not favor thrombosis [22]. These plaques have been defined as vulnerable plaques. Vulnerable plaques are those with some distinctive features that include several features, including the presence of high degree luminal stenosis. Luminal stenosis however is not the sole and necessarily the most important aspect of a plaque prone to rupture. Positive remodeling of the vessel, a large necrotic core, a thin fibrous cap, inflammatory cells, calcium spots and other aspects are frequently encountered in those plaques that rupture causing an ACS [22, 23].

Recently, the results of the PROSPECT trial [3] have shown that among the several features examined that could predict a new major CV event the simple presence of a relevant amount of coronary plaques was associated to a HR of 5.3 compared, as an example, to lesions with a thin cap fibroatheroma that showed a HR of 3.35. As cardiac CT (CCT) represents the most accurate noninvasive technique for detecting coronary atherosclerosis [24], this field of application may be particularly fruitful.

29.7 Therapeutic Choices for Patients at High CV Risk

The demonstration of atherosclerotic lesions represents a sign of a propensity for developing CV events. As already stated, in spite of the efforts to detect qualitative aspects that may predict plaque rupture, at the moment there is a growing evidence that the demonstration of subclinical atherosclerosis per se rather than the aspect or quality of the plaques represent relevant information for risk prediction.

Dealing with the coronary arterial bed, recent clinical data show that the invasive treatment of severely angiographic lesions causing ischemia may not improve survival with respect to medical therapy alone, at least in the chronic setting [25]. This and other data suggest that treating atherosclerosis rather than the coronary lesions may indeed favorably modify prognosis. However, the presence and extent of coronary atherosclerosis may predict a worse outcome [26] per se: the more the atherosclerotic burden the worse the prognosis.

29.8 Role of Cardiac CT

The constant development of technology has already made possible CCT with a very low effective radiation dose for the patient. Although at present calcium score is the only recommended CT based technique in primary prevention, one can foresee a very different position in the future [27]. By using CCT alone or in combination with calcium scoring it is possible to evaluate the vessel wall and therefore describe the presence, extent and some characteristics of the atherosclerotic plaques. Among these, positive vascular remodeling and low Hounsfield units have been demonstrated to help in identifying those plaques that subsequently will cause ACS [28]. Whether data from CCT will add more information or not to the calcium score is currently under investigation. However, in a context where invasive coronary angiography is traditionally the only tool able to provide anatomic information from the coronary vessels, it is easy to foresee a wide application of noninvasive coronary angiography for identifying patients with high risk of CAD and CV events.

29.9 Conclusions

The correct identification of patients at risk of CV events is a difficult and challenging task. While risk score charts are available to evaluate the population risk at any level of traditional risk factors, individual risk can only be imprecisely derived from the collection and analysis of traditional risk factors and a large proportion of the population fall in the intermediate risk. The use of biomarkers and/or imaging may offer an opportunity to reclassify the individual risk and allow the identification of patients that would not benefit from evidence based preventive measures. With regard to imaging, the 2011 AHA/ACC guidelines have implemented its use for the assessment of CV risk of asymptomatic adults. Subclinical atherosclerosis is a very interesting field of application for several imaging techniques. Both calcium score and coronary plaques detected by CT hold a prognostic impact. Noninvasive coronary angiography will be a major tool for identifying the CV risk of events and the risk of ACS over the traditional practice.

References

1. Roger VL, Go AS, Lloyd-Jones DM et al (2011) Heart disease and stroke statistics–2011 update: a report from the American Heart Association. Circulation 123:e18-e209
2. Fuster V, Stein B, Ambrose JA et al (1990) Atherosclerotic plaque rupture and thrombosis. Evolving concepts. Circulation 82:II47-II59
3. Stone GW, Maehara A, Lansky AJ et al (2011) PROSPECT Investigators A prospective natural-history study of coronary atherosclerosis. N Engl J Med 364:226-235
4. – (2002) Third Report of the National Cholesterol Education Program (NCEP) export Panel on Detection, Evaluation, and Treatment of High Blood Cholesterol in Adults (Adult Treatment Panel III) Final Report. Circulation 106:3143-3421
5. Lloyd-Jones DM (2010) Cardiovascular Risk Prediction Basic Concepts, Current Status, and Future Directions. Circulation 121:1768-1777
6. Conroy RM, Pyorala K, Fitzgerald AP et al (2003) Estimation of ten-year risk of fatal cardiovascular disease in Europe: the SCORE project. Eur Heart J 24:987-1003
7. Assmann G, Cullen P, Schulte H (2002) Simple scoring scheme for calculating the risk of acute coronary events based on the 10-year follow-up of the Prospective Cardiovascular Munster (PROCAM) study. Circulation 105:310-315
8. Lloyd-Jones DM, Larson MG, Beiser A, Levy D (1999) Lifetime risk of developing coronary heart disease. Lancet 353:89 -92
9. Eagle KA, Ginsburg GS, Musunuru K et al (2010) Identifying patients at high risk of a cardiovascular event in the near future: current status and future directions: report of a national heart, lung, and blood institute working group. Circulation 121:1447-1454
10. Rose G (1992) The Strategy of Preventive Medicine. New York, NY: Oxford University Press
11. Pasternak RC, Abrams J, Greenland P et al (2003) 34th Bethesda Conference: Task force #1-Identification of coronary heart disease risk: is there a detection gap? J Am Coll Cardiol 41:1863-1874
12. Getz L, Sigurdsson JA, Hetlevik I et al (2005) Estimating the high risk group for cardiovascular disease in the Norwegian HUNT 2 population according to the 2003 European guidelines: modelling study. BMJ 331:551
13. U.S. Preventive Services Task Force (2009) Using Nontraditional Risk Factors in Coronary Heart Disease Risk Assessment: U.S. Preventive Services Task Force Recommendation Statement. Ann Intern Med 151:474-482
14. Pearson TA, Mensah GA, Alexander RW et al (2003) Centers for Disease Control and Prevention. Markers of inflammation and cardiovascular disease: application to clinical and public health practice: A statement for healthcare professionals from the Centers for Disease Control and Prevention and the American Heart Association. Circulation 107:499-511
15. National Heart Lung and Blood Institute, National Cholesterol Education Project (2002) Third Report of the Expert Panel on Detection, Evaluation, and Treatment of High Blood Cholesterol in Adults (Adult Treatment Panel III). Bethesda, MD: National Institutes of Health
16. Helfand M , Buckley DI , Freeman M et al (2009) Emerging Risk Factors for Coronary Heart Disease: A Summary of Systematic Reviews Conducted for the U.S. Preventive Services Task Force. Ann Intern Med 151:496-507
17. D'Agostino RB Sr, Grundy S, Sullivan LM, Wilson P, for the CHD Risk Prediction Group (2001) Validation of the Framingham coronary heart disease prediction scores: results of a multiple ethnic groups investigation 286:180-187
18. Akosah K, Schaper A, Cogbil C, Schoenfeld P (2003) Preventing myocardial infarction in the young adult in the first place: how do the National Cholesterol Education Panel III guidelines perform? J Am Coll Cardiol 41:1475-1479
19. Brindle P, Emberson J, Lampe F et al (2003) Predictive accuracy of the Framingham coronary risk score in British men: prospective cohort study. BMJ 327:1267
20. Naghavi N, Falk E, Hecht HS for the SHAPE et al (2006) Task Force.From Vulnerable Plaque to Vulnerable Patient-Part III:Executive Summary of the Screening for Heart Attack Prevention and Education (SHAPE) Task Force Report. Am J Cardiol 98:2-15
21. Greenland P, Alpert JS, Beller GA et al; American College of Cardiology Foundation; American Heart Association (2010) 2010 ACCF/AHA guideline for assessment of cardiovascular risk in asymptomatic adults: a report of the American College of Cardiology Foundation/American Heart Association Task Force on Practice Guidelines. J Am Coll Cardiol 56:50-103
22. Falk E (2006) Pathogenesis of Atherosclerosis. J Am Coll Cardiol 47:7-12
23. Naghavi M, Libby P, Falk E et al (2003) From vulnerable plaque to vulnerable patient: a call for new definitions and risk assessment strategies: Part I. Circulation 108:1664-1672
24. Velzen JE, Schuijf JD, de Graaf FR et al (2011) Diagnostic performance of non-invasive multidetector computed tomography coronaryangiography to detect coronary artery diseaseusing different endpoints: detection of significantstenosis vs. detection of atherosclerosis European Heart Journal 32:637-645
25. Boden WE, O'Rourke RA, Teo KK et al (2007) Optimal medical therapy with or without PCI for stable coronary disease. N Engl J Med 356:1503-1516
26. Min JK, Dunning A, Lin FY et al; CONFIRM Investigatore (2011) Age- and Sex-Related Differences in All-Cause Mortality Risk Based on Coronary Computed Tomography Angiography Findings Results From the International Multicenter CONFIRM (Coronary CT Angiography Evaluation for Clinical Outcomes: An International Multicenter Registry) of 23,854 Patients Without Known Coronary Artery Disease. J Am Coll Cardiol 58:849-860
27. Ferencik M (2010) Assessment of coronary claque burden by computed tomography: getting closer step by step. Heart 96: 75-576
28. Motoyama S, Sarai M, Harigaya H et al (2009) Computed tomographic angiography characteristics of atherosclerotic plaques subsequently resulting in acute coronary syndrome. J Am Coll Cardiol 54:49-57

Thoracic Aortic Diseases

30

Vincenzo Russo, Francesco Buia, Giovanni Rinaldi, Giangaspare Mineo, and Rossella Fattori

30.1 Introduction

In the past decades conventional angiography was the exclusive available test for diagnosis and anatomic definition of thoracic aortic diseases. With the advent of non-invasive imaging modalities such as computed tomography (CT), magnetic resonance and echocardiography the role of such invasive testing was significantly and progressively reduced.

Of the various noninvasive modalities, CT offers the greatest versatility and is widely used. In particular, the development of multidetector CT (MDCT) in the late 1990s was the most significant advance in CT technology. Thinner collimations, faster gantry rotation times, large detector arrays, powered x-ray tubes and increased table speed dramatically improved image quality and expanded the applications and indications of CT noninvasive vascular imaging. MDCT angiography provides an efficient and cost-effective evaluation of the arterial vascular system, allowing greater vessel length and smaller diameter to be visualized. Today, a very high quality submillimeter scanning of the whole thoracic-abdominal vasculature has become possible within comfortable (4-8 s) breath-hold duration, enabling high quality vascular imaging with 2D-3D artifact-free reconstructions from virtually any angle and in any desirable plane [1-6]. Moreover, in a single study, information of the vessel lumen and wall may be obtained together with extra-vascular information [7].

Another very important feature of MDCT is the capability of having an ECG gating of the scan sequence [8-10]. This allows the acquisition of thoracic vascular data to be synchronised with the cardiac cycle achieving a good temporal resolution (80-200 ms) which minimizes any motion artifact, especially in the ascending aorta.

V. Russo (✉)
Cardio-Thoraco-Vascular Department,
Cardiovascular Radiology Unit,
"Sant'Orsola" University Hospital,
Bologna, Italy

In the evaluation of aortic diseases the more frequently used CT post-processing techniques are multiplanar reconstruction (MPR), maximum intensity projection (MIP) and volume rendering (VR) [3, 11, 12]. MPR re-format image datasets to alternate 2D planes, in general sagittal, coronal or oblique. With thinner slices the aorta is not completely visualized in a single image due to the aortic curvature which cannot be reduced to any single plane. However, with current software it is possible to thicken any selected plane (MPR thick or MIP thin) and look at the entire vessel. MIP is a technique closer to digital subtraction angiography: it shows aortic contrast-enhancement and caliber, but may provide only endoluminal information. Similar to a threshold technique, density values below that of contrast such as plaques or thrombus and above that of contrast such calcifications are difficult to discriminate; MIP images will not allow depth perception or understanding of inter-structural relationships. VR is a powerful method for 3D reconstruction. With high fidelity to the original dataset all tissues are represented based on their density/intensity values so that, unlike a threshold technique, simultaneous depiction of different kind of tissues is possible in a 3D view. With this feature, combined with adequate filters, metallic stents or surgical clips do not present a problem and both calcifications and thrombus can be discriminated from the vessel lumen.

30.2 CT of Thoracic Aortic Disease

30.2.1 Aortic Dissection

Aortic dissection is characterized by a laceration of the aortic intima and inner layer of the aortic media that allows blood to course through a false lumen in the outer third of the media. Dissection can occur throughout the length of the aorta. One of the most used classifications of aortic dissection is the Stanford classification: type A is defined as an aortic dissection irrespective of the site of the entry tear if the ascending aorta is involved,

F. Cademartiri, G. Casolo, M. Midiri (eds.), *Clinical Applications of Cardiac CT*,
© Springer-Verlag Italia 2012

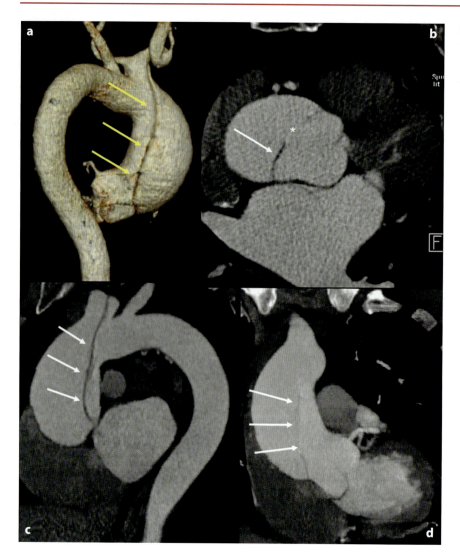

Fig. 30.1 Type A aortic dissection. ECG-gated MDCT VR (**a**), and MPR axial, oblique sagittal and coronal (**b-d**) images showing the intimal flap (*arrow*) and also the entry tear (*)

whereas in type B the ascending aorta is spared. The Stanford classification is fundamentally based on prognostic factors: type A dissection requires urgent surgical repair whereas most of type B dissections can be successfully managed with medical therapy. The anatomic characteristics of the dissection indicate the type of surgical technique, and affect both the surgical success rate and long term results. Therefore, in dissection the diagnostic goal, regardless of the imaging modality used, is a clear delineation not only of the intimal flap and its extension but also of entry and re-entry sites, presence and degree of aortic insufficiency and flow in the aortic branches [13].

CT allows diagnosis of acute aortic dissection with a sensitivity and specificity rates respectively of 83-94% and 87-100% for single detector CT [14-16] and close to 100% for MDCT. Imaging of dissection requires a volume of coverage from the supra-aortic branches to the femoral arteries, and MDCT can acquire this extent in a few seconds. Imaging sensitivity is enhanced by greater temporal resolution and ECG gating sequences, which minimize pulsation artifacts at the aortic root (Fig. 30.1). Unenhanced CT is able to visualize the internal displacement of intimal calcifications and this finding could be confused with an aneurysm with calcified mural thrombus. High attenuation of the false lumen at unenhanced CT may help differentiate between the two conditions [17]. The main and characteristic finding of aortic dissection on contrast enhanced CT scan is an intimal flap separating the true from the false lumen. This usually appears as a thin linear luminal filling defect and its appearance is determined by the circumference and length of dissection, the relative lumen flow and aortic pulsation. The slender linear areas of low attenuation that occasionally appear in the false lumen on CT images, known as the cobweb sign, are specific to the false lumen and may aid in its recognition. These findings correspond to residual ribbons of the media which are incompletely

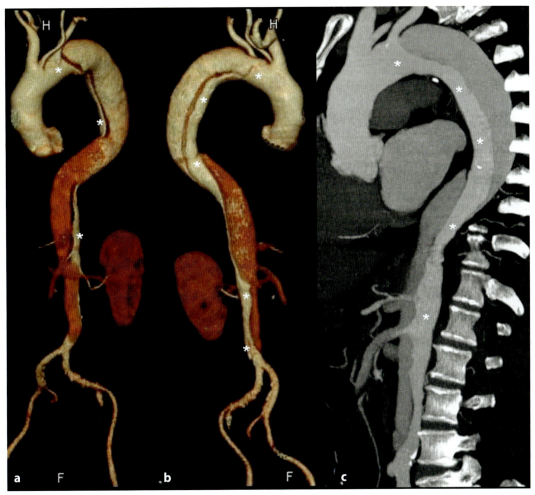

Fig. 30.2 VR (**a**, **b**) and MIP thin (**c**) MDCT images of type B aortic dissection showing the anatomy of the true lumen (*) and its continuation with an undissected portion of the ascending aorta/aortic arch (*)

sheared away during the dissection process [18]. However, on most contrast enhanced CT scans the true lumen may be identified by its continuity with an undissected portion of the aorta (Fig. 30.2). One unusual type of aortic dissection is the intimo-intimal intussusception produced by circumferential dissection of the intimal layer, which subsequently invaginates like a wind sock; CT scan may shows one lumen wrapped around the other lumen in the aortic arch, with the inner lumen invariably being the true one [19, 20]. Sometimes an aortic aneurysm with intraluminal thrombus may be difficult to distinguish from a dissection with a thrombosed false lumen. A useful feature is the fact that dissection generally has a spiral shape, whereas a thrombus tends to maintain a constant circumferential relationship with the aortic wall and, furthermore, a mural thrombus usually has a smooth internal border. Calcifications in aneurysm are typically located at the periphery of the aorta [21]. Visceral and supra-aortic vessel involvement can account for high mortality and MDCT has the spatial and contrast resolution to reliably diagnose branch vessel involvement and document true or false lumen supply (Fig. 30.3).

Apart from axial images and MPR, which provide an overall view of the aortic dissection and demonstrate the anatomic relationships between the flap and adjacent great vessels, VR is preferred to MIP for dissection 3D post-processing as it preserves the variable enhancement patterns of the lumina and is more sensitive for the visualization of the flap. The accurate localization of entry and re-entry sites remains a difficulty for all imaging techniques, but the high resolution of submillimeter MDCT acquisitions with cardiac gating may be reliable enough to depict them, together with possible coronary artery involvement.

30.2.2 Intramural Hematoma

Intramural hematoma (IMH) was first described in 1920 as "dissection without intimal tear" [22], but it was

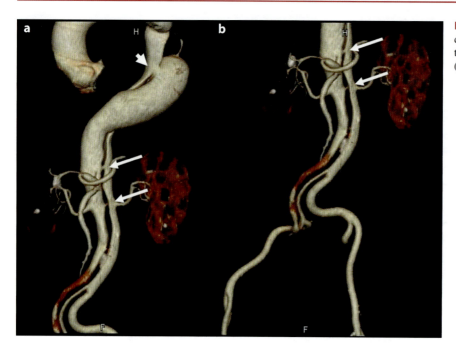

Fig. 30.3 MDCT images of type B aortic dissection: VR images showing the dissection and the entry (*arrowhead*) and re-entry (*arrows*) tears

rarely recognized in the clinical setting before the advent of high resolution imaging modalities. Spontaneous rupture of aortic vasa vasorum of the media layer is considered the initiating process, which is confined in the aortic wall without intimal tear. This results in a circumferentially oriented blood containing space seen on tomographic imaging studies. IMH may occur spontaneously or as a consequence of penetrating aortic ulcer (PAU) in intrinsically diseased media; it has also been described following blunt chest trauma [23].

The diagnosis of IMH relies on the visualization of intramural blood manifested as localized thickened aortic wall. The abnormal wall thickness, symmetric or asymmetric, can vary in dimension from 3 mm to more than 1 cm. The mural involvement can encompass the entire aortic circumference. However, with all the imaging modalities IMH can be confused with clot or plaque especially if localized in the descending aorta.

A typical finding of IMH at unenhanced CT is a crescent shaped area of hyperdensity in the aortic wall or circumferential wall thickening, corresponding to a hematoma in the medial layer which extends cranially and caudally beneath a displaced calcified intima, with constant relations to the wall (subintimal location) [24-28] (Fig. 30.4a). It is important to perform unenhanced CT as the first imaging evaluation, because contrast agent within the vessel may obscure IMH. Unlike the false lumen in typical aortic dissection, the crescent shaped area of IMH remains unenhanced after contrast material administration, and no intimal tear is seen on contrast-enhanced CT scan (Fig. 30.4b). Aortic dilatation could be present. One useful observation that may help differentiate intramural hematoma from thrombosed false lumen of a classic intimal dissection is that the latter tends to longitudinally spiral around the aorta, whereas the former tends to maintain a constant circumferential relationship with aortic wall.

Axial images alone will suffice for detection of IMH or penetrating ulcers in most cases, but 3D review is useful to discriminate both from irregular mural thrombus and to map the full extent of the IMH.

30.2.3 Penetrating Atherosclerotic Ulcer

In 1934 Shennan [29] was the first to describe penetrating atheromatous ulcers of the thoracic aorta. Aortic ulcer is characterized by rupture of an atheromatous plaque disrupting the internal elastic lamina. Extension of the ulcerated atheroma into the media may result in an intramural hematoma as well as localized intramedial dissection, or the plaque may break through to the adventitia and form a saccular pseudoaneurysm. The adventitia may also rupture and in that case only the surrounding mediastinal tissues contain the hematoma. Aortic ulcers occur almost only in the descending aorta but location in the aortic arch or in the ascending aorta have occasionally been reported.

At unenhanced CT, the plaque rupture and disruption of the internal elastic lamina appears as extensive atherosclerosis and IMH of variable extent. Frequently the IMH is focal, due to medial fibrosis caused by atherosclerosis

30 Thoracic Aortic Diseases

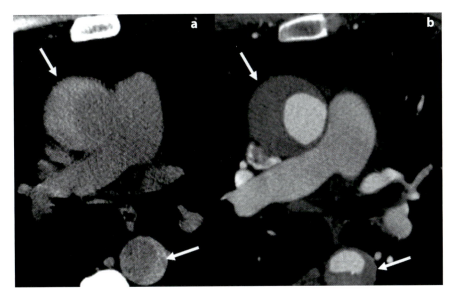

Fig. 30.4 IMH. a Unenhanced CT axial image showing a bright crescent shaped area of attenuation in the aortic wall (*arrows*) in ascending and descending thoracic aorta. b After contrast media administration the abovementioned area is not enhanced and no tears are present (*arrows*)

[30]. Displaced intimal calcifications are also often seen. On CTA, penetrating ulcer appears as a discrete "collar button" contrast filled ulceration, similar to that of a peptic ulcer. (Fig. 30.5) [24-28, 31]. Lesions can be single or multiple. It appears more eccentric than irregular mural thrombus and may be associated with wall thickening and enhancement, pseudoaneurysms, dissection or rupture [26]. CT has the advantage, as well as in IMH, of being able to visualize dislodgment of the intimal calcifications which are very frequently observed in aortic ulcers. MDCT can also depict small penetrating atherosclerotic ulcers and can demonstrate complex spatial relationships, mural abnormalities and extraluminal pathologic conditions, which may offset this weakness [32].

30.2.4 Aortic Aneurysm

Aortic aneurysm is a localized or diffuse dilation involving all layers of the aortic wall, exceeding the expected aortic diameter by a factor of 1.5 or more. MDCT can easily detect aneurysms and facilitate surgical planning by delineating the extent of the aneurysm and the involvement of aortic branches (Fig. 30.6) with 100% of accuracy.

Due to the tortuosity and curvature of the thoracic aorta, aneurysm sizing is performed most accurately when double-oblique tomograms are generated perpendicular to the aortic flow lumen, but to date, information concerning the risk of aneurysm rupture (significant for

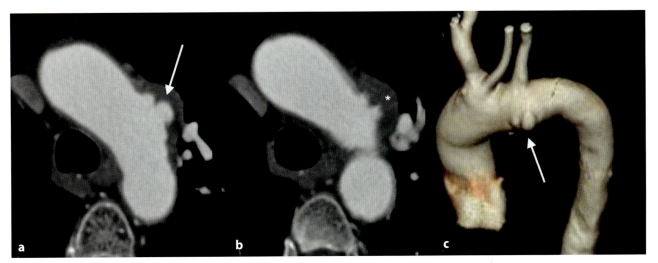

Fig. 30.5 MDCT axial (a, b) and VR (c) images of a penetrating atherosclerotic ulcers (*arrow*) with intramural hematoma (*) of the aortic arch (*arrow*)

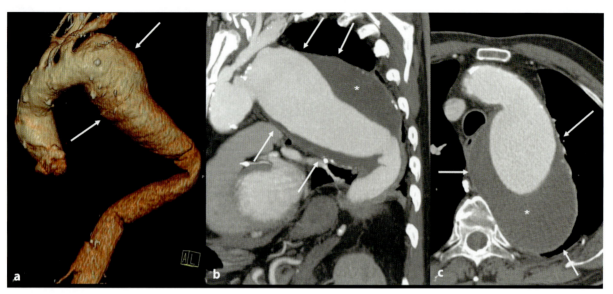

Fig. 30.6 MDCT VR (**a**) and oblique sagittal-axial MPR (**b, c**) images of a large aneurysm of the proximal descending aorta (*arrows*) with partial lumen thrombosis (*)

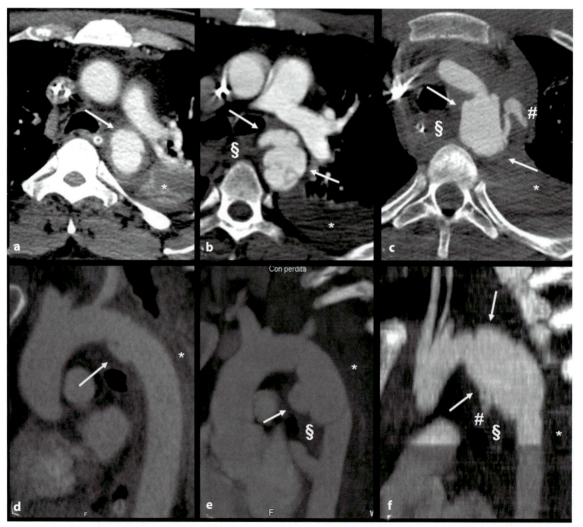

Fig. 30.7 MPR axial (**a-c**) and MIP oblique sagittal (**d-f**) CT images of 3 different traumatic aortic lesions (**a/d, b/e, c/f**) showing the aortic injury (*arrows*) with pleural effusion (*), periaortic mediastinal hematoma (§) and acute thoracic-mediastinal hemorrhage (#)

Table 30.1 Presley trauma center CT grading system: grades and CT findings. (Modified from [41])

Grade	Subgrade	CT Findings
Grade I - Normal aorta	Ia	Normal thoracic aorta No mediastinal hematoma
	Ib	Normal thoracic aorta Mediastinal hematoma (para-aortic)
Grade II - Minimal aortic injury	IIa	Small (<1cm) pseudoaneurysm Indeterminate <1cm intimal flap or thrombus No mediastinal hematoma
	IIb	Small (usually <1cm) pseudoaneurysm Indeterminate <1cm intimal flap or thrombus Mediastinal hematoma (para-aortic)
Grade III - Confined thoracic aortic injury	IIIa	> 1cm regular, well defined pseudoaneurysm Intimal flap or thrombus No ascending aorta, arch or great vessel involvement Mediastinal hematoma
	IIIb	> 1cm regular, well defined pseudoaneurysm Intimal flap or thrombus Ascending aorta, arch or great vessel involvement Mediastinal hematoma
Grade IV - Total aortic disruption	IV	Irregular, poorly defined pseudoaneurysm Intimal flap or thrombus Mediastinal hematoma and/or thoracic hemorrhage

aortic size of 5.5 cm or more) and expansion rate is based upon measurements made from transverse sections, where true diameters can be overestimated.

MDCT and 3D volume rendering can help the assessment of caliber, length, angle, calcification and burden of mural thrombus, as well as length, shape and angle of the aneurysm necks [33, 34].

30.2.5 Aortic Trauma

A traumatic aortic rupture is a lesion caused by trauma extending from the intima to the adventitia. The aortic segment subjected to the greatest strain by rapid deceleration forces is just beyond the isthmus, where the relatively mobile thoracic aorta is joined by the ligamentum arteriosus: aortic rupture occurs at this site 90% of the time in clinical series. In the ascending aorta the segment close to the innominate artery or the proximal segment immediately superior to the aortic valve may be involved. Other less common locations of trauma are the distal segments of the descending aorta or the abdominal infrarenal segment. When a laceration is present it may extend through the media into the adventitia with the formation of false aneurysm; periaortic hemorrhage occurs irrespective of the type of lesion.

CT scanning for the detection of aortic injury is widely employed, especially in emergency due to the availability and speed of this technique. CT is not operator dependent or significantly influenced by patient habitus, nor is it invasive and the patient can be easily monitored while in the scanner. In addition, CT allows quick assessment of not only the aorta, but also the entire thorax and abdomen. CTA has been found to be effective and efficient in emergency post-traumatic aortic evaluation [35-37]. Traumatic injuries could manifest on CT as frank contrast agent extravasation, aortic contour abnormality (representing intima and media disruption), focal caliber change and pseudoaneurysm or dissection flap (Fig. 30.7) [37, 38]. CTA is also widely applied in the setting of acute chest trauma providing vessel information and a review of the chest wall, lungs, airways and mediastinum [39]. It is considered to have high sensitivity and specificity (close to 100%) and good negative and positive predictive value for aortic injury [40-42]. In 1999 Gavant [41] proposed a useful helical CT traumatic aortic injuries grading system in which, for each grade of aortic injury, CT findings and triage/clinical management were considered. There are four grade of injury: normal aorta, minimal aortic injury, confined thoracic aortic injury and total aortic disruption (Table 30.1).

References

1. Rubin GD, Shiau MC, Leung AN et al (2000) Aorta and iliac arteries: single versus multiple detector-row helical CT angiography. Radiology215:670-676
2. Rubin GD (2003) MDCT imaging of the aorta and peripheral vessels. Eur J Radiol 45:42-49

3. Lawler LP, Fishman EK (2001) Multi-detector row CT of thoracic disease with emphasis on 3D volume rendering and CT angiography. Radiographics 21:1257-1273
4. Lawler LP, Fishman EK (2003) Multidetector row computed tomography of the aorta and peripheral arteries. Cardiol Clin 21607-629
5. Wintersperger BJ, Nikolaou K, Becker CR (2004) Multidetector-row CT angiography of the aorta and visceral arteries. Semin Ultrasound CT MR 2525-40
6. Wintersperger BJ, Herzog P, Jakobs T et al (2002) Initial experience with the clinical use of a 16 detector row CT system. Crit Rev Comput Tomogr 43:283-316
7. Katz DS, Jorgensen MJ, Rubin GD (1999) Detection and follow-up of important extra-arterial lesions with helical CT angiography. Clin Radiol 54:294-300
8. Fuchs T, Kachelriess M, Kalender WA (2000) Technical advances in multi-slice spiral CT. Eur J Radiol 36:69-73
9. Flohr T, Ohnesorge B (2001) Heart rate adaptive optimization of spatial and temporal resolution for electrocardiogram-gated multislice spiral CT of the heart. J Comput Assist Tomog 25:907-923
10. Flohr T, Stierstorfer K, Bruder H et al (2003) Image reconstruction and image quality evaluation for a 16-slice CT scanner. Med Phys 30:832-845
11. Fishman EK (1997) High-resolution three-dimensional imaging from subsecond helical CT data sets: applications in vascular imaging. AJR Am J Roentgenol 169:441-443
12. Kirchgeorg MA, Prokop M (1998) Increasing spiral CT benefits with postprocessing applications. Eur J Radiol 1:39-54
13. Cigarroa JE, Isselbacher EM, De Sanctis RW, Eagle KA (1993) Diagnostic imaging in the evaluation of suspected aortic dissection. Old standard and new direction. N Engl J Med 328:35-43
14. Small JH, Dixon AK, Coulden RA et al (1996) Fast CT for aortic dissection Br J Radiol 69:900-905
15. Chung JW, Park JH, Im JG (1996) Spiral CT angiography of the thoracic aorta Radiographics 16:811-824
16. Sebastia C, Pallisa E, Quiroga S et al (1999) Aortic dissection: diagnosis and follow-up with helical CT. Radiographics 19:45-60
17. Fisher RG, Chasen MH, Lamki N (1994) Diagnosis of injuries of the aorta and brachiocephalic arteries caused by blunt chest trauma: CT vs aortography. AJR Am J Roentgenol 162:1047-1052
18. Williams MP, Farrow R (1994) Atypical patterns in the CT diagnosis of aortic dissection. Clin Radiol 49:686-689
19. Nelsen KM, Spizarny DL, Kastan DJ (1994) Intimointimal intussusception in aortic dissection: CT diagnosis. AJR Am J Roentgenol 162:813-814
20. Karabulut N, Goodman LR, Olinger GN (1998) CT diagnosis of an unusual aortic dissection with intimointimal intussusception: the wind sock sign. Comput Assist Tomogr 22:692-693
21. Rubin GD (1997) Helical CT angiography of the thoracic aorta. J Thorac Imaging 12:128-149
22. Krukemberg E (1920) Beiträge zur Frage des Aneurysma dissecans. Beitr Pathol Anat Allg Pathol 67:329-351
23. Fattori R, Bertaccini P, Celletti F et al (1997) Intramural posttraumatic hematoma of the ascending aorta in a patient with a double aortic arch. Eur Radiol 7:51-53
24. Keren A, Kim CB, Hu BS et al (1996) Accuracy of multiplane transesophageal echocardiography in diagnosis of typical acute aortic dissection and intramural hematoma. J Am Coll Cardiol 28:627-636
25. Quint LE, Williams DM, Francis IR et al (2001) Ulcerlike lesions of the aorta: imaging features and natural history. Radiolo 218:719-723
26. Kazerooni EA, Bree RL, Williams DM (1992) Penetrating atherosclerotic ulcers of the descending thoracic aorta: evaluation with CT and distinction from aortic dissection. Radiology 183:759-765
27. Sueyoshi E, Matsuoka Y, Imada T et al (2002) New development of an ulcerlike projection in aortic intramural hematoma: CT evaluation. Radiology 224:536-541
28. Castaner E, Andreu M, Gallardo X et al (2003) CT in nontraumatic acute thoracic aortic disease: typical and atypical features and complications. Radiographics 23:93-110
29. Shennan T Dissecting aneurisms. Medical Research Council Special Report series no 193:1934
30. Welch TJ, Stanson AW, Sheedy PF 2nd et al (1990) Radiologic evaluation of penetrating aortic atherosclerotic ulcer. Radiographics 10:675-685
31. Sawhney NS, DeMaria AN, Blanchard DG (2001) Aortic intramural hematoma: an increasingly recognized and potentially fatal entity. Chest 120:1340-1346
32. Chung JW, Park JH, Im JG et al (1996) Spiral CT angiography of the thoracic aorta. Radiographics 16:811-824
33. Rydberg J, Kopecky KK, Lalka SG et al (2001) Stent grafting of abdominal aortic aneurysms: pre-and postoperative evaluation with multislice helical CT. J Comput Assist Tomogr 25580-586
34. Bortone AS, De Cillis E, D'Agostino D, de Luca Tupputi Schinosa L (2004) Endovascular treatment of thoracic aortic disease: four years of experience. Circulation 110:I262-I267
35. Mirvis SE, Kostrubiak I, Whitley NO et al (1987) Role of CT in excluding major arterial injury after blunt thoracic trauma. AJR Am J Roentgenol 149:601-605
36. Mirvis SE, Shanmuganathan K, Miller BH et al (1996) Traumatic aortic injury: diagnosis with contrast-enhanced thoracic CT–five-year experience at a major trauma center. Radiology 200:413-422
37. Creasy JD, Chiles C, Routh WD, Dyer RB (1997) Overview of traumatic injury of the thoracic aorta. Radiographics 17:27-45
38. Marotta R, Franchetto AA (1996) The CT appearance of aortic transection. AJR Am J Roentgenol 166:647-651
39. Kuhlman JE, Pozniak MA, Collins J, Knisely BL (1998) Radiographic and CT findings of blunt chest trauma: aortic injuries and looking beyond them. Radiographics 18:1085-1106
40. Gavant ML, Menke PG, Fabian T et al (1995) Blunt traumatic aortic rupture: detection with helical CT of the chest. Radiology 197:125-133
41. Gavant ML (1999) Helical CT grading of traumatic aortic injuries. Impact on clinical guidelines for medical and surgical management. Radiol Clin North Am 37:553-574
42. Dyer DS, Moore EE, Mestek MF et al (1999) Can chest CT be used to exclude aortic injury? Radiology 213:195-202

Clinical Indications of Cardiac CT

31

Erica Maffei, Chiara Martini, Sara Seitun, and Filippo Cademartiri

31.1 Introduction

Cardiac computed tomography (CCT) is undoubtedly one of the most inspiring of the recent innovations in cardiologic imaging [1-16]. The introduction of the latest generation multislice CT systems (64 slices [9-11, 13-16]) and dual source systems [17-20] capable of elevated spatial and temporal resolution has established noninvasive coronary artery imaging in clinical practice. The correct use of the procedure however cannot be divested from knowledge of its limitations and advantages with respect to other diagnostic techniques.

The precise role CCT will play with respect to conventional coronary artery angiography (CAG) and other imaging modalities in cardiology is still not altogether clear. There are many distinctive features of CCT: the noninvasiveness of the procedure, the possibility of visualizing the coronary wall and vascular lumen and therefore identifying atheromatous coronary plaques, and the ability to investigate the spatial relations between the cardiac structures thanks to three-dimensional reconstructions. All of these can prove useful in the clinical setting by providing complementary information with respect to traditional diagnostic modalities. CCT has already proved to be a reliable clinical tool for the assessment of obstructive coronary artery disease (CAD) and the full implementation of low radiation dose techniques will make of CCT the primary tool for CAD assessment.

31.2 Suspected CAD

Numerous studies have to date been published validating CCT in comparison with CAG. The gradual technologic improvement with the introduction of 16- and 64-slice

E. Maffei (✉)
Cardiovascular Imaging Unit,
"Giovanni XXIII" Hospital,
Monastier di Treviso (TV), Italy

scanners has led to an improvement in diagnostic accuracy and a reduction in the number of non-evaluable segments due to spatial resolution limitations or residual motion artifacts. In the evaluation of coronary artery segments, the data in the literature report values of sensitivity ranging from 72% to 95% and specificity from 86% to 98% with 16-slice CCT [1-8, 12], while with 64-slice scanners the figures are sensitivity 93-99%, specificity 95-97% and negative predictive value 99% [9-11, 13-16] (Table 31.1). The difference in terms of sensitivity and specificity between the various studies is due to the different populations of patients enrolled (patients with different prevalence of disease), different presence and distribution of calcifications, different heart rates and other factors able to influence the performance of the technique (modality of intravenous contrast agent administration, use of sublingual nitrates, etc.).

Diagnostic accuracy is in general high, especially if we consider that exercise testing has a sensitivity and specificity for the diagnosis of CAD in the range of 70-80% while the figures for myocardial SPECT and stress echocardiography are 90% and 75-80% in patient populations with an elevated pretest probability.

A recent study prospectively compared exercise testing and CCT in 80 patients with suspected coronary heart disease (CHD) (pretest probability 75% and prevalence of disease 55%), reporting sensitivity and specificity for CT of 91% and 83%, respectively, compared with 73% and 31% for exercise testing [21]. The study also underlined that CT was considerably more expensive (in Germany) than exercise testing (175 vs. 33) [21]. It should however also be borne in mind that the studies carried out to date were done only in select patient populations and prevalently in patients with an intermediate-high pretest probability of CAD, as demonstrated by the elevated prevalence of obstructive disease in these series (on average 60-85%).

Despite the elevated sensitivity of CCT in identifying coronary artery plaques, the accurate quantification of the degree of stenosis is still limited. Recent studies indicate that the quantitative analysis of stenoses at CCT

F. Cademartiri, G. Casolo, M. Midiri (eds.), *Clinical Applications of Cardiac CT*,
© Springer-Verlag Italia 2012

Table 31.1 Diagnostic accuracy of CT in the study of native coronary arteries

Study	No. pts	NE	Sensitivity (%)	Specificity (%)	PPV (%)	NPV (%)
16 slices						
Nieman et al. [1]	59	7	95	86	80	97
Ropers et al. [2]	77	12	92	93	79	97
Kuettner et al. [3]	60	AS>1000	98	98	-	-
Martuscelli et al. [3]	64	16	89	98	90	97
Mollet et al. [5]	128	-	92	95	79	98
Mollet et al. [12]	51	-	95	98	87	99
Hoffmann et al. [6]	103	6	95	98	99	87
Achenbach et al. [7]	50	5	93	95	69	99
Garcia et al. [8]	238	29	94	67	13	99
64 slices						
Raff et al. [9]	70	12	95	86	66	98
Leschka et al. [10]	67	-	94	97	87	99
Mollet et al. [11]	57	3	99	95	76	99
Fine et al. [13]	66	-	95	96	97	92
Ropers et al. [14	84	3	93	97	56	100
Nikolaou et al. [15]	72	6	97	79	86	96
Schuijf et al. [16]	61	1	85	97	82	99

Sensitivity, specificity, positive predictive value (PPV) and negative predictive value (NPV) of CT coronary angiography (given in percentages) compared with conventional coronary angiography for the detection of significant stenosis (reduction of lumen diameter ≥50%). *AS*, Agatston score; *No. pts*, number of patients enrolled; *NE*, nonevaluable segments.

only moderately correlates with quantitative CAG [9, 14]. This is largely due to the lower spatial resolution of CCT compared with CAG.

It is still not precisely clear what the optimal role of CCT in clinical practice should be. The high negative predictive value (97-99%) which has been confirmed across the board in all the published studies suggests the use of CCT to rule out the presence of CAD. In this setting CCT could be the technique of choice in patients with a low or intermediate probability of CHD and atypical chest pain, or it could be used as a second-level diagnostic technique in patients who have already undergone stress testing with equivocal or indeterminate findings [22-24].

CCT could be implemented in all patients whose clinical and instrumental findings are not sufficient to warrant CAG. The current guidelines of the European Society of Cardiology (ESC 2006) for the evaluation of patients with suspected stable angina place CCT in class IIb in patients with low pretest probability of CAD and equivocal stress test [22]. CCT cannot be seen as an alternative to the traditional stress test, but rather as an integration and/or a further level of stratification. CCT is in fact an anatomic/morphologic imaging modality which is able to directly visualize CAD, but unable to provide functional information, such as the presence and extent of ischemia [25].

It is likely that in patients with a certain diagnosis or high probability of CHD there already exists a direct indication for CAG, so the functional study should be favored in view of myocardial revascularization. In patients with a low or intermediate probability the integration of anatomic and functional findings can prove useful: CCT could be used to identify those patients with atherosclerosis, and in patients testing positive a stress test (SPECT or stress echocardiography) could be performed to identify myocardial ischemia. The identification of atherosclerosis without associated ischemia can still prove useful in patient risk stratification and in implementing aggressive primary prevention.

31.3 Known CAD: Stents

The evaluation of stents with CCT is encumbered by further technical difficulties: the blooming artifact caused by the metal mesh of the stent tends to impair the correct visualization of the stent lumen [26-29]. Several recent studies have however reported significant improvements in detecting in-stent restenosis largely due to the improved spatial resolution of the latest generation CT systems. Although promising, the performance of 16-slice scanners is still inadequate for a potential clinical use, with 78% sensitivity and 100% specificity in the

Table 31.2 Diagnostic accuracy of CT in the evaluation of in-stent restenosis

Study	No. patients	No. stents	Diameter (mm)	Evaluable (no.)	Sensitivity (%)	Specificity (%)
4 slices						
Kruger et al. [26]	20	32	-	32	-	-
Maintz et al. [27]	29	47	3.0-5.0	38	100	100
Ligabue et al. [28]	48	72	-	72	100	100
16 slices						
Schuijf et al. [29]	22	68	2.25-5.0	50	78	100
Gilard et al. [30]	29	29	-	27	100	92
Gilard et al. [31]	143	232	≥3.5	126	86	100
		86	<3.5	40	54	100
Cademartiri et al. [32]	51	76	>2.0	74	84	99
Cademartiri et al. [33]	50	47	-	47	50	100
Ohnuki et al. [34]	16	20	>3.0	19	75	88
40 slices						
Gaspar et al. [35]	65	111	3.3≥0.5	106	74	83
64 slices						
Rixe et al. [36]	64	102	>2.5	59	86	98
Ehara et al. [37]	81	125	2.5-4.5	110	92	81
Rist et al. [38]	25	46	-	45	75	92
Cademartiri et al. [39]	95	106	>2.5	102	93	89

Studies published reporting the results of diagnostic accuracy in the assessment of in-stent restenosis (reduction of the in-stent lumen ≥50%). Different patency criteria have been used, particularly in the early phases (4- and 16-slice scanners). With the advent of 40-slice scanners direct visualization of the in-stent lumen has become the diagnostic criterion.

evaluation of stent patency and 75% sensitivity and 96% specificity in the identification of intimal hyperplasia [29-34]. Consistent improvements in diagnostic performance have however been demonstrated by 64-slice scanners (Table 31.2) [35-39].

A recent 64-slice CCT study in 81 patients (125 stents), however, reported values of sensitivity, specificity, positive predictive value and negative predictive value of 92%, 81%, 54% and 98%, respectively, with approximately 12% of stented segments nonevaluable due to artifacts [37]. Van Mieghem et al. studied the possibility of using CCT to monitor the patency of stents implanted in the left main coronary artery. They reported a diagnostic accuracy of 93% in identifying in-stent restenosis and a sensitivity and negative predictive value of 100% [40]. The accuracy of CCT is directly correlated with the size of the stent studied and the type of stent in use (material, mesh size) [41]. Currently only stents positioned in the proximal coronary tracts can be evaluated with relative reliability, nonetheless there are still insufficient data available to support a widespread clinical application of the technique.

31.4 Known CAD: Bypass Grafts

In the setting of patients with known and revascularized CHD, consistent data have been obtained regarding CCT in the study of venous and arterial grafts. The good diameter of coronary artery bypass grafts (CABG) and their relative immobility offer the possibility of an accurate evaluation with noninvasive imaging (Table 31.3) [42-51]. In a population of 51 patients (131 bypass grafts) studied with 16-slice CCT, Schlosser et al. reported sensitivity of 95%, specificity of 95%, positive predictive value of 81% and negative predictive value of 99% for the detection of graft disease (occlusion and/or restenosis) [46]. Even better results have been reported with 64-slice scanners: 97.8% sensitivity, 89.3% specificity, positive predictive value of 90% and negative predictive value of 97.7% [50]. Global diagnostic accuracy is significantly greater, in that 94% of distal anastomoses proved evaluable with the 64-slice scanner compared with 74% in the study by Schlosser [46, 50].

The limitations of CCT in the study of bypass grafts include the presence of metal clips which can generate

Table 31.3 Diagnostic accuracy of CT in the evaluation of stenosis and occlusion of bypass grafts

				Graft stenosis		Graft occlusion	
Study	No.patients	Arterial grafts	Venous grafts	Sensitivity	Specificity	Sensitivity	Specificity
4 slices							
Ropers et al. [42]	65	20	162	75	92	97	98
Nieman et al. [43]	24	18	23	83	90	100	98
Marano et al. [44]	57	57	27	92	96	93	98
16 slices							
Martuscelli et al. [45]	84	85	166	90	100	100	100
Schlosser et al. [46]	51	40	91	96	95	-	-
Chiurlia et al. [47]	52	49	117	96	100	100	100
64 slices							
Malagutti et al. [48]	52	45	64	99	96	-	-
Ropers et al. [49]	50	37	101	100	94	-	-
Pache et al. [50]	31	23	73	98	89	-	-
Meyer et al. [51]	138	147	259	97	97	-	-

Studies published reporting the results of diagnostic accuracy in the assessment of stenosis and occlusion of bypass grafts. Different patency criteria have been used, particularly in the early phases (4- and 16-slice scanners). With the advent of 40-slice scanners direct visualization of the bypass graft lumen has become the diagnostic criterion.

beam hardening artifacts and/or the blooming effect, and the difficulty in visualizing distal anastomoses. It should also be borne in mind that alongside an accurate visualization of the grafts, the study of the native coronary arteries can prove extremely difficult due to the extensive presence of atheromatous plaques, prior multiple angioplasties/stenting and calcifications.

A recent study has reported an improvement in diagnostic accuracy even in the study of the native coronary arteries with the use of a 64-slice scanner [48]: the reported sensitivity and specificity for graft disease are 99% and 96%, respectively, while the figures for the diagnosis of significant stenosis of the native arteries are 97% and 86% [48]. CCT however tends to overestimate the presence of disease in distal and particularly calcified vessels.

Given these limitations the current clinical utility of CCT in the study of CABG patients, where an accurate evaluation of both the grafts and the native coronary arteries distal to the graft anastomoses or of the non-bypassed vessels, should be carefully assessed on a case-by-case basis. The classic example could be the patient with recurrent but atypical symptoms who should undergo a study of the arterial graft as a prognostic element. CCT however does have a role to play in the integration with CAG, in that it can be used to guide the angiographic procedure in the mapping of bypass grafts in patients in whom the precise surgical procedure performed is unknown. Alternatively it can complete the evaluation in the event of technical difficulty in selecting or visualizing the grafts.

31.5 Coronary Plaque Imaging

CCT distinguishes itself from CAG in its ability to directly visualize the vascular wall as well as the coronary lumen [52-61]. CCT is able to detect the presence of atheromatous coronary plaque and describe its location and extension. CCT can also classify plaques as calcified, noncalcified (fibrofatty) and mixed, thanks to their different densities (attenuation) given in Hounsfield units (Table 31.4). The realistic applications of plaque imaging are at present based only on ancillary evidence, and therefore requiring codification. Support for a clinical application of the technique would require validation studies of its prognostic power in relation to hard endpoints such as mortality and acute myocardial infarction, which to date are lacking.

A possible integration of CAG and CCT which exploits the ability of the latter to study the vascular wall is in the study of chronic coronary artery occlusions [62]. In this specific field CCT can provide additional information regarding the length of the occlusion, the course (tortuous, angle) of the occluded coronary, and the presence of calcifications, which can be useful in the planning of percutaneous reopening of the vessel.

31.6 Chest Pain Triage

In cases of chest pain whose origin cannot be rapidly identified with the most common diagnostic tools (ECG,

Table 31.4 Diagnostic accuracy of CT in detecting and characterizing coronary artery plaques

	Achenbach [56] (n = 22)			Leber [53] (n = 37)
Cardiac CT	Sensitivity	IVUS		Sensitivity
Mixed	78% (35/45)	Hypoechoic		78% (62/80)
Noncalcified	53% (8/15)	Hyperechoic		78% (87/112)
Calcified	94% (33/36)	Calcified		95% (150/158)
All plaques	82% (41/50)	All plaques		86% (299/350)
Exclusion of plaques (specificity)	88% (29/33)	Exclusion of plaques (specificity)		92% (484/525)

The diagnostic accuracy of CT for the detection and characterization of coronary plaques as reported by the two main studies on the topic [53, 56]. In the first study [56], the analysis was performed per segment with no patient excluded. In the second study [53], the analysis was performed on 3 mm sections and 9 patients were excluded. In the heading in parentheses is the number of patients evaluated. In parentheses next to the sensitivity and specificity values are the original numbers. *n*, no of patients; *IVUS*, intravascular ultrasound (the criterion standard used for comparison).

biochemical markers, blood-gas analysis, CRX) it would be highly desirable to have available a diagnostic technique capable of ruling out the presence of the three most dangerous causes of chest pain: acute coronary syndrome, aortic dissection and pulmonary thromboembolism.

The possibility of performing the *triple rule-out* with a single diagnostic test has enormous clinical advantages in the setting of emergency medicine. These include a fast and accurate diagnosis and consequent appropriate treatment in cases which would otherwise likely be misinterpreted or require much longer and numerous diagnostic tests, and the possible safe discharge of a broad group of patients which would otherwise require hospitalization and more-or-less complex and invasive procedures. Incidentally, with the acquisition of the entire lung field, alternative not immediately life-threatening diagnoses could also be identified such as pleural or pulmonary diseases (a hypothetical quintuple rule-out).

An emerging application of CCT is the evaluation of patients with chest pain of uncertain origin [63-68]. Included in this category are patients with suspected CAD. The first comparative studies on the subject appeared towards the end of 2006 and at the beginning of 2007. This is largely due to the fact that this patient population is characterized by greater clinical heterogeneity which translates into greater difficulty in indicating the patients for CCT, given the limitations regarding heart rate. Following a preliminary, purely descriptive analysis [63], recent studies have been performed in a clinical setting with the clinical and/or CAG criterion standard (evaluation of major cardiovascular events at follow-up) [64-68]. The studies see CCT being employed in the evaluation of chest pain with suspected coronary origin [64, 66-70]. Non-STEMI type pain can be investigated with CCT with two advantages: on the one hand the technique offers the possibility of a broad differential diag-

nosis (aortic and pulmonary artery disease) and on the other has a very high negative predictive value with regard to obstructive coronary disease [64, 66]. In addition there are lower costs and the rapidity of the diagnostic pathway compared with traditional procedures [67]. Adequate clinical trials are required to confirm and strengthen these observations. In addition, the management of CCT in the setting of chest pain poses a number of complex problems both at the technologic level and in terms of training and internal quality control. This is even more so given that ionizing radiation is used and the technique requires the intravascular injection of iodinated contrast material.

31.7 Prognostic Value of CCT

There are currently no large population studies on the predictive value of CCT. Although this information is widely available for techniques such as scintigraphy, several years will pass before the same can be said for CCT. A number of ancillary studies have assessed the prognostic value of a negative CCT in patients with chest pain [66, 67, 71]. At one year the prognostic value of a negative CCT reported in a heterogeneous and limited population is 100%. Large multicenter registries (e.g. CONFIRM) are delivering the same results in large patient populations.

Another application on the border between risk stratification and prognostic evaluation regards preoperative screening [72, 73]. In the case of cardiac valve disease CCT could substitute a CAG performed routinely in patients with low probability of CAD (e.g. patients with mitral valve disease). In the case of major noncardiac surgery the technique can be used to stratify coronary risk (currently based on surrogates similar to those adopted for epidemiologic studies; see metabolic equiva-

Table 31.5 Current indications for CCT [91]

Type	Description	Evidence
Coronary artery	Suspected CAD at low/intermediate risk	Major
	Suspected CAD at low/intermediate risk with equivocal or indeterminate or not feasible stress test	
	Suspected CAD with typical/atypical chest pain and conflicting stress tests	
	Suspected CAD with typical chest pain with negative stress test	
	Acute chest pain with negative/nondiagnostic ECG and negative Troponin or no curve	
	Acute chest pain with equivocal stress tests	
	Differential diagnosis dilative cardiomyopathy	
	New onset heart failure	
	Preoperative screening in cardiac valve surgery and major noncardiac surgery	
	Screening in TAVI patients	
	Follow-up of revascularized patient with atypical symptoms and/or altered functional tests	
	Study of coronary artery anomalies in adults	
	Study of myocardial volumes and function in patients with indeterminate MR/TEE or unable to perform	
	Study of cardiac masses and pericardial disease in patients with indeterminate MR/TEE or unable to perform	
	Preoperative mammary artery mapping in candidates for CABG	
	Study/characterization of coronary plaques	Minor
	Preangioplasty evaluation of chronic total occlusions	
	Preoperative screening in major non-cardiac surgery	
	Study of resting myocardial viability Study of myocardial perfusion	Investigative
Other	Diagnosis/rule-out of pulmonary thromboembolism	Major
	Diagnosis/rule-out of aortic dissection	
	Preoperative pulmonary vein mapping prior to ablation	
	Preliminary cardiac vein mapping prior to biventricular pacemaker implantation	

CCT, cardiac computed tomography angiography; *ECG*, electrocardiogram; *MR*, magnetic resonance; *TEE*, transesophageal echocardiography; *CABG*, coronary artery bypass grafting surgery; *TAVI*, transfemoral aortic valve intervention.

lents, MET) in patients scheduled to undergo surgery with significant hemodynamic risk (e.g. abdominal aortic aneurysm, total hip replacement, etc.) in order to implement the best interventional and anesthetic strategies for the prevention of perioperative events.

31.8 Further Applications

The noncoronary applications of 64-slice CCT also includes the evaluation of ventricular function [74-80], the preoperative evaluation of the left atrium and pulmonary veins and follow-up of radiofrequency catheter ablation, the evaluation of the venous circulation prior to biventricular pacemaker implantation [81, 82], the evaluation of resting myocardial viability via delayed enhancement [83-88] and first-pass perfusion scan [89, 90]. These emerging applications are not supported by solid evidence in the literature, although they will become of considerable importance in the future given the relative simplicity of the CCT study.

31.9 Summary and Future Scenarios

The indications and current recommendations of CCT are summarized in Table 31.5, which reveals a broad spectrum of indications and recommendations for the use of CCT [91]. These indications/recommendations are the result of repeated observations, validation and clinical studies including multicenter trials. The prognostic value has been defined with large numbers in a prospective international multicenter registry named CONFIRM [92].

Several investigators have proposed a real paradigm shift in the diagnostic algorithm for risk stratification in the patient with suspected CAD. In contrast to the current paradigm which sees the first information sought regarding signs of inducible or prior myocardial ischemia, the proposed paradigm suggests that morphologic imaging could constitute the first diagnostic level capable of immediately stratifying patients as normal, with nonobstructive CAD and with obstructive CAD

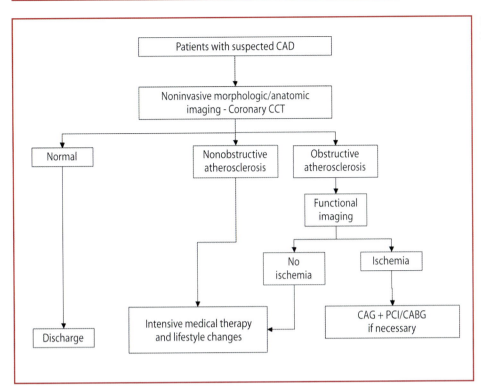

Fig. 31.1 Potential diagnostic algorithm in patients with suspected CAD

(Fig. 31.1). The next step should then be the functional study of the ischemia induced by the morphologic alterations detected. This approach is based on the concept of the individual stratification of the presence/absence and extent of CAD. To date this information could be extrapolated from epidemiologic data (Framingham score) or methods such as the calcium score. The latter, however, only shows slight independence in the stratification of cardiovascular risk with respect to previous epidemiologic data.

31.10 Conclusions

CCT is a noninvasive imaging modality for the diagnosis of CAD which is growing both in geographical distribution and clinical indications. In the future the clinical applications of the technique are likely to increase hand in hand with technologic developments and growing evidence in the literature. The reliability and accuracy of the technique will increase by the introduction of new solutions, such as dual-source, allowing the technique to be implemented in the field of acute chest pain. To be effective in the current setting, CCT should be used in specialist areas by personnel with all-embracing training.

References

1. Nieman K, Cademartiri F, Lemos PA et al (2002) Reliable noninvasive coronary angiography with fast submillimeter multislice spiral computed tomography. Circulation 106:2051-2054
2. Ropers D, Baum U, Pohle K et al (2003) Detection of coronary artery stenoses with thin-slice multi-detector row spiral computed tomography and multiplanar reconstruction. Circulation 107:664-666
3. Kuettner A, Trabold T, Schroeder S et al (2004) Noninvasive detection of coronary lesions using 16-detector multislice spiral computed tomography technology: initial clinical results. J Am Coll Cardiol 44:1230-1237
4. Martuscelli E, Romagnoli A, D'Eliseo A et al (2004) Accuracy of thin-slice computed tomography in the detection of coronary stenoses. Eur Heart J 25:1043-1048
5. Mollet NR, Cademartiri F, Nieman K et al (2004) Multislice spiral computed tomography coronary angiography in patients with stable angina pectoris. J Am Coll Cardiol 43:2265-2270
6. Hoffmann MH, Shi H, Schmitz BL et al (2005) Noninvasive coronary angiography with multislice computed tomography. JAMA 293:2471-2478
7. Achenbach S, Ropers D, Pohle FK et al (2005) Detection of coronary artery stenoses using multi-detector CT with 16 x 0.75 collimation and 375 ms rotation. Eur Heart J 26:1978-1986
8. Garcia MJ, Lessick J, Hoffmann MH (2006) Accuracy of 16-row multidetector computed tomography for the assessment of coronary artery stenosis. JAMA 296:403-411
9. Raff GL, Gallagher MJ, O'Neill WW, Goldstein JA (2005) Diagnostic accuracy of noninvasive coronary angiography using 64-slice spiral computed tomography. J Am Coll Cardiol 46:552-557

10. Leschka S, Alkadhi H, Plass A et al (2005) Accuracy of MSCT coronary angiography with 64-slice technology: first experience. Eur Heart J 26:1482-1487

11. Mollet NR, Cademartiri F, van Mieghem CA et al (2005) High-resolution spiral computed tomography coronary angiography in patients referred for diagnostic conventional coronary angiography. Circulation 112:2318-2323

12. Mollet NR, Cademartiri F, Krestin GP et al (2005) Improved diagnostic accuracy with 16-row multi-slice computed tomography coronary angiography. J Am Coll Cardiol 45:128-132

13. Fine JJ, Hopkins CB, Ruff N, Newton FC (2006) Comparison of accuracy of 64-slice cardiovascular computed tomography with coronary angiography in patients with suspected coronary artery disease. Am J Cardiol 97:173-174

14. Ropers D, Rixe J, Anders K et al (2006) Usefulness of multidetector row spiral computed tomography with 64- x 0.6-mm collimation and 330-ms rotation for the noninvasive detection of significant coronary artery stenoses. Am J Cardiol 97:343-348

15. Nikolaou K, Knez A, Rist C et al (2006) Accuracy of 64-MDCT in the diagnosis of ischemic heart disease. AJR Am J Roentgenol 187:111-117

16. Schuijf JD, Pundziute G, Jukema JW et al (2006) Diagnostic accuracy of 64-slice multislice computed tomography in the noninvasive evaluation of significant coronary artery disease. Am J Cardiol 98:145-148

17. Scheffel H, Alkadhi H, Plass A et al (2006) Accuracy of dual-source CT coronary angiography: first experience in a high pre-test probability population without heart rate control. Eur Radiol 16:2739-2747

18. Achenbach S, Ropers D, Kuettner A et al (2006) Contrast-enhanced coronary artery visualization by dual-source computed tomography-initial experience. Eur J Radiol 57:331-335

19. Flohr TG, McCollough CH, Bruder H et al (2006) First performance evaluation of a dual-source CT (DSCT) system. Eur Radiol 16:256-268

20. Johnson TR, Nikolaou K, Wintersperger BJ et al (2006) Dual-source CT cardiac imaging: initial experience. Eur Radiol 16:1409-1415

21. Dewey M, Dubel HP, Schink T et al (2007) Head-to-head comparison of multislice computed tomography and exercise electrocardiography for diagnosis of coronary artery disease. Eur Heart J 28:2485-2490

22. Fox K, Garcia MA, Ardissino D et al (2006) Guidelines on the management of stable angina pectoris: executive summary: the Task Force on the Management of Stable Angina Pectoris of the European Society of Cardiology. Eur Heart J 27:1341-1381

23. Hendel RC, Patel MR, Kramer CM et al (2006) ACCF/ACR/SCCT/SCMR/ASNC/NASCI/ SCAI/SIR 2006 appropriateness criteria for cardiac computed tomography and cardiac magnetic resonance imaging: a report of the American College of Cardiology Foundation Quality Strategic Directions Committee Appropriateness Criteria Working Group, American College of Radiology, Society of Cardiovascular Computed Tomography, Society for Cardiovascular Magnetic Resonance, American Society of Nuclear Cardiology, North American Society for Cardiac Imaging, Society for Cardiovascular Angiography and Interventions, and Society of Interventional Radiology. J Am Coll Cardiol 48:1475-1497

24. Ghostine S, Caussin C, Daoud B et al (2006) Non-invasive detection of coronary artery disease in patients with left bundle branch block using 64-slice computed tomography. J Am Coll Cardiol 48:1929-1934

25. Schuijf JD, Wijns W, Jukema JW et al (2006) Relationship between noninvasive coronary angiography with multi-slice computed tomography and myocardial perfusion imaging. J Am Coll Cardiol 48:2508-2514

26. Kruger S, Mahnken AH, Sinha AM et al (2003) Multislice spiral computed tomography for the detection of coronary stent restenosis and patency. Int J Cardiol 89:167-172

27. Maintz D, Grude M, Fallenberg EM et al (2003) Assessment of coronary arterial stents by multislice- CT angiography. Acta Radiol 44:597-603

28. Ligabue G, Rossi R, Ratti C et al (2004) Noninvasive evaluation of coronary artery stents patency after PTCA: role of multislice computed tomography. Radiol Med (Torino) 108:128-137

29. Schuijf JD, Bax JJ, Jukema JW et al (2004) Feasibilit y of assessment of coronary stent patency using 16-slice computed tomography. Am J Cardiol 94:427-430

30. Gilard M, Cornily JC, Rioufol G et al (2005) Noninvasive assessment of left main coronary stent patency with 16-slice computed tomography. Am J Cardiol 95:110-112

31. Gilard M, Cornily JC, Pennec PY et al (2006) Assessment of coronary artery stents by 16-slice computed tomography. Heart 92:58-61

32. Cademartiri F, Mollet N, Lemos PA et al (2005) Usefulness of multislice computed tomographic coronary angiography to assess in-stent restenosis. Am J Cardiol 96:799-802

33. Cademartiri F, Marano R, Runza G et al (2005) Non-invasive assessment of coronary artery stent patency with multislice CT: preliminary experience. Radiol Med (Torino) 109:500-507

34. Ohnuki K, Yoshida S, Ohta M et al (2006) New diagnostic technique in multi-slice computed tomography for in-stent restenosis: pixel count method. Int J Cardiol 108:251-258

35. Gaspar T, Halon DA, Lewis BS et al (2005) Diagnosis of coronary in-stent restenosis with multidetector row spiral computed tomography. J Am Coll Cardiol 46:1573-1579

36. Rixe J, Achenbach S, Ropers D et al (2006) Assessment of coronary artery stent restenosis by 64-slice multi-detector computed tomography. Eur Heart J 27:2567-2572

37. Ehara M, Kawai M, Surmely JF et al (2007) Diagnostic accuracy of coronary in-stent restenosis using 64-slice computed tomography comparison with invasive coronary angiography. J Am Coll Cardiol 49:951-959

38. Rist C, von Ziegler F, Nikolaou K et al (2006) Assessment of coronary artery stent patency and restenosis using 64-slice computed tomography. Acad Radiol 13:1465-1473

39. Cademartiri F, Palumbo A, La Grutta L et al (2007) Diagnostic accuracy of 64-slice CT in the evaluation of coronary stents. Radiol Med (Torino) 112:526-537

40. Van Mieghem CA, Cademartiri F, Mollet NR et al (2006) Multislice spiral computed tomography for the evaluation of stent patency after left main coronary artery stenting: a comparison with conventional coronary angiography and intravascular ultrasound. Circulation 114:645-653

41. Maintz D, Seifarth H, Raupach R et al (2005) 64-slice multidetector coronary CT angiography: in vitro evaluation of 68 different stents. Eur Radiol 16:818-826

42. Ropers D, Ulzheimer S, Wenkel E et al (2001) Investigation of aortocoronary artery bypass grafts by multislice spiral computed tomography with electrocardiographic-gated image reconstruction. Am J Cardiol 88:792-795

43. Nieman K, Pattynama PM, Rensing BJ et al (2003) Evaluation of patients after coronary artery bypass surgery: CT angiographic assessment of grafts and coronary arteries. Radiology 229:749-756

44. Marano R, Storto ML, Maddestra N, Bonomo L (2004) Non-invasive assessment of coronary artery bypass graft with retrospectively ECG-gated four-row multi-detector spiral computed tomography. Eur Radiol 14:1353-1362

45. Martuscelli E, Romagnoli A, D'Eliseo A et al (2004) Evaluation of venous and arterial conduit patency by 16-slice spiral computed tomography. Circulation 110:3234-3238

46. Schlosser T, Konorza T, Hunold P et al (2004) Noninvasive visualization of coronary artery bypass grafts using 16-detector row

47. Chiurlia E, Menozzi M, Ratti C et al (2005) Follow-up of coronary artery bypass graft patency by multislice computed tomography. Am J Cardiol 95:1094-1097

48. Malagutti P, Nieman K, Meijboom WB et al (2006) Use of 64-slice CT in symptomatic patients after coronary bypass surgery: evaluation of grafts and coronary arteries. Eur Heart J 28:1879-1885

49. Ropers D, Pohle FK, Kuettner A et al (2006) Diagnostic accuracy of noninvasive coronary angiography in patients after bypass surgery using 64-slice spiral computed tomography with 330-ms gantry rotation. Circulation 114:2334-2341; quiz 2334

50. Pache G, Saueressig U, Frydrychowicz A et al (2006) Initial experience with 64-slice cardiac CT: non-invasive visualization of coronary artery bypass grafts. Eur Heart J 27:976-980

51. Meyer TS, Martinoff S, Hadamitzky M et al (2007) Improved noninvasive assessment of coronary artery bypass grafts with 64-slice computed tomographic angiography in an unselected patient population. J Am Coll Cardiol 49:946-950

52. Leber AW, Knez A, White CW et al (2003) Composition of coronary atherosclerotic plaques in patients with acute myocardial infarction and stable angina pectoris determined by contrast-enhanced multislice computed tomography. Am J Cardiol 91:714-718

53. Leber AW, Knez A, Becker A et al (2004) Accuracy of multidetector spiral computed tomography in identifying and differentiating the composition of coronary atherosclerotic plaques: a comparative study with intracoronary ultrasound. J Am Coll Cardiol 43:1241-1247

54. Achenbach S, Ropers D, Hoffmann U et al (2004) Assessment of coronary remodeling in stenotic and nonstenotic coronary atherosclerotic lesions by multidetector spiral computed tomography. J Am Coll Cardiol 43:842-847

55. Caussin C, Ohanessian A, Ghostine S et al (2004) Characterization of vulnerable nonstenotic plaque with 16-slice computed tomography compared with intravascular ultrasound. Am J Cardiol 94:99-104

56. Achenbach S, Moselewski F, Ropers D et al (2004) Detection of calcified and noncalcified coronary atherosclerotic plaque by contrast-enhanced, submillimeter multidetector spiral computed tomography: a segment-based comparison with intravascular ultrasound. Circulation 109:14-17

57. Leber AW, Knez A, von Ziegler F et al (2005) Quantification of obstructive and nonobstructive coronary lesions by 64-slice computed tomography: a comparative study with quantitative coronary angiography and intravascular ultrasound. J Am Coll Cardiol 46:147-154

58. Hoffmann U, Moselewski F, Nieman K et al (2006) Noninvasive assessment of plaque morphology and composition in culprit and stable lesions in acute coronary syndrome and stable lesions in stable angina by multidetector computed tomography. J Am Coll Cardiol 47:1655-1662

59. Ferencik M, Chan RC, Achenbach S et al (2006) Arterial wall imaging: evaluation with 16-section multidetector CT in blood vessel phantoms and ex vivo coronary arteries. Radiology 240:708-716

60. Caussin C, Larchez C, Ghostine S et al (2006) Comparison of coronary minimal lumen area quantification by sixty-four-slice computed tomography versus intravascular ultrasound for intermediate stenosis. Am J Cardiol 98:871-876

61. Leber AW, Becker A, Knez A et al (2006) Accuracy of 64-slice computed tomography to classify and quantify plaque volumes in the proximal coronary system: a comparative study using intravascular ultrasound. J Am Coll Cardiol 47:672-627

62. Mollet NR, Hoye A, Lemos PA et al (2005) Value of preprocedure multislice computed tomographic coronary angiography to predict the outcome of percutaneous recanalization of chronic total occlusions. Am J Cardiol 95:240-243

63. White CS, Kuo D, Kelemen M et al (2005) Chest pain evaluation in the emergency department: can MDCT provide a comprehensive evaluation? AJR Am J Roentgenol 185:533-540

64. Gallagher MJ, Ross MA, Raff GL et al (2006) The diagnostic accuracy of 64-slice computed tomography coronary an giography compared with stress nuclear imaging in emergency department low-risk chest pain patients. Ann Emerg Med 49:125-136

65. Hoffmann U, Pena AJ, Moselewski F et al (2006) MDCT in early triage of patients with acute chest pain. AJR Am J Roentgenol 187:1240-1247

66. Rubinshtein R, Halon DA, Gaspar T et al (2007) Usefulness of 64-slice cardiac computed tomographic angiography for diagnosing acute coronary syndromes and predicting clinical outcome in emergency department patients with chest pain of uncertain origin. Circulation 115:1762-1768

67. Goldstein JA, Gallagher MJ, O'Neill WW et al (2007) A randomized controlled trial of multi-slice coronary computed tomography for evaluation of acute chest pain. J Am Coll Cardiol 49:863-871

68. Johnson TR, Nikolaou K, Wintersperger BJ et al (2007) ECG-gated 64-MDCT angiography in the differential diagnosis of acute chest pain. AJR Am J Roentgenol 188:76-82

69. Hoffmann U, Nagurney JT, Moselewski F et al (2006) Coronary multidetector computed tomography in the assessment of patients with acute chest pain. Circulation 114:2251-2260

70. Meijboom WB, Mollet NR, van Mieghem CA et al (2007) 64-slice computed tomography coronary angiography in patients with non-ST elevation acute coronary syndrome. Heart 96:1386-1392

71. Pundziute G, Schuijf JD, Jukema JW et al (2007) Prognostic value of multislice computed tomography coronary angiography in patients with known or suspected coronary artery disease. J Am Coll Cardiol 49:62-70

72. Reant P, Brunot S, Lafitte S et al (2006) Predictive value of noninvasive coronary angiography with multidetector computed tomography to detect significant coronary stenosis before valve surgery. Am J Cardiol 97:1506-1510

73. Meijboom WB, Mollet NR, Van Mieghem CA et al (2006) Pre-operative computed tomography coronary angiography to detect significant coronary artery disease in patients referred for cardiac valve surgery. J Am Coll Cardiol 48:1658-1665

74. Juergens KU, Grude M, Maintz D et al (2004) Multi-detector row CT of left ventricular function with dedicated analysis software versus MR imaging: initial experience. Radiology 230:403-410

75. Juergens KU, Grude M, Fallenberg EM et al (2002) Using ECG-gated multidetector CT to evaluate global left ventricular myocardial function in patients with coronary artery disease. AJR Am J Roentgenol 179:1545-1550

76. Schuijf JD, Bax JJ, Jukema JW et al (2006) Assessment of left ventricular volumes and ejection fraction with 16-slice multi-slice computed tomography; comparison with 2D-echocardiography. Int J Cardiol 116:201-205

77. Henneman MM, Schuijf JD, Jukema JW et al (2006) Comprehensive cardiac assessment with MSCT: evaluation of LV function and perfusion in addition to coronary anatomy in patients with previous myocardial infarction. Heart 92:1779-1783

78. Henneman MM, Bax JJ, Schuijf JD et al (2006) Global and regional left ventricular function: a comparison between gated SPECT, 2D echocardiography and multi-slice computed tomography. Eur J Nucl Med Mol Imaging 33:1452-1460

79. Schuijf JD, Bax JJ, Salm LP et al (2005) Noninvasive coronary imaging and assessment of left ventricular function using 16-slice computed tomography. Am J Cardiol 95:571-574

80. Salm LP, Schuijf JD, de Roos A et al (2005) Global and regional left ventricular function assessment with 16-detector row CT: comparison with echocardiography and cardiovascular magnetic resonance. Eur J Echocardiogr 7:308-314

81. Jongbloed MR, Lamb HJ, Bax JJ et al (2005) Noninvasive visual-

ization of the cardiac venous system using multislice computed tomography. J Am Coll Cardiol 45:749-753

82. V an de Veire NR, Schuijf JD, De Sutter J et al (2006) Non-invasive visualization of the cardiac venous system in coronary artery disease patients using 64-slice computed tomography. J Am Coll Cardiol 48:1832-1838

83. Mahnken AH, Koos R, Katoh M et al (2005) Assessment of myocardial viability in reperfused acute myocardi al infarction using 16-slice computed tomography in comparison to magnetic resonance imaging. J Am Coll Cardiol 45:2042-2047

84. Baks T, Cademartiri F, Moelker AD et al (2006) Multislice computed tomography and magnetic resonance imaging for the assessment of reperfused acute myocardial infarction. J Am Coll Cardiol 48:144-152

85. Lardo AC, Cordeiro MA, Silva C et al (2006) Contrast-enhanced multidetector computed tomography viability imaging after myocardial infarction: characterization of myocyte death, microvascular obstruction, and chronic scar. Circulation 113:394-404

86. Gerber BL, Belge B, Legros GJ et al (2006) Characterization of acute and chronic myocardial infarcts by multidetecto r computed tomography: comparison with contrast-enhanced magnetic resonance. Circulation 113:823-833

87. Baks T, Cademartiri F, Moelker AD et al (2007) Asse ssment of acute reperfused myocardial infarction with delayed enhancement 64-MDCT. AJR Am J Roentgenol 188:W135-W137

88. Habis M, Capderou A, Ghostine S et al (2007) Acute myocardial infarction early viability assessment by 64-slice computed tomography immediately after coronary angiography: comparison with low-dose dobutamine echocardiography. J Am Coll Cardiol 49:1178-1185

89. Nikolaou K, Sanz J, Poon M et al (2005) Assessment of myocardial perfusion and viability from routine contrast-enhanced 16-detector-row computed tomography of the heart: preliminary results. Eur Radiol 15:864-871

90. Nikolaou K, Knez A, Sagmeister S et al (2004) Assessment of myocardial infarctions using multidetector-row computed tomography. J Comput Assist Tomogr 28:286-292

91. Taylor AJ, Cerqueira M, Hodgson JM et al (2010) ACCF/SCCT/ACR/AHA/ASE/ASNC/NASCI/SCAI/SCMR 2010 appropriate use criteria for cardiac computed tomography. A report of the American College of Cardiology Foundation Appropriate Use Criteria Task Force, the Society of Cardiovascular Computed Tomography, the American College of Radiology, the American Heart Association, the American Society of Echocardiography, the American Society of Nuclear Cardiology, the North American Society for Cardiovascular Imaging, the Society for Cardiovascular Angiography and Interventions, and the Society for Cardiovascular Magnetic Resonance. J Am Coll Cardiol 56:1864-1894.

92. Min JK, Dunning A, Lin FY, et al (2011) Age- and Sex-Related Differences in All-Cause Mortality Risk Based on Coronary Computed Tomography Angiography Findings Results From the International Multicenter CONFIRM (Coronary CT Angiography Evaluation for Clinical Outcomes: An International Multicenter Registry) of 23,854 Patients Without Known Coronary Artery Disease. J Am Coll Cardiol 58:849-860

Section VI

Other Diagnostic Modalities

Stress ECG

32

Pompilio Faggiano, Giacomo Faden, and Livio Dei Cas

32.1 Introduction

Exercise stress testing is a noninvasive procedure widely used to evaluate patients with known or suspected cardiovascular (CV) disease. It is mainly used to obtain diagnostic and prognostic information and to evaluate individual's functional capacity and exercise tolerance.

32.2 Exercise Protocols

Three types of muscular activity can be applied as a stress to the cardiovascular system: isometric (static), isotonic (dynamic) and resistance (a combination of isometric and isotonic) [1, 2]. Dynamic exercise protocols are most commonly used to evaluate cardiac reserve, and the optimal duration for diagnostic and prognostic information should be 6-12 minutes [3]. The protocol should also include an initial warm-up (low load) and a recovery period.

32.2.1 Cycle Ergometry

Cycle ergometry is the standard method for testing in much of Europe. Two types of stationary bicycles are used for testing: mechanically braked and electrically braked. Work rate is calculated in watts (W) or kilopond-meters (Kpm/min): 1 W is equivalent to ≈ 6 kpm/min. Work intensity can be adjusted by varying the resistance and the cycling rate. The highest values of body oxygen uptake (VO$_2$) and heart rate (HR) are obtained during a symptom-limited test at a pedaling speed of 50 to 80 row-per-minute (rpm). Usually most protocols start with 10-25 W/minute followed by a progressive workload increase of 25-30 W every 2-3 minutes. In young and trained subjects it is possible to use a 50 W step protocol [1, 4]. Care must be taken to prevent isometric or resistance exercise of the arms while grasping the handle bars. Maximum oxygen uptake is 5% to 20% lower on a cycle ergometer than on a treadmill. It is convenient to express oxygen uptake in multiples of sitting/resting requirements. One metabolic equivalent (MET) is a unit of sitting/resting oxygen uptake (≈ 3.5 mL O$_2$ per kilogram of body weight per minute). Table 32.1 lists the approximate oxygen cost in METs for cycle ergometry relative to weight [5].

32.2.2 Treadmill

A treadmill should be electrically driven and should have front and/or side rails to aid in subject stability. Several treadmill protocols are in use and are defined according to treadmill speed, grade, stage duration and estimated METs [1, 5]. The most commonly used are the Bruce protocol and the modified Bruce protocol [1, 6]. The advantage of the Bruce protocol (3-minute step) is the possibility to acquire submaximal data. Its disadvantages are large interstage increments in work that can make estimation of VO$_{2max}$ less accurate. Furthermore, in elderly patients it might be necessary to use different protocols such as ramp protocols that starts at a relatively low treadmill speed which is gradually increased, or protocols such as Naughton and Weber [7].

32.3 Electrocardiographic Recording

A suitable electrocardiographic recording system is needed for continuous monitoring of heart rhythm and evaluation of ischemic electrocardiographic changes during exercise and recovery. The instrument should meet the specifications set by the AHA [8]. Since a high quality 12-lead electrocardiogram (ECG), essential for an accurate interpretation of ischemic changes and arrhythmias, cannot be obtained with electrodes placed

P. Faggiano (✉)
Department of Cardiology,
Spedali Civili University Hospital,
Brescia, Italy

F. Cademartiri, G. Casolo, M. Midiri (eds.), *Clinical Applications of Cardiac CT,*
© Springer-Verlag Italia 2012

Table 32.1 Approximate energy requirements in METs (1 MET= 3.5 mL/kg/min) during bicycle ergometry

Body weight (Kg)	Power output (Watts)			
	50	100	150	200
50	5.1	8.2	11.3	14.3
60	4.6	7.1	9.7	12.3
70	4.2	6.4	8.6	10.8
80	3.9	5.9	7.8	9.7
90	3.7	5.4	7.1	8.9

on limbs, other electrode placements have been used. The most commonly used is the Mason-Likar adaptation (Fig. 32.1) [1, 4, 9]. A standard 12 lead ECG should be performed before placement of the final limb leads since the Mason-Likar system may alter the inferior lead complexes to either mimic or hide previous Q waves. Furthermore it determines a rightward deviation of cardiac axis.

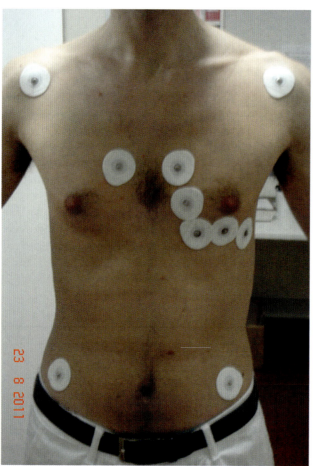

Fig. 32.1 Mason-Likar placement of 12-lead ECG electrodes

32.3.1 Abnormal ECG Responses

32.3.1.1 ST Segment Changes

The ST level is measured relatively to the P-Q junction. Ideally three consecutive beats in the same leads with a stable baseline should be identified and the average displacement determined. The three fundamental measurements are identification of the P-Q junction (isoelectric line), the J point (QRS end and ST segment beginning), and 60-80 ms after the J point. Exercise-induced myocardial ischemia can result in one of the following three ST segment alterations: depression, elevation or normalization (Fig. 32.2) [1, 7, 9].

ST Segment Depression

ST segment depression is the most common manifestation of exercise induced ischemia, as a consequence of abnormal myocardial perfusion. The standard criterion for this abnormal response is horizontal or downsloping ST segment depression of ≥.10 mV (1 mm) for 80 ms (60 ms if ventricular rate >130 beat per minute). Downsloping ST segment depression is considered to be a more specific change than horizontal or upsloping depression (Fig. 32.3). However, other factors are related to the probability and severity of coronary artery disease (CAD) such as the extent of this change, time of appearance, duration, number of leads with ST segment alteration [1, 3, 7, 9]

ST Segment Elevation

ST segment elevation is defined as a J point elevation of ≥10 mV (1 mm) that is persistently elevated at 60 ms after J point and may occur both in an infarct territory or in a non infarct territory. It occurs in approximately 30% of subjects with anterior myocardial infarction (MI) and 15% of subjects with inferior MI and it seems to be related to the presence of severe hypokinetic or akinetic left ventricular (LV) segmental wall motion. In patients with prior MI and Q waves ST segment elevation should

32 Stress ECG

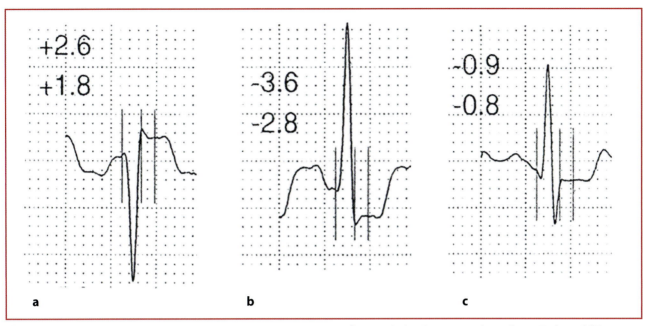

Fig. 32.2 Exercise induced ST segment alterations. **a** ST segment elevation. **b** Downsloping ST segment depression. **c** Horizontal ST segment depression

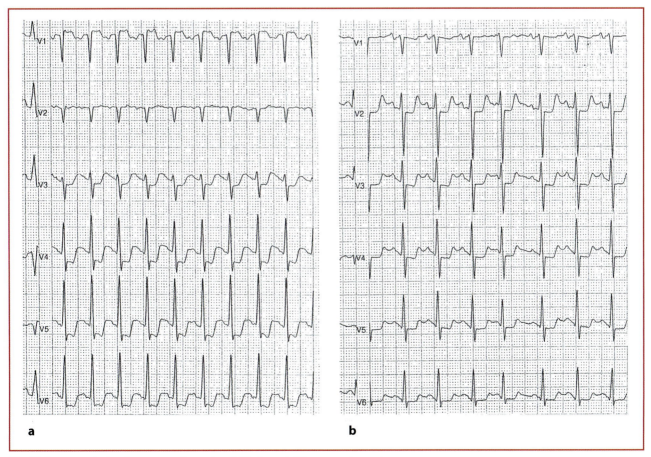

Fig. 32.3 a Downsloping ST segment depression. **b** Horizontal ST segment depression

not be considered a sign of exercise induced ischemia. However, the appearance of a ST segment elevation in patients without prior MI or in leads without pathologic Q waves should be considered as an abnormal response induced by coronary vasospasm or severe CAD. In those situations ST segment elevation frequently localizes the site of severe transient ischemia [1, 3, 7, 9].

32.3.1.2 T Wave Changes

T wave morphology is influenced by body position, respiration, hyperventilation, drug therapy, and myocardial ischemia/necrosis. In patient populations with low CAD prevalence, normalizing of T waves during a stress test should not be considered a sign of ischemia [1, 3, 9]. However, in patients with known CAD this finding may be related to myocardial ischemia and further investigations are required [10].

32.3.1.3 Other ECG Findings

Athens QRS Score

The "Athens QRS score" is a new index proposed to increase the sensitivity of ST segment alterations. It is based only on changes of Q, R and S waves during exercise. In order to calculate the "Athens QRS score" physicians should subtract Q and S waves from the R wave in aVF and V5 leads at rest and sum the two values. The same operation should be done at peak exercise:

Athens QRS score (mm): (DR-DQ-DS) aVF + (DR-DQ-DS) V5

A value ≤5 mm is considered abnormal and negative values are almost always associated with CAD [11].

Left Bundle Branch Block

Diagnosis of myocardial ischemia from the exercise is usually impossible when left bundle branch block is present (LBBB). However the appearance of LBBB during the exercise test can be a sign of myocardial ischemia. In fact a LBBB that occurs at a HR <125 beats/min (bpm) in subjects with typical angina is frequently associated with CAD, whereas a LBBB at HR >125 bpm occurs more frequently in subjects with normal coronary arteries [1, 12].

Second-Degree AV Block

The occurrence of Wenckebach-Mobitz type I atrioventricular (AV) block during exercise is rare. On the other hand, a new onset of a Mobitz type II AV block can be both a rate-related phenomenon or the reflex of a more critical underlying system disease. The exercise test should therefore be terminated in the case of Mobitz type II AV block development [1, 7].

Ventricular Arrhythmias

Exercise may induce cardiac arrhythmias under several conditions, including concomitant diuretic and digitalis therapy. Furthermore, exercise induced myocardial ischemia can predispose to ventricular ectopy, though it seems that ischemia with ST depression is not as arrhythmogenic as ischemia with ST elevation [1]. However, exercise-induced ventricular arrhythmias (EIVAs) are not an established criterion for diagnosis of CAD in the absence of ST segment depression [7]. Nevertheless, they do have a prognostic role since EIVAs and premature ventricular contractions (PVCs) are associated with a modest increase in mortality and CV events, especially in patients with known CAD [13]. Data suggest that EIVAs tend to be more frequent during recovery because of the high catecholamine levels associated with generalized vasodilation and the decreased vagal tone; in addition, peripheral arterial dilation induced by exercise and reduced cardiac output, resulting from diminished venous return, may lead to a reduction in coronary perfusion while HR is still elevated [1]. Moreover, 5-year mortality is higher in patients with frequent PVCs and EIVAs in the recovery phase compared with patients who present arrhythmias only during exercise [14].

Supraventricular Arrhythmias

Supraventricular arrhythmias can occur in either normal or diseased hearts. Exercise induced atrial fibrillation (AF) and flutter occur in <1% of patients who undergo exercise testing. Paroxysmal AV junctional tachycardia is observed during exercise only rarely. Exercise-induced supraventricular arrhythmias alone are not usually related to CAD but rather to older age, pulmonary disease and caffeine or alcohol ingestion [1, 15].

32.4 Non-electrocardiographic Findings

32.4.1 Blood Pressure Response During Exercise

In normal subjects systolic blood pressure (SBP) tends to increase greatly with a peak exercise value between 160 and 230 mmHg (higher values can be observed in elderly male patients), whereas diastolic blood pressure (DBP) usually shows only a slight increase, thus leading to an approximately 40% increase in mean arterial pressure [2, 16]. On the other hand, several different responses can be noticed in subjects affected by different heart diseases.

32.4.1.1 Exercise-induced Hypotension

Exercise induced hypotension (EIH) is most frequently defined as either (1) a drop in exercise SBP below resting value or (2) an initial increase followed by a subsequent drop of ≥ 20 mmHg while exercising [17].

Different studies have established a reliable association in men between hypotension accompanying the onset of exertional angina and multivessel CAD, as well as LV dysfunction. EIH seems to have the highest positive predictive value among middle-aged men with known CAD (positive predictive value 70%) [17-19]. Although less studied, women tend to experience EIH more than men, but this finding does not seem to be associated with a higher incidence of CAD [20].

Despite being a marker of poor prognosis and a relative indication to terminate an exercise test, the validity of EIH as a sign of significant CAD is still limited. Physicians should firstly exclude other possible mechanisms of EIH (e.g. dynamic intraventricular flow obstruction, severe aortic stenosis, bradycardia etc) [21].

32.4.1.2 Low Maximal Exercise Systolic Blood Pressure

There is no recommended definition for low maximal exercise SBP since most criteria and cutpoint used in literature have been arbitrarily chosen. Its corrected prevalence is therefore unknown. In population based studies, lower SBP have often been associated with a more severe CAD, reduced ejection fraction, or both. Furthermore, in populations with known CAD, a relatively low SBP at peak exercise is independently associated with severe CAD and worse CV outcomes [17, 22, 23].

32.4.2 Double Product

The double-product (DP = maximal SBP x peak hear rate) reflects myocardial oxygen uptake and has been used as an estimate of the maximal performance of LV performance. In healthy subjects DP ranges between 20 and 35 mmHg/beat/min x 10^{-3}, whereas it is usually <25 mmHg/beat/min x 10^{-3} in subjects affected by CAD. However, this threshold value has progressively been abandoned because of technical limitations in its reproducibility and possible interactions with cardiac therapies [7, 17, 24].

32.4.3 Heart Rate Response

The immediate response of the cardiovascular system to exercise is an increase in HR due to a decrease in vagal tone. This increase is followed by an increase in sympathetic outflow to the heart and the systemic blood vessels. An accelerated heart rate response to standardized workload is observed in various situations, i.e. physical deconditioning due to prolonged bed rest, atrial fibrillation, anemia, hypovolemia [1, 7].

On the other hand, some patients are unable to increase properly HR during exercise. Many studies have shown a relation between this inability and a greater risk of adverse cardiac events both in asymptomatic men and symptomatic referral population [25, 26]. Chronotropic incompetence is defined as the inability to achieve at least 85% of age predicted maximum-heart rate or as an abnormal heart rate reserve (HRR) which is the difference between maximal predicted HR and resting HR [27].

Another marker of abnormal heart rate response is the chronotropic index, which is an expression of the inability to use the whole HRR. Chronotropic index is measured as: % HRR = (HR_{max} – $HR_{resting}$) / (220-age-$HR_{resting}$). A threshold value of 80% has been identified for chronotropic incompetence [28]. However chronotropic incompetence should not be considered in patients receiving beta-blockers.

HR response abnormalities can be observed also in the recovery period. Heart rate recovery (HRR^1) is defined as difference between maximum HR and HR after 1 or 2 min in the recovery phase ($HRR^1 = HR_{max} - HR_{1\text{-}2 \text{ min}}$) and is considered abnormal when inferior to 12 beats after 1 minute or 22 beats after 2. Some studies have demonstrated a strong relation between impaired HRR^1 and worse prognosis [29, 30].

32.4.4 Angina and Dyspnea

Typical myocardial ischemia related symptoms (i.e. angina and dyspnea) induced by the exercise test are predictive of CAD. Angina and dyspnea should therefore be assessed with a 1-to-4 scale (Table 32.2) and both the exact time of onset and symptom progression should be registered [1, 31]. Usually exertional angina follows the onset of ST segment ischemic abnormalities. However, in some patients it may be the only sign of CAD presence [7].

32.5 Indications for Exercise Testing

The most common indications for exercise testing are CAD diagnosis, evaluation of functional capacity and prognostic stratification in order to help physicians to adopt the best strategies for every cardiac patient. According to current guidelines, the most striking indi-

Table 32.2 Angina and dyspnea scales

Angina scale	
Level 1	Onset of discomfort, mild but recognized as the usual angina-of-effort pain or discomfort
Level 2	Moderate, definitely uncomfortable but still tolerable
Level 3	Moderately severe angina pain. The subject will wish to stop
Level 4	Severe; most intense pain ever felt
Dyspnea scale	
Level 1	Mild, noticeable to patient but not to the observer
Level 2	Mild, some difficulty, noticeable to the observer
Level 3	Moderate difficult but the subject can continue
Level 4	Severe difficulty, the subject will wish to stop

cations are evaluation of subjects at intermediate probability of CAD based on age, sex and symptoms (Table 32.3), evaluation of patients with chronic stable angina, evaluation of patients with previous percutaneous coronary intervention (PCI) or coronary artery by-pass graft (CABG). Exercise testing is not indicated as a screening test in asymptomatic subjects, probably except for those affected by diabetes mellitus, who are planning to start vigorous exercise as shown in Table 32.4. [9, 32-35].

32.6 Diagnostic Value of Exercise Testing

There are several reports and meta-analyses concerning the performance of exercise ECG for the diagnosis of CAD. Using exercise ST depression >1 mm to define a positive test the reported sensitivity and specificity for the detection of CAD range between 23-100% (mean 68%) and 17-100% (mean 77%). Excluding patients with prior MI the mean sensitivity was 67% and specificity 72% [9, 36, 37]. In subjects affected by single-vessel disease sensitivity range between 25-71%, while in patients with multivessel disease mean sensitivity is 81% and

mean specificity is 66% [7]. False-positive results are more frequent in patients with resting ECG abnormalities due to various causes (Table 32.5). Furthermore exercise ECG testing is less sensitive and less specific in women [38]. In subjects with normal resting ECG the most useful leads are V_4-V_6.

Interpretation of exercise ECG findings (see Table 32.6 for positiveness criteria) requires a Bayesian approach to diagnosis. This approach uses clinicians' pre-test estimates of disease along with the results of diagnostic tests to generate individualized post-test disease probability [33]. Along with ECG abnormalities other parameters should be evaluated during exercise testing in order to assess the presence and severity of CAD thus enabling risk stratification (see Table 32.7).

It should be emphasized that positivity of exercise stress test for CAD detection appears to be limited to the recognition of a hemodynamically significant coronary artery stenosis, but it does not allow to identify mild non-significant disease. Accordingly, the role of stress test in risk stratification of asymptomatic subjects and in detection of subclinical coronary atherosclerosis is limited [39].

32.7 Prognostic Value of Exercise Testing

Stress ECG is not only a diagnostic tool but is also useful to obtain prognostic information in different clinical settings. It is fundamental to underline the importance of integrating the results of exercise testing with other clinical data available, i.e. risk factors, CAD extension, comorbidities, electrical instability, etc.

32.7.1 Asymptomatic Subjects

Routine screening of asymptomatic individuals with exercise testing is not recommended [9, 34] though different studies have shown an increased risk of CV events

Table 32.3 Pre-test probability of CAD (%) based on age, sex, and symptom classification

Age (yrs)	Typical Angina		Atypical Angina		Non-anginal chest pain	
	Male	Female	Male	Female	Male	Female
30-39	Intermediate (69.7 ± 3.2)	Intermediate (25.8 ± 6.6)	Intermediate (21.8 ± 2.4)	Very Low 4.2 ± 1.3	Low (5.2 ± 0.8)	Very Low (0.8 ± 0.3)
40-49	High (87.3 ± 1.0)	Intermediate (55.2 ± 6.5)	Intermediate (46.1 ± 1.8)	Low (13.3 ± 2.9)	Intermediate (14.1 ± 1.3)	Very Low (2.8 ± 0.7)
50-59	High (92 ± 0.6)	Intermediate (79.4 ± 2.4)	Intermediate (58.9 ± 1.5)	Intermediate (32.4 ± 3.0)	Intermediate (21.5 ± 1.7)	Low (8.4 ± 1.2)
60-69	High (94.3 ± 0.4)	High (90.1 ± 1.0)	Intermediate (67.1 ± 1.3)	Intermediate (54.4 ± 2.)	Intermediate (28.1 ± 1.9)	Intermediate (18.6 ± 1.9.)

32 Stress ECG

Table 32.4 Recommendations for exercise testing [9, 32-35]

Class I recommendations	Class II a recommendations
CAD diagnosis and initial risk evaluation in patients at intermediate pre-test probability according to age, sex and symptoms, including those with right bundle branch block or less than 1mm of resting ST depression	CAD detection in patients with vasospastic angina
	After discharge for activity counseling and/or exercise training as a part of cardiac rehabilitation in patients who have undergone PCI or CABG after MI
Patients with suspected or known CAD, previously evaluated, now presenting with significant change in clinical status	Asymptomatic persons with diabetes mellitus who plan to start vigorous exercise
Assessment of functional capacity after NSTEMI/unstable angina	
In patients with NSTEMI/unstable angina without recurrence of pain, normal ECG findings, and negative troponin, before discharge	4 to 7 weeks after discharge (if technically feasible) in patients with NSTEMI/unstable angina
In patients with recent MI for prognostic assessment, activity prescription, evaluation of medical therapy, and cardiac rehabilitation: • Before discharge (submaximal at about 4 to 6 days) • Early after discharge if the early exercise test was not done (symptom limited; about 14 to 21 days) • Later after discharge if the early exercise test was submaximal (symptom limited; about 3 to 6 weeks)	
Detection of myocardial ischemia before any planned revascularization procedure	
Evaluation of patients referring symptoms suggestive for myocardial ischemia after revascularization	

Table 32.5 Non-coronary causes of ST segment depression

Severe aortic stenosis
Left ventricular hypertrophy
Digoxin therapy
Hypokalemia
Right bundle branch block
Anemia
Ventricular pre-excitation
Severe volume overload (e.g. secondary to valve regurgitation)
Underlying dilated or hypertrophic cardiomyopathy
Severe hypoxia

Table 32.6 Positivity criteria for exercise testing

New flat or downsloping ST segment depression ≥1 mm below the baseline, at least 60-80 ms after the J point in multiple leads
ST segment elevation >1 mm in leads without Q waves (other than V1 or aVR)
New ST segment depression at the start of exercise (within 3 minutes)
Fall in SBP >20 mmHg or >10 mmHg with evidences of ischemia
Typical Angina pectoris
Inability to exercise more than 2 min on a cardiac basis

in asymptomatic patients with abnormal ECG response to exercise. In fact, there is no demonstration of its value for improving long-term stratification [40]. According to current guidelines, exercise testing in asymptomatic subjects should be performed only in people with diabetes who are contemplating an exercise program [9, 34].

32.7.2 Symptomatic Subjects

Exercise testing provides valuable information in outpatients with chronic ischemic heart disease. Patients with excellent exercise tolerance usually have a good prognosis regardless of anatomical extent of CAD. [1]

The prognostic exercise testing markers include exercise capacity (measured in METs), blood pressure response, exercise-induced ischemia (clinical and ECG) as shown in Table 32.7 [33]. In order to obtain a better a risk stratification Mark et al. developed a treadmill score (Duke treadmill score) that divides patients into low risk (1-year mortality <0.25%), intermediate risk (1-year mortality 1.25%) and high risk (1-year mortality >5.25 %). Duke treadmill score (DTS) is calculated as follow: DTS = exercise time in minutes – (5 x ST depression in mm) – (4 x angina index). Angina index has a value of '0' if no angina occurs, '1' if angina occurs and '2' if it is the reason for stopping the test. Patients at low risk have a DTS >5 whereas patients at high risk have a DTS <-11 [41].

Table 32.7 Exercise parameters linked to poor prognosis and multi-vessels disease

Low working capacity (<5METs) and angina
Low maximal SBP (≤120mmhg) or SBP drop >10mmHg or below resting levels despite an increase in workload
ST segment depression >2mm or downsloping ST segment depression appearing at low workload (<5METs) in 5 or more leads that persists at least 5 minute after recovery.
ST segment elevation
Sustained ventricular tachycardia or symptomatic ventricular tachycardia.
Systemic diseases (pulmonary embolisms, aortic dissection)
Duke Treadmill Score <-11
Athens QRS score ≤0

Table 32.8 Complication during exercise tests

Cardiac
• Brady- and tachyarrhythmias
• Acute coronay syndromes
• Acute Heart Failure
• Hypotension, syncope, and shock
• Aortic dissection
• Stroke
• Death
Non cardiac
• Musculoskeletal trauma
• Soft-tissue injury
• Severe fatigue
• Dizziness

Table 32.9 Emergency equipment and drugs for exercise testing

Equipment
Automated external defibrillator
Oxygen tank
Nasal cannula, Ventimask, nonrebreathing mask O_2 mask.
Bag-valve-mask (Ambu Bag)
Suction apparatus and supplies (eg. gloves, tubing)
Syringes, needles, adhesive tape
Oral and nasal airways
Drugs
Antiarrhythmic drugs: Amiodarone, Diltiazem, Adenosine, Verapamil, Lidocaine, Intravenous Metoprolol, Atropine
Inotropic drugs: Dobutamine, Dopamine, Vasopressin, Epinephrine
Chewable or intravenous aspirin
Sublingual nitroglycerin

32.7.3 Silent Myocardial Ischemia

In subjects with known CAD the onset of ST segment depression during exercise testing is associated with a higher risk of CV events even in the absence of angina [42, 43]. It is therefore necessary to detect silent ischemia since recent studies have demonstrated the effectiveness of aggressive medical treatment in patients with stable CAD [44]. More controversial is the prognostic role of silent myocardial ischemia in subjects without known CAD, though recent data suggests that asymptomatic ST segment depression is a strong predictor of sudden cardiac death (SCD) [45]. Nevertheless, current guidelines do not recommend exercise testing in asymptomatic subjects without known CAD [9, 34].

32.7.4 Risk Stratification in the Emergency Department

Patients who present to the emergency department are a heterogeneous population with a large range of pretest risk for CAD. According to current guidelines, people presenting to the emergency department for chest pain/unstable angina should be evaluated with a stress test before discharge when resting ECG is not diagnostic and provided there is no pain, no signs of heart failure, and normal biomarkers [32, 35, 46]. This is due to the high negative predictive value of stress test [47] and the safety of this approach has been demonstrated in different studies [48, 49].

32.8 Safety of Exercise Testing

Table 32.8 lists the main complications secondary to exercise tests. Although exercise testing is a very safe procedure, the risk of testing varies with the patient population being tested. In unselected population mortality is below 0.01% and morbidity is below 0.05% with a slightly higher risk in case of early testing after acute myocardial infarction [50]. In a large study Gibbons et al. evaluated 34,295 patients for a total number of 71,914 maximal exercise tests; the overall cardiac complication rate in men and women was 0.8 complication per 10,000 test [51]. Furthermore exercise testing has been proved to be safe also in patients with stable chronic heart failure [52]. Nevertheless in order to minimize the risk of com-

32 Stress ECG

Table 32.10 Absolute and relative contraindications to exercise testing [9]

Absolute contraindications	Relative contraindications
Acute MI (<2 days)	Left main coronary stenosis or its equivalent
High risk unstable angina	Moderate stenotic valvular heart disease
Acute decompensated heart failure	Electrolyte abnormalities
Uncontrolled cardiac arrhythmias causing symptoms or hemodynamic instability.	Tachyarrhythmias (including AF with uncontrolled ventricular rate), bradyarrhythmias or high degree AV block.
Acute myocarditis, pericarditis or active endocarditis	Hypertrophic cardiomyopathy or outflow obstruction
Severe symptomatic aortic stenosis	Uncontrolled arterial hypertension: SBP>200 mmHg or DBP >100 mmHg
Systemic diseases (e.g. acute pulmonary embolus, pulmonary infarction, aortic dissection, acute renal failure, thyrotoxicosis)	Complete left bundle branch block and pre-excitation (Wolff-Parkinson-White) syndrome

Table 32.11 Reasons to terminate exercise testing [9, 33]

Absolute indications	Relative Indications
ST segment elevation >1mm in leads without Q waves (other than V1 or aVR)	ST segment horizontal or downsloping depression >2mm or marked axis shift
ST segment depression ≥4 mm	Symptom limitation: Fatigue, shortness of breath, leg cramps
Moderate to severe angina	Increasing chest pain
Drop in systolic blood pressure >10 mmHg or below baseline despite an increase in workload when associated to other evidences of ischemia	Drop in systolic blood pressure >10mmHg or below baseline despite an increase in workload without other evidences of ischemia
Sustained ventricular tachycardia Subjects request to stop	Arrhythmia other than sustained ventricular tachycardia (e.g. advanced AV block, AF, bradyarrhythmias)
Signs of poor perfusion (cyanosis or pallor) or central nervous system symptoms (e.g. dizziness, vertigo, near syncope)	Hypertensive response SBP >250 mmhg and/or DBP >115 mmHg
Technical difficulties in ECG or blood pressure monitoring	Achievement of maximum predicted heart rate at the discretion of the supervising physician

plication exercise, all testing laboratories must have the equipment, drugs, and personnel trained to deliver appropriate emergency care in accordance with current guidelines (Table 32.9) [4].

Moreover, physicians should examine carefully each subject in order to detect possible contraindication to stress testing (Table 32.10); finally, they should strictly attain to guidelines for the interruption criteria (Table 32.11) [1].

When all requirements are met and the stress test is administered by well-trained personnel the risk for complications is minimum and the quantity of useful data maximum.

References

1. Fletcher GF, Balady GJ, Amsterdam EA et al (2001) Exercise standards for Testing and Training: A statement for healthcare Professionals from the American Heart Association. Circulation 104:1694-1740
2. Mac Dougall J. (1994) Blood Pressure responses to resistive static and dynamic exercise. In: Fletcher G ed. Cardiovascular Response to Exercise. Mount Kisko, NY: Futura Publishing Co, Inc; pp 155-173
3. Froelicher VF, Myers J (2006) Exercise and the Heart. 5th ed. Philadelphia, Pa: WB Saunders.
4. Myers J, Arena R, Balady GJ et al (2009) Recommendations for clinical exercise laboratories: a scientific statement from the American Heart Association. Circulation 119:3144-3161
5. American College of Sports Medicin (2010) ACSM's guidelines for exercise testing and prescription. Philadelphia, Pa: Lippincot Wiliams & Wilkins.
6. Kaminsky LA, Whaley MH (1998) Evaluation of a new standardized ramp protocol: the BSU/Bruce ramp protocol. J Cardiopulm Rehabil 18:438-444
7. Braunwald E, Bonow RO, Libby P, Zipes DP. (2007) Braunwald's Heart Disease, 7th ed. Elsevier
8. Kligfield P, Gettes LS , Bailey JJ et al (2007) Recommendations for the standardization and interpretation of electrocardiogram: part 1: the electrocardiogram and its technology: a scientific statement from the American Heart Association Electrocardiograpy and Arrhytmias Committee, Council on Clinical Cardiology: the American College of Cardiology Foundation; and the Heart rhythm Society. Circulation 115:1306-1324
9. Gibbons RJ, Baldy GJ, Smith SC et al (2002) ACC/AHA 2002 guideline update for exercise testing. Summary article: A report of the ACC/AHA task force on practice guidelines (Committee to update the 1997 exercise testing guidelines). J Am Coll Cardiol 40:1531-1540
10. Mobilia G, Zanco P, Desideri A et al (1998) T wave normalization in infarct-related electrocardiographic leads during exercise testing for detection of residual viability: Comparison with positon emission tomography. J Am Coll Cardiol 32:75-82

11. Michaelides AP, Triposkiadis FK, Boudalas H et al (1990) New coronary artery disease index based on exercise-induced QRS changes. Am Heart J 120:292-302
12. Vasey C, O'Donnel J, Morris S et al (1985) Exercise-induced left bundle branch block and its relation to coronary artery disease. Am J Cardiol 56:892-895
13. Partington S, Myers J, Cho S et al (2003) Prevalence and prognostic value of exercise-induced ventricular arrhythmias. Am Heart J 145:139-146
14. Frolkis JP, Pothier CE, Lauer MS et al (2003) Frequent ventricular ectopy after exercise as a predictor of death. N Engl J Med 348:781-790
15. Atwood JE, Myers J, Sullivan M et al (1988) Maximal exercise testing and gas exchange in patients with chronic atrial fibrillation. J Am Coll Cardiol 11:508-513
16. Myers JN (1994) The physiology behind exercise testing. Prim Care 21:415-437
17. Le VV, Mitiku T, Sungar G et al (2008) The blood pressure response to dynamic exercise testing: a systematic review. Prog Cardiovasc Dis 51:135-160
18. Dubach P, Froelicher VF, Klein J et al (1988) Exercise induced hypotension in a male population. Criteria, causes and prognosis. Circulation 78:1380-1387
19. Sanmarco ME, Pontius S, Selvester RH (1980) Abnormal blood pressure response and marked ischemic St-segment depression ad predictors of severe coronary artery disease. Circulation 61:572-578
20. Morrow K, Morris CK, Froelicher VF et al (1993) Prediction of cardiovascular death in men undergoing noninvasive evaluation for coronary artery disease. Ann Intern Med 118:689-695
21. Gleim GW, Stachefeld NS, Coplan NL et al (1991) Gender differences in the systolic blood pressure response to exercise. Am Heart J 121:524-530
22. Irving JB, Bruce RA, Derouen TA (1977) Variation in and significance of systolic pressure during maximal exercise (treadmill) testing. Am J Cardiol 39:841-848
23. Gupta MP, Polena S, Coplan N et al (2007) Prognostic significance of systolic blood pressure increases in men during exercise stress testing. Am J Cardiol 100:1609-1613
24. Crea F, Margonato Am, Kaski JC et al (1986) Variability of results during repeat exercise stress testing in patients with stable angina pectoris: role of dynamic coronary flow reserve. Am Heart J 112:249-254
25. Jouven X, Empan JP, Schwarts PJ et al (2005) Heart-rate profile during exercise as predictor if sudden death. N Engl J Med 352:1951-1958
26. Savonen KP, Lakka TA, Laukkanen JA et al (2006) Heart rate response during exercise test abìnd cardiovascular mortality in middle-aged men. Eur Heart J 27:582-588
27. Laure MS, Francis G, Okin PM et al (1999) Impaired chronotropic response to exercise stress testing as a predictor of mortality. JAMA 281:524-529
28. Azarbal B, Hayes SW, Lewin HC et al (2004) The incremental prognostic value of percentage heart rate reserve achieved over myocardial perfusion single photon emission computed tomography in the prediction of cardiac death and all-cause mortality: superiority over 85% of maximal age-predicted heart rate. J Am Coll Cardiol 44:423-430
29. Myers J, Tan SY, Froelicher VF et al (2007) Comparison of the chronotropic response to exercise and heart rate recovery in predicting cardiovascular mortality. Eur J Cardiovasc Prev Rehabil 14:215-221
30. Vivekananthan DP, Blackstone EH, Pothier CE et al (2003) Heart rate recovery after exercise is a predictor of mortality, independent of the angiographic severity of coronary disease. J Am Coll Cardiol 42:831-838

31. Myers JN (1994) Perception of chest pain during exercise testing in patients with coronary artery disease. Med Sci Sport Exerc 26:1082-1086
32. Erhardt L, Herlitz J, Bossaert L et al (2002) Task force on the management of chest pain. Eur Heart J 23:1153-1176
33. Fox K, Garcia MA, Ardissino D et al (2006) Guidelines on the management of stable angina pectoris: full text. Eur Heart J doi:10.1093/eurheartj/ehl002
34. Lauer M, Froelicher ES, Williams m et al (2005) Exercise testing in asymptomatic adults. A statement for professionals from the American Heart Association council on clinical cardiology, subcommittee on exercise, cardiac rehabilitation, and prevention. Circulation 112:771-776
35. Hamm CW, Ardissino D, Boersma E et al (2007) Guidelines for the diagnosis and treatment of non-ST-segment elevation acute coronary syndromes. Eur Heart J 28:1598-1660
36. Gianrossi R, Detrano R, Mulvihill D et al (1989) Exercise-induced ST depression in the diagnosis of coronary artery disease. A meta-analysis. Circulation 80:87-98
37. Ashley EA, Myers J, Froelicher V (2000) Exercise testing in clinical medicine. Lancet 356:1592-1597
38. Hung J, Chaitman Br, Lam J et al (1984) Noninvasive diagnostic test choices for the evaluation of coronary artery disease in women: a multivariate comparison of cardiac fluoroscopy, exercise electrocardiography and exercise thallium myocardial perfusion scintigraphy. J Am Coll Cardiol 4:8-16
39. Amsterdam EA, Kirk JD, Blemke DA et al (2010) Testing of low-risk patients presenting to the emergency department with chest pain: a scientific statement from the American Heart Association. Circulation 122:1756-1776
40. Fowler-Brown A, Pignone M, Pletcher M et al (2004) U.S. Preventive task force. Exercise tolerance testing to screen for coronary heart disease: a systematic review for the technical support for the U.S. Preventive Service Task Force. Ann Intern Med 140:W 9-24
41. Mark DB, Shaw L, Harrel FE Jr et al (1991) Prognostic value of a treadmill exercise score in outpatients with suspected coronary artery disease. N Engl J Med 325:849-853
42. Stone PH, Chaitman BR, Forman S et al (1997) Prognostic significance of myocardial ischemia detected by ambulatory electrocardiogram, exercise treadmill testing, and resting electrocardiogram to predicts cardiac events by 1 year (the Asymptomatic Cardiac Ischemia Pilot [ACIP] study). Am J Cardiol 80:1395-1401
43. Dagenais GR, Rouleau JR, Hochart P et al (1988) Survival with painless strongly positive exercise electrocardiogram. Am J Cardiol 62:892-895
44. Boden WE, O'Rourke RA, Teo KK et al (2007) Optimal medical therapy with or without PCI for stable coronary disease. N Engl J Med 356:1503-1516
45. Laukkanen JA, Makikallio TH, Rauramaa R et al (2009) Ayimptomatic ST-segment depression during exercise testing and the risk of sudden cardiac death in middle-aged men: a population-based follo-up study. Eur Heart J 30:558-565
46. Stein R, Chaitman B, Balady GJ et al (2000) Safety and utility of exercise testing in emergency room chest pain centers: an advisory from the committee on exercise, rehabilitation, and prevention, Council on clinical cardiology, American Heart Association. Circulation 102:1463-1467
47. Nyman I, Wallentin L, Areskog NH et al (1993) Risk stratification by early exercise testing after an episode of unstable coronary artery disease. The RISC study group. Int J Cardiol 39:131-142
48. Nichol G, Walls R, Goldman L et al (1997) A critical pathway for management of patients with acute chest pain who are at low risk for myocardial ischemia: recommendations and potential impact. Ann Intern Med 127:996-1005
49. Amsterdam EA, Kirk JD, Diercks DB et al (2002) Immediate exercise testing to evaluate low-risk patients presenting to the emer-

gency department with chest pain. J Am Coll Cardiol 40:251-256

50. Stuart RJ, Ellestad MH (1980) National Survey exercise stress testing facilities. Chest 77:94-97

51. Gibbons L, Blair SN, Kohl HW et al (1989) The safety of maximal exercise testing. Circulation 80:846-852

52. Tristani FE, Hughes CV. Archibald DG et al (1987): Safety of graded symptom-limited exercise testing in patients with congestive heart failure. Circulation 76:VI 54-58

Rest and Stress Echocardiography

33

Fausto Rigo, Lauro Cortigiani, Elisabetta Grolla, and Eugenio Picano

33.1 Introduction

In 1935, for the first time Tennant and Wiggers showed how a coronary occlusion results in instantaneous abnormality of wall motion of the left ventricle [1]. Forty years later an experimental study with two-dimensional ultrasound on a canine model highlighted that during acute ischemia and infarction reductions in regional flow are closely mirrored by reductions in contractile function, opening the road for the clinical use of ultrasound as gatekeeper for ischemic heart disease [2]. Stress echocardiography combines 2D echocardiography with a physical, pharmacologic or electrical stress for assessing the presence, localization and extent of myocardial ischemia. Stress-induced wall motion abnormality is the early and specific marker of ischemia. Identification of viable myocardium and evaluation of severity of valvular heart disease are additional recognized applications of stress echocardiography. The wide availability of echocardiographic equipment in all medical centers has been a factor of paramount importance for the diffusion of the technique, especially in the light of its limited costs and resource consumption.

33.2 Pathophysiology of Ischemia

Myocardial ischemia is the final common pathway of various morphologic and functional substrates. Coronary flow reserve is the capacity of the coronary arteriolar bed to dilate in response to increased metabolic demand. In normal conditions, arteriolar vasodilation can determine a four-to-six fold increment of coronary blood flow, leading to global increase in left ventricular contractility. In the presence of coronary stenosis between 75% and 95% coronary flow reserve reduces progressively [3], and a

transient imbalance between oxygen demand and supply occurs. This results in a typical *cascade* of ischemic events in which the various markers are ranked in a well-defined temporal sequence. Regional malperfusion is the forerunner of ischemia, followed by regional systolic dysfunction, and only at a later stage by electrocardiographic changes and angina [4] (Fig. 33.1). Ischemia tends to occur centrifugally with respect to the ventricular cavity, involving earlier the subendocardial layer, whereas the subepicardial layer is affected only at a later stage if ischemia persists. In fact, extravascular pressure is higher in the subendocardial than in the subepicardial layer; this provokes a higher metabolic demand (wall tension being among the main determinants of myocardial oxygen consumption) and an increased resistance to flow. The impairment of systolic function correlates with the severity of flow reduction. In fact, a 20% reduction in subendocardial flow produces a 15-20% decrease in left ventricular wall thickening; a 50% reduction in subendocardial flow decreases regional wall thickening by about 40%, and when subendocardial flow is reduced by 80%, akinesia occurs. When the flow deficit is extended to the subepicardial layer, dyskinesia appears [5].

33.2.1 Mechanisms of Ischemia

Cardiovascular stress can induce ischemia by means of different mechanisms that may either act by enhancing myocardial oxygen consumption, or by reducing oxygen supply, through an inappropriate arteriolar vasodilation, with subsequent flow maldistribution, or coronary artery spasm.

33.2.1.1 Increased Demand

In resting conditions, myocardial oxygen consumption is dependent mainly on heart rate, inotropic state, and the left ventricular wall stress (which is proportional to the systolic blood pressure). During exercise, the increase in heart rate, blood pressure, and inotropic state accounts for the overall increase in myocardial oxygen consump-

F. Rigo (✉)
Cardiology Division, "dell'Angelo" Hospital,
Mestre-Venice, Italy

F. Cademartiri, G. Casolo, M. Midiri (eds.), *Clinical Applications of Cardiac CT*,
© Springer-Verlag Italia 2012

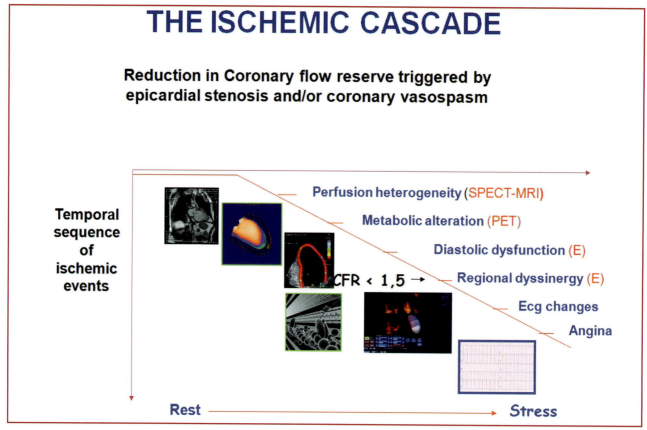

Fig. 33.1 The ischemic cascade, triggered by a coronary stenosis and/or vasospasm. The various markers are usually ranked according to a well-defined time sequence

tion [5] (Fig. 33.2). To a lesser degree, pacing and dobutamine also increase myocardial oxygen demand. During pacing, the increase is mainly due to the increased heart rate [5]. Dobutamine stimulates adrenoreceptors, markedly increasing contractility and heart rate [5] (Table 33.1). Following dipyridamole or adenosine administration, only a mild increase in myocardial oxygen consumption, due to a slight increase in contractility and heart rate, can be observed. Greater myocardial oxygen consumption due to heart rate increase occurs with co-administration of atropine with dobutamine and dipyridamole [5].

33.2.1.2 Flow Maldistribution

In the presence of a fixed coronary atherosclerosis, arteriolar dilation can paradoxically produce detrimental effects on regional myocardial perfusion, causing overperfusion of myocardial layers or regions already well perfused in resting conditions at the expense of layers or regions with a precarious flow balance in resting conditions [5]. In *vertical steal* the anatomic requisite is the presence of an epicardial coronary stenosis and the subepicardium *steals* blood from the subendocardial layers. In fact, the administration of a coronary vasodilator causes a fall in post-stenotic pressure, and therefore a critical fall in subendocardial perfusion pressure, which in turn provokes a fall in absolute subendocardial flow, even with subepicardial overperfusion. Regional thickening is closely related to subendocardial rather than transmural flow, and this explains the apparent paradox of regional asynergy, with ischemia in spite of a regionally increased transmural flow [5]. *Horizontal steal* requires the presence of collateral circulation between two vascular beds; the victim of the steal is the myocardium fed by the more stenotic vessel. After vasodilation, the flow in the collateral circulation is reduced relative to resting conditions, since the arteriolar bed of the donor vessel competes with the arteriolar bed of the receiving vessel, whose vasodilatory reserve was already exhausted in resting conditions [5]. The biochemical effector of this hemodynamic mechanism is the inappropriate accumulation of adenosine, which is the main physiologic modulator of arteriolar vasodilation by stimulating A_{2a} adenosinergic receptors present on the

33 Rest and Stress Echocardiography

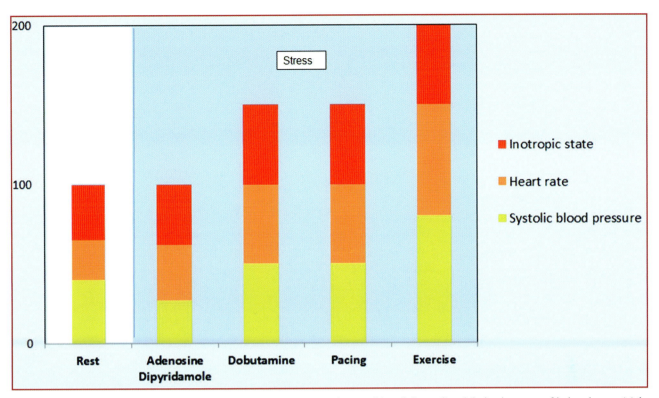

Fig. 33.2 Major determinants of myocardial oxygen consumption in resting condition (*left panel*) and during instances of induced stress (*right panel*) commonly employed with echocardiography. The relative contributions of systolic blood pressure, heart rate, and inotropic state to myocardial oxygen demand are represented

Table 33.1 Pharmacologic stressors

	Vasodilatator			Dobutamine		
Stress	Dipyridamole (adenosine)			Dobutamine		
Receptor target	A1	A₂ a	A₂ b	α 1	β 1	β 2
Pharmacodynamics						
Myocardium	Decreased chronotropy and dromotropy			Increased inotropy	Increased chronotropy and inotropy	
Vasculature		Coronary arteriolar vasodilation	Conductance vessel vasodilation	Vasoconstriction		Vasodilation
Hemodynamic mechanisms	Reduces supply			Increases supply		
Physiologic targets	Coronary arterioles			Myocardium		
Cellular targets	Smooth muscle cells			Myocytes		
Antidote	Aminophylline			β-blockers		
Contraindications	Asthma, bradyarrhythmias			Tachyarrhythmias, hypertension		

endothelial and smooth muscle cells of coronary arterioles (Table 33.1). Flow maldistribution plays a key role in myocardial ischemia induced by adenosine or dipyridamole (which act by blocking the uptake of endogenous adenosine into the cells), while it is likely to have a minor role in exercise- or pacing-induced ischemia.

33.2.1.3 Vasospasm

The mechanisms of coronary spasm are still unclear. The smooth muscle cell in the medial layer of coronary epicardial arteries reacts to several vasoconstrictive stimuli, coming from the adventitial layer (such as α-mediated vasoconstriction) or centrifugally from the intima-blood

Table 33.2 Classifications and clinical implications of stress echo responses. Modified from the American Society of Echocardiography guidelines

Classification	Rest	Stress	Implication
Normal	Normal	Hyperdynamic	No ischemia
Ischemia	Normal	Abnormal	Ischemia induced
Scar	Abnormal	No change	Post myocardial infarct No inducible ischemia
Viability	Abnormal	Improvement	Hibernation, stunning

Table 33.3 Left ventricle regional wall function

	Systolic thickening	Endocardial motion
Hyperkinesia	Increased	Increased
Normokinesia	10-80%	4-10 mm
Hypokinesia	Reduced	Reduced
Akinesis	Abolished	Abolished
Dyskinesia	Systolic thinning	Outward systolic movement

interface (such as endothelin and serotonin). Clinically, coronary vasospasm can be elicited by ergonovine, which exerts a direct constrictive effect on vascular smooth muscle by stimulating both β-adrenergic and serotoninergic receptors. Exercise and dobutamine can also induce an increase in coronary tone, sometimes up to complete vasospasm, through α-adrenergic stimulation [4]. Interruption of dipyridamole test by aminophylline (blocking adenosine receptors but also stimulating α-adrenoreceptors) can evoke vasospasm in one third of patients with variant angina [4].

33.3 Diagnostic Criteria

All stress echocardiographic diagnoses can be summarized into four categories centered on regional wall function and describing the fundamental response patterns: normal, ischemic, necrotic, and viable (Tables 33.2-33.4).

Normal response. A segment is normokinetic at rest and normal or hyperkinetic during stress.

Ischemic response. The function of a segment worsens during stress from normokinesia to hypokinesia (decrease of endocardial movement and systolic thickening), akinesia (absence of endocardial movement and systolic thickening), or dyskinesia (paradoxical outward movement and possible systolic thinning). However, a resting akinesia becoming dyskinesia during stress reflects a purely passive phenomenon of increased intraventricular pressure developed by normally contracting walls and should not be considered true active ischemia [4].

Necrotic response. A segment with resting dysfunc-

tion remains fixed during stress.

Viability response. A segment with resting dysfunction may show either a sustained improvement during stress indicating a non-jeopardized myocardium (stunned) or improve during early stress with subsequent deterioration at peak (biphasic response). The biphasic response is suggestive of viability and ischemia, with jeopardized myocardium fed by a critically coronary stenosis [4].

33.4 Methodology of Stress-Echo

33.4.1 General Test Protocol

During stress echo, a 12-lead electrocardiogram and pressure cuff are used to make blood pressure recordings in resting condition and at each minute throughout the examination. Echocardiographic imaging is performed from the conventional parasternal and apical views. Images are recorded in resting conditions from all views and captured digitally [6]. A quad-screen format is used for comparative analysis. Echocardiography is then continuously monitored and intermittently stored. In the presence of dyssynergy, a complete echo examination is performed and recorded from all employed approaches to allow optimal documentation of the presence and extent of myocardial ischemia [6]. These same projections are obtained and recorded during the recovery phase, after cessation of stress (exercise or pacing) or administration of the antidote (aminophylline for dipyridamole, beta-blocker for dobutamine, nitroglycerine for ergonovine). Analysis of the study is usually performed using a 16- or

Table 33.4 Stress echocardiography in four equations

Rest	+	Stress	=	Diagnosis
Normokinesia	+	Normo-hyperkinesia	=	Normal
Normokinesia	+	Hypo-, a-, dyskinesia	=	Ischemia
Akinesis	+	Hypo-, normokinesia	=	Viable
A-, dyskinesia	+	A-, dyskinesia	=	Necrosis

Table 33.5 Exercise versus pharmacologic stress

Parameter	Exercise	Pharmacologic
Intravenous line required	No	Yes
Diagnostic utility of heart rate and blood pressure response	Yes	No
Use in deconditioned patients	No	Yes
Use in physically limited patients	No	Yes
Level of echocardiography imaging difficulty	High	Low
Safety profile	High	Moderate
Clinical role in valvular disease	Yes	No
Clinical role in pulmonary hypertension	Yes	No
Fatigue and dyspnea evaluation	Yes	No

17-segment model of the left ventricle [6]. Regional wall motion is semiquantitatively graded from 1 to 4 as follows: 1=normal; 2=hypokinetic; 3=akinetic; 4=dyskinetic. Dividing the sum of individual segment scores by the number of interpretable segments derived the wall motion score index [6]. Diagnostic endpoints of stress echocardiography include maximum workload (for exercise testing) or maximum dose (for pharmacologic), achievement of target heart rate, echocardiographic positivity (akinesis of ≥ 2 left ventricular segments), severe chest pain, or electrocardiographic positivity (>2 mV ST-segment shift). Submaximal nondiagnostic endpoints are nontolerable symptoms or asymptomatic side effects such as hypertension (systolic blood pressure >220 mmHg or diastolic blood pressure >120 mmHg), symptomatic hypotension (>40 mmHg drop in blood pressure), supraventricular arrhythmias (supraventricular tachycardia or atrial fibrillation), and complex ventricular arrhythmias (ventricular tachycardia or frequent, polymorphic premature ventricular beats).

33.4.2 Specific Test Protocols

The most frequent stressor agents currently adopted for echocardiographic test are exercise, dobutamine, and dipyridamole. There are distinct advantages and disadvantages to exercise versus pharmacologic stress, which are outlined in Table 33.5.

33.4.2.1 Exercise
Exercise echocardiography can be performed using either a treadtablemill or bicycle protocol. When a tread-

mill test is performed, scanning during exercise is quite difficult, so most protocols rely on post-exercise imaging. It is imperative to complete post-exercise imaging as soon as possible. To accomplish this, the patient is moved immediately from the treadmill to an imaging table so that imaging may be completed within 1-2 min. This technique assumes that regional wall motion abnormalities will persist long enough into recovery to be detected. When abnormalities recover rapidly, false-negative results occur [6]. Information on exercise capacity, heart rate response, and rhythm and blood pressure changes are analyzed and, together with wall motion analysis, become part of the final interpretation [6]. Bicycle exercise echocardiography is performed during either an upright or a recumbent posture. Unlike treadmill test, bicycle exercise allows images to be obtained during the various levels of exercise. The patient pedals against an increasing workload (escalated in a stepwise fashion) while imaging is performed. In the supine posture, using a bed-ergometer, it is relatively easy to record images from multiple views during graded exercise. In the upright posture, imaging is generally limited to apical views [5].

33.4.2.2 Dobutamine
The standard dobutamine stress protocol consists of continuous intravenous infusion of dobutamine in 3 min increments, starting with 5 µg/kg/min and increasing to 10, 20, 30, and 40 µg/kg/min. If no endpoint is reached, atropine (up to 1 mg) is added to the 40 µg/kg/min dobutamine infusion [6].

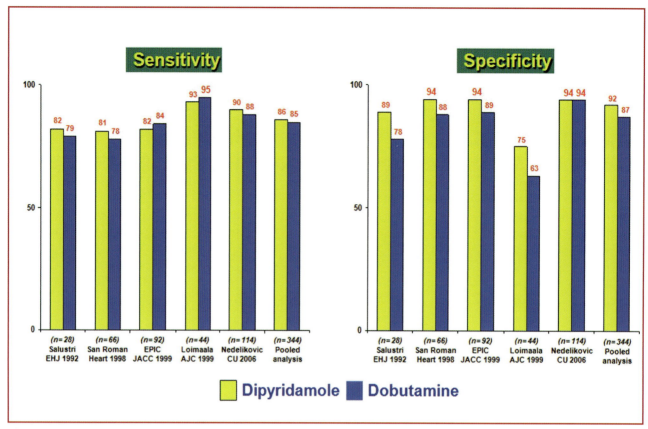

Fig. 33.3 Summary of a metanalysis of the values of sensitivity and specificity obtained with the two main pharmacologic stress tests: dipyridamole and dobutamine

33.4.2.3 Dipyridamole

The standard dipyridamole protocol consists of an intravenous infusion of 0.84 mg/kg over 10 min, in two separate infusions: 0.56 mg/kg over 4 min, followed by 4 min of no dose and, if still negative, an additional 0.28 mg/kg over 2 min. If no endpoint is reached, atropine (up to 1 mg) is added. The same overall dose of 0.84 mg/kg can be given in fast injection, over 6 min [5], and this protocol is very useful for assessing coronary flow reserve. Aminophylline should be available for immediate use in case an adverse dipyridamole-related event occurs and routinely infused at the end of the test regardless of the result.

33.4.2.4 Adenosine

Adenosine is usually infused at a maximum dose of 140 g/kg/min over 6 min [6]. When side-effects are intolerable, down-titration of the dose is also possible.

33.4.2.5 Pacing

The presence of a permanent pacemaker can be exploited to conduct a pacing stress test in a totally noninvasive manner by externally programming the pacemaker to increasing frequencies. Pacing is started at 100 bpm and increased every 2 min by 10 bpm until the target heart rate or other standard endpoints are achieved [6]. A limiting factor is, however, that several pacemakers cannot be programmed to the target heart rate.

33.4.2.6 Ergonovine

A bolus injection of ergonovine (50 g) is administered intravenously at 5 min intervals until a positive response is obtained or a total dose of 0.35 mg is reached [6]. Positive criteria for the test include the appearance of ST-segment elevation or depression >0.1 mV (ECG criteria) or wall motion abnormality (echocardiographic criteria). An intravenous bolus injection of nitroglycerin is administered as soon as an abnormal response is detected; sublingual nifedipine is also recommended to counter the possible delayed effects of ergonovine [6].

33.5 Diagnostic Value

The accuracy of stress echocardiography for the detection of angiographically significant coronary artery dis-

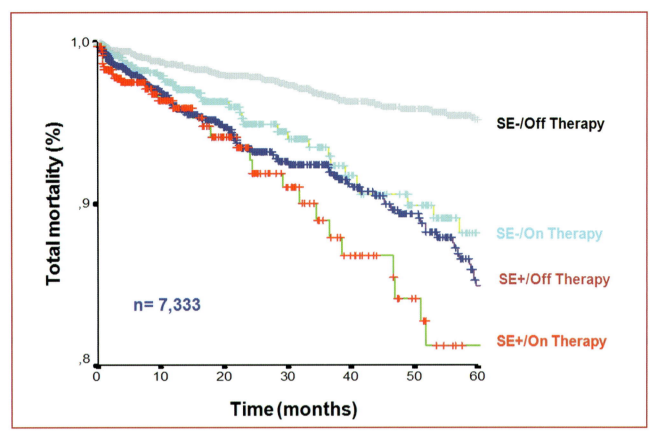

Fig. 33.4 Kaplan-Meier survival curves in patients stratified according to presence (SE+) or absence (SE-) of myocardial ischemia at pharmacologica stress echocardiography on and off antianginal medical therapy. Best survival is observed in patients with no inducible ischemia off therapy; worst survival is seen in patients with inducible ischemia on therapy. (Modified from [27])

ease is high, regardless of the stress employed. Recently, a meta-analysis of 55 studies with 3,714 patients, exercise, dobutamine, dipyridamole, and adenosine echocardiography showed a sensitivity, respectively, of 83%, 81%, 72%, and 79%, and a specificity of 84%, 84%, 95%, and 91% [7]. In another meta-analysis of 5 studies adopting state-of-the-art protocols for dipyridamole (fast or atropine-potentiated) and dobutamine (atropine-potentiated) test, the two stresses had identical sensitivity (84%) and comparable specificity (92% vs 87%) [8] (Fig. 33.3). Good diagnostic results have also been reported with pacing stress echocardiography (70% sensitivity, 90% specificity) using external programming of the pacemaker [9]. Ergonovine stress echocardiography provided >90% sensitivity and specificity for assessing variant angina [10].

Anti-ischemic therapy lowers sensitivity of either exercise [11] or pharmacologic stress echocardiography [11, 12]. However, therapy lowers the sensitivity of dipyridamole more than that of dobutamine [11]. Additionally, β-blockers are more effective than calcium antagonists and long-acting nitrates in decreasing test sensitivity [12].

When compared to standard exercise electrocardiography, stress echocardiography has a particularly impressive advantage in terms of specificity [13]. Compared to nuclear perfusion imaging, stress echocardiography at least has similar accuracy, with a moderate sensitivity gap that is more than balanced by a markedly higher specificity [8].

33.6 Prognostic Value

The results of a large number of studies enrolling thousands of patients have highlighted capability by exercise [14-16] or pharmacologic stress echocardiography [16-20] to allow effective risk assessment in patients with known or suspected coronary artery disease (Fig. 33.4). While the ischemic or necrotic pattern are associated with markedly increased risk of death or myocardial infarction, a normal test is predictive of a generally favorable outcome particularly in nondiabetic patients [19]. The ischemic threshold can be further stratified with additive stress echo parameters, such as the extent of inducible wall motion abnormalities and the work-

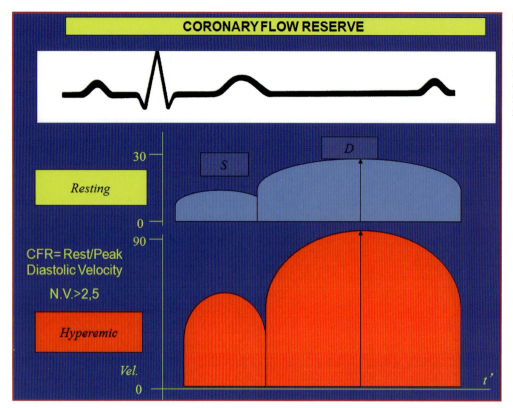

Fig. 33.5 Schematic representation of coronary flow velocity profile obtained with transthoracic Doppler of mid-distal left anterior descending coronary artery: in diastole the flow velocity is higher than in systole

load/dose. The higher the wall motion score index and the shorter the ischemia-free stress time are, the lower is the survival rate [14, 19]. Particularly appealing is the very high negative predictive value of the test in patients with suspected coronary artery disease. In a meta-analysis on 3,021 patients, a normal exercise echo yielded 0.5% yearly hard event-rate [21]. Stress echocardiography maintains a high prognostic value also in an angiographically benign subset such as that of single-vessel disease [22]. Furthermore, the result of the test has shown capability to predict which patients can obtain the maximal beneficial effect by coronary revascularization. In fact, ischemia at stress echo was the only independent prognostic indicator in medically treated patients among clinical, angiographic and echocardiographic parameters. Moreover, coronary revascularization was effective to improve the infarction-free survival in subjects with ischemia but not in those without ischemia [22]. A similar prognostic value has been reported for the different pharmacologic stress modalities such as dobutamine and dipyridamole [23]. Anti-ischemic therapy heavily modulates the prognostic impact of pharmacologic stress echocardiography [24]. Inducible myocardial ischemia in patients on medical therapy identifies the subset of patients at highest risk of death. At the opposite end, the incidence of death in patients with a negative test off medical therapy is very low. At intermediate risk are those patients with a negative test on medical therapy or a positive test off medical therapy [24] (Fig. 33.4). Table 33.6 and Table 33.7 summarize the established prognostic parameters of a stress echocardiography test positive and negative for ischemia.

33.7 Coronary Flow Reserve

In the last decade the evaluation of coronary flow reserve by combining transthoracic Doppler assessment of coronary flow velocities with vasodilator stress entered the echo lab as an effective modality for both diagnostic and prognostic purposes.

33.7.1 Methodology

The coronary flow velocity profile recorded with pulsed-wave Doppler, under color-Doppler guide, is biphasic, with a lower peak during systole and a higher peak during diastole (Fig. 33.5). In fact, the myocardial extravascular resistance is higher in systole and lower in diastole due to the effect of myocardial contraction. The flow velocity variations are proportional to the total blood

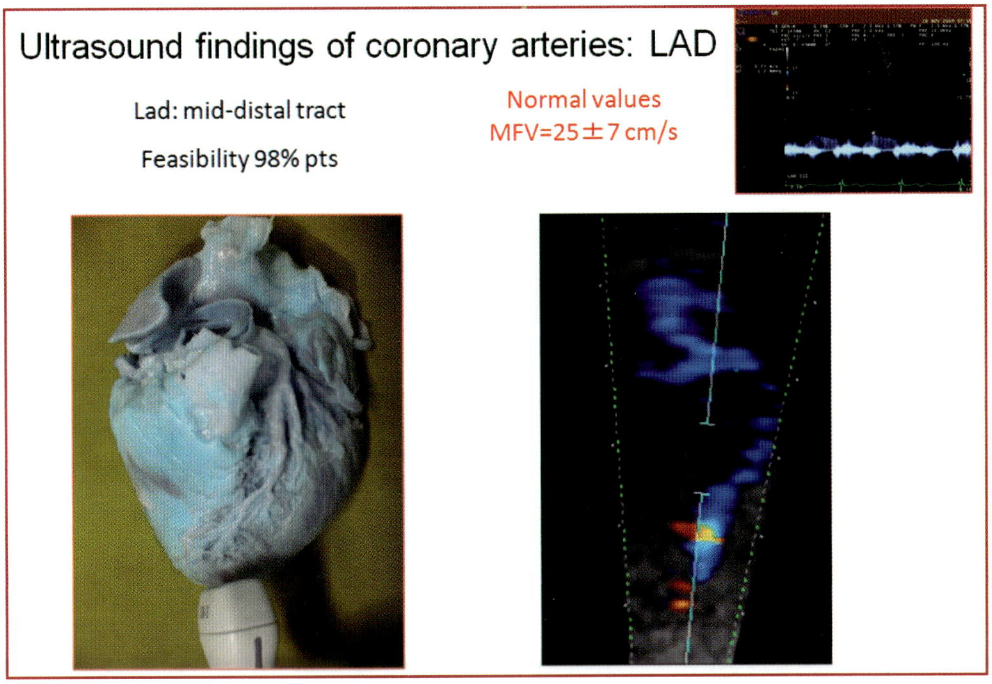

Fig. 33.6 Anatomic and color Doppler reference obtained by transthoracic ultrasound of the whole left anterior descending coronary artery (LAD)

Table 33.6 Stress echocardiography risk titration of a positive test result

One year- risk (hard events)	Intermediate (1-3% year)	High (> 10 % year)
Dose/workload	High	Low
Resting EF	>50%	< 40%
Anti-ischemic therapy	Off	On
Coronary territory	RCA/LCx	LAD
Peak WMSI	Low	High
Recovery	Fast	Slow
Positivity or baseline dyssynergy	Homozonal	Heterozonal
CFR	>2.0	< 2.0

Table 33.7 Stress echocardiography risk titration of a negative test result

One year-risk (hard events)	Very low (< 0,5% year)	Low (1-3% year)
Stress	Maximal	Submaximal
Resting EF	>50%	< 40%
Anti-ischemic therapy	Off	On
CFR	>2.0	<2.0

flow if the vessel lumen is kept constant. This assumption is reasonable with vasodilators such as adenosine or dipyridamole [4], and less valid with dobutamine. The coronary flow velocity variation between baseline and peak effect of a coronary vasodilator makes it possible to derive an index of coronary flow reserve. Peak diastolic flow variation is the simplest and the easiest parameter to obtain (Fig. 33.6). Moreover, it is the most reproducible and the one with the closest correlation to coronary perfusion reserve measured with Doppler flow wire [25] and positron emission tomography [26]. Only the employment of vasodilators can guarantee a full recruitment of coronary flow reserve and minimize the factors conditioning image quality. Among vasodilators, dipyridamole

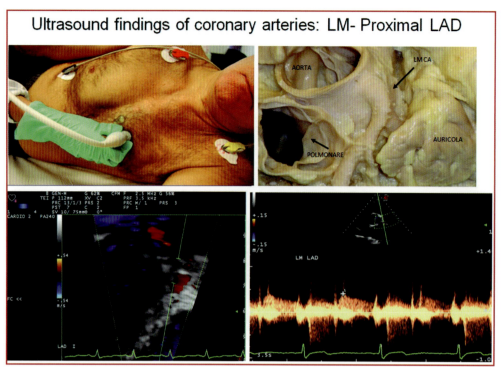

Fig. 33.7 Anatomic projections for transthoracic imaging of proximal tract of left anterior descending coronary artery (LAD)

is better tolerated subjectively than adenosine, induces less hyperventilation, costs much less in most countries, and has a longer-lasting vasodilatory effect, which is more convenient for dual flow and function imaging. A broadband transducer (2-7 MHz) or two transducers (with low-frequency imaging of wall motion and high-frequency imaging of left anterior descending artery flow) should be used, allowing an integrated evaluation of coronary flow velocity and wall motion [27-30] (Figs. 33.6-33.8). The mid-distal portion of the left anterior descending coronary artery can be highlighted from a modified apical 3-chamber view under the guidance of color Doppler flow mapping, with a feasibility of about 95% [29]. The posterior descending coronary artery can also be imaged using a modified apical 2-chamber view, but with greater difficulty and a success rate of about 50% [28]. A value of coronary flow velocity reserve ≤2 is generally considered abnormal [28-30].

33.7.2 Diagnostic Value

The use of coronary flow reserve as a stand-alone diagnostic criterion suffers from two main limitations. Firstly, only the left anterior descending coronary artery is sampled with very high success rate to be proposed widely in the clinical arena. Secondly, coronary flow reserve cannot distinguish between microvascular and macrovascular coronary disease (Figs. 33.9-33.15). Precisely for this reason it is much more useful to assess the additional diagnostic value of CFR over conventional wall motion analysis. Considering the available papers on the diagnostic role of dipyridamole stress echocardiography, it becomes clear that by adding the evaluation of coronary flow reserve to wall motion analysis we significantly increase the sensitivity of the test with only a modest loss of specificity [29-30]. In a meta-analysis of 5 studies on 741 patients, test sensitivity improved from 67% to 90% after the addition of flow information, while specificity reduced from 93% to 86% [29-36]. The superior sensitivity of coronary flow reserve compared to wall motion analysis can be attributed to two main causes. First, a coronary stenosis can reduce flow reserve producing, however, no effect on systolic function. In fact, the detection of a regional dysfunction by 2D echocardiography requires a critical ischemic mass of at least 20% of transmural wall thickness and about 5% of the total myocardial mass [4]. Second, the flow information is relatively unaffected by anti-ischemic therapy [34], which markedly reduces sensitivity of ischemia-dependent regional wall motion abnormality [5, 12, 29].

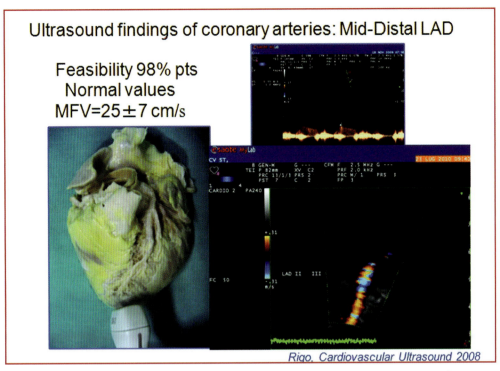

Fig. 33.8 Anatomic projections for transthoracic imaging of mid-distal tract of left anterior descending coronary artery (LAD)

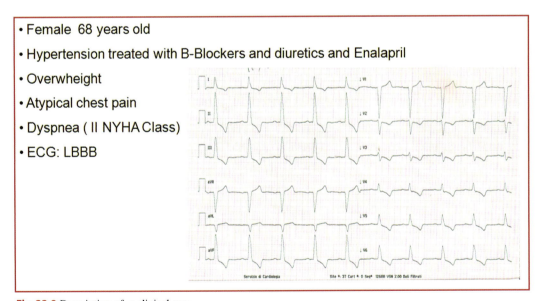

Fig. 33.9 Description of a clinical case

33.7.3 Prognostic Value

Coronary flow velocity reserve on the left anterior descending artery has provided additional prognostic value over stress echo results in patients with known or suspected coronary artery disease [31-36], allowing a better risk stratification in several cryptic situations such as in negative wall motion stress tests, in intermediate coronary stenosis [31], in diabetic patients [31], in patients with normal or near normal coronary arteries [37] as well as in non-ischemic condition such as dilated and hypertrophic cardiomyopathy. In fact, a coronary flow reserve ≤2.0 represents an additional prognostic marker in stratifying those patients with a negative test for wall motion criteria during dipyridamole stress echocardiography [31]. However, the spectrum of prog-

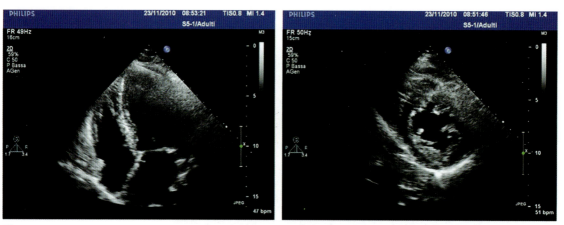

Fig. 33.10 Imaging of resting echocardiography: a four chamber view (*left*), a short axis view (*right*)

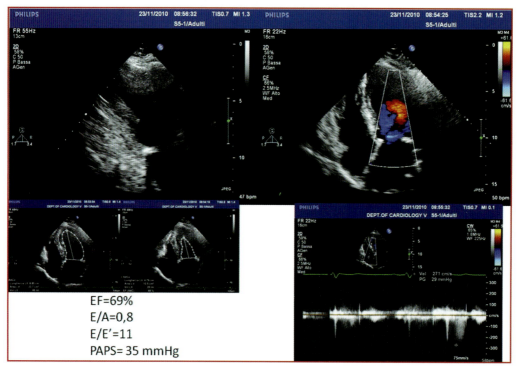

Fig. 33.11 Echocardiographic parameters. *EF*, ejection fraction; *E/A*, transmitral flow: early diastolic/end diastolic ratio; *E/E'*, early diastolic filling/early diastolic deformation; *PAPS*, pulmonary artery pressure systolic

nostic stratification is expanded if the response is titrated according to a continuous scale rather than artificially dichotomized. Indeed, the analysis of quartiles of coronary flow reserve has revealed that a value ≤1.80 is a strong and independent predictor of death or myocardial infarction in patients with known or suspected coronary artery disease, while a value between 1.81 to 2.16 is associated with intermediate risk, and a value ≥2.17 is predictive of a better prognosis [38]. A similar prognostication is obtained also when the group with no stress-induced ischemia is separately analyzed [38]. Importantly is the fact that anti-ischemic medication at the time of testing does not modulate the prognostic value of coronary flow reserve, which is per se a prognostic marker independent of therapy [34]. Starting from these perspectives, the European guidelines suggest that, whenever possible, we should perform an integrated stress-echo including both coronary flow velocity reserve and wall motion response [39].

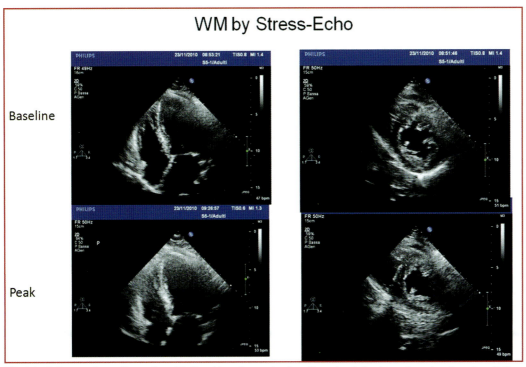

Fig. 33.12 Stress echocardiography with dipyridamole: rest/peak wall motion behavior: a four chamber view (*left*) and a short axis view (*right*)

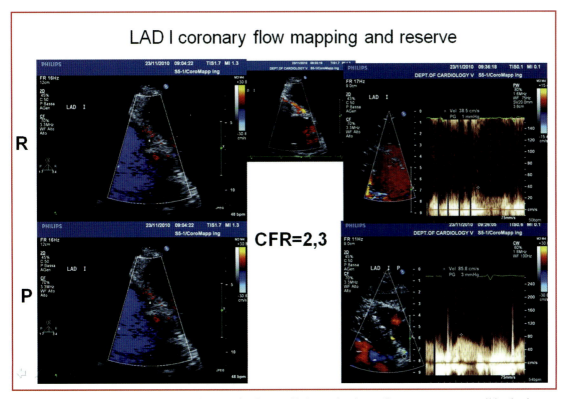

Fig. 33.13 Coronary flow reserve detected on proximal tract of left anterior descending coronary artery: mild reduction

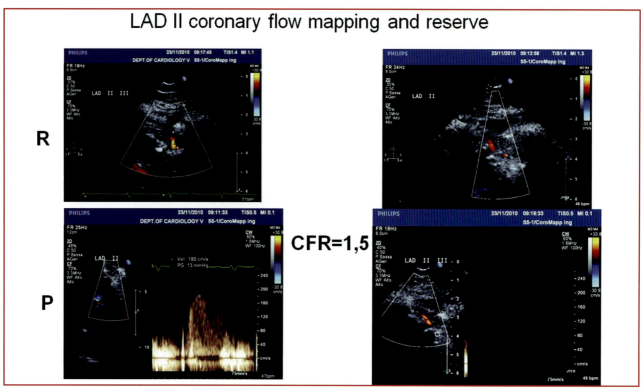

Fig. 33.14 Coronary flow reserve detected on mid tract of left anterior descending coronary artery: pathologic reduction

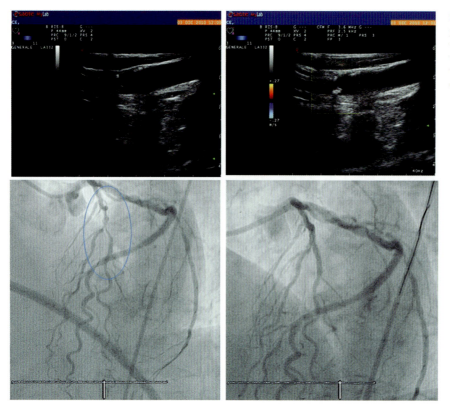

Fig. 33.15 Presence of pathologic plaques on carotid artery (*top*). Coronary angiography highlighted the presence of a critical stenosis in the mid tract of left anterior descending coronary artery (*bottom*)

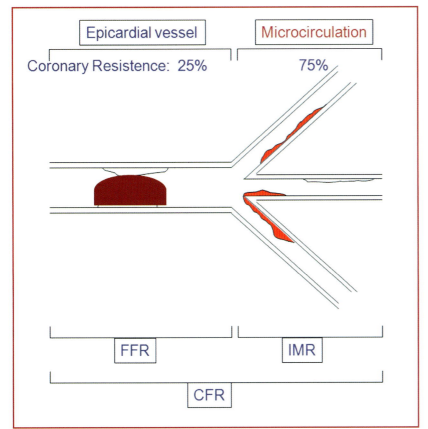

Fig. 33.16 Schematic representation of coronary artery tree. Coronary flow reserve represents the hyperaemic response to metabolic stimulus of the entire coronary circulation. A CFR reduction can be due to an epicardial stenosis as well as to a microvascular dysfunction. Only by applying an invasive assessment in cath-lab is possible to highlight the exact mechanism of a CFR impairment, evaluating two parameters. *FFR*, Fractional flow reserve; *IMR*, microvascular resistance

33.8 Diagnostic Work-flow in Daily Practice

Exercise electrocardiography still remains the first-line tool for screening patients with known or suspected coronary artery disease due to the high feasibility, excellent safety, ease of application, low cost, and high negative predictive value, similar to that of stress echocardiography [5, 10]. Accordingly, no further imaging test is warranted in low-risk patients with a maximal negative exercise electrocardiography test result (Figs. 33.16-33.19). At the other end of the spectrum, a high-risk ischemic response at exercise electrocardiography (i.e. positivity with an exercise time <4 min, positivity with recovery >8 min, >3 mm of ST-segment depression, ST-segment elevation in the absence of Q waves, global ST-segment changes, associated hypotension, malignant arrhythmias) warrants direct coronary angiography without any further investigations. In patients unable to exercise, with negative exercise testing at a submaximal workload or with uninterpretable or ambiguous electrocardiogram such as those with left bundle branch block or paced rhythm, and those with ST-segment depression >1 mm, an imaging technique is indicated and stress echocardiography has to be preferred for logistic and economic reasons. Stress echocardiography is also indicated in patients with exercise electrocardiography positivity at intermediate to high load [35], patients with negativity in the presence of chest pain, and patients in whom ST-segment changes during exercise can often occur in the absence of true ischemia. Stress echocardiography test positivity identifies a group of patients at higher risk in whom coronary angiography is warranted. Stress echocardiography test negativity makes the presence of prognostically important organic coronary disease unlikely and identifies a group of patients at low-risk [14-20]. In these patients, further effective prognostic results can be obtained from the analysis of coronary flow reserve in the left anterior descending artery [30-35].

33.9 Myocardial Viability

33.9.1 Pathophysiology

When the local supply-demand balance of the cell is critically endangered, the cell minimizes expenditure of energy

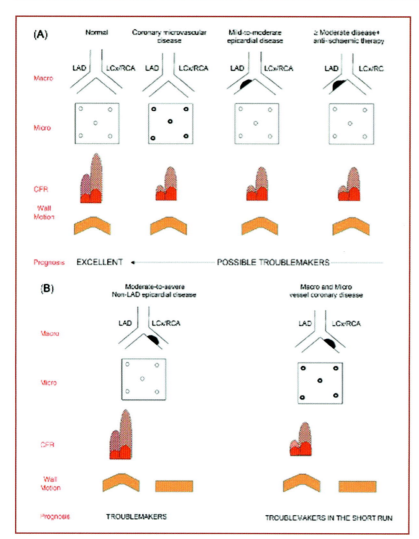

Fig. 33.17 Pathophysiologic and prognostic heterogeneity behind normal (*left*) and abnormal (*right*) wall motion response. From left to right we can see the behavior in normal coronary artery to moderate and severe coronary LAD disease, and effective anti-ischemic therapy. All four situations represent different pathophysiological conditions with negative wall motion response in all cases. The abnormal coronary flow reserve response is present in the second, third and fourth column. In the last two conditions, in the right part, CFR can be normal in spite of wall motion abnormality when the anterior descending artery is not significantly involved and microcirculatory level is not impaired

used for the development of contractile force and utilizes whatever is left for the maintenance of cellular integrity. The echocardiographic counterpart of this cellular strategic choice is the regional asynergy of viable segments. Both viable and necrotic segments show a depressed resting function, but the segmental dysfunction of viable regions can be transiently normalized by inotropic stimulus. Hibernation and stunning are the two pathophysiologic forms of viable myocardium which may be detected, respectively, in ischemic cardiomyopathy and acute coronary syndromes. In the hibernating myocardium, myocardial perfusion is chronically reduced (for months or years), although it remains beyond the critical threshold indispensable to keep the tissue viable, and recovery of function occurs after revascularization [4, 5]. In the stunned myocardium, persistent but reversible ischemia causes a metabolic alteration and imbalance between energy supply and work produced; recovery of function occurs spontaneously within hours, days, and even weeks after restoration of flow [5].

33.9.2 Dobutamine Stress Echocardiography

In patients with dysfunctional but viable myocardium, regional function can be improved by the inotropic effect of low-dose (5-10 μg/kg/min) dobutamine stress echocardiography [5]. Sensitivity and specificity of low-dose dobutamine test are, respectively, 86% and 90% for predicting spontaneous functional recovery after an acute myocardial infarction (stunning) [40], and 84% and 81% for predicting functional recovery following revascularization in patients with chronic coronary artery disease (hibernation) [41]. Dobutamine stress echocardiography compared with nuclear techniques shows lower sensitivity, higher specificity, with similar overall accuracy regarding recovery of function [41].

33.9.2.1 Prognostic Value

In patients with a poor left ventricular function, the presence of substantial contractile reserve is associated with

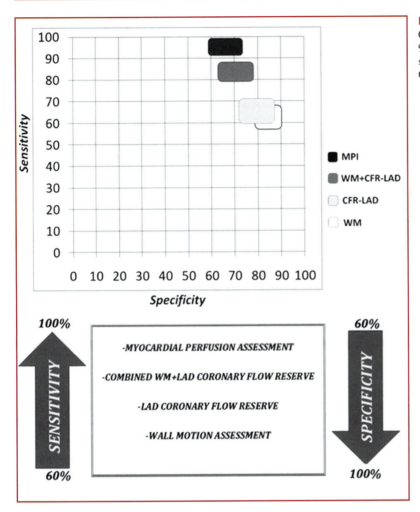

Fig. 33.18 Sensitivity and specificity to detect CAD >50% for all tested parameters, with their 95% confidence intervals (*Top*); Inverse relationship between sensitivity and specificity to detect CAD >50% for all tested parameters (*Bottom*)

significantly better survival compared with patients with smaller or absent myocardial viability [42, 43]. On the other hand, viability has no impact on survival in patients with preserved or just moderately depressed left ventricular function; in this case, it can rather predict the occurrence of acute coronary events, representing a substrate for unstable ischemic episodes [44].

In those patients with a severe left ventricular impairment at rest (ejection fraction <35%) and chronic coronary artery disease the finding of a large amount of viable myocardium (at least four segments or 20% of the total left ventricle) by stress-echocardiography is associated with a lower mortality rate in revascularized patients than in medically treated patients [45-48]). Viability highlighted by dobutamine stress echocardiography predicts a good outcome following revascularization. No measurable performance difference for predicting revascularization benefit between stress echocardiography and nuclear methods has been reported [49].

The detection of viable myocardium at dobutamine test also predicts responders to resynchronization therapy. In fact, patients with contractile reserve show a favorable clinical and reverse left ventricular remodeling response to resynchronization therapy [50].

33.10 Contrast Stress Echocardiography

About 40 years ago contrast agents were introduced in the Echo-Lab fundamentally to improve the image quality of transthoracic echo in several clinical settings and particularly in obese subjects and patients with lung disease. Contrast agents are encapsulated microbubbles filled with either air or high-molecular-weight gas that resonate when excited by diagnostic ultrasound frequencies, producing an increasing echo-backscatter from the blood. Currently three agents are commercially available: Sonovue (Bracco, Italy), Definity or Luminity (Bristol-Meyers Squibb, US) and Optison (GE, US) that are licensed for left ventricular opacification and endocardial definition [51]. In fact, the conventional role of contrast agents is to improve endocardial resolution

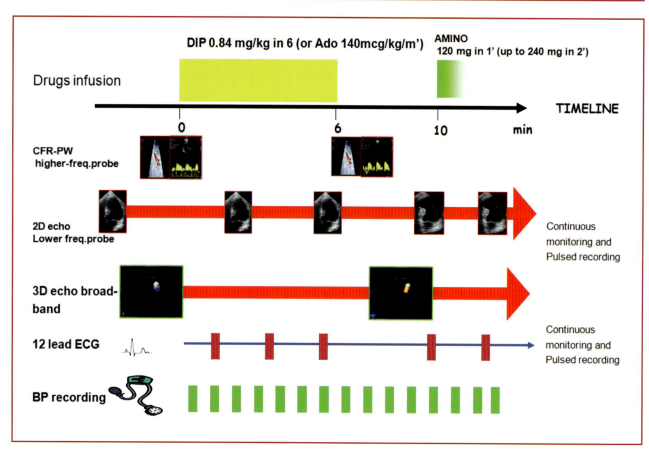

Fig. 33.19 Currently adopted protocol for dipyridamole stress echocardiography

facilitating concordant test interpretation with a diagnostic benefit especially for less-expert readers [52, 53]. The application of myocardial contrast echocardiography has led to an improvement in the accuracy of stress echocardiography [54]. Recently, it has been demonstrated how myocardial perfusion imaging performed during a vasodilator stress echo guarantees the highest values of sensitivity and accuracy for the detection of coronary stenosis >50% in comparison with the assessment of coronary flow reserve on the left anterior descending coronary artery and of wall motion assessment [54]. Regarding the prognostic value of MPI, it has been emphasized how the detection of abnormal perfusion adds significant incremental value to clinical analysis, resting and stress wall motion assessment [55-57]. The routine utilization of contrast agents has been hampered by several factors such as technical experience of the operators, costs, the difficulty in objectively quantifying perfusion defects and safety [58]. The risk-benefit ratio of contrast use strongly favors its utilization in appropriate patients and probably in the past the risks were clearly overstated in the original 2007 FDA warning [4, 58].

33.11 Diastolic Stress Echocardiography

The assessment of left ventricular diastolic function at rest has independent and additive prognostic value over resting and stress-induced systolic dysfunction [59]. The ratio of transmitral E wave (peak early diastolic velocity) to pulse tissue Doppler-derived e' of the mitral annulus can be used to estimate LV filling pressure at rest and during exercise. Patients with impaired LV relaxation develop an increase in LV filling pressure with exercise as a result of tachycardia and shortened diastolic filling time. Accordingly, transmitral peak E velocity increases. However, given the minimal effect of preload on annular e in the presence of impaired relaxation, annular e' remains reduced. Therefore, the E/e' ratio increases with exercise in patients with diastolic dysfunction [4, 60]. Diastolic stress echocardiography has been demonstrated to be feasible using supine bicycle exercise based on the assumption that the ratio of early diastolic transmitral velocity to early diastolic tissue velocity correlates with invasively measured LVDP during exercise [60, 61]. The algorithms to interpret the rest/stress variation of the E/e' can be summarized as follows: normal rest/normal stress, normal rest/altered stress and altered in both conditions [4]. The methodological approach during stress is less clearly standardized and issues remain on feasibility, accuracy and prognostic value.

According to the ASE guidelines on stress test diastolic stress echocardiography might be useful "for the evaluation of patients with dyspnea of possible cardiac origin" [61]. This evaluation is extremely important in those patients without inducible wall motion abnormalities, in whom these symptoms could represent an angina equivalent, and where to add diastolic information to pulmonary artery pressure assessed by flow velocity on tricuspid valve could reveal the underlying pathophysiologic mechanism responsible for dyspnea [4].

33.12 Three-dimensional Echocardiography

Over the last decade real time 3-dimensional echocardiography (3D) has sought to overcome the limitations of 2D echocardiography [4]. The major advantage of this technique over more conventional 2D echocardiography is the improvement in the accuracy of the evaluation of cardiac chamber volumes, which is achieved by eliminating the need for geometric modeling and the errors caused by foreshortened views [62]. Potentially, this new technique should be faster to learn, easier to implement, and less operator-dependent in the interpretation, also based on a robust quantitative package of excursion, synchronicity, shape, and volumes [5]. Fundamentally, two types of imaging modes - full-volume and multiplanar mode - can be used to acquire and analyze stress echocardiography. The multiplanar mode is suitable for regional wall motion analysis, since regional function can be represented as a function of time, and a series of plots is obtained representing the change in volume for each segment throughout the cycle. A complete 3D cardiac ultrasound image acquisition can be obtained in a shorter time than 2D echocardiography and this is a valuable advantage, especially when imaging children and adults during stress [63]. However, in spite of its exciting potential, the overall accuracy of 3D stress echocardiography is at present no better, and the feasibility lower, than 2D echocardiography [64]. In fact, the 3D application has a lower spatial resolution than 2D, and the resolution becomes even worse when needed more, at faster heart rates during stress test (3D = frame rates of 40 fps - 2D = frame rate of 100 fps) [63]. However, the 3D evaluation of volumes is ideally suited to quantitative and accurate calculation of a set of parameters allowing a complete characterization of cardiovascular hemody-

namics and improving the global wall motion analysis [5, 64, 65] (Figs. 33.20, 33.21). For the near future it is expected that the technology will improve the current critical areas of the technique, such as the need for only one transducer for both applications, 2D and 3D at the same time, with higher frequencies, smaller footprints, full Doppler capabilities, and higher frame rates, especially important for stress echocardiography applications.

33.13 Feasibility and Safety of Stress Echocardiography

33.13.1 Exercise

The safety of exercise stress is witnessed by decades of experience with electrocardiographic testing and stress imaging. Also in stress echocardiography registries, exercise was safer than pharmacologic stress [66]. Death occurs at an average in 1 in 10,000 tests, according to the American Heart association statements on exercise testing based on a review of more than 1,000 studies on millions of patients [67]. Major life-threatening effects, including myocardial infarction, ventricular fibrillation, sustained ventricular tachycardia, and stroke, were reported in about 1 in 6,000 patients with exercise in the international stress echocardiography registry [66].

33.13.2 Dobutamine

Minor but limiting side effects preclude the achievement of maximal dobutamine stress in about 10% of patients [68]. The history of systemic hypertension is an independent predictor of cumulative adverse effects, lowering test feasibility [68]. In order of frequency, limiting side effects during dobutamine stress include complex ventricular tachyarrhythmias, hypotension, atrial fibrillation, hypertension, and bradyarrhythmia [67]. Both the patients and the physician should be aware of the rate of major complications that may occur in 1 in 300 cases during dobutamine stress [66-69]. Tachyarrhythmias are the most frequent complications, which are independent of ischemia in many cases and can also develop at low-dose dobutamine regimen. The mechanism of their onset can be attributed to the direct adrenergic arrhythmogenic effect of dobutamine, through myocardial β-receptor stimulation [1]. Significant hypotension, sometimes associated with bradyarrhythmias, including asystole, is another frequent adverse reaction during dobutamine echocardiography. In some cases these findings have been attributed to dynamic intraventricular obstruction

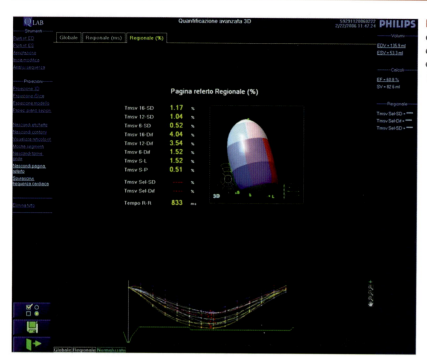

Fig. 33.20 3D echocardiography imaging of a patient with a critical stenosis of left anterior descending coronary artery: baseline imaging of left ventricle in pre-test with normal values in terms of parametric indexes

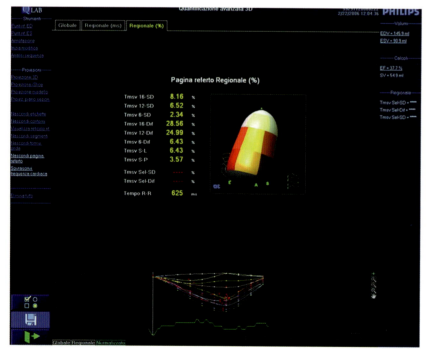

Fig. 33.21 Same case after dipyridamole injection that induced an abnormal wall motion response In left anterior coronary territory, highlighted by the appearance of abnormal parametric indexes with 3D echocardiography

provoked by inotropic action of dobutamine, especially in hypertrophic hearts [4]. A vasodepressor reflex triggered by left ventricular mechanoreceptor stimulation (Bezold-Jarish reflex) due to excessive inotropic stimulation may be an alternative mechanism [4]. Late and long-lasting transmural myocardial ischemia, with persistent ST-elevation, is probably due to the coronary vasoconstrictive effect of dobutamine, through α-receptor stimulation.

33.13.3 Dipyridamole

Limiting side effects occur in 3% of patients tested with dipyridamole [68]. In order of frequency, they include hypotension, supraventricular tachycardia, general malaise, headache, dyspnea, and atrial fibrillation [68]. Major life-threatening complications, such as myocardial infarction, third-degree atrioventricular block, cardiac asystole, sustained ventricular tachycardia, or pulmonary edema, occur in about 1 in 1,000 cases with high-dose dipyridamole stress [66]. Accordingly, the test induces major complications three times less frequently than dobutamine.

33.13.4 Adenosine

Side effects are very frequent and are limiting in up to 20% of patients investigated with adenosine stress echocardiography [70]. They include high-degree atrioventricular block, hypotension, intolerable chest pain (possibly induced by direct stimulation of myocardial A1 adenosine receptors), shortness of breath, flushing, and headache. Although side effects are frequent, the incidence of life-threatening complications, such as myocardial infarction, ventricular tachycardia, and shock, has been shown to be very low, with only one fatal myocardial infarction in approximately 10,000 cases [70]. Among pharmacologic stress tests, adenosine is probably the least well tolerated subjectively, but at the same time possibly the safest.

33.14 Appropriateness

An appropriate imaging study is one in which the expected incremental information, combined with clinical judgment, exceeds any expected negative consequences by a sufficiently wide margin for a specific indication that the procedure is generally considered acceptable care and a reasonable approach for the indication [71]. Negative consequences include the risks of the procedure itself (i.e. radiation) and the downstream impact of poor performance such as delay in diagnosis (false-negative results) or inappropriate diagnosis (false-positive results). According to recent estimates, more that 30% of cardiac stress imaging studies, including stress echocardiography [43], are unnecessary. This implies potential harm for patients undergoing imaging (who take the risks of the technique without a commensurate benefit), excessive delay in the waiting lists for other patients needing the examination, and an exorbitant cost for society. Every test has a cost and a risk. Compared with the treadmill exercise test, the cost of stress echocardiography is 2.1 times higher, myocardial perfusion imaging is 5.7 times higher, and coronary angiography is 21.7 times higher [72].

All forms of stress echocardiography are inappropriately applied as a first-line test in lieu of exercise electrocardiography. As a rule, the less informative the exercise testing is, the stricter the indication to stress echocardiography. Indications for stress echocardiography can be grouped in very broad categories, which encompass the majority of patients [73-76]:

1. diagnosis of coronary artery disease in patients in whom exercise electrocardiography is contraindicated, not feasible, uninterpretable, nondiagnostic, or gives ambiguous result;
2. risk stratification in patients with established diagnosis;
3. preoperative risk assessment (high-risk nonemergent, poor exercise tolerance);
4. evaluation after revascularization (not in the early post-procedure period, with change in symptoms);
5. search for viability in patients with ischemic cardiomyopathy eligible for revascularization;
6. coronary artery disease of unclear significance at angiography or computed tomography;
7. evaluation of valvular heart disease severity.

Pharmacologic stress echocardiography is the choice for patients in whom exercise is unfeasible or contraindicated. The choice of dobutamine or dipyridamole should depend on specific contraindications of either of the drugs, patient characteristics, local drug cost, and the physician's preference. It is important for all stress echocardiography laboratories to become familiar with all stresses to achieve a flexible and versatile diagnostic approach that enables the best stress to be tailored to individual patient needs.

33.15 Competence

Interpretation of stress echocardiography requires extensive experience in echocardiography and should be performed only by physicians with specific training in the technique [5]. The basic skills required for imaging the heart under resting conditions are not substantially different from those required for imaging the same heart during stress. Furthermore, the echocardiographic signs of ischemia are basically the same as those during myocardial infarction. The diagnostic accuracy of an experienced echocardiographer who is an absolute beginner in stress echocardiography is equivalent to that achieved by tossing a coin [77]. However, 100 stress echocardiography studies are sufficient to build the individual learning curve and reach the plateau of diagnostic accuracy [78]. After 15-30 days of exposure to a high-volume stress echocardiography laboratory, the physician begins to accumulate his or her own experience with a stepwise approach, starting from more innocuous and simple stresses (such as vasodilator tests) and moving up to more technically demanding ones (such as dobutamine and exercise). Maintenance of competence requires at least 15 stress echo exams per month [79]. The use of stresses is associated with the possibility of life-threatening complications. Therefore, the cardiologist and the attendant nurse should be certified in Basic and Advanced Life Support [79].

33.16 Comparison with Other Imaging Techniques

When compared with perfusion scintigraphy, stress echocardiography has an advantage in terms of specificity, versatility, cost, and risk [5]. The advantages of stress perfusion imaging include less operator-dependence, higher technical success rate, higher sensitivity, better accuracy when multiple resting left ventricular wall motion abnormalities are present, and a more extensive database for the evaluation of prognosis [5]. The ESC Guidelines on stable angina conclude that 'On the whole, stress echocardiography and stress perfusion scintigraphy, whether using exercise or pharmacological stress (inotropic or vasodilator), have very similar applications. The choice as to which is employed depends largely on local facilities and expertise. Advantages of stress echocardiography include its being free of radiation' [78]. On the basis of the large body of evidence assessing the comparable accuracy of stress echocardiography and perfusion scintigraphy, the choice of one test over the other will depend on the overall biological risk related to the use of radiation [5]. European law (Euratom directive 97/43) states that a radiologic (and nuclear medicine) examination can be performed only 'when it cannot be replaced by other techniques that do not employ ionizing radiation' and it should always be justified (Article 3: 'if an exposure cannot be justified it should be prohibited'). At the patient level, the effective dose of a single nuclear cardiology stress imaging examination ranges from 10 mSv (corresponding to 500 chest X-rays) for a technetium-MBI scan to 25 mSv (corresponding to 1,250 chest X-rays) from a thallium scan [78]. According to the latest estimation of BEIR VII (2006), this exposure corresponds to an extra-lifetime risk of cancer per examination ranging from 1 in 1,000 (sestamibi) to 1 in 500 (thallium). The risk is greatest in special subsets particularly vulnerable to the damaging effects of ionizing radiation, such as reproductive-age

women and children [78-80]. Therefore, in an integrated risk–benefit balance, stress echocardiography has advantages when compared with perfusion scintigraphy and should be preferred.

Cardiac magnetic resonance has higher costs, higher time of image acquisition, and lower availability when compared with echocardiography. Therefore, it represents an excellent option only when stress echocardiography is inconclusive or not feasible [4, 5].

References

1. Tennant R,Wiggers CJ (1935) The effect of coronary occlusion on myocardial contraction. Am J Physiol 112:351-61
2. Theorux P, Franklin D, Ross J jr et al (1974) Regional myocardial function during acute coronary artery occlusion and its modification by pharmachological agents in dog. Circ Res 4:896-908
3. Kerber RE, Abboud FM (1973) Echocardiographic detection of regional myocardial infarction. An experimental study. Circulation 47:997-1005
4. Picano E (2009) Stress Echocardiography. 5th ed. Heidelberg: Springer-Verlag
5. Picano E (1992) Stress echocardiography: from pathophysiological toy to diagnostic tool. Point of view. Circulation 85:1604-1612
6. Sicari R, Nihoyannopoulos P, Evangelista A et al (2008) Stress echocardiography expert consensus statement. Eur J Echocardiogr 9:415-437
7. Heijenbrok-Kal MH, Fleischmann KE, Hunink MG (2007) Stress echocardiography, stress single-photon-emission computed tomography and electron beam computed tomography for the assessment of coronary artery disease: a meta-analysis of diagnostic performance. Am Heart J 54:415-23
8. Picano E, Molinaro S, Pasanisi E (2008) The diagnostic accuracy of pharmacological stress echocardiography for the assessment of coronary artery disease: a meta-analysis. Cardiovasc Ultrasound 6:30
9. Picano E, Alaimo A, Chubuchny V et al (2002) Noninvasive pacemaker stress echocardiography for diagnosis of coronary artery disease: a multicenter study. J Am Coll Cardiol 40:1305-1310
10. Song JK, Lee SJ, Kang DH et al (1996) Ergonovine echocardiography as a screening test for diagnosis of vasospastic angina before coronary angiography. J Am Coll Cardiol 27:1156-1161
11. San Roman JA, Vilacosta I, Castillo JA et al (1996) Dipyridamole and dobutamine-atropine stress echocardiography in the diagnosis of coronary artery disease. Comparison with exercise stress test, analysis of agreement, and impact of antianginal treatment. Chest 110:1248-1254
12. Lattanzi F, Picano E, Bolognese L et al (1991) Inhibition of dipyridamole-induced ischemia by antianginal therapy in humans. Correlation with exercise electrocardiography. Circulation 83:1256-1262
13. Severi S, Picano E, Michelassi C et al (1994) Diagnostic and prognostic value of dipyridamole echocardiography in patients with suspected coronary artery disease. Comparison with exercise electrocardiography. Circulation 89:1160-1173
14. Marwick TH, Case C, Vasey C et al (2001) Prediction of mortality by exercise echocardiography: a strategy for combination with the duke treadmill score. Circulation 103:2566-2571
15. Arruda-Olson AM, Juracan EM, Mahoney DW et al (2002) Prognostic value of exercise echocardiography in 5,798 patients: is there a gender difference? J Am Coll Cardiol 39:625-631
16. Shaw LJ, Vasey C, Sawada S et al (2005) Impact of gender on risk

stratification by exercise and dobutamine stress echocardiography: long-term mortality in 4234 women and 6898 men. Eur Heart J 26:447-456

17. Picano E, Severi S, Michelassi C et al (1989) Prognostic importance of dipyridamole-echocardiography test in coronary artery disease. Circulation 80:450-459

18. Poldermans D, Fioretti PM, Boersma E et al (1999) Long-term prognostic value of dobutamine-atropine stress echocardiography in 1737 patients with known or suspected coronary artery disease: A single-center experience. Circulation 99:757-762

19. Sicari R, Pasanisi E, Venneri L et al (2003) Stress echo results predict mortality: a large scale multicenter prospective international study. J Am Coll Cardiol 41:589-595

20. Cortigiani L, Bigi R, Sicari R et al (2006) Prognostic value of pharmacological stress echocardiography in diabetic and mondiabetic patients with known or suspected coronary artery disease. J Am Coll Cardiol 47:605-610

21. Metz LD, Beattie M, Hom R et al (2007) The prognostic value of normal exercise myocardial perfusion imaging and exercise echocardiography: a meta-analysis. J Am Coll Cardiol 49:227-237

22. Cortigiani L, Picano E, Landi P et al (1998) Value of pharmacologic stress echocardiography in risk stratification of patients with single-vessel disease: a report from the Echo-Persantine and Echo-Dobutamine International Cooperative Studies. J Am Coll Cardiol 32:69-74

23. Pingitore A, Picano E, Varga A et al (1999) Prognostic value of pharmacological stress echocardiography in patients with known or suspected coronary artery disease: a prospective, large scale, multicenter, head-to-head comparison between dipyridamole and dobutamine test. J Am Coll Cardiol 34:1769-1777

24. Sicari R, Cortigiani L, Bigi R et al (2004) The prognostic value of pharmacologic stress echo is affected by concomitant anti-ischemic therapy at the time of testing. Circulation 109:1428-1431

25. Caiati C, Montaldo C, Zedda N et al (1999) New noninvasive method for coronary flow reserve assessment: contrast-enhanced transthoracic second harmonic echo Doppler. Circulation 99:771-778

26. Beattie WS, Abdelnaem E, Wijeysundera DN, Buckley DN (2006) A meta-analytic comparison of preoperative stress echocardiography and nuclear scintigraphy imaging. Anesth Analg 102:8-16

27. Boersma E, Poldermans D, Bax JJ et al; DECREASE Study Group (Dutch Echocardiographic Cardiac Risk Evaluation Applying Stress Echocardiogrpahy) (2001) Predictors of cardiac events after major vascular surgery: Role of clinical characteristics, dobutamine echocardiography, and beta-blocker therapy. JAMA 285:1865-1873

28. Rigo F (2005) Coronary flow reserve in stress-ecgho lab:from pathophysiologic toy to diagnostic tool. Cardiovascular Ultrasound 3:8

29. Rigo F, Richieri M,Pasanis E et al (2003) Usefulness of coronary flw reserve over regional wall motion when added to dual-imaging dipyridamole echocardiography. Am J Cardiol 91:269-273

30. Rigo F, Murer B, Ossena G, Favaretto G (2008) Transthoracic echocardiographic imaging of coronary arteries: tips, tricks and pitfalls. Cardiovascular Ultrasound pp 6-7

31. Cortigiani L, Rigo F, Gherardi S et al (2007) Additional prognostic value of coronary flow reserve in diabetic and nondiabetic patients with negative dipyridamole stress echocardiography by wall motion criteria. J Am Coll Cardiol 50:1354:1361

32. Cortigiani L, Rigo F, Sicari R et al (2009) Prognostic correlates of combined coronary flow reserve assessment on left anterior descending and right coronary artery in patients with negative stress echocardiography by wall motion criteria. Heart 95:1423-1428

33. Rigo F, Gherardi S, Galderisi M, Cortigiani L (2006) Coronary flow reserve evaluation in stress-echo lab. J Cardiovasc Med 7:472-479

34. Sicari R, Rigo F, Gherardi S et al (2008) The prognostic value of

Doppler echocardiographic-derived coronary flow reserve is not affected by concomitant antiischemic therapy at the time of testing. Am Heart J 156:573-579

35. Rigo F, Sicari R, Gherardi S et al (2008) The additive prognostic value of wall motion abnormalities and coronary flow reserve during dipyridamole stress echo. Eur Heart J 29:79-88

36. Rigo F, Sicari R, Gherardi S et al (2007) Prognostic value of coronary flow reserve in medically treated patients with left anterior descending coronary disease with stenosis 51%-75% in diameter. Am J Cardiol 100:1527-1531

37. Sicari R, Rigo F, Cortigiani L et al (2009) Long-term survival of patients with chest pain syndrome and angiographically normal or near normal coronary arteries: the additional prognostic value of coronary flow reserve. Am J Cardiol 103:626-631

38. Cortigiani L, Rigo F, Gherardi S et al (2010) Prognostic implication of the continuous sprectrum of doppler echocardiographic derived coronary flow reserve on left anterior descending artery. Am J Cardiol 105:158-162

39. Sicari R, Nihoyannopulos P, Evangelista A et al (2008) Stress echocardiography expert consensus statement (EAE) Eur Heart J 9:415-437

40. Smart SC, Sawada S, Ryan T et al (1993) Low-dose dobutamine echocardiography detects reversible dysfunction after thrombolytic therapy of acute myocardial infarction. Circulation 88:405-415

41. Bax JJ, Wijns W, Cornel JH et al (1997) Accuracy of currently available techniques for prediction of functional recovery after revascularization in patients with left ventricular dysfunction due to chronic coronary artery disease: comparison of pooled data. J Am Coll Cardiol 30:1451-1460

42. Baumgartner H, Porenta G, Lau YK et al (1998) Assessment of myocardial viability by dobutamine echocardiography, positron emission tomography and thallium-201 SPECT: correlation with histopathology in explanted hearts. J Am Coll Cardiol 32:1701-1708

43. Picano E, Sicari R, Landi P et al (1998) The prognostic value of myocardial viability in medically treated patients with global ventricular dysfunction early after an acute uncomplicated myocardial infarction: a dobutamine stress echocardiographic study. Circulation 98:1078-1784

44. Sicari R, Picano E, Landi P et al (1997) Prognostic value of dobutamine-atropine stress echocardiography early after acute myocardial infarction. J Am Coll Cardiol 29:54-60

45. Mezulin J, Cerny J, Frelich M et al (1998) Prognostic value of the amount of dysfunctional but viable myocardium in revascularized patients with coronary disease and left ventricular dysfunction. J Am Coll Cardiol 32:912-920

46. Senior R, Kaul S, Lahiri A (1999) Myocardial viability on echocardiophiy predicts long-term survival after revascularization in patients with ischemic congestive heart failure. J Am coll cardiol 33:1848-1854

47. Sicari R, Picano E, Cortigiani L et al (2003) Prognostic value of myocardial viability recognized by low-dose dobutamine echocardiography in chronic ischwemic left ventricular dysfunction. Am J Cardiol 92:1263-1266

48. Cortigiani L, Sicari R, Desideri A et al (2007) Stress echocardiography and the effect of revascularization on outcome of diabetic and nondiabetic patients with chronic ischemic left ventricular dysfunction. Eur Heart Fail 9:138-143

49. Allman KC, Shaw LJ, Hacchamoviitch R, Udelson JE (2002) Myocardial viability testing and impact of revascularization on prognosis in patients with coronary artery disease and left ventricular dysfunction: a meta-analysis. J Am Coll cardiol 39:1151-1158

50. Ciampi Q, Pratali l, Citro R et al (2009) Identification of responders to cardiac resynchronization therapy by contractile reserve during stress echocardiography. Eur J Heart fail 11:489-496

51. Bhatia VK, Senior R (2008) Contrast echocardiography: evidence for clinical use. J Am Soc Echocardiogr 21:409-416

52. Hundley WG, Kizilbash AM, Afridi I et al (1999) Effect of contrast enhancement on transthoracic echocardiographic assessment of left ventricular regional wall motion. Am J Cardiol 84:1365-1369
53. Dolan MS, Riad K, El-Shafei A et al (2001) Effect of intravenous contrast for left ventricle opacification border definition on sensitivity and specificity of dobutamine stress echocardiography compared with coronary angiography in technically difficult patients. Am Heart J 142:908-915
54. Gaibazzi N, Rigo F, Reverberi C (2010) Detection of coronary artery disease by combined assessment of wall motion, myocardial perfusion and coronary flow reserve: a multiparamentric contrast stress-echocardiographic study. J Am Soc Echocardiograph 23:1242-1250
55. Moir S, Haluska BA, Jenkins C (2004) Incremental benefit of myocardial contrast to combined dipyridamole-exercise stress echocardiography for the assessment of coronary artery disease. Circulation 110:1108-113
56. Tsutsui JM, Elhendy A, Anderson J R (2005) Prognostic value of dobutamine stress myocardial contrast perfusion echocardiography. Circulation 112:1444-1450
57. Marwick TH (2005) Contrast stress echocardiography: completing the picture from image enhancement to improved accuracy and prognostic insight. Circulation 112:1382-1383
58. Lester SJ, Miller FA, Khandheria BK (2008) Contrast echocardiography: beyond a black box warning? J Am Soc Echocardiogr 21:417-418
59. Agricola E, Oppizzi M, Pisani M. (2004) Stress Echocardiography in heart failure. Cardiovasc Ultrasound 2:11-16
60. Ha JW, Oh JK, Pellikka PA (2005) Diastolic stress echocardiography: a novel non invasive diagnostic test for diastolic dysfunction using supine bicycle exercise Doppler echocardiography 8: 63-68
61. Burgess MI, Jenkins C, Sharman JE (2006) Diastolic stress echocardiography: hemodynamic validation and clinical significance of estimation of ventricular filling pressure with exercise. J Am Coll Cardiol 47:1891-1900
62. Takeuchi M, Lang RM (2007) Three dimensional stress testing: volumetric acquisitions. Cardiol Clin 25:267-272
63. Hung J, Lang R, Flachskamp F et al (2007) 3D echocardiography: a review of the current status and future directions. J Am Soc Echocardiogr 20:213-233
64. Matsumara Y, Hozumi T, Arai K et al (2005) Non-invasive assessment of myocardial ischemia using new real time three-dimensional dobutamine stress echocardiography: comparison with two-dimensional methods. Eur Heart J 26:1625-1632
65. Badano LP, Muraru D, Rigo F et al (2010) High volume rate three-dimensional echocardiography to assess myocardial ischemia: a feasibility study. J Am Soc Echocardiogr 23:628-635
66. Varga A, Garcia MA, Picano E (2006) Safety of stress echocardiography (from the International Stress Echo Complication Registry). Am J Cardiol 98:541-543
67. Fletcher GF, Balady GJ, Amsterdam EA et al (2001) Exercise standards for testing and training: a statement for healthcare professionals from the American Heart Association. Circulation 104:1694-740
68. Cortigiani L, Zanetti L, Bigi R et al (2002) Safety and feasibility of dobutamine and dipyridamole stress echocardiography in hypertensive patients. J Hypertens 20:1423-1429
69. Picano E, Mathias W Jr, Pingitore A et al on behalf of the EDIC study group (1999) Safety and tolerability of dobutamine-atropine stress echocardiography: a prospective, large scale, multicenter trial. Lancet 344:1190-1192
70. Cerqueira MD, Verani MS, Schwaiger M et al (1999) Safety profile of adenosine stress perfusion imaging: results from the Adenoscan Multicenter Trial Registry. J Am Coll Cardiol 23:384-389
71. Patel MR, Spertus JA, Brindis RG et al (2005) American College of Cardiology Foundation. ACCF proposed method for evaluating the appropriateness of cardiovascular imaging. J Am Coll Cardiol 46:1606-1613
72. Gibbons RJ, Abrams J, Chatterjee K et al (2003) American College of Cardiology; American Heart Association Task Force on practice guidelines (Committee on the Management of Patients With Chronic Stable Angina). ACC/AHA 2002 guideline update for the management of patients with chronic stable angina--summary article: a report of the American College of Cardiology/American Heart Association Task Force on practice guidelines (Committee on the Management of Patients With Chronic Stable Angina). J Am Coll Cardiol 41:159-168
73. Douglas PS, Khandheria B, Stainback RF (2008) American College of Cardiology Foundation Appropriateness Criteria Task Force; American Society of Echocardiography; American College of Emergency Physicians; American Heart Association; American Society of Nuclear Cardiology; Society for Cardiovascular Angiography and Interventions; Society of Cardiovascular Computed Tomography; Society for Cardiovascular Magnetic Resonance. ACCF/ASE/ACEP/AHA/ASNC/SCAI/SCCT/SCMR 2008 appropriateness criteria for stress echocardiography: a report of the American College of Cardiology Foundation Appropriateness Criteria Task Force, American Society of Echocardiography, American College of Emergency Physicians, American Heart Association, American Society of Nuclear Cardiology, Society for Cardiovascular Angiography and Interventions, Society of Cardiovascular Computed Tomography, and Society for Cardiovascular Magnetic Resonance: endorsed by the Heart Rhythm Society and the Society of Critical Care Medicine. Circulation 117:1478-1497
74. Picano E, Pasanisi E, Brown J, Marwick TH (1991) A gatekeeper for the gatekeeper: inappropriate referrals to stress echocardiography. Am Heart J 154:285-290
75. Picano E, Lattanzi F, Orlandini A et al (1991) Stress echocardiography and the human factor: the importance of being expert. J Am Coll Cardiol 17:666-669
76. Popp R, Agatston A, Armstrong W et al (1998) Recommendations for training in performance and interpretation of stress echocardiography. Committee on Physician Training and Education of the American Society of Echocardiography. J Am Soc Echocardiogr 11:95-96
77. Fox K, Garcia MA, Ardissino D et al (2006) Task Force on the Management of Stable Angina Pectoris of the European Society of Cardiology; ESC Committee for Practice Guidelines (CPG). Guidelines on the management of stable angina pectoris: executive summary: The Task Force on the Management of Stable Angina Pectoris of the European Society of Cardiology. Eur Heart J 27:1341-1381
78. Picano E (2003) Stress echocardiography: a historical perspective. Special article. Am J Med 114:126-130
79. Picano E (2004) Informed consent and communication of risk from radiological and nuclear medicine examinations: how to escape from a communication inferno. Education and debate. BMJ 329:849-851
80. Picano E (2004) Sustainability of medical imaging. Education and debate. BMJ 328:578-580

Nuclear Medicine – SPECT/PET

34

Alberto Cuocolo

34.1 Introduction

In current clinical practice the assessment of myocardial perfusion with radiotracers is an integral component of the evaluation of patients with suspected or known coronary artery disease (CAD) and it has been successfully performed for over 30 years. More than 10 million studies per year are executed worldwide with a rich literature confirming both high diagnostic and prognostic values of this approach. Its strengths include standardized protocols, ease of use, and well-established guidelines [1] and, over these years, considerable technologic advancement has been made to improve image quality and optimize acquisition protocols.

The first historical attempts to perform cardiac perfusion imaging with potassium-43 and rubidium-81 in the early 1970s, despite a wide number of technical limitations, provided a conceptual framework for future developments in this field [2, 3]. The introduction of thallium-201 (Tl-201) in the mid 1970s marked a milestone in the development and widespread clinical use of myocardial perfusion imaging [4]. Indeed this radiotracer had a great impact on diagnostic evaluation, risk stratification, and therapeutic decision-making in patients with CAD over the next two decades. However, Tl-201 has important limitations, like a relatively low energy of emitted photons, a physical half-life of 73 hours, and an unfavorable biodistribution in testes and kidneys. These restrictions affect the amount of administrable dose to approximately 150 MBq, limiting image quality, in association with a relatively high-absorbed dose and thereby stimulating the search for better myocardial perfusion imaging agents.

When technetium-99m (Tc-99m) labeled compounds, such as methoxyisobutyl isonitrile (sestamibi) and 1,2-bis[bis(2-ethoxyethyl)phosphino] ethane (tetro-

fosmin) were approved for clinical use in the early 1990s, there was a rapid adoption of these radiopharmaceuticals [5]. Despite a lower first-pass extraction in the myocardium and higher uptake in bowel and liver in comparison to Tl-201, these tracers have relatively higher energy photons, a shorter physical half-life (6 hours) and can be used in much higher doses limiting attenuation artifacts with superior single-photon emission computed tomography (SPECT) image quality and providing a lower radiation burden than that achieved through Tl-201 imaging. Another major advantage of Tc-99m labeled agents over Tl-201 is that, in addition to perfusion data, simultaneous assessment of left ventricular function (motion, thickening, and ejection fraction) can be accurately determined with ECG-triggered acquisition (gated-SPECT) using one injection and one imaging sequence. By providing this additional information gated-SPECT helps to significantly increase both specificity and prognostic value of myocardial scintigraphy [6]. However, despite the success of cardiac single-photon tracers, there is still the room for further improvement in myocardial perfusion imaging. In particular the presence of diffuse disease in all three main coronary arteries may decrease the sensitivity of conventional SPECT images for each individual vessel, and *balanced ischemia* may mask or minimize the presence of disease [7].

In this context, myocardial perfusion positron emission tomography (PET) offers many theoretical advantages over traditional single-photon techniques. These advantages include higher spatial and contrast resolution, resulting in higher image quality and improved diagnostic accuracy. Moreover, the possibility of quantifying myocardial perfusion in absolute terms (i.e. milliliters per gram per minute), which allows the noninvasive evaluation of coronary microcirculation and the identification of three-vessel disease, represents the major goal of PET. Despite the fact that clinical value of cardiac PET imaging was demonstrated more than 30 years ago [8], its use has been minimal because of several reasons. The main ones are the need for an on-site cyclotron, high costs of PET scanners, lack of reimbursement, and limit-

A. Cuocolo (✉)
Departments of Biomorphological and Functional Sciences,
University of Naples "Federico II",
Naples, Italy

F. Cademartiri, G. Casolo, M. Midiri (eds.), *Clinical Applications of Cardiac CT*,
© Springer-Verlag Italia 2012

ed availability of user-friendly software for cardiac image processing and display [9]. Nowadays, however, the increasing availability of PET facilities in a large number of nuclear medicine centers worldwide is rapidly changing many of these issues.

34.2 SPECT

The most widely available nuclear technique to assess myocardial perfusion is SPECT using diffusible radio-tracers [10]. SPECT imaging is performed at rest and during stress to produce images of regional myocardial blood flow. During maximal exercise or vasodilator stress, myocardial blood flow is typically increased three- to five-fold compared to rest. In the presence of a significant coronary stenosis, myocardial perfusion will not increase appropriately in the territory supplied by the artery with the stenosis, creating heterogeneous uptake. In patients who are unable to exercise, coronary vasodilator agents such as dipyridamole or adenosine may be used to increase blood flow [11]. In some circumstances, dobutamine might be used as an alternative, although it does not increase blood flow to the same degree. The capabilities of radionuclide techniques to assess myocardial perfusion in the presence of coronary artery stenosis are related to the relationship between myocardial distribution of a perfusion tracer and corresponding regional blood flow.

The principal characteristics of the currently used SPECT perfusion tracers are illustrated in Table 34.1. The available SPECT flow agents are characterized by a rapid myocardial extraction and by a cardiac uptake proportional to blood flow [12-15]. Although Tl-201 has been the most used tracer to assess myocardial blood flow, its physical characteristics are suboptimal. The energy level (69 to 83 KeV) is marginally suitable for imaging with conventional gamma camera and creates some problems for attenuation within the body. The relatively long physical half-life (73 hours) and biological half-life (10 days) lead to a radiation dose to the kidneys

and only a small amount (74 to 111 MBq) of Tl-201 can be administered. The energy level (140 KeV) of Tc-99m labeled tracers is ideal for imaging with conventional gamma camera, decreasing problems for tissue attenuation. Moreover, the half-life (6 hours) means that larger dose can be administered to the patient than with Tl-201 [12]. It has also been shown that both sestamibi and tetrofosmin tomography yield images of comparable quality and produce similar results in the identification of patients with CAD and in the detection of the individual stenotic coronary vessels [16].

Although SPECT is very sensitive, specificity is relatively low [17]. One of the causes of reduced specificity is the occurrence of artifacts due to soft tissue attenuation. Dedicated hardware and software programs have been developed to allow direct reconstruction of attenuation-corrected images based on measurements of the attenuation distribution profile [18]. In addition, the use of ECG-gated imaging, allowing simultaneous assessment of myocardial perfusion and ventricular function, has led to further improvement of the diagnostic accuracy of SPECT. The most recent nuclear medicine computer systems allow complex procedures, such as image reconstruction, quantification and display, to be performed rapidly. Because the tomographic projections are easily-standardized from patient to patient, quantification of myocardial tomograms and comparison to normal limits, established in population of healthy subjects, can be accomplished. Quantification makes it possible to document objectively specific patterns of abnormal perfusion or soft-tissue attenuation, suspected from subjective image interpretation. A further advantage of the quantification approach is the standardization of image interpretation resulting in a reduction of intra- and interobserver variability, as shown by data from our laboratory (Table 34.2). A potential limitation of SPECT tracers is that absolute myocardial blood flow in mL/min/kg cannot be measured. In addition, nuclear imaging methods have the intrinsic disadvantage of requiring the use of radioactive materials. It has been documented that radionuclide myocardial perfusion imaging is safe, particularly in

Table 34.1 Principal characteristics of currently used SPECT and PET blood flow tracers

	Production	Physical half-life	Energy (keV)	Extraction fraction (%)
SPECT tracers				
201Tl	Cyclotron	72 hours	80, 165	80
99mTc-sestamibi	Generator	6 hours	140	65
99mTc-tetrofosmin	Generator	6 hours	140	60
PET tracers				
13N-ammonia	Cyclotron	10 min	511	95
82Rb	Generator	1.3 min	511	50
15O-water	Cyclotron	2.1 min	511	100

Table 34.2 Intraobserver and interobserver reproducibility of segmental score analysis for stress myocardial perfusion SPECT in patients with coronary artery disease

	Intraobserver reproducibility	Interobserver reproducibility
Intraclass coefficient of correlation	0.98	0.97
Confidence intervals	0.97 - 0.99	0.95 - 0.99
F value	55.9	27.0
p value	<0.001	<0.001

Table 34.3 Sensitivity and specificity of stress myocardial perfusion SPECT in detecting coronary artery disease (≥50% stenosis) in 1459 patients

Study	Patients (n)	Tracer	Stress test	Sensitivity (%)	Specificity (%)
Mahmarian [19]	360	Tl-201	Exercise	87	87
Berman [20]	170	Sestamibi/Tl-201	Exercise	96	82
Van Train [21]	160	Sestamibi	Exercise	97	67
Palmas [22]	70	Sestamibi	Exercise	91	75
Taillefer [23]	78	Sestamibi	Exercise	72	81
Acampa [16]	32	Sestamibi	Exercise	92	71
Acampa [16]	32	Tetrofosmin	Exercise	96	86
Watanabe [24]	140	Tl-201	Dipyridamole	83	72
Taillefer [23]	37	Sestamibi	Dipyridamole	72	100
Iskandrian [25]	132	Tl-201	Adenosine	92	88
Cuocolo [26]	26	Tetrofosmin	Adenosine	88	100
Amanullah [27]	222	Sestamibi	Adenosine	93	73
Mean ± SD				88 ≥ 8	82 ≥ 11

comparison with invasive procedures. In particular, no significant adverse medical effects have been documented resulting from the use of radioactive agents in standard diagnostic nuclear medicine procedures.

The diagnostic applications of myocardial perfusion imaging are based on the ability to detect a hemodynamically significant anatomic endpoint: a flow-limiting coronary stenosis. Sensitivity and specificity of SPECT in detecting CAD, using different tracers and different forms of stress [16, 19-27] are shown in Table 34.3. By current guidelines, the use of stress imaging should be preceded by the assessment of the pre-test likelihood of CAD [28]. Specifically, before stress testing, the likelihood of CAD should be assessed by Bayesian analyses of patient age, sex, risk factors, and symptoms [29]. Beyond risk stratification, perfusion imaging by SPECT can identify patients who are likely to benefit from revascularization procedures [30]. In the setting of no or only mild ischemia, patients undergoing medical therapy as their initial treatment have been shown to have survival superior to that of patients referred for revascularization. On the other hand, when moderate-to-severe ischemia is detected, patients undergoing revascularization have an increased survival benefit over those undergoing medical

therapy. Furthermore, a recent study demonstrated in patients who underwent serial SPECT that adding percutaneous coronary intervention to optimal medical therapy resulted in greater reduction in ischemia compared with optimal medical therapy alone [31]. The findings also suggest a treatment target of ≥5% of ischemia reduction at SPECT imaging with optimal medical therapy with or without coronary revascularization.

34.3 PET

PET has many advantages over SPECT, including higher spatial resolution and the ability to provide absolute quantitative measurements of physiologic parameters, such as regional myocardial blood flow and coronary flow reserve (Fig. 34.1). The most common tracers used for the assessment of myocardial perfusion with PET are nitrogen-13 (N-13) ammonia, rubidium-82 (Rb-82) and oxygen-15 (O-15) water chloride [10]. The principal characteristics of these tracers are illustrated in Table 34.1.

N-13 ammonia is the most commonly used perfusion tracer with PET. When injected, N-13 ammonia is extracted by myocardial tissue with a very high extrac-

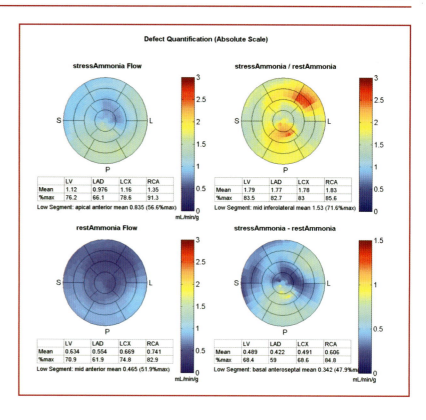

Fig. 34.1 Example of myocardial blood flow quantification with stress (dipyridamole) and rest N-13 ammonia PET imaging in a patient with nonischemic dilated cardiomyopathy: 17-segment model polar maps of rest blood flow (lower left, color scale: 0-3.0 mL/min/g), stress blood flow (upper left; scale: 0-3.0 mL/min/g), flow reserve (upper right; scale: 0-3.0), and flow difference (lower right; scale: 0-1.5) which demonstrate a global impairment (absolute and percentage values are displayed in the tables below)

tion fraction where it is converted to N-13 glutamine [32]. The clearance half time of ammonia activity from the myocardium is slow enough that one can wait until blood pool activity is significantly lower than myocardial activity. N-13 ammonia myocardial extraction is nonlinear and inversely related to blood flow. N-13 ammonia provides excellent quality images of the myocardium, because of the high single-pass extraction (approximately 70% to 80% at physiologic flow rates), the relatively prolonged retention of tracer by the heart (biological half-life of 80 to 400 min) after intravenous administration and the rapid blood-pool clearance (Fig. 34.2). Imaging with N-13 ammonia requires either an on-site cyclotron or proximity to a regional positron radiopharmaceutical source center.

Rb-82 is a cation and its uptake depends on myocardial perfusion. An advantage of Rb-82 over N-13 ammonia is the production by a generator without the need for a costly cyclotron. The single-pass extraction of Rb-82 by the myocardium is inversely and nonlinearly related to coronary blood flow [33]. The quality of images obtained after intravenous administration of Rb-82 depends on the tracer infusion duration and imaging protocol. Although disappearance of tracer from arterial blood is rapid, infusion system with prolonged administration time results in high myocardial blood-pool activity.

O-15 water is a freely diffusible tracer with a short physical half-life (2.1 minutes) requiring an on-site cyclotron. To effectively obtain myocardial images, O-15 (because of its short half-life) requires administration with rapid data acquisition. Because water is distributed in both the vascular space and myocardium, visualization of myocardial activity with this tracer requires correction for activity in the vascular compartments, which makes the images difficult to interpret visually. The correction is accomplished by acquiring a separate scan that identifies either the intravascular or the myocardial compartments [34].

PET has a high sensitivity and specificity for the detection of myocardial ischemia. Many studies that compared perfusion imaging with PET and SPECT in the assessment of CAD found PET to be superior to SPECT in terms of sensitivity, specificity and predictive accuracy [35-39]. Myocardial perfusion PET is particularly useful in reducing the number of false-positive SPECT studies due to attenuation artifacts. The higher sensitivity of PET can also be useful in the evaluation of quantitative myocardial blood flow. Gated PET may provide additional information regarding ventricular function similar to gated SPECT. Patients in whom stress imaging with exercise is neither required nor feasible, and patients with a high likelihood of false positive or false negative studies by SPECT are likely to benefit from PET imaging. This includes obese individuals and women with large breasts, where SPECT imaging is less effective due to attenuation artifacts [40]. Many patients

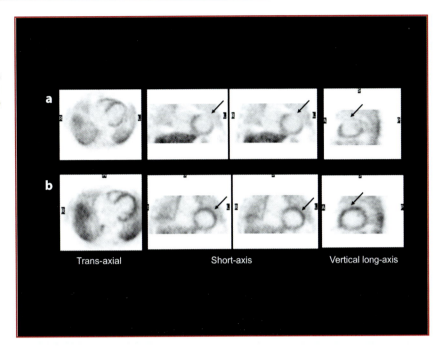

Fig. 34.2 Transaxial, short-axis, and long-axis images of PET myocardial perfusion obtained at stress (dipyridamole) and at rest with N-13 ammonia in a patient with ischemic dilated cardiomyopathy and atypical chest pain. There is a moderately large flow deficit in the lateral and anterolateral walls (*arrows*) with stress (**a**) that is normal at rest (**b**)

with end-stage renal and liver disease have edema, ascites, and high-elevated diaphragms, sometimes with pericardial effusions, which may lead to non-uniform attenuation abnormalities [41]. Furthermore, patients with equivocal results with other noninvasive tests or conflicting results can benefit from PET imaging.

34.4 Hybrid imaging

PET and SPECT scanners have now been linked to computed tomography (CT) scanners, which are digital radiologic systems that acquire data in the axial plane, producing images of internal organs at high spatial and contrast resolution. The combination of PET or SPECT and CT as a single unit provides spatial and pathologic correlation of the abnormal functional and/or metabolic activities, allowing images from both systems to be obtained by a single instrument in one examination procedure with optimal co-registration of images. The resulting fusion images facilitate the most accurate interpretation of both PET or SPECT and CT studies. CT attenuation maps from these integrated systems are used for rapid and optimal attenuation correction of the PET or SPECT images. In addition, PET-CT and SPECT-CT images are used to guide intervention. This process of integration of imaging systems has progressed to magnetic resonance [42, 43]. The major advantage of the integrated approach to the diagnosis of CAD is the added sensitivity of PET or SPECT and CT angiography. As not all coronary artery stenoses are flow limiting, PET or SPECT stress perfusion imaging complements the anatomic CT data by providing functional information on the hemodynamic significance of such stenoses, thus allowing more appropriate selection of patients who may benefit from revascularization procedures [42, 43]. While the principle may be the same, each modality has its specific benefits. Earlier studies conducted with three-dimensional image fusion of CT and SPECT showed promising results [44-47]. One of the major uses of SPECT/CT is the production of better attenuation correction. Apparent perfusion defects occur most often in the anterior wall in women and in the inferior wall in men, and soft-tissue attenuation can also shift between resting and stress images. Interpreting these examinations requires clinicians to recognize any attenuation artifacts and allow for them in evaluating the underlying perfusion pattern [48]. In addition, to being intuitively convincing, these images provide a panoramic view of the myocardium, the regional myocardial perfusion and the coronary artery tree, thus eliminating uncertainties in the relationship of perfusion defects and stenotic coronary arteries in watershed regions. This may be particularly helpful in patients with multiple perfusion abnormalities and complex CAD [49]. Similarly, the integration of PET and CT scanners enables detection and quantification of the burden of calcified and noncalcified plaques, quantification of vascular reactivity and endothelial health, identification of flow limiting coronary stenosis. Integrated PET/CT offers an opportunity to assess the presence and magnitude of sub-clinical atherosclerotic disease burden and to measure myocardial blood flow as a marker of endothelial health and atherosclerotic disease activity. Because not all coronary stenoses detected by CT are flow limiting, the stress myocardial perfusion PET data complement the CT anatomic information by providing instant readings about the clinical significance of such stenosis [50]. Further studies are needed to refine these technologies, address the issue of cost-effectiveness, and validate a range of clinical applications in large-scale clinical trials. Lastly, it should be stressed that although these new multimodality imaging systems carry enormous potential for rapid and efficient diagnosis, they also challenge established patterns of professional practice and patient care.

34.5 Conclusions

Available data indicate that cardiac imaging using advanced noninvasive modalities is useful in the assessment of coronary anatomy and myocardial perfusion in patients with known or suspected CAD. Given the rapid evolution of technologies, evaluation of their integration in clinical practice is ongoing and guidelines for clinical use will require regular updates. Lastly, optimal use of these approaches will require proper training and a joint effort among specialties is recommended.

References

1. Hendel RC, Berman DS, Di Carli MF et al (2009) ACCF/ASNC/ACR/AHA/ASE/SCCT/SCMR/SNM 2009 appropriate use criteria for cardiac radionuclide imaging: a report of the American College of Cardiology Foundation Appropriate Use Criteria Task Force, the American Society of Nuclear Cardiology, the American College of Radiology, the American Heart Association, the American Society of Echocardiography, the Society of Cardiovascular Computed Tomography, the Society for Cardiovascular Magnetic Resonance, and the Society of Nuclear Medicine. Circulation 119:e561-e587
2. Zaret BL, Strauss HW, Martin ND et al (1973) Noninvasive evaluation of regional myocardial perfusion with radioactive potassium: study of patients at rest, exercise, and during anginal pectoris. N Engl J Med 288:809-812
3. Berman DS, Salel AF, DeNardo GL et al (1975) Noninvasive detection of regional myocardial ischemia using rubidium-81 and the scintillation camera: comparison with stress electrocardiography in patients with arteriographically documented coronary stenosis. Circulation 52:619-626
4. Kaul S, Boucher CA, Newell JB et al (1986) Determination of the quantitative thallium imaging variables that optimize detection of coronary artery disease. J Am Coll Cardiol 7:527-537
5. Maddahi J, Kiat H, Berman DS (1991) Myocardial perfusion imaging with technetium-99m-labeled agents. Am J Cardiol 67:27D-34D

6. Cuocolo A, Petretta M, Acampa W et al (2010) Gated SPECT myocardial perfusion imaging: the further improvements of an excellent tool. Q J Nucl Med Mol Imaging 54:129-144
7. Aarnoudse WH, Botman KJ, Pijls NH (2003) False-negative myocardial scintigraphy in balanced three-vessel disease, revealed by coronary pressure measurement. Int J Cardiovasc Intervent 5:67-71
8. Gould KL, Schelbert H, Phelps M et al (1979) Noninvasive assessment of coronary stenoses with myocardial perfusion imaging during pharmacologic coronary vasodilatation. V. Detection of 47 percent diameter coronary stenosis with intravenous nitrogen-13 ammonia and emission-computed tomography in intact dogs. Am J Cardiol 43:200-208
9. Cuocolo A, Breatnach E (2010) Multimodality imaging in Europe: a survey by the European Association of Nuclear Medicine (EANM) and the European Society of Radiology (ESR). Eur J Nucl Med Mol Imaging 37:163-167
10. Cuocolo A, Acampa W, Imbriaco M et al (2005) The many ways to myocardial perfusion imaging. Q J Nucl Med Mol Imaging 49:4-18
11. Cuocolo A, Nicolai E, Soricelli A et al (1996) Technetium 99m-labeled tetrofosmin myocardial tomography in patients with coronary artery disease: comparison between adenosine and dynamic exercise stress testing. J Nucl Cardiol 3:194-203
12. DePuey EG, Berman DS, Garcia EV (1996) Cardiac SPECT imaging. Philadelphia: Lippincott-Raven
13. Leppo J, Meerdink D (1989) Comparison of the myocardial uptake of a technetium-labeled isonitrile analog and thallium. Circ Res 65:632-639
14. Sinusas AJ, Shi Q, Saltzberg MT et al (1994) Technetium-99m-tetrofosmin to assess myocardial blood flow: experimental validation in an intact canine model of ischemia. J Nucl Med 35:664-671
15. Higley B, Smith FW, Smith T et al (1993) Technetium-99m-1,2 bis (bis(2-ethoxyethyl)phosphino) ethane: human biodistribution, dosimetry and safety of a new myocardial perfusion imaging agent. J Nucl Med 34:30-38
16. Acampa W, Cuocolo A, Sullo P et al (1998) Direct comparison of technetium 99m-sestamibi and technetium 99m-tetrofosmin cardiac single photon emission computed tomography in patients with coronary artery disease. J Nucl Cardiol 3:265-274
17. Underwood SR, Anagnostopoulos C, Cerqueira M et al (2004) Myocardial perfusion scintigraphy: the evidence. Eur J Nucl Med Mol Imaging 261-291
18. Bateman TM, Cullom SJ (2005) Attenuation correction single-photon emission computed tomography myocardial perfusion imaging. Semin Nucl Med 1:37-51
19. Mahmarian JJ, Boyce TM, Goldberg RK, et al (1990) Quantitative exercise thallium-201 single photon emission computed tomography for the enhanced diagnosis of ischemic heart disease. J Am Coll Cardiol 15:318-329
20. Berman DS, Kiat H, Friedman JD et al (1993) Separate acquisition rest thallium-201/stress technetium-99m sestamibi dual-isotope myocardial perfusion single-photon emission computed tomography: a clinical validation study. J Am Coll Cardiol 22:1455-1464
21. Van Train KF, Areeda J, Garcia EV et al (1993) Quantitative same-day rest-stress technetium-99m-sestamibi SPECT: definition and validation of stress normal limits and criteria for abnormality. J Nucl Med 34:1494-1502
22. Palmas W, Friedman JD, Diamond GA et al (1995) Incremental value of simultaneous assessment of myocardial function and perfusion with technetium-99m sestamibi for prediction of extent of coronary artery disease. J Am Coll Cardiol 25:1024-1031
23. Taillefer R, DePuey EG, Udelson JE et al (1997) Comparative diagnostic accuracy of Tl-201 and Tc-99m sestamibi SPECT imaging (perfusion and ECG-gated SPECT) in detecting coronary artery disease in women. J Am Coll Cardiol 29:69-77

24. Watanabe K, Sekiya M, Ikeda S et al (1997) Comparison of adenosine triphosphate and dipyridamole in diagnosis by thallium-201 myocardial scintigraphy. J Nucl Med 38:577-581

25. Iskandrian AS, Heo J, Nguyen T et al (1991) Assessment of coronary artery disease using single-photon emission computed tomography with thallium-201 during adenosine-induced coronary hyperemia. Am J Cardiol 67:1190-1194

26. Cuocolo A, Sullo P, Pace L et al. (1997) Adenosine coronary vasodilation in coronary artery disease: technetium-99m tetrofosmin myocardial tomography versus echocardiography. J Nucl Med 38:1089-1094

27. Amanullah AM, Berman DS, Kiat H et al (1997) Usefulness of hemodynamic changes during adenosine infusion in predicting the diagnostic accuracy of adenosine technetium-99m sestamibi single-photon emission computed tomography (SPECT). Am J Cardiol 79:1319-1322

28. Gibbons RJ, Abrams J, Chatterjee K et al (2003) ACC/AHA 2002 guideline update for the management of patients with chronic stable angina: summary article - a report of the American College of Cardiology/American Heart Association Task Force on Practice Guidelines (Committee on the Management of Patients With Chronic Stable Angina). Circulation 107:149-158

29. Diamond GA, Forrester JS (1979) Analysis of probability as an aid in the clinical diagnosis of coronary-artery disease. N Engl J Med 300:1350-1358

30. Hachamovitch R, Hayes SW, Friedman JD et al (2003) Comparison of the short-term survival benefit associated with revascularization compared with medical therapy in patients with no prior coronary artery disease undergoing stress myocardial perfusion single photon emission computed tomography. Circulation 107:2900-2907

31. Shaw LJ, Berman DS, Maron DJ et al (2008) Optimal medical therapy with or without percutaneous coronary intervention to reduce ischemic burden: results from the Clinical Outcomes Utilizing Revascularization and Aggressive Drug Evaluation (COURAGE) trial nuclear substudy. Circulation 117:1283-1291

32. Tamaki N, Senda M, Yonekura Y et al (1985) Dynamic positron computed tomography of the heart with a high sensitivity positron camera and nitrogen-13 ammonia. J Nucl Med 26:567-575

33. Selwyn AP, Allan RM, L'Abbate A et al (1982) Relation between regional myocardial uptake of rubidium-82 and perfusion: absolute reduction of cation uptake in ischemia. Am J Cardiol 50:112-121

34. Bergmann SR, Fox KA, Rand AL et al (1984) Quantification of regional myocardial blood flow in vivo with 0-15 water. Circulation 70:724-733

35. Bergmann SR. Imaging of the heart with positron emission tomography (1994) Am J Card Imaging 8:181-188

36. Schwaiger M (1994) Myocardial perfusion imaging with PET. J Nu-

37. Stewart RE, Schwaiger M, Molina E et al (1991) Comparison of Rb-82 PET and Tl-201 SPECT imaging for detection of CAD. Am J Cardiol 67:1303-1310

38. Go RT, Marwick TH, MacIntyre WJ et al (1990) A prospective comparison of Rb-82 PET and Tl-201 SPECT myocardial perfusion imaging utilizing a single stress in the diagnosis of CAD. J Nucl Med 31:1899-1905

39. Tamaki N, Yonekura Y, Senda M et al (1988) Value and limitation of stress thallium-201 single-photon emission computed tomography: comparison with nitrogen-13 ammonia positron tomography. J Nucl Med 29:1181-1188

40. Araujo W, DePuey EG, Kamran M et al (2000) Artifactual reverse redistribution pattern in myocardial perfusion SPECT with technetium-99m sestamibi. J Nucl Cardiol 7:633-638

41. Tallaj JA, Kovar D, Iskandrian AE (2000) The use of technetium-99m sestamibi in a patient with liver cirrhosis. J Nucl Cardiol 6:722-723

42. Bax JJ, Beanlands RS, Klocke FJ et al (2007) Diagnostic and clinical perspectives of fusion imaging in cardiology: is the total greater than the sum of its parts? Heart 93:16-22

43. Bischof Delaloye A, Carrio I, Cuocolo A et al (2007) White paper of the European Association of Nuclear Medicine (EANM) and the European Society of Radiology (ESR) on multimodality imaging. Eur J Nucl Med Mol Imaging 34:1147-1151

44. Kalki K, Blankespoor SC, Brown JK et al (1997) Myocardial perfusion imaging with a combined x-ray CT and SPECT system. J Nucl Med 10:1535-1540

45. Wallis JW, Miller TR, Koppel P (1995) Attenuation correction in cardiac SPECT without a transmission measurement. J Nucl Med 3:506-512

46. Schindler TH, Magosaki N, Jeserich M et al (1999) Fusion imaging: combined visualization of 3D reconstructed coronary artery tree and 3D myocardial scintigraphic image in coronary artery disease. Int J Card Imaging 15:357-368

47. Schindler TH, Magosaki N, Jeserich M et al (2000) 3D assessment of myocardial perfusion parameter combined with 3D reconstructed coronary artery tree from digital coronary angiograms. Int J Card Imaging 16:1-12

48. Faber TL, Santana CA, Garcia EV et al (2004) Three-dimensional fusion of coronary arteries with myocardial perfusion distributions: clinical validation. J Nucl Med 45:745-753

49. Nakaura T, Utsunomiya D, Shiraishi S et al (2005) Three-dimensional cardiac image fusion using new CT angiography and SPECT methods. AJR Am J Roentgenol 185:1554-1557

50. Di Carli MF, Dorbala S, Curillova Z et al (2007) Relationship between CT coronary angiography and stress perfusion imaging in patients with suspected ischemic heart disease assessed by integrated PET-CT imaging. J Nucl Cardiol 14:799-809

cl Med 35:693-688

Cardiac Magnetic Resonance

35

Erica Maffei, Chiara Martini, Carlo Tedeschi, Andrea I. Guaricci, Giuseppe Tarantini, Giancarlo Casolo, and Filippo Cademartiri

35.1 Introduction

Magnetic resonance (MR) has become a consolidated imaging modality in the field of cardiology. The technique is characterized by enormous operative versatility ranging from pure morphology to myocardial tissue spectroscopy. Cardiac MR is probably the most complete diagnostic technique available today and is the reference standard in the majority of clinical applications (except noninvasive coronary angiography).

Nonetheless, for many years the technique has been the sole prerogative of extremely expert operators and has been unable to become as widespread as its performance could allow. This is due to a number of reasons, the most important being the relatively limited availability of scanners, both in terms of number and machine time.

In fact most MR diagnostic activity involves neurologic and osteoarticular studies. Secondary factors with a not insignificant impact on the distribution of MR include the relative scarcity of appropriately trained operators, the fact that the technique cannot be performed at the patient's bedside (unlike echocardiography), the fact that it is a technique with elevated costs, etc.

The introduction of cardiac computed tomography (CCT) is one of the major innovations in the field of cardiac imaging [1-16]. The rapid diffusion of scanners for coronary CCT should prompt an internal reorganization of diagnostic imaging departments capable of guaranteeing the integration between noninvasive modalities (CT, MR, Nuclear Medicine) aimed at optimizing diagnostic algorithms (appropriateness and less redundancy) and rationalizing resources (the best diagnostic procedure to those who need it).

35.2 Main Applications of Cardiac MR

MR imaging of coronary heart disease (CHD) has come up against technical problems related to the motion of the heart and the diaphragm, the synchronization of the sequences with the intrinsic duration of the cardiac cycle and the specific diseases of this organ.

35.2.1 Morphofunctional Study

The morphologic study of the myocardium consists in the evaluation of the appearance of the cardiac chambers and the intrathoracic vessels and the signal characteristics that the tissues produce in the standard sequences. The ventricular myocardium can be described both in terms of anatomy (trabeculae, presence or otherwise of an infundibular component) and spatial distribution of thickness or signal.

With the use of appropriate sequences pathologic conditions can be evaluated, such as edema, acute necrosis or the presence of scarring.

The functional (or cine) study in contrast is used to evaluate cardiac chamber volumes and myocardial contractility. All the functional parameters of the myocardium can be extracted after accurate segmentation of the epicardial and endocardial surfaces with dedicated software.

35.2.2 Left Ventricular Tagging

Myocardial tagging is applied to the functional evaluation of the left ventricle and can demonstrate segmental changes in the pattern of ventricular contraction. This technique can help to directly distinguish the functionally compromised areas from areas with abnormal wall motion exclusively as a result of lying adjacent to other diseased areas. By way of analogy, tagging in MR corresponds to strain/strain-rate imaging in Doppler echocardiography.

E. Maffei (✉)
Cardiovascular Imaging Unit,
"Giovanni XXIII" Hospital,
Monastier di Treviso (TV), Italy

F. Cademartiri, G. Casolo, M. Midiri (eds.), *Clinical Applications of Cardiac CT*,
© Springer-Verlag Italia 2012

35.2.3 Perfusion Study

Myocardial perfusion imaging is based on a dynamic scan at multiple levels, generally in the short axis, during the administration of an intravenous bolus of gadolinium chelate contrast agent. With this sequence the nonperfused or hypoperfused areas of the left ventricle display lower signal intensity than the remaining normally perfused areas. Quantification can be performed by relating the intensity curve of the normal ventricle and the left ventricular lumen with the intensity curve of the infarcted myocardium using dedicated software. The most important application is undoubtedly the perfusion study during pharmacologic stress. A comparison of images obtained during stress and those obtained at rest can reveal regions with reduced perfusion reserve which correspond to myocardial regions distal to obstructive coronary lesions. In this way ischemic regions can be identified, thus assigning an important functional implication to the MR examination.

35.2.4 Phase-contrast Study

Dedicated sequences can be used in MR to perform evaluations similar to those traditionally performed with Doppler or color-Doppler. However, thanks to phase-contrast velocity mapping, the signal intensity in the images corresponds to the absolute velocity. Therefore, stenosis and valvular insufficiency, shunt and output can be identified and quantified. With appropriate sequences and dedicated software the analysis almost becomes quantitative, unlike the evaluation with Doppler. The same principles can be applied to the individual vessels, the coronary arteries and bypass grafts.

35.2.5 Delayed Enhancement

Delayed enhancement (DE) indicates necrotic myocardial impairment. This is based on the extravascular diffusion of contrast material 5-15 min after IV administration. The areas of DE correspond to nonviable myocardium and appear hyperintense due to the presence of gadolinium in the extracellular compartment.

35.2.6 MR Coronary Angiography

MR coronary angiography is able to study the coronary arteries in much the same way as coronary CCT. However, there are a number of limitations, and the comparative studies and meta-analyses on the subject reveal a superiority of CCT 16-slice scanners and above. The limitations of MR in the study of the coronary arteries are essentially technical in nature and they allow the adequate analysis of only the proximal tracts of the coronary circulation. Currently MR coronary angiography is mainly used in the demonstration of coronary anomalies, thus avoiding techniques with a greater relative risk in patients of a generally young age.

35.2.7 Spectroscopy

Myocardial spectroscopy is one of the most advanced applications of cardiac MR and is generally based on phosphorous. The applications are yet to be introduced in the clinical setting, but the potential of this technique in providing the myocardial energy profile is high.

35.2.8 General Considerations on MR in Coronary Heart Disease

MR exploits nonionizing radiation to provide practically all the information required for the evaluation of the patient indicated for myocardial revascularization. Ventricular function can be qualitatively evaluated with dynamic (cine) images or quantitatively evaluated with dedicated segmentation software or tagging. Chronic transmural infarctions display a reduction/lack of myocardial wall thickening in systole and a reduction in myocardial wall thickness. Morphologic images can reveal areas of reduced signal intensity which correspond to areas of post-infarction scarring.

Cardiac MR is able to study acute and chronic infarction and can differentiate between viable and nonviable tissue. Several studies of acute myocardial infarction have reported an increased signal in T2-weighted sequences (edema). The most reliable signal, however, is myocardial wall thinning. In this setting distinguishing areas of subendocardial signal changes from flow-related artifacts can prove difficult. A more reliable technique is DE. In patients with acute myocardial infarction the maximum signal intensity has been observed within a week of the event. The signal remains high and recognizable in these patients for at least six weeks. By combining perfusion and DE, information regarding myocardial viability and the possibility of functional recovery can be obtained. In fact nonperfused or hypoperfused areas which do not display DE are those considered stunned or hibernating which could benefit from revascularization.

35.2.9 Advanced Applications

The most advanced applications of cardiac MR are myocardial spectroscopy and the implementation of 3-Tesla scanners. Spectroscopy provides information on the metabolism of phosphates and therefore on myocardial viability. The implementation of 3-Tesla scanners, on the other hand, may improve spatial resolution and/or reduce scan times.

35.3 Integration between CT and MR

35.3.1 Cardiomyopathies

The tissue evaluation of cardiomyopathies has long been dominated by MR. Nonetheless, CCT has recently been used for the differential diagnosis of dilative cardiomyopathy [17]. The investigators of the study suggested CCT be used to distinguish between idiopathic and ischemic forms on the basis of the evaluation of coronary circulation. In this setting, however, CCT is complementary or a substitute to conventional coronary angiography rather than to MR. In all other cardiomyopathies MR should be considered the criterion standard.

35.3.2 Congenital Anomalies

MR plays a fundamental role after echocardiography in the detection and characterization of congenital anomalies. The question of radiation protection in this category of patients is in fact highly relevant. In addition, the possibility of using MR to study flow parameters and pressure gradients makes it the criterion standard for the diagnosis and follow-up in these patients.

35.3.3 Suspected Coronary Artery Disease

Currently the optimal role of CCT in the clinical setting is not completely clear. The high negative predictive value of CCT suggests its use as a technique for ruling out the presence of coronary artery disease (CAD). In this context CCT could be the technique of choice in patients with a low or intermediate risk of CHD presenting with atypical chest pain, or it could be used as a second-phase diagnostic technique in patients with an equivocal stress test [18-20].

MR and CT could therefore be integrated in completing the morphofunctional picture of the suspected CHD patient, thus enabling an informed decision on whether to proceed or not with conventional coronary angiography (Figs. 35.1, 35.2). Which imaging modality should be used as first choice is debatable and current diagnostic algorithms and guidelines define the demonstration of inducible ischemia as the crucial factor for the definition of CHD. In this setting, however, MR is in "competition" with many other less complex (and also much less versatile) techniques such as exercise ECG, stress echocardiography and myocardial scintigraphy. It is therefore perhaps more appropriate to establish which functional test should be used in which patients.

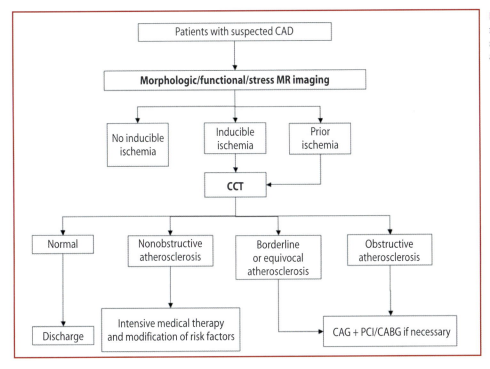

Fig. 35.1 Proposed current diagnostic algorithm in patients with suspected CAD with integrated CT and MR

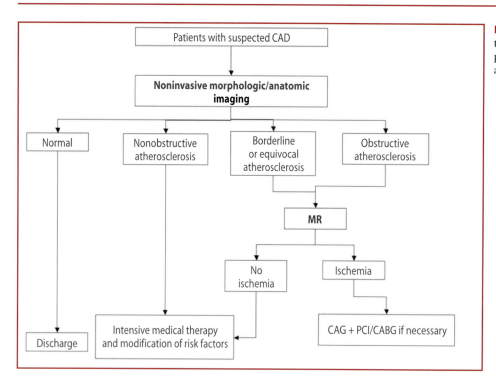

Fig. 35.2 Potential future diagnostic algorithm in patients with suspected CAD with integrated CT and MR

35.3.4 Known Coronary Heart Disease

Nonrevascularized known CHD can be characterized by several main clinical features: unstable angina, stable angina, prior nonrevascularized myocardial infarction, prior myocardial infarction as incidental finding, myocardial infarction with healthy coronary arteries or without critical stenoses. These clinical features are essentially derived from clinical practice. In these patients a range of diagnostic information is required which may not be easily obtained or quantified.

In unstable angina the role of CT and MR is undoubtedly limited by the patient's need for conventional coronary angiography. In some cases, however, the condition is misinterpreted due to the relatively atypical symptoms, and such patients undergo different diagnostic tests according to the clinical specialist and/or examining physician. In such cases the information which CCT can provide is similar to that obtained from conventional coronary angiography and includes the presence, location and degree of coronary artery stenosis. MR, on the other hand, is often used in situations of an uncertain presentation which comes into the differential diagnosis of other heart diseases such as myocarditis, pericarditis, endocarditis and syndrome X.

In these doubtful or spurious cases the diagnostic pathway often cannot be determined a priori. In the case of stable angina the guidelines clearly outline the procedures to be performed, and despite its great potential, MR is not considered as a first option technique. In these patients inducible ischemia and response to pharmacologic treatment determine the diagnostic technique of choice. CCT is used to quantify the degree and extent of CAD and MR to quantify its ability to cause ischemia.

In prior nonrevascularized myocardial infarction MR definitely plays a leading role in the evaluation and quantification of residual myocardial viability. Nonetheless, the majority of patients currently undergo other tests such as stress echocardiography and stress myocardial scintigraphy.

When prior myocardial infarction is an incidental finding, like the other morphofunctional techniques MR is essential for immediately establishing infarction site, residual function and viability. CCT in these cases can easily identify the culprit lesion even when it is not critical at the time of the examination. Included in this context are also the acute coronary syndromes (STEMI/NSTEMI) in which conventional coronary angiography is unable to identify a culprit lesion. These clinical conditions are superimposed with those of other diseases such as takotsubo cardiomyopathy or coronary thromboembolism. In these situations conventional coronary angiography is able to provide a surrogate of IVUS, with the identification even of *vulnerable* lesions which do not cause critical stenosis, but which can cause a transitory occlusion of the vascular lumen. In these conditions MR is fundamental for the evaluation of edema and myocardial scarring which can then have a significant impact not only on diagnosis but also on prognosis.

35.3.5 Revascularized Coronary Tree

Cardiac CT for the evaluation of stents is still not a robust technique. It can be adequate in the case of stents implanted in the left main branch or at the ostium of the right coronary artery. The size, the material and the position of the stent are significant factors in deciding whether or not to perform CCT on a patient. As with other previously described cases, MR instead is able to accurately assess the functional parameters, inducible residual ischemia and residual viability in these patients and thus suggest the best treatment options to adopt.

In the setting of coronary artery bypass grafts (CABG), on the other hand, the integration between CT and MR is more practicable due to the excellent performance of coronary CCT. The decision to proceed with angioplasty and stenting, additional bypass grafting or medical therapy in CABG patients can be fully supported by the combination of these two techniques. The previous considerations regarding the prognostic role of MR functional parameters are also valid here.

35.3.6 Coronary Plaque Imaging

At present coronary CCT is the only method capable of performing a routine evaluation of coronary wall atherosclerosis. Nonetheless, MR is equipped with a much greater potential in terms of tissue characterization and the possible characterization of the lipid core. A future scenario could see these two imaging modalities in a diagnostic algorithm whereby CCT provides the panoramic assessment of the coronary circulation and the *road map* for the characterization of the vulnerability of the lesions by MR. The latter could therefore be highly focused on the lesions identified by CCT.

35.4 Conclusions

The integration of CT and MR is definitely favored by the fact that the former is a prevalently morphologic technique especially capable of providing an evaluation of the coronary arteries, whereas the latter is a prevalently functional technique.

The majority of cardiologic conditions could receive a complete diagnostic algorithm with the integration of these *two heavy* imaging modalities. Clearly the filter for the evaluation should remain clinical assessment and should make use of other *light* techniques, but the future of cardiovascular imaging lies in the integration of these two modalities.

References

1. Nieman K, Cademartiri F, Lemos PA et al (2002) Reliable noninvasive coronary angiography with fast submillimeter multislice spiral computed tomography. Circulation 106:2051-2054
2. Ropers D, Baum U, Pohle K et al (2003) Detection of coronary artery stenoses with thin-slice multi- detector row spiral computed tomography and multiplanar reconstruction. Circulation 107:664-666
3. Kuettner A, Trabold T, Schroeder S et al (2004) Noninvasive detection of coronary lesions using 16-detector multislice spiral computed tomography technology: initial clinical results. J Am Coll Cardiol 44:1230-1237
4. Martuscelli E, Romagnoli A, D'Eliseo A et al (2004) Accuracy of thin-slice computed tomography in the detection of coronary stenoses. Eur Heart J 25:1043-1048
5. Mollet NR, Cademartiri F, Nieman K et al (2004) Multislice spiral computed tomography coronary angiography in patients with stable angina pectoris. J Am Coll Cardiol 43:2265-2270
6. Hoffmann MH, Shi H, Schmitz BL et al (2005) Noninvasive coronary angiography with multislice computed tomography. JAMA 293:2471-2478
7. Achenbach S, Ropers D, Pohle FK et al (2005) Detection of coronary artery stenoses using multidetector CT with 16 x 0.75 collimation and 375 ms rotation. Eur Heart J 26:1978-1986
8. Garcia MJ, Lessick J, Hoffmann MH (2006) Accuracy of 16-row multidetector computed tomographyfor the assessment of coronary artery stenosis. JAMA 296:403-411
9. Raff GL, Gallagher MJ, O'Neill WW, Goldstein JA (2005) Diagnostic accuracy of noninvasive coronary angiography using 64-slice spiral computed tomography. J Am Coll Cardiol 46:552-557
10. Leschka S, Alkadhi H, Plass A et al (2005) Accuracy of MSCT coronary angiography with 64-slice technology: first experience. Eur Heart J 26:1482-1487
11. Mollet NR, Cademartiri F, van Mieghem CA et al (2005) High-resolution spiral computed tomography coronary angiography in patients referred for diagnostic conventional coronary angiography. Circulation 112:2318-2323
12. Mollet NR, Cademartiri F, Krestin GP et al (2005) Improved diagnostic accuracy with 16-row multi-slice computed tomography coronary angiography. J Am Coll Cardiol 45:128-132
13. Fine JJ, Hopkins CB, Ruff N, Newton FC (2006) Comparison of accuracy of 64-slice cardiovascular computed tomography with coronary angiography in patients with suspected coronary artery disease. Am J Cardiol 97:173-174
14. Ropers D, Rixe J,Anders K et al (2006) Usefulness of multidetector row spiral computed tomography with 64- x 0.6-mm collimation and 330-ms rotation for the noninvasive detection of significant coronary artery stenoses. Am J Cardiol 97:343-348
15. Nikolaou K, Knez A, Rist C et al (2006) Accuracy of 64-MDCT in the diagnosis of ischemic heart disease. AJR Am J Roentgenol 187:111-117
16. Schuijf JD, Pundziute G, Jukema JW et al (2006) Diagnostic accuracy of 64-slice multislice computed tomography in the noninvasive evaluation of significant coronary artery disease. Am J Cardiol 98:145-148
17. Andreini D, Pontone G, Pepi M et al (2007) Diagnostic accuracy of multidetector computed tomography coronary angiography in patients with dilated cardiomyopathy. J Am Coll Cardiol 49:2044-2050
18. Fox K, Garcia MA,Ardissino D et al (2006) Guidelines on the management of stable angina pectoris: executive summary: the Task Force on the Management of Stable Angina Pectoris of the European Society of Cardiology. Eur Heart J 27:1341-1381

19. Hendel RC, Patel MR, Kramer CM et al (2006) ACCF/ACR/SC-CT/SCMR/ASNC/NASCI/SCAI/SIR 2006 appropriateness criteria for cardiac computed tomography and cardiac magnetic resonance imaging: a report of the American College of Cardiology Foundation Quality Strategic Directions Committee Appropriateness Criteria Working Group, American College of Radiology, Society of Cardiovascular Computed Tomography, Society for Cardiovascular Magnetic Resonance, American Society of Nuclear Cardiology, North American Society for Cardiac Imaging, Society for Cardiovascular Angiography and Interventions, and Society of Interventional Radiology. J Am Coll Cardiol 48:1475-1497

20. Ghostine S, Caussin C, Daoud B et al (2006) Non-invasive detection of coronary artery disease in patients with left bundle branch block using 64-slice computed tomography. J Am Coll Cardiol 48:1929-1934

Invasive Imaging of Coronary Atherosclerotic Plaques

36

Francesco Prati, Michele Occhipinti, and Luca Di Vito

36.1 Imaging Modalities

36.1.1 Coronary Angiography

Coronary angiography depicts lumen narrowings caused by the encroachments of atherosclerotic plaques and thus provides a lumen cast of the coronary tree. A major limitation of angiography is its inability to study mild plaques that fail to reduce the coronary lumen, due to the Glagov phenomenon. Indeed, the vast majority of acute coronary syndromes (ACS) are due to acute thrombus formation at plaque sites that are not significant at angiography. On the other hand severe stenoses are less likely to cause major events.

36.1.2 Intravascular Ultrasound

Intravascular ultrasound (IVUS) images are obtained with intravascular transducers that have a diameter less than 6 F and a resolution of 150-200 μm IVUS is able to provide a gross evaluation of atherosclerotic components and distinguish calcific components from soft ones and fibrotic tissue [1-4]. Identification of lipid necrotic pools is non optimal and not surprisingly the IVUS term *soft tissue*, which has nothing to do with the morphology of a plaque, is widely adopted to describe components that may comprise lipid tissue. Calcium, on the other hand can be easily identified, although the shadowing effect caused by calcific deposits does not permit the measurement of their thickness. Thrombus is very difficult to see at IVUS; this is because the acoustic properties of thrombus resemble those of lipid tissue. IVUS can address the whole thickness of atherosclerotic plaques and therefore enables the assessment of vessel remodeling, which is now a recognized factor of vulnerability [5] (Fig. 36.1).

F. Prati (✉)
Interventional Cardiology Unit,
"San Giovanni" Hospital,
Rome, Italy

36.1.3 Virtual Histology

Virtual histology has been extensively used in the attempts to better characterize coronary plaque components [6]. The method is based on the radiofrequency analysis of IVUS backscatter. The use of a color-coding technique enables a fast definition of tissue components. Fibrotic components are generally in dark green, fibro-fatty in light green, calcium in white and lipid necrotic core in red.

36.1.4 Palpography

Palpography is an adjunctive IVUS derived imaging modality that measures plaque strain during the cardiac cycle. In patients with ACS, plaques exhibit a greater strain than those with stable angina [7].

36.1.5 Angioscopy

Angioscopy contributed to the understanding of pathophysiology of ACS [8]. The technique enables an accurate assessment of vessel endothelium and superficial plaque components. Plaque ulcerations and thrombus encroachments can be easily appreciated by angioscopy [9]. Plaques at higher risk of rupture, characterized by a large superficial lipid pool and a thin fibrous cap appear yellow and translucid at angioscopy. Unfortunately angioscopy is unable to study the plaque components beneath the endothelium and does not allow quantitative assessment. This drawback and the complexity in its use have limited the widespread use of angioscopy, confining its use to Japan.

36.1.6 Optical Coherence Tomography

Optical coherence tomography (OCT) is an imaging modality that uses light instead of sound and offers significantly improved resolution as compared to IVUS

F. Cademartiri, G. Casolo, M. Midiri (eds.), *Clinical Applications of Cardiac CT*,
© Springer-Verlag Italia 2012

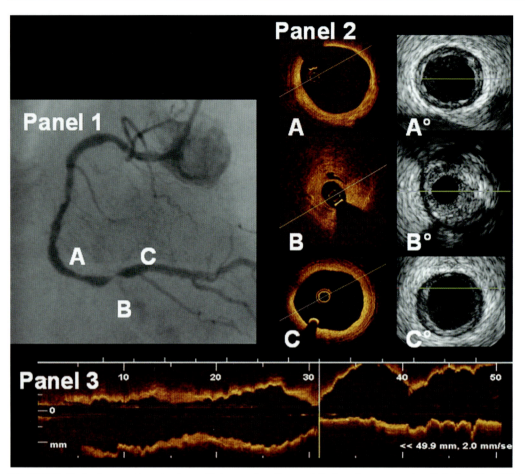

Fig. 36.1 Optical coherence tomography and intravascular ultrasound findings in a severe stenotic lesion. **Panel 1** Angiogram of right coronary artery shows a severe stenosis located in the distal tract of the artery. *A* and *C* indicate reference segments characterized by normal appearing vessel structure. *B* indicates the stenosis. **Panel 2** Optical coherence tomography findings are shown (*A*, *B* and *C*). *A* and *C* show the characteristic bright appearance of superficial cap. A severe fibrotic lesion is shown (*B*). Intravascular ultrasound findings are shown (*A°*, *B°* and *C°*). IVUS is able to identify deeper vessel layers but it has a lower capability to characterize the superficial vessel layer. **Panel 3** Longitudinal OCT view

[10-17]. In fact, OCT resolution is about ten times higher than that of IVUS, being in the range of 10-15 μm, as a result of the very short wavelength of the imaging light [10, 15]. Cross-sectional images are generated by measuring the echo time delay and intensity of light that is reflected or back-scattered from internal structures in the tissue [10-14]. Unlike angiography or IVUS, OCT is able to identify lipid necrotic pools and thrombi with high accuracy. Problems in plaque assessment and quantification mainly derive from the mild penetration of infrared light.

36.1.7 Intracoronary Thermography

Intracoronary thermography can be used to address the presence of inflammation, measured by local changes in the temperature of atherosclerotic plaques. Casscells et al. showed a positive significant correlation between carotid atherosclerotic plaques and macrophage content [18]. The increase in temperature of atherosclerotic lesions is also partially related to the extension of lipid components [19]. The widespread use of this technique is limited by the fact that thermography assessment of local temperature is hampered by the cooling effect of blood.

Other techniques that are being investigated include infrared spectroscopy, a promising solution for studying the chemical composition of coronary plaques. One recently developed algorithm combines infrared spectroscopy with IVUS.

36.2 Normal Coronary Arteries

Normal angiograms or angiograms with minimal irregularities are found in around 10% to 15% of patients undergoing coronary angiography for suspected coronary artery disease [20]. IVUS and OCT can confirm the absence of significant atherosclerosis or indicate the degree of subclinical atherosclerotic lesion formation.

As a well known concept, the media gets thinner at the site of atherosclerosis and vessel wall tends to bulge outwards. This so called Glagov phenomenon tends to occur in the early stages of atherosclerosis and preserves the lumen area until the plaque burden exceeds 40% of the original area. As a consequence the term *normal vessels* at angiography should be adopted only in presence of a smooth vessel contour, without those irregularities that indicate the presence of atherosclerosis.

IVUS and OCT are two valid solutions for ruling out the presence of atherosclerosis. IVUS, with its optimal penetration, is an ideal method for the study of vessel remodeling whilst the limited penetration of OCT does not consistently enable the study of vessel remodeling.

In normal vessels and at the sites of thin plaques, with thicknesses not exceeding 1.2 mm, the coronary artery wall appears as a 3-layer structure in OCT images. Unlike IVUS, OCT can clearly distinguish the intimal from the medial layer of the coronary artery wall, and measure its thickness, which lies between 125 μm to 350 μm (mean 200 μm) [21, 22].

Nearly all coronary arteries of adults show some grade of intimal thickness as it increases with age. However the identification of pathologic neointimal growth is limited by the lack of an established cut-off value. Despite this limitation OCT, compared with IVUS [20, 22, 23], detects even the earliest stages of intimal thickening, depicted as a bright, homogeneous thin rim of tissue having a texture similar to fibrous plaque components. A comparative study between OCT and integrated backscatter IVUS (IB-IVUS) showed that both methods detect intimal hyperplasia with high specificity (100% vs. 99%) but OCT is more sensitive (86% vs. 67%) [21].

36.3 Evaluation of Intermediate Stenoses and Ambiguous Lesions

Suboptimal angiographic visualization impairs the accurate assessment of stenosis severity. This may happen in the presence of intermediate lesions of uncertain severity, very short lesions, pre- or post-aneurysmal lesions, ostial or left main stem stenoses, disease at branching sites, sites with focal spasm, or angiographically hazy lesions.

IVUS and OCT can quantify lesion severity more accurately than quantitative coronary angiography. The measurement of a minimal lumen area of 2.4–3.0 mm^2 is considered the significant cut-off threshold for a clinically significant flow-limiting stenosis in appropriately sized (>3 mm) vessels excluding the left main coronary artery [24]. Further validation studies may be needed to corroborate this issue, in particular with the use of OCT. Comparison of the minimal lumen area with reference lumen areas is an alternative method for assessment of the degree of stenosis.

In particular, OCT is indicated for the assessment of angiographically hazy lesions and focal vessel spasm. In angiographically hazy lesions OCT often detects ruptured plaques with thrombus attached to the rupture site of the fibrous cap over a partially emptied lipid pool. In such cases the decision to proceed with treatment is based on morphologic observations and not on absolute measurement of lumen area.

The relatively small size of OCT imaging catheters compared to IVUS catheters may reduce the incidence of catheter wedging and coronary spasm [25].

A limitation of frequency-domain OCT (FD-OCT) is that plaque located at the very ostium of the left or right coronary arteries cannot be accurately imaged [14]. Unlike IVUS, OCT assessment requires blood displacement with contrast or a different solution (dextran or ringer lactate). This requires the firm engagement of the coronary ostium with a guiding catheter. As infrared light is unable to penetrate the partially metallic structure of guide catheters, the structures beneath cannot be visualized by OCT.

Previous studies using IVUS to guide interventional procedures in the presence of ambiguous and intermediate angiographic lesions, reported a modification of the overall revascularization strategy in 40% of patients, with aborted planned revascularizations in a high percentage of patients and promising clinical outcome [26]. As for IVUS, preliminary data indicate that OCT can change the operator's intention-to-treat, thus avoiding unnecessary interventional procedures or modifying the strategy in some cases [25].

Assessment of target lesions by IVUS is frequently a demanding issue as IVUS probes tend to occlude the lumen in tight lesions during the time required to acquire pull-back images at a relatively low pull-back speed (1 mm/sec). Symptoms of myocardial ischaemia may therefore develop during IVUS acquisition.

36.3.1 Assessment of Atherosclerosis

It is well known that angiography has poor sensitivity in the detection of calcific deposits, especially when they have a radial extension less than 180° [20]. Infrared light penetrates calcium better than IVUS, but calcific components with a thickness greater than 1-1.3 mm can prove impossible to penetrate. Therefore calcium deposits with a deep intra-plaque location may be missed with OCT. Compared to IVUS, OCT leads to a more precise measurement of the thickness of the fibrous cap, and improves the study of structures located behind superficial macro-calcification [14]. Furthermore, OCT is highly accurate in the identification of tissue components such as intimal hyperplasia and lipid-rich plaques [14]. Unlike angiography or IVUS, OCT holds promises in identifying thrombi, measuring their dimensions and guiding their removal [27, 28]. This is of utmost importance for detection of culprit lesions in patients with ACS [29, 30].

36.3.1.1 Plaque Vulnerability

One of the future challenges in the field of interventional cardiology is the characterization of the vulnerable plaque and how to best manage it. Vulnerable plaques are typically characterized by a thin fibrous cap, a large superficial lipid pool and inflammatory cells. Furthermore, plaque vulnerability is related to positive remodeling [31]. Some of these aspects can be studied with IVUS [31, 32]; in fact, vessel remodeling is easily addressed and the application of radiofrequency analysis with virtual histology to IVUS backscatter enhances visualization of plaque lipid components [31, 33]. A number of IVUS studies based on gray-scale assessment or signal radiofrequency analysis of IVUS backscatter have attempted to characterize the appearance of vulnerable plaques containing superficial necrotic-lipid cores. Recently the PROSPECT trial showed for the first time that IVUS is capable of characterizing the risk different plaque types have of causing an event, or of remaining stable for up to three years. Angiographically mild lesions with certain morphologic features on grayscale and virtual histology IVUS such as lesion severity, as detected by lumen area measurement, plaque burden and thin fibrous atheroma, conferred a 3 year higher risk of cardiac events [34].

OCT has the potential to study the features that are indicative of plaque vulnerability. As OCT penetration through superficial *necrotic lipid pools* is less than that through calcified and fibrous tissues, in the majority of lesions lipid pool thickness cannot be measured [35, 36]. However OCT enables the measurements of the *thickness of the fibrous cap,* delimiting superficial lipid pools. Fibrous-cap thickness can be obtained either as a single measurement at the cross-section where the fibrous cap thickness is considered minimal [37, 38] or as the average of multiple (three or more) samples [1]. Superficial microcalcifications are small calcific deposits that form an angle less than 90 degrees and are separated from the

lumen by a rim of tissue less than 100 μm thick [35, 36]. The arc (in degrees) and the longitudinal extent of a superficial necrotic lipid pool can be measured, analogous to the semiquantitative grading of calcium [35, 36, 39].

OCT has the potential to identify *inflammatory cells* such as clusters of lymphocytes and macrophages. Streaks of macrophages or foam cells are appreciated as bands of high reflectivity in OCT images. When located in a plaque with a lipid pool, macrophage streaks appear within the fibrous cap covering the lipid pool. However, the interface between the fibrous cap and the lipid pool produces a bright OCT appearance that can be difficult to distinguish from tightly packed foam cells [40, 41]. Previous studies showed that application of OCT algorithm can identify inflammatory cells with high specificity and sensitivity. Off-line use of these dedicated algorithms may be instrumental in identifying and possibly quantifying plaque inflammation.

However, the limited penetration of OCT may pose some problems in the identification of lesion components and, as a consequence, in the recognition of plaque vulnerability. For this reason the utility of a combined approach based on the use of OCT and virtual histology IVUS has been proposed [42, 43].

Angioscopy has great potential in the identification of superficial tissue components. In vivo comparative studies between OCT and angioscopy showed that the plaque color observed at angioscopy is strongly associated with the thickness of the fibrous cap, whilst correlation with the size of the lipid core is lower [44].

The combined used of IVUS and thermography is a solution for merging morphologic and functional characteristics. In fact, ruptured plaques with expansive remodeling are associated with increased local inflammatory activation, as demonstrated by increased temperature difference [26-45]. Furthermore, the development of algorithms capable of detecting plaque deformation or calculating shear stress using OCT would provide an excellent combination of morphologic and functional imaging with the use of a single catheter.

Identification of *erosion* as a mechanism of plaque instability is a challenge even for a technique with a resolution below 20 μm such as OCT. Thrombosis with apparently normal endothelial lining underneath may be indicative of erosion. Despite its complexity angioscopy appears to be the only method capable of addressing anatomic features such as the absence of a endothelial lining. Validation studies combining OCT with techniques providing a functional assessment of the endothelium may be able to give us more information on vessel thrombosis induced by erosion.

36.3.2 Pathophysiology of Acute Coronary Syndromes

Angiography shows a high specificity and a low sensitivity for the identification of plaque ulcerations; therefore mild plaque rupture cannot be addressed at angiography. Despite a non optimal resolution, IVUS is able to identify signs of plaque rupture and the presence of thrombus. OCT is so far the most accurate technique for identifying acute plaque ulceration and thrombosis. Rupture can be easily detected by OCT as a ruptured fibrous cap that connects the lumen with the lipid pool. These ulcerated or ruptured plaques may occur with or without a superimposed thrombus. When signs of ulceration are present without evidence of thrombosis, the lesion cannot be defined as a "culprit" with certainty, unless clinical criteria provide some evidence that the lesion is responsible for the acute events. Use of thrombolysis, IIb-IIIa glycoprotein inhibitors or other anti-thrombotic drugs facilitate clot degradation and in some circumstances may lead to complete disappearance (Fig. 36.2).

36.4 Progression/Regression of Atherosclerosis

According to Ambrose [46] lesions with complex appearance and irregular borders and or an appearance indicative of thrombosis tend to progress more rapidly. Complex lesions exhibit a progression rate of 11% whilst simple ones progress at a rate of 1.5% [47].

IVUS gained attention as a method for measuring serial changes in plaque volume during progression/ regression studies. IVUS addresses plaque volume (measured as plaque plus media) by subtracting the lumen area from the area delimited by the external elastic membrane.

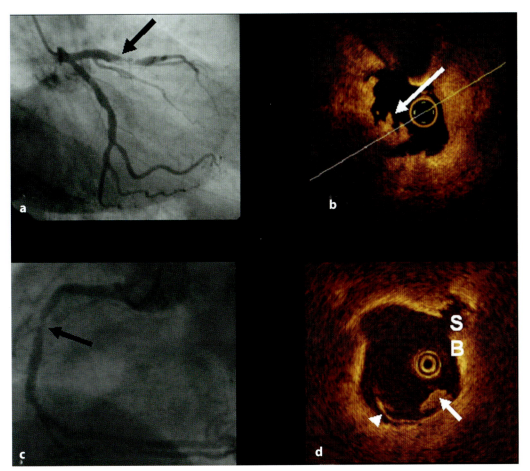

Fig. 36.2 Culprit coronary lesion as assessed by optical coherence tomography and angiography. A sub occlusive lesion is located in the mid portion of left descending coronary artery (**a**). OCT shows a ruptured plaque with an overlying thrombus (**b**). Another type of culprit lesion is shown (**c**) in the proximal tract of right coronary artery. OCT shows a linear superficial dissection and luminal thrombus (**d**)

OCT is potentially capable of studying serial changes in plaque composition, such as fibrous cap thickness or lipid pool extension. However validation studies are needed for such an application.

36.4.1 Post-intervention Assessment

Many studies have addressed the ability to reduce restenosis and thrombosis with IVUS guided expansion. Results have been conflicting but meta-analyses indicate a potential advantage, particularly in complex lesions [48]. In particular left main stenting benefits from an IVUS guided approach, producing a significant decrease in mortality when compared with simple angiographic guidance. Intravascular imaging modalities also play a role in tackling the occurrence of thrombosis, as suggested by recent IVUS data obtained in a large propensity-score matched population after drug eluting stent deployment [49]. In the presence of a drug eluting stent a threshold of absolute minimal lumen cross-sectional area within the stent of at least 5.0–5.5 mm^2 has been advocated as the target minimum stent area necessary to prevent failure [48].

Most of the IVUS guided criteria for stent expansion used at the time of bare metal stent are based on a comparison with the lumen area in the reference segments [48]. The optimal resolution of OCT further facilitates the assessment of optimal stent expansion by comparing minimal stent area and reference areas.

Unlike IVUS OCT has sufficient resolution to perform a per-strut analysis, revealing mild levels of malapposition, small intrastent thrombotic formations and mild dissection at the stent edges [50, 51]. Although the clinical significance of this finding is still unknown, it is possible that the presence of thrombus after stenting elevates the risk of acute and subacute stent thrombosis. Randomized studies are needed to validate these concepts.

References

1. Mintz GS, Nissen SE, Anderson WD et al (2001) ACC Clinical Expert Consensus Document on Standards for the acquisition, measurement and reporting of intravascular ultrasound studies: a report of the American College of Cardiology Task Force on Clinical Expert Consensus Documents (Committee to Develop a Clinical Expert Consensus Document on Standards for Acquisition, Measurement and Reporting of Intravascular Ultrasound Studies [IVUS]. J Am Coll Cardiol 37:1478-1492
2. Gussenhoven EJ, Essed CE et al (1989) Arterial wall characteristics determined by intravascular ultrasound imaging: an in vitro study. J Am Coll Cardiol 14:947-952
3. Nissen SE, Gurley JC, Grines CL et al (1991) Intravascular ultrasound assessment of lumen size and wall morphology in normal subjects and patients with coronary artery disease. Circulation 84:1087-1099
4. Prati F, Arbustini E, Labellarte A et al (2000) Intravascular ultrasound insights into plaque composition. Z Kardiol 89:117-123
5. Prati F, Mallus MT, Parma A et al (1998) Incidence of compensatory enlargement and paradoxical shrinkage of coronary arteries in presence of atherosclerotic lesions: an intracoronary ultrasound study based on multiple cross-section analysis per artery. G Ital Cardiol 28:1063-1071
6. Nasu K, Tsuchikane E, Katoh O et al (2006) Accuracy of in vivo coronary plaque morphology assessment: a validation study of in vivo virtual histology compared with in vitro histopathology. J Am Coll Cardiol 47:2405-2412
7. Schaar JA, van der Steen AF, Mastik F et al (2006) Intravascular palpography for vulnerable plaque assessment. J Am Coll Cardiol 47:86-91
8. Nesto RW, Waxman S, Mittleman MA et al (1998) Angioscopy of culprit coronary lesions in unstable angina pectoris and correlation of clinical presentation with plaque morphology. Am J Cardiol 81:225-228
9. Masumura Y, Ueda Y, Matsuo K et al (2011) Frequency and location of yellow and disrupted coronary plaques in patients as detected by angioscopy. Circ J 75:603-612
10. Huang D, Swanson EA, Lin CP et al (1991) Optical coherence tomography. Science 254:1178-1181
11. Brezinski ME, Tearney GJ, Bouma BE et al (1996) Optical coherence tomography for optical biopsy properties and demonstration of vascular pathology. Circulation 93:1206-1213
12. Fujimoto JG, Schmitt JM (2006) Handbook of Optical Coherence Tomography in Cardiovascular Research. E Regar, TG van Leeuwen and P Serruys Eds, pp 19-33
13. Jang IK, Bouma BE, Kang DH et al (2002) Visualization of coronary atherosclerotic plaques in patients using Optical Coherence Tomography: comparison with intravascular ultrasound. J Am Coll Cardiol 39:604-609
14. Prati F, Regar E, Mintz GS et al, for the Expert's OCT Review Document (2010) Expert review document on methodology and clinical applications of OCT. Physical principles, methodology of image acquisition and clinical application for assessment of coronary arteries and atherosclerosis. Eur Heart J 31:401-415
15. Tearney GJ, Waxman S, Shishkov M et al (2008) Three-dimensional coronary artery microscopy by intracoronary Optical Frequency Domain Imaging. J Am Coll Cardiol Img 1:752-761
16. Takarada S, Imanishi T, Liu Y et al (2010) Advantage of next-generation frequency-domain optical coherence tomography compared with conventional time-domain system in the assessment of coronary lesion. Catheter & Cardiovasc Interv 75:202-206
17. Jang IK, Tearney GJ, MacNeill B et al (2005) In vivo characterization of coronary atherosclerotic plaque by use of Optical Coherence Tomography. Circulation 111:1551-1555
18. Casscells W, Hathorn B, David M et al (1996) Thermal detection of cellular infiltrates in living atherosclerotic plaques: possible implications for plaque rupture and thrombosis. Lancet 347:1447-1449
19. Verheye S, De Meyer GRY, Van Langenhove G et al(2002) In vivo temperature heterogeneity of atherosclerotic plaques is determined by plaque composition. Circulation 105:1596-1601
20. Germing A, Lindstaedt M, Ulrich S et al (2005) Normal angiogram in acute coronary syndrome-preangiographic risk stratification, angiographic findings and follow-up. Int J Cardiol 99:19-23
21. Kawasaki M, Bouma BE, Bressner J et al (2006) Diagnostic accuracy of optical coherence tomography and integrated backscatter intravascular ultrasound images for tissue characterization of human coronary plaques. J Am Coll Cardiol 48:81-88
22. Kume T, Akasaka T, Kawamoto T et al (2005) Assessment of coronary intima-media thickness by Optical Coherence Tomography. Comparison with intravascular ultrasound. Circ J 8:903-907

23. Rieber J, Meissner O, Babaryka G et al (2006) Diagnostic accuracy of optical coherence tomography and intravascular ultrasound for the detection and characterization of atherosclerotic plaque composition in ex-vivo coronary specimens: a comparison with histology. Coron Artery Dis 17:425-433

24. Gonzalo N, Garcia-Garcia HM, Regar E et al (2009) In vivo assessment of high-risk coronary plaques at bifurcations with combined intravascular ultrasound and optical coherence tomography. JACC Cardiovasc Imaging 2:473-482

25. Imola F, Mallus MT, Ramazzotti V et al (2010) Safety and feasibility of frequency domain Optical Coherence Tomography to guide decision making in percutaneous coronary intervention. EuroInterv 6:575-581

26. Toutouzas K, Synetos A, Stefanadis E et al (2007) Correlation between morphologic characteristics and local temperature differences in culprit lesions of patients with symptomatic coronary artery disease. J Am Coll Cardiol 49:2264-2271

27. Prati F, Cera M, Ramazzotti V et al (2007) Safety and feasibility of a new non-occlusive technique for facilitated intracoronary optical coherence tomography (OCT) acquisition in various clinical and anatomical scenarios. EuroInterv 3:365-370

28. Kume T, Akasaka T, Kawamoto T et al (2005) Assessment of coronary intima-media thickness by Optical Coherence Tomography. Comparison with intravascular ultrasound. Circ J 8:903-907

29. Prati F, Cera M, Ramazzotti V et al (2008) From bench to bed side: A novel technique to acquire OCT images. Circ J 72:839-843

30. Toutouzas K, Karanasos A, Tsiamis E (2011) New insights by optical coherence tomography into the differences and similarities of culprit ruptured plaque morphology in non-ST-elevation myocardial infarction and ST-elevation myocardial infarction. Am Heart J 161:1192-1199

31. von Biergelen C, Klinkhart W, Mintz GS et al (2001) Mechanical and structural characteristics of vulnerable plaques: analysis by coronary angioscopy and intravascular ultrasound. J Am Coll Cardiol 38:934-940

32. Prati, F, Arbustini, E & Labellarte A et al (2001) Correlation between high frequency intravascular ultrasound and histomorphology in human coronary arteries. Heart 85:567-570

33. Rodriguez-Granillo GA, García HM, Valgimigli M (2006) Global characterization of coronary plaque rupture phenotype using three-vessel intravascular ultrasound radiofrequency data analysis. Eur Heart J 27:1921-1927

34. Chia S, Raffel OC, Takano M et al (2008) Comparison of coronary plaque characteristics between diabetic and non-diabetic subjects: An in vivo optical coherence tomography study. Diabetes Res Clin Pract 81:155-160

35. Kawase Y, Hoshino K, Yoneyama R et al (2005) In vivo volumetric analysis of coronary stent using optical coherence tomography with a novel balloon occlusion-flushing catheter: a comparison with intravascular ultrasound. Ultrasound Med Biol 31:1343-1349

36. Kubo T, Imanishi T, Takarada S et al (2007) Assessment of culprit lesion morphology in acute myocardial infarction: ability of Optical Coherence Tomography compared with intravascular ultrasound and coronary angioscopy. J Am Coll Cardiol 50:933-939

37. Kume T, Akasaka T, Kawamoto T et al (2006) Assessment of coronary arterial thrombus by Optical Coherence Tomography. Am J Cardiol 97:1713–1717

38. Takano M, Jang IK, Inami S et al (2008) In Vivo Comparison of Optical Coherence Tomography and Angioscopy for the Evaluation of Coronary Plaque Characteristics. Am J Cardiol 101:471-478

39. Hayden H, Renu V, Hesham Y, Burke AP (2001) The Impact of Calcification on the Biomechanical Stability of Atherosclerotic plaques Circulation 10:1051-1056

40. Tanaka A, Tearney G, Bouma BE (2010) Challenges on the frontier of intracoronary imaging: atherosclerotic plaque macrophage measurement by optical coherence tomography. J Biomed Opt 15:011104

41. Kume T, Akasaka T, Kawamoto T et al (2006) Measurements of the thickness of the fibrous cap by optical coherence tomography. Am Heart J 152:755.e1-4

42. Takarada S, Imanishi T, Kubo T et al (2009) Effect of statin therapy on coronary fibrous-cap thickness in patients with acute coronary syndrome: assessment by optical coherence tomography study. Atheroscler 202:491-497

43. Peterson CL, Schmitt JM (2006) Design of an OCT imaging system for intravascular applications. Handbook of Optical Coherence Tomography in Cardiovascular Research. E Regar, TG van Leeuwen and P Serruys Eds pp 35-42

44. Stone GW, Maehara A, Lansky AJ et al (2011) for the PROSPECT Investigators. A prospective natural-history study of coronary atherosclerosis. N Engl J Med 364:226-235

45. Stefanadis C, Toutouzas K, Tsiamis E (2001) Increased local temperature in human coronary atherosclerotic plaques: an independent predictor of clinical outcome in patients undergoing a percutaneous coronary intervention J Am Coll Cardiol 37:1277-1283

46. Ambrose JA (1991) Prognostic implications of lesion irregularity on coronary angiography. J Am Coll Cardiol 18:675-676

47. Ambrose JA, Tannenbaum MA, Alexopoulos D et al (1988) Angiographic progression of coronary artery disease and the development of myocardial infarction. J Am Coll Cardiol 12:56-62

48. Chester MR, Chen L, Tousoulis D et al (1995) Differential progression of complex and smooth stenoses within the same coronary tree in men with stable coronary artery disease. J Am Coll Cardiol 25:837-842

49. Rogowska J, Patel NA, Fujimoto JG, Brezinski ME (2004) Optical coherence tomographic elastography technique for measuring deformation and strain of atherosclerotic tissues. Heart 90:556-562

50. Kang Y, Mintz GS. IVUS vs. FFR for the assessment of intermediate lesions. Circ Card Interv, in press

51. Abizaid AS, Mintz GS, Mehran R et al (1999) Long-term follow-up after percutaneous transluminal coronary angioplasty was not performed based on intravascular ultrasound findings: importance of lumen dimensions. Circulation 100:256-261

Future Developments in Cardiac CT

37

Filippo Cademartiri, Erica Maffei, Chiara Martini, Sara Seitun, and Giuseppe Tarantini

37.1 Present State of Technologic Development

Coronary artery imaging is the major challenge for the current noninvasive imaging modalities. Although giant steps have already been made, many problems still need to be solved before coronary CT is accepted as a valid substitute for invasive coronary angiography. Most digital angiographic systems in fact have a 512x512 pixel resolution at 8-bit gray scale, with the possibility of acquiring up to 30 frames per second. This produces a spatial resolution in the order of 0.2-0.3 mm, and in the case of a 1024x1024 matrix 0.1-0.15 mm, and a temporal resolution of approximately 8 ms. To approach these levels, therefore, further development is required in terms of temporal and spatial resolution, since the most recent CT scanners have a temporal resolution of 83 ms and spatial resolution of 0.3-0.4 mm [1].

Many avenues are still open for the improvement of noninvasive imaging through the development of all the parameters which play a role in image formation. Scanner manufacturers are currently focusing their efforts on a constant improvement in spatial and temporal resolution. At present, technologic development is essentially aimed at cardiac imaging, where a temporal resolution of 50 ms is desirable, and at the study of organ perfusion, which requires the coverage in the z-axis of a volume markedly larger than can currently be achieved.

37.2 Emerging Solutions

Developmental efforts are being directed in a number of areas. One of these is a change in the geometry of the scanner [2]. Scanner design is in fact an important element capable of significantly influencing important technical parameters such as resolution, signal-to-noise ratio, scanner performance in relation to radiation dose delivered and artifacts.

The reduction of temporal resolution to the hypothetic threshold of 50 ms is anything but a simple problem, due not only to purely mechanical factors (the gantry would need to sustain centrifugal forces much greater than 30 g, which is beyond the capacity of current technology), but also to the necessary increase in power that the radiation sources would need to sustain in a reduced temporal space. The construction of systems capable of rotating even faster and providing more than 200 kW to the tubes seems a long way off.

One favorable approach sees the combination of more than one tube-detector systems so as to significantly influence temporal resolution. The approach is not altogether new, since it was first proposed in the 1970s. Temporal resolution will therefore improve proportionally to the number of tube-detector systems inserted into the gantry. This modification in scanner geometry was recently achieved by Siemens with the introduction of dual source CT equipped with two tube-detector systems mounted on a single gantry at an angle of 90°, thus reducing temporal resolution to 83 ms. Although it only reached the prototype stage and was only used on animal subjects, the Monster CT was a system equipped with 28 pairs of tube-detectors mounted in parallel within a gantry to improve the temporal resolution, with the aim of simultaneously acquiring a thicker section [3]. Other manufacturers are experimenting in different directions. For example, Toshiba is seeking to improve spatial resolution with a further increase in the number of detectors/slices, up to 256 which promises a spatial resolution of 0.47 mm with a 512x512 matrix [4-8].

Still in the prototype phase are flat panel systems which aim to offer a marked increase in spatial resolution, a fundamental parameter in the study of stents. Flat panel detectors can in fact achieve higher spatial resolution than conventional detectors, thus providing excellent image quality especially in high-contrast structures. The spatial resolution of the first prototypes is 0.25 mm,

F. Cademartiri (✉)
Cardiovascular Imaging Unit,
"Giovanni XXIII" Hospital,
Monastier di Treviso (TV), Italy

F. Cademartiri, G. Casolo, M. Midiri (eds.), *Clinical Applications of Cardiac CT*,
© Springer-Verlag Italia 2012

although this is achieved against a temporal resolution of 20 s to cover a 30 cm section in the z-axis with a collimation of 0.75 mm, values which are insufficient for cardiac imaging [9, 10].

In current CT systems the sizes of the focal spot and the detectors are typically in the order of millimeters or slightly less than the millimeter. The integration of micro-CT technology could bring substantial improvements to spatial resolution. Characterized by a spatial resolution of 60-100 μm, i.e. a three- to fivefold improvement over the current standard, these systems at present are only used for research purposes in animal studies. However, they could further reduce the focal spot to values of 0.1-0.2 mm, but at the cost of a significant increase in radiation dose to the patient. These sources would also need to be coupled with flat panel detectors, which represent the state of the art in the sector, such that a development in this direction is impossible at present and unlikely in the near future.

The increase in contrast resolution is another step forward in the development of cardiac imaging. At present all intravenous contrast agents are iodine-based. Unlike in magnetic resonance imaging, where new molecules have been recently developed for a variety of purposes, especially in hepatic imaging, there has been no similar development in CT. Therefore the use of new molecules capable of producing images with better contrast resolution and without the side effects of iodine-based compounds is desirable.

One possible solution in patients with renal insufficiency or allergic to iodinated contrast agents is the use of gadolinium. Widely used in MR, gadolinium does not have the characteristic nephrotoxicity of the compounds used in CT. At equivalent concentrations gadolinium is able to guarantee 50% more vascular attenuation than iodine. Due to its higher atomic number it produces a K-edge of 50.2 keV against the 33.2 keV of iodine. Gadolinium is therefore able to promote better contrast resolution than iodine for energies above 50.2 keV. In clinical reality, however, gadolinium is used in low concentrations and therefore promotes low enhancement. The optimization of the intravenous administration of contrast material with the use of a bolus chaser has proven capable of producing an intravascular enhancement similar to that achieved with iodinated compounds. The introduction to the base compounds of additional molecules of gadolinium to strengthen contrast resolution has not met with success for the moment, as this approach is encumbered not only by the instability of the molecule, but also by the increase in osmolarity. Even the synthesis of new compounds based on other atoms belonging to the Lanthanide series like gadolinium is for the moment an area of research unlikely to produce practical applications in the near future.

In addition to improving contrast resolution, in the future contrast agents could be used for drug delivery, e.g. compounds capable of preventing restenosis during angioplasty. The therapeutic effect of contrast agents in radiotherapy could be a further advantage, modifying for example the progression of atherosclerosis. Even though the diameter of stents is not less than the diameter of native vessels, even with the latest generation of CT scanners the evaluation of their lumen is a challenge. The recent developments in stent design have led to an increase in clinical advantages and long-term results. The enormous success of stenting alongside the increasingly marginal use of bypass grafting has prompted manufactures to develop a variety of stents. To date some 40 models have appeared on the market, all of which however create difficulties for CT. The recent introduction of bioabsorbable stents (substituting metal alloy with bioabsorbable polymer) has on the one hand provided short-term clinical advantages in terms of treatment, while minimizing the long-term disadvantages of metal stents. On the other, the absence of radiopaque material is advantageous for CT by enabling the correct visualization of the lumen. In the near future, alongside stents of this type will be part-metal part-polymer stents, such as the magnesium alloy stent which can provide mechanical support to the vessel in the short term and be absorbed in the long-term.

There is still the significant problem of the elevated radiation dose delivered to the patient by the scanners currently in use. The effective dose for men and women varies between 7.6 and 13 mSv for a 4-slice scanner, and 11-16 mSv for a dual-source CT system. The effective dose can at any rate be reduced by approximately 50% using a protocol of ECG-dependent dose modulation, so that the peak dose is delivered only during the diastolic phase, which is the ideal moment for image acquisition, and a much lower dose is delivered during systole, a phase in which no useful data for image reconstruction are acquired.

The use of multiple source scanners implies the advantage of the combined use of two radiation tubes with different voltages, enabling the characterization of tissue on the basis of their different attenuation coefficients. This allows the possibility of performing a direct subtraction of the vascular or calcified component within the volume acquired. In the near future it will therefore be possible to obtain additional information regarding plaque, or subtract the calcium content in the vascular wall, thus overcoming the current problem of beam hardening artifacts.

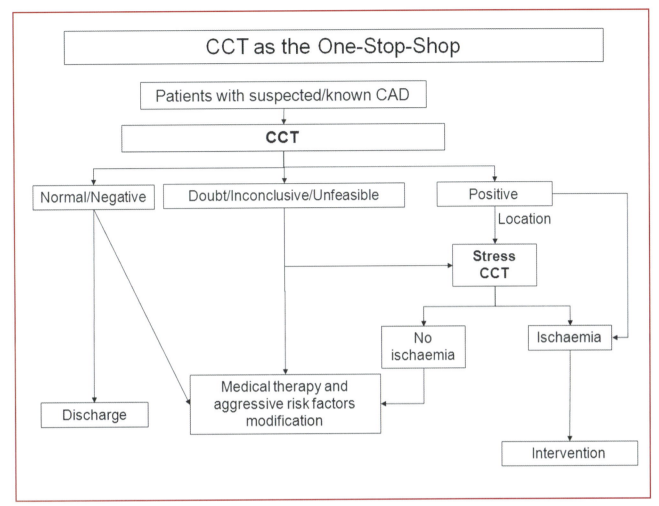

Fig. 37.1 One Stop Shop with CCT

37.3 Functional Imaging

While a limitation of CT to date has been its use prevalently for the study of organ morphology, new prospects are opening up for its use in the study of organ function.

The idea of combining the two types of information to obtain the "one-stop-shop" will be possible through the union with other techniques in the field of functional/molecular imaging (Fig. 37.1) [11]. This will lead to a real CT revolution, freeing it definitively from the Hounsfield unit.

Fusion imaging, i.e. the combination of different systems to obtain complementary information, is already available in PET-CT systems, the performance of which in the study of the heart is currently under evaluation. With PET-CT imaging the precise fusion of functional data obtained by PET and morphologic data obtained by CT is possible in a single image. The evaluation of these hybrid images is of particular importance in oncologic imaging for limiting the number of false positives. In cardiac imaging the hybrid technique can be used to study patients with reduced ventricular function or post-infarction patients in the evaluation of post-infarction reperfusion and contractile reserve.

The measurement of tissue density, on which CT is based, can in theory also be used to obtain information on the type of plaque and its morphology. In vivo and in vitro studies have demonstrated that fibrous, calcified and soft plaques have different attenuation values [12]. The detection and evaluation of plaque morphology in the preclinical and clinical phase at different stages of its development could become one of the most important applications of cardiac imaging. It has however been found that the data obtained from fibrous plaques and soft plaques are similar to the point of it not being possible to characterize plaques as either stable or vulnerable.

Another important advantage of the combination of CT and PET systems is the fact that they both use ionizing radiation and therefore only require a single detector for both the combined techniques. Perfusion imaging is already an example, and PET–CT systems are used in routine clinical practice. Another prospect capable of providing additional functional information is delayed enhancement. The latest generation multislice scanners are already able to perform a delayed enhancement study of infarcted patients. One advantage this technique has over MR is the greater spatial resolution, thus allowing the study of transmural differentiation of viable and non-viable myocardium. The combined use of multiple source systems and new contrast agents, or even the combination of several different contrast agents will be important developments in the evaluation of the perfused myocardium.

37.4 CT Perfusion and CT Fractional Flow Reserve

Current technology development has led to equipments able to perform stress perfusion imaging with CCT. At present few validation studies have been published in the international literature, although they all clarify that the integration between morphologic CCT and functional CCT determines an increased specificity and positive predictive value.

This concept holds true also for a recent technology breakthrough referred to as fractional flow reserve (FFR) with CCT. Undergoing trials (i.e. DISCOVER-FLOW and De-FACTO) presented preliminary results in which the Authors were able to calculate FFR of the coronary tree by using CCT dataset (at rest). This may appear an impossible task, but results are promising and the scientific community is waiting to see the widespread implementation of this technology. If the technology behind FFR CT holds the promise, in the near future we may be able to collect all the morphologic and functional information from CCT without pharmacologic stress.

37.5 Conclusions

CCT is the most important advancement in the evaluation of coronary atherosclerosis in clinical practice and offers a broad range of possible developments and implementations in cardiac applications. The simultaneous evaluation of cardiac function and morphology, cardiac perfusion and the complex interactions of the pulmonary cir-

culation will enable this technique to establish itself even more firmly among noninvasive imaging modalities. These significant aspects will influence routine clinical practice by increasing the number of examinations, prompting the need for automated or semiautomated detection software for the morphologic and functional study. Ideally these approaches will assist the operators in performing a more accurate and thorough global evaluation of the patient, enabling them to save time and healthcare costs.

References

1. Bashore TM, Bates ER, Berger PB et al (2001) American College of Cardiology/Society for Cardiac Angiography and Interventions Clinical Expert Consensus Document on cardiac catheterization laboratory standards.A report of the American College of Cardiology Task Force on Clinical Expert Consensus Documents. J Am Coll Cardiol 37:2170-2214
2. Redington RW (1981) Possible direction in CT scanner design. Adv Neurol 30:63-66
3. Block M, Bove AA, Ritman EL (1984) Coronary angiographic examination with the dynamic spatial reconstructor. Circulation 70:209-216
4. Mori S, Gibson G, McTiernan CF (2006) Differential expression of MMPs and TIMPs in moderate and severe heart failure in a transgenic model. J Card Fail 12:314-325
5. Mori S, Obata T, Kishimoto R et al (2005) Clinical potentials for dynamic contrast-enhanced hepatic volumetric cine imaging with the prototype 256-MDCT scanner. AJR Am J Roentgenol 185:253-256
6. Mori S, Kondo C, Suzuki N et al (2006) Volumetric coronary angiography using the 256-detector row computed tomography scanner: comparison in vivo and in vitro with porcine models. Acta Radiol 47:186-191
7. Mori S, Nishizawa K, Ohno M, Endo M (2006) Conversion factor for CT dosimetry to assess patient dose using a 256-slice CT-scanner. Br J Radiol 79:888-892
8. Mori S, Obata T, Nakajima N et al (2005) Volumetric perfusion CT using prototype 256-detector row CT scanner: preliminary study with healthy porcine model.AJNR Am J Neuroradiol 26:2536-2541
9. Mahnken AH, Seyfarth T, Flohr T et al (2005) Flat-panel detector computed tomography for the assessment of coronary artery stents: phantom study in comparison with 16-slice spiral computed tomography. Invest Radiol 40:8-13
10. Nikolaou K, Flohr T, Stierstorfer K et al (2005) Flat panel computed tomography of human ex vivo heart and bone specimens: initial experience. Eur Radiol 15:329-333
11. Ben-Haim S, Israel O (2006) PET/CT for atherosclerotic plaque imaging. Q J Nucl Med Mol Imaging 50:53-60
12. Pohle K, Achenbach S, Macneill B et al (2007) Characterization of non-calcified coronary atherosclerotic plaque by multidetector row CT: comparison to IVUS. Atherosclerosis 190:174-180

Index

The letters which may be seen accompanying the page number indicate the positioning of a word within a figure or table (f, figure; t, table).

A
ACCURACY trial, 281
ACS (Acute Coronary Syndrome), 29, 35
  classification of, 39, 40f
Acute Coronary Syndrome (ACS), 29, 35
  pathophysiology of, 367
Acute myocardial infarction, 4
  incidence, 5
  prevalence, 5
  prognosis, 5
Adenosine, 330, 345
Adult Treatment Panel III (ATP III), 15
Agatston, 118
AHA (American Heart Association), 96, 123
  classification, 96
ALARA, 235
Anatomy, cardiac, 93
Aneurysm, 106
Angina pectoris, 4, 317
  classification of, 31t
  incidence, 4
  prevalence, 4
Angiograms, coronary, 140f
Angiography
  conventional coronary, 141
  invasive coronary, 139
Angioscopy, 363
Anomalies, congenital, 359
ANP (Atrial Natriuretic Peptide), 74
Aortic
  aneurysm, 297
  atherosclerosis, model of, 56f
  dissection, 293
  trauma, 299
  valve bicuspid, 98f
  valve tricuspid, 96f
Applications of cardiac MR, 357
Appropriateness, 235
Arrhythmias, 271, 316
Arteries
  carotid, 20
  coronary, *see* coronary arteries
Artery
  coronary, non obstructive disease, 13
  coronary, right, 101
  disease, paracrine mediators in coronary, 12
  gastroepiploic, right, 155
  human coronary, 53f, 54f
  inferior epigastric, 155, 157
  internal thoracic, 156
  left coronary, 101, 110f
  unprotected LM coronary, 150
Artifact

beam hardening, 267
  cone, 275
  helical (windmill), 275
  ring, 275
Artifacts, MDCT, *see* MDCT artifacts
ASCOT (Anglo-Scandinavian Cardiac Outcomes Trial), 16
ASSIGN (Assessing Cardiovascular Risk to Scottish Intercollegiate
  Guidelines Network), 18
  risk score, 18
Asymptomatic, 318
Atherosclerosis, 365
  model of aortic, 56f
  pathophysiology, 115
  progression/regression of, 367
Atherosclerotic
  disease, 47
  plaques, histologic sections of human, 51f
  plaques, histological classification of coronary, 123t
  ulcer, penetrating, 296
ATP III (Adult Treatment Panel III), 15, 16
Atrial fibrillation, 82f, 83f, 84f
  treatment of, 83
Atrial Natriuretic Peptide (ANP), 74
Atrium, electroanatomic reconstruction of the left, and the pulmonary
  veins, 86f
Automatic exposure control, 251
Axial images, 231

B
BARI classification, 101t
  coronary artery segments, 101
Bayes theorem, 141
Beam hardening artifacts, 267
Benzodiazepine, 237, 239
Beta-blockers, 237, 257
Bicuspid aortic valve, 98f
Biomarkers of cardiac necrosis, 37, 38t
Blood
  flow, coronary, 8
  pressure
    response during exercise, 316
    systolic, exercise, 317
Blooming effect, 147
BNP (Brain Natriuretic Peptide), 74
Bolus
  chaser, 242
  geometry for CCT, 241
  geometry, parameters influencing, CCT, 242
  tracking, 243
Bruce protocol, 313
Bypass
  grafts, 303
  triple coronary, 156f, 158f

C

CABG (Coronary Artery Bypass Grafting surgery), 153, 180f
CAC (Coronary Artery Calcium), 119, 120f
CAD (Coronary Artery Disease), 29
  diagnostic accuracy in detecting significant, 281
  medical therapy of, 31
  suspected, 301
Calcified
  nodules,131
  plaque, 55f
    multiple, 126f
Calcium
  antagonists, 237, 239
  score, standardized categories for the, 101f
Canadian Cardiovascular Society (CCS), 37
Cardiac
  anatomy,93
  biomarkers of necrosis, 38t
  cycle, 176f
  geometry,74
  incidental findings, 204
  necrosis, biomarkers of, 37
  output, 70
  veins, 79,106, 186
    main, 186f
Cardiac Computed Tomography (CCT), 141
Cardiac CT (CCT), 213, 291
  angiography, 22
    technology, spatial resolution, 93
    technology, temporal resolution, 93
  contrast resolution, 261
  spatial resolution, 260
  temporal resolution, 260
Cardiac Magnetic Resonance (CMR), 59, 64, 75, 215f, 346
  applications of, 375
Cardiac Resynchronization Therapy (CRT), 71, 79
Cardiomyopathies, 359
Cardiovascular risk, 17t
Carotid arteries, 20
Carotid
  artery intima-media thickness (CIMT), 20
  ultrasonography, prognostic value, 21
CARTO-MERGE, 85, 197
Cascade, ischaemic, 30f
CCS (Canadian Cardiovascular Society), 37
CCT (Cardiac Computed Tomography), 141
  chronic total occlusion, 143
  contrast, material and radiation dose reduction, 243
  hardware requirements for, 248t
  image formation in, 219
    collimation, 219
    convolution filter (kernel), 223
    effective slice thickness, 220
    feed, 219
    field of view (FOV), 220
    matrix, 220
    pitch, 219
    reconstruction increment, 220
    rotation time, 220
  images:
    evaluation, 231
    iterative reconstructions, 233
  implementation of, 213, 215
  limitations of, 233
  low radiation dose, 257

parameter optimization, 248
parameters influencing bolus geometry, 242
patient preparation in, 235
  appropriateness, 235
  borderline situations, 236
  exclusion criteria, 236
  inclusion criteria, 235
  patient selection, 235
  pharmacologic management, 237
perfusion and delayed enhancement, 243
plaque burden, 143
prognostic value of, 305
protocols, 220t
  general principles for the optimization of, 247
radiation dose, 248
  reduction, 251
remodeling index, 143
retrospective gating, 228
scan parameters for, 228
stenosis grading in, 143t
training in, 213
with >64-slice spiral scanners, 224
with 16-slice spiral scanners, 223
with 64-slice spiral scanners, 223
with single-slice spiral scanners, 223
CFR (Coronary Flow Reserve), 11, 60, 139, 332
  see Coronary Flow Reserve
CHD (Coronary Heart Disease), 3, 47, 357
  see Coronary Heart Disease (CHD)
Chest pain, 304
Chronic total occlusion, 143
CIMT (carotid artery intima-media thickness), 20
CK-MB, 37
Classification
  BARI, 101t
  of ACS, 39, 40f
  of angina pectoris, 31t
  of coronary artery segments, 100f
  of coronary segments, 96
Collimation, 219
Computed Tomography (CT), 19
  64-slice, 227
Cone
  artifact, 275
  beam, 275
CONFIRM registry, 306
Congenital anomalies, 359
Contractility, myocardial, 8
Contrast
  resolution, 261
  stress echocardiography, 341
Convolution
  filter (kernel), 223
  kernels, 149
Coronary
  angiograms, 140f
  angiography, MR, 358
    conventional, 141
    invasive, 139
  arteries, 7
    anatomic variants of the, 102
    anomalies, 104, 106f
  atherosclerosis, 124f
  atherosclerotic plaque, 123
  blood flow, 8
  calcium, 120

Index 377

disease, obstructive, 12
fistula, 112f
map, 99f
plaque
characteristics of, 130f
evaluation of, 123
imaging, 304
revascularization,155
segments, classification, 96
stenosis, 139
tree, 109f
map of the, 100f
Coronary artery
Bypass Grafting surgery (CABG), 153, 180f
disease, non obstructive, 13
deft, 101, 110f
right, 101
segments
BARI classification, 101
classification of, 100f
Coronary Calcium Score (CCS), 19
Coronary Flow Reserve (CFR), 11, 60, 139, 332
diagnostic value, 334
prognostic value, 335
Coronary Heart Disease (CHD), 3, 47, 357
incidence, 3
prevalence, 3
risk factors, 4
mortality, 3
MR in, 358
COURAGE trial, 31
CRT (Cardiac Resynchronization Therapy), 71, 79
CT (Computed Tomography), 19
and MR, integration between, 359
Dual Energy, 172
dual-source, 274
fractional flow reserve, 374
image reconstruction in, 255
images, 259
perfusion, 374
scanners, dual-source, 274
Culprit plaque, 49
CV risk, 290
Cycle
cardiac, 176f
ergometry, 313

D
De-FACTO, 374
DECT (Dual Energy CT), 172
DES (Drug-Eluting Stent), 150
Diagnostic
accuracy in detecting significant CAD, 281
value, 330, 334
of exercise testing, 318
Diastole, 69
ventricular, 70
Diastolic
dysfunction, 71
stress echocardiography, 342
Dipyridamole, 330, 345
DISCOVER-FLOW, 374
Dobutamine, 329, 343
stress echocardiography, prognostic value, 340
Double product, 317
Drug-Eluting Stent (DES), 150

Dual energy, 149
source, 115
source CT, 274
scanners, 274
Dual Energy CT (DECT), 172
Duke probability risk score, 30t
Dyspnea, 317

E
EBCT (Electron-Beam Computed Tomography), 16, 54, 115, 117, 230, 254
ECG
abnormal responses, 314
gating, retrospective, 254
triggering
high pitch spiral prospective, 255
prospective, 254, 230
triggered, prospective, current modulation, 251
Echocardiography
contrast stress, 341
diastolic stress, 342
dobutamine stress, 340
feasibility and safety of stress, 343
three-dimensional, 343
EF (Ejection Fraction), 70
Electron-Beam Computed Tomography (EBCT), 16, 54, 115, 117, 230, 254
scanner, 117f
Electrophysiologic studies, 185
Epigastric artery, inferior, 155, 157
Ergonovine, 330
Euro Heart Survey, 4
European Systematic Coronary Risk Evaluation (SCORE), 289
Exercise, 329
blood pressure, response during, 316
capacity, 74
protocols, 313
systolic blood pressure, 317
exercise testing
diagnostic value of, 318
prognostic value of, 318
asymptomatic subjects, 318
silent myocardial ischemia, 320
symptomatic subjects, 319
safety of, 320
induced hypotension, 317

F
Feed, 219
FFR (Fractional Flow Reserve), 12, 13, 140, 374
Fibrillation, mechanisms of, 82
Filters, 267
FOV (Field Of View), 220
Framingham
heart study, 3, 4, 16, 290
risk score, 16, 120
score, 307
Functional imaging, 373

G
Gastroepiploic artery, right, 155
Gating, retrospective, 228
Geometric remodeling, 75f
Geometry, cardiac, 74
GRACE score, 41t, 42t
Gradient echo, 189

GUSTO-IIB trial, 5

H
Hardware requirements for CCT, 248t
Heart, 94f, 95f, 99f
  rate, 7
    control, 149
    response, 317
  study, Framingham, 3, 4, 16, 290
Helical (windmill) artifact, 275
Hematoma, intramural, 295
High pitch spiral prospective ECG triggering, 255
Histologic
  characteristics of plaque, 51
  sections of human atherosclerotic plaques, 51f
Histological classification of coronary atherosclerotic plaques, 123t
Histology, virtual, 363
Human coronary artery, 53f, 54f
Hypertrophy, left ventricular, 73, 75f
Hypotension, exercise-induced, 317

I
ICD (Implantable Cardiovector Defibrillator), 71
Images
  axial, 231
  evaluation, CCT, 231
  iterative reconstructions, CCT, 233
  reconstruction, CCT, 230
Incidence of coronary heart disease, 3t
Inferior epigastric artery, 155, 157
Interpolation, 267
Iodine, 242
Ischaemic cascade, 30f
Ischemia, 325
  mechanisms of, 325
  repetitive, 61f
  silent myocardial, 320
  transient, 59
Ischemic heart disease, mortality from, in European regions, 4f
Iterative reconstructions, 233, 255
Ivabradine, 237, 239
IVUS (intravascular ultrasound), 363

K
K-edge, 241
Kilovoltage, 254

L
Left
  atrium, 96f
  ventricle, 69, 81f
  ventricular contractility, 70
Left ventricular
  hypertrophy, 73, 75f
  mass, 72
Limitations of CCT, 233
LITA, 155
Luminity, 341
LVEF (Left Ventricular Ejection Fraction), 70, 175

M
Map of the coronary tree, 100f
Mass, left ventricular, 72
Maximum Intensity Projections (MIP), 232
MBF (Myocardial Blood Flow), 59
MDCT (multidetector computed tomography), 93

artifacts
  cone artifact, 275
  cone beam effect, 275
  helical (windmill) artifact, 275
  ring artifact, 275
  stair-step and zebra artifact, 276
coronary angiography, 261
  beam hardening artifacts, 267
  contrast agent artifacts, 269
    speed, 269
    volume, 269
  filters, 267
  interpolation, 267
  motion artifacts, 263
  noise, 264
  partial volume effects, 266
Mechanisms of
  fibrillation, 82
  ischemia, 325
Medical therapy of CAD, 31
MESA (Multi-Ethnic Study of Atherosclerosis), 20
MET (metabolic equivalent), 313
MIP (Maximum Intensity Projections), 232
Mitral valve, 96f
Mortality from ischemic heart disease in European regions, 4f
MPR (multiplanar reconstructions), 231
MR (Magnetic Resonance), 293, 357
  coronary angiography, 358
  in coronary heart disease, 358
  integration between CT and, 359
MRI (Magnetic Resonance Imaging), 19, 54, 115, 175
Multi-Ethnic Study of Atherosclerosis (MESA), 20
Multiplanar reconstructions (MPR), 231
Myocardial Blood Flow (MBF), 59
Myocardial
  bridging, 100f, 106
  contractility, 8
  CT perfusion (CTP), 172f
    imaging, 165
  infarction, 180f
  ischemia silent, 320
  oxygen demand and supply, relation between, 62f
  viability, 60, 339
Myocardium, fully viable, 64

N
National Cholesterol Education Program, 15
Near infrared spectroscopy (NIRS), 52, 125
Necrosis, cardiac biomarkers of, 38t
NHLBI ARIC (National Heart, Lung, and Blood Institute–Atherosclerosis Risk In Communities), 4
NIRS (near infrared spectroscopy), 52, 125
Nitrates, 237, 239
Nitrogen-13 (N-13) ammonia, 351
Noise, 264
Non obstructive coronary artery disease, 13
NSTE (non ST-segment elevation), 35
NSTEMI (non ST Elevation MI), 5, 59
Nuclear stress myocardial perfusion imaging-MPI, 165
NYHA, 79
  class, 81

O
Obstructive coronary disease, 12
OCT (Optical Coherence Tomography), 52, 55, 125, 363
OPERA registry, 5

Index 379

Optison, 341
Output, cardiac, 70
Oxygen demand and supply, relation between myocardial, 62f

P
Pacing, 330
Pain, chest, 304
Palpography, 363
Paracrine mediators in coronary artery disease, 12
Parameter optimization, 248
Partial volume effects, 266
Perfusion, 358
  and delayed enhancement, CCT, 243
PET (Positron Emission Tomography), 59, 351
PET/CT, 65, 353
Pitch, 219
Plaque
  burden, 143
    CCT, 143
  coronary, characteristics of, 130f
  culprit, 49
  evaluation of coronary, 123
  histologic characteristics of, 51
  vulnerable, definition of, 49t
Plaques
  histologic sections of human atherosclerotic, 51f
  histological classification of coronary atherosclerotic, 123t
  multiple calcified, 126f
  types of vulnerable, 48f
Post-test probability, 282
Pre-test probability, 282
Probability risk score, Duke, 30t
PROCAM (prospective cardiovascular munster), 289
Prognostic value, 305, 318, 331, 335
  carotid ultrasonography, 21
  coronary calcium scanning, 21
  of CCT, *see* CCT
  of exercise testing, *see* exercise
PROSPECT, 366
Prospective
  ECG triggering, 254, 230
  ECG-triggered current modulation, 251
Pulmonary vein ablation, 198f
Pulmonary veins, 81, 84, 85f, 86f, 189
  electroanatomic reconstruction of the left atrium and the, 86f

Q
QCA (quantitative coronary angiography), 153
QRISK (QRESEARCH cardiovascular risk algorithm), 18
  risk score, 18

R
Radial artery, 155, 157
Radiation dose, 248
  CCT, 248
  low, CCT, 257
  reduction, CCT, 251
Raman spectroscopy, 125
Reconstruction increment, 220
Reconstructions, iterative, 233, 255
Remodeling
  vascular, 132f
  index, 143
    CCT, 143
Repetitive ischemia, 61f
Retrospective

ECG gating, 254
  gating, 228
    CCT, 228
Reynolds risk score, 18
Right
  coronary artery, 101
  gastroepiploic artery, 155
  ventricle, 69
  ventricular dysfunction, 72
Ring artifact, 275
Risk:
  cardiovascular, 17t
  CV, 290
  score
    ASSIGN, 18
    Duke probability, 30t
    Framingham, 16, 120
    Reynolds, 18
  stratification, 41
RITA, 155
Rotation time, 220
Rubidium-82, 351

S
Safety of exercise testing, 320
Saphenous vein, 156
Scan parameters for CCT, 228
SCORE (Systematic COronary Risk Evaluation), 16, 289
  project, 16
Score
  Framingham, 307
  GRACE, 41t, 42t
SHAPE (Screening for HeartAttack Prevention and Education), 22, 290
Silent myocardial ischemia, 320
Simpson's rule, 178f
Slice thickness, effective, 220
Spatial resolution, 93, 260
SPECT (Single Photon Emission Computed Tomography), 59, 350
SPECT/CT, 353
Spectroscopy, 358
Speed, 269
SSFP (Steady-State Free Precession), 189
STEMI (ST elevation MI), 5
STEMI/NSTEMI, 360
Stenosis
  grading, 143t
    in CCT, 143t
  severity, 283
Stents, 302
Stress echocardiography
  diagnostic value, 330
  feasibility and safety of, 343
  pharmacologic stressors, 327
  prognostic value, 331
  vasospasm, 327
Stress magnetic resonance imaging-MRI, 165
Stressors, 327f
Symptomatic, 319
Systole, 69
  ventricular, 69
Systolic blood pressure exercise, 317

T
Tagging, 357
TCFA (thin-cap fibroatheroma), 130

Temporal resolution, 93, 260
Test bolus, 243
Thermography, intracoronary, 364
Thoracic artery, internal, 156
TIMI score, 41t
Training in CCT, 213
Transient ischemia, 59
Treadmill, 313
Tricuspid aortic valve, 96f
Troponin T, 37

U
UA (Unstable Angina), 35
UA/NSTEMI, 41t
Ulcer, penetrating atherosclerotic, 296
USPIO (Ultra Small Particles of Iron Oxide), 55

V
Valve
  aortic, tricuspid, 96f
  mitral, 96f

Vascular remodeling, 132f
Vasospasm, 327
Vein, saphenous, 156
Veins
  cardiac, 79, 106, 185
  electroanatomic reconstruction of the left atrium and the pulmonary, 86f
  main cardiac, 186f
  pulmonary, 81, 84, 85f, 86f, 189
Ventricle, right, 69
Ventricular
  diastole, 70
  dysfunction, right, 72
  left, contractility, 70
  left, hypertrophy, 73, 75f
  left, mass, 72
  systole, 69
Virtual histology, 363
Volume, 242, 269
Voxel, 93
Vulnerable plaque, 49, 128, 366
  definition of, 49t
  types of, 48f

Printed in November 2011